THIRD EDITION

INTRODUCTION TO
GLOBAL
HEALTH

Kathryn H. Jacobsen, MPH, PhD

George Mason University

Fairfax, Virginia

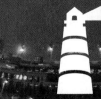

JONES & BARTLETT
LEARNING

World Headquarters
Jones & Bartlett Learning
5 Wall Street
Burlington, MA 01803
978-443-5000
info@jblearning.com
www.jblearning.com

Jones & Bartlett Learning books and products are available through most bookstores and online booksellers. To contact Jones & Bartlett Learning directly, call 800-832-0034, fax 978-443-8000, or visit our website, www.jblearning.com.

Substantial discounts on bulk quantities of Jones & Bartlett Learning publications are available to corporations, professional associations, and other qualified organizations. For details and specific discount information, contact the special sales department at Jones & Bartlett Learning via the above contact information or send an email to specialsales@jblearning.com.

12396-8

Production Credits

VP, Product Management: David D. Cella
Director of Product Management: Michael Brown
Product Specialist: Carter McAlister
Production Manager: Carolyn Rogers Pershouse
Director of Vendor Management: Amy Rose
Vendor Manager: Molly Hogue
Senior Marketing Manager: Sophie Fleck Teague
Manufacturing and Inventory Control Supervisor: Amy Bacus
Composition: codeMantra U.S. LLC

Project Management: codeMantra U.S. LLC
Cover Design: Scott Moden
Director of Rights & Media: Joanna Gallant
Rights & Media Specialist: Robert Boder
Media Development Editor: Shannon Sheehan
Cover Image (Title Page, Chapter Opener):
    © Xinzheng. All Rights Reserved/Moment/Getty
Printing and Binding: LSC Communications
Cover Printing: LSC Communications

Library of Congress Cataloging-in-Publication Data

Names: Jacobsen, Kathryn H., author.
Title: Introduction to global health / Kathryn H. Jacobsen.
Description: Third edition. | Burlington, MA: Jones & Bartlett Learning, [2019] | Includes bibliographical references and index.
Identifiers: LCCN 2017044502 | ISBN 9781284123890 (paperback: alk. paper)
Subjects: | MESH: Global Health | Communicable Diseases | Health Promotion | Social Determinants of Health | Health Transition
Classification: LCC RA441 | NLM WA 530.1 | DDC 362.1—dc23
LC record available at https://lccn.loc.gov/2017044502

6048

Printed in the United States of America
22 21 20 19 18   10 9 8 7 6 5 4 3 2 1

Contents

Chapter 18 Promoting Neonatal, Infant, Child, and Adolescent Health. 410

Chapter 19 Promoting Healthy Adulthood and Aging 425

Chapter 20 Global Health Careers. 436

Preface

The first and second editions of *Introduction to Global Health* were written during the Millennium Development Goals (MDG) era of global health. The MDGs spelled out an ambitious plan for significantly reducing global poverty between 2000 and 2015. They were wildly successful. The number of people living on less than $1 per day dropped substantially during the first 15 years of the 21st century. As a growing number of global health partnerships set agendas for change and financed action plans, significant progress was made toward alleviating hunger, preventing maternal and child mortality, and controlling HIV/AIDS and malaria.

The next generation of global goals—the Sustainable Development Goals (SDGs)—were launched at the end of 2015. They spell out 17 goals for enhancing human flourishing by 2030, including targets related to poverty reduction, hunger, health, education, gender equality, clean water and sanitation, affordable and clean energy, decent work, infrastructure and technology development, human rights, sustainable urbanization, responsible production and consumption, climate and environment, peace, and governance. The SDGs seek to promote prosperity while upholding human rights, protecting the planet, and fostering peace and security. All of the goals are interdependent, and all are inextricably tied to health. Improvements in any of the 17 areas will yield benefits for population health, and improvements in public health will enable other SDGs to be achieved.

Most of the MDGs were targeted at improving quality of life among the world's poorest people. The SDGs retain those aims but add a lengthy list of objectives that apply to countries across the income spectrum. For example, the SDGs include targets for preventing new hepatitis B virus infections; reducing the number of adults who die from cardiovascular diseases, cancers, and other noncommunicable diseases before their 70th birthdays; reducing the suicide mortality rate; increasing access to treatment for substance use disorders; and reducing deaths from road traffic injuries and violence. These conditions affect people in every country, and all countries have the opportunity under the SDGs to track their progress toward improving health metrics related to these concerns.

This third edition of *Introduction to Global Health* is a book for the SDG era. The socioeconomic and environmental determinants of health are presented in the context of the SDGs. The shifting landscape for financing and implementing global health initiatives is described in expanded chapters on payers and players. Chapters on infectious diseases, reproductive health, and nutrition are complemented by new chapters on noncommunicable diseases, mental health, and injuries. The similarities and differences in the conditions that cause illness and death in featured countries representing diverse world regions and income levels are illustrated with estimates from the Global Burden of Disease (GBD) project, which now produces annually updated profiles of health status in every country. (Disclosure: the author is a GBD collaborator.) The global health agenda has expanded to cover all of the world's people, and this book provides a positive, forward-looking perspective on the numerous actions that are helping promote the health, well-being, and security of people across the lifespan and across the globe.

New to This Edition

The third edition of *Introduction to Global Health* has been significantly expanded to include more comprehensive coverage of the full spectrum of topics that now constitute part of the global health agenda.

Chapter 1 presents a new model for identifying global health issues—one that incorporates populations, action, cooperation, equity, and security—and it introduces the key concepts of prevention science, health transitions theory, globalization, and global health security.

Chapter 2 introduces the new Sustainable Development Goals (SDGs) that will guide international development efforts through 2030 and describes the most commonly used global health metrics.

Chapters 3 and 4 use the SDGs as a framework for exploring the social and environmental determinants of health. Chapter 3 describes the connections between health and economics, education, gender, employment, culture, migration, and governance. Chapter 4 examines the links between health and water, sanitation, energy, air quality, occupational and industrial health, urbanization, sustainability, and climate change.

Chapter 5 uses the SDGs and the Universal Declaration of Human Rights to highlight some of the major ethical issues in global health, including questions about the right to have access to healthcare services and medicines, humanitarian responsibilities after natural disasters and during times of conflict, and the rights of people in prison, people with disabilities, and other special populations.

Chapter 6 is a new chapter that describes the health system models used in various countries and explains the funding mechanisms used to pay for global health activities. Chapter 7 features the diversity of entities involved in implementing and evaluating global health interventions, including governmental and intergovernmental agencies, nonprofit organizations, and for-profit corporations.

Chapters 8 through 17 present the health conditions that account for the greatest burden of disease globally. Each chapter begins with a section that explains why the featured topic is considered to be a global health issue, and each chapter emphasizes the interventions that can reduce the impact of adverse health conditions on individuals and populations. Health metrics from the Global Burden of Disease (GBD) collaboration are used to illustrate the populations affected by each condition.

Chapter 8 describes the global threats posed by HIV/AIDS, tuberculosis, and antimicrobial resistance. Chapter 9 discusses the heavy toll that child mortality from diarrheal diseases and pneumonia takes on low-income countries and describes the tools that are available to contain outbreaks of influenza and other vaccine-preventable infections. Chapter 10 describes the burden from malaria and neglected tropical diseases in low-income countries and the global threats associated with emerging infectious diseases. Chapter 11 highlights a diversity of reproductive and sexual health issues, including family planning, infertility, pregnancy, maternal mortality, neonatal health, men's health, and sexual minority health. Chapter 12 describes the nutrition transition and the challenges associated with undernutrition, overnutrition, and food safety.

A series of new chapters describe the opportunities for global health initiatives to address the noncommunicable diseases (NCDs), mental health disorders, and injuries that are among the leading causes of death worldwide. Chapter 13 focuses on cancer, Chapter 14 focuses on cardiovascular disease, and Chapter 15 focuses on chronic respiratory diseases and diabetes. The principles of behavior change, tobacco control, and other methods for prevention and management of NCDs are highlighted. Chapter 16 describes the diversity of mental health conditions that contribute to global disease burden and emphasizes the need for greater access to mental health services. Chapter 17 discusses injury prevention and control methods.

Two chapters synthesize the core messages of the book through the lens of health promotion across the lifespan. Chapter 18 presents the major improvements in neonatal, infant, child, and adolescent health that were achieved under the MDGs and the opportunities for continued progress under the SDGs. Chapter 19 describes the emerging challenges associated with aging populations and the opportunities for promoting healthy adulthood and aging.

Chapter 20 is a new chapter that describes the links between diverse educational and career pathways and global health, and emphasizes the opportunities for everyone to be involved in making communities and the world a healthier place for current and future generations.

More than 350 figures and tables highlight key material, and nearly all of these are new for the third edition. All of the statistics in the book have been updated. Data from eight of the world's largest countries, which collectively are home to half of the world's people, are used to illustrate the patterns of health status in high-income, middle-income, and low-income countries: Brazil, China, Ethiopia, Germany, India, Iran, Nigeria, and the United States. A new glossary provides definitions for more than 780 key terms in global health.

About the Author

Kathryn H. Jacobsen, MPH, PhD, is professor of epidemiology and global health at George Mason University. She is the author of more than 150 scientific articles as well as *Introduction to Health Research Methods: A Practical Guide*, also published by Jones & Bartlett Learning.

She is also a contributor to the Global Burden of Disease project and frequently provides commentary for print and television media.

CHAPTER 1

Global Health Transitions

Global health is a multidisciplinary, multisectoral field in which diverse partners from around the world act together to improve population and environmental health. Scientific advances during the last century have reduced infant and child death rates, increased the number of infectious diseases that can be prevented or cured, and provided new tools for managing the chronic diseases associated with aging. Global health activities can also be effective for promoting security, stimulating economic growth, fostering justice, and achieving other shared goals.

▶ 1.1 Defining Global Health

Health is often defined as the absence of disease or injury, but this is an incomplete explanation because the focus is on what health is not, rather than on what health is. Some definitions of health try to focus on the essence of health by emphasizing health as the ability to conduct normal daily activities. But that type of statement is also limited because the definition of "normal" varies from person to person. For example, some people assume that it is normal for an older person to have limited mobility and forgetfulness, but that is not true. Many older people are very active and mentally sharp, and many of those who have joint pain or memory loss could be helped by therapy and medication. Similarly, in many parts of the world, parents think it is normal for their children to have intestinal worms. This belief is also not true, and untreated worm infections significantly reduce the health, growth, and school performance of millions of children worldwide.

A more comprehensive definition of health addresses both physical and mental health as well as the presence of a social system that facilitates health. The Constitution of the World Health Organization (WHO), written in 1948, defines **health** as "a state of complete physical, mental, and social well-being and not merely the absence of disease or infirmity." This definition recognizes that health is not just a function of biology. Health stems from biology, psychology, sociology, and a host of other factors. Although there is almost no one in the world today who would be classified as having "complete" health according to the WHO statement,[1] this definition provides a target for medical and public health systems as they work together to promote the improved health status of individuals and communities.

An ideal health trajectory begins with a consenting adult becoming pregnant and that pregnancy leading to an uneventful full-term delivery of a healthy newborn. After birth,

1

the ideal health trajectory continues with that healthy infant growing into adulthood without experiencing serious infections, injuries, or illnesses, and that adult remaining healthy and active for many decades. Because everyone eventually dies, the ideal health trajectory ends in very old age with a gentle death that is not preceded by months or years of disability and pain. However, few people achieve this ideal pathway (**FIGURE 1–1A**). In very low-income communities, a large proportion of children are born with low birthweight and struggle with repeated bouts of infectious diseases like pneumonia and malaria, and many young women die in childbirth (**FIGURE 1–1B**).

No matter where a person lives, a combination of happenstance and health behaviors may reduce health status at various time periods over the life span. A healthy child may develop permanent physical impairments due to a serious car crash in adolescence, then have reduced health status from alcohol abuse in middle adulthood, and die from a heart attack before reaching retirement age (**FIGURE 1–1C**). Even when people live to be very old, they usually experience a

gradual decline in function and loss of independence prior to dying (**FIGURE 1–1D**). A diversity of medical, behavioral, social, economic, environmental, and other interventions and changes can help people make progress toward long, healthy life trajectories. Some of these actions are taken by individuals to improve their own health status, some are communal activities by families and neighborhoods, and some are large-scale initiatives that take place on a national or international scale.

Global health refers to the collaborative actions taken to identify and address transnational concerns about the exposures and diseases that adversely affect human populations. There are many different lenses that are used to identify global health issues (**FIGURE 1–2**). Epidemiologists and health economists may evaluate global health metrics and select the conditions that cause the majority of deaths, disability, and lost productivity worldwide. Physicians, nurses, and other clinical practitioners may see suffering that could easily be prevented or relieved and feel compelled to find ways to scale up the delivery of cost-effective solutions

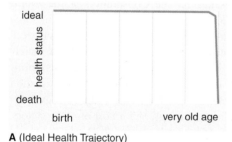

A (Ideal Health Trajectory)

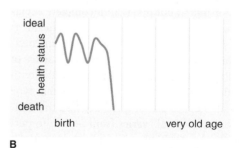

B

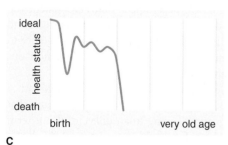

C

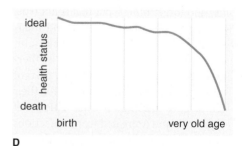

D

FIGURE 1–1 Examples of health trajectories.

Populations	A focus on the exposures and diseases that cause the greatest public health burden and affect large numbers of people in diverse geographic regions
Action	A focus on effective, low-cost interventions that prevent illness and injury, diagnose and treat diseases, and alleviate suffering
Cooperation	A focus on the health concerns that must be addressed through worldwide efforts to share knowledge, tools, and resources
Equity	A focus on helping the global poor and addressing social, environmental, and health inequalities
Security	A focus on addressing the health issues most likely to contribute to political and economic instability and conflict

FIGURE 1–2 PACES: Defining global health.

to people in need, no matter where those people live. Environmental health scientists may observe how quickly some pathogens and toxins cross international borders and recognize that international partnerships are necessary in order to mitigate those threats to health. Health promoters and others whose work is guided by a social justice perspective may focus on calling attention to the health needs of the most vulnerable people around the world. Security experts may zero in on the factors that contribute to instability and conflict. All of these global health lenses—ones focused on populations, action, cooperation, equity, and security (PACES)—emphasize transnational health issues, but

different global health priorities will emerge when different lenses are applied (**FIGURE 1–3**). These varied perspectives are why so many different environmental concerns, a broad range of diseases, and a diversity of special populations have been targeted by global health initiatives.

▶ 1.2 Health Interventions

Etiology is the study of the causes of disease, including both intrinsic (internal) causes, such as genetics and psychological factors, and extrinsic (external) causes, such as infectious disease and environmental exposures. A person's health status at a given age is a function of his or her experiences throughout the life course.[2] These biological, behavioral, and other exposures occur in particular natural and built environments, and they are also a function of a broad set of social, political, cultural, economic, occupational, and other factors.[3] The diversity of contributors to disease means that a considerable diversity of changes can improve health.

Humans have long recognized the environment's role in disease etiology. For many centuries before microscopes allowed people to observe bacteria, communities recognized that some illnesses were linked to environmental exposures, and they took care to dispose of human waste, protect water sources, and bury the carcasses of diseased animals. During most of the 19th century, the term **miasma** was used to describe the pungent odors of poorly managed waste, and the prevailing theory of disease causation in Western countries was that epidemics were spontaneously generated in places with poor sanitation.[4] When cholera outbreaks occurred in England in the mid-1800s, investigators found a higher infection rate in places of low altitude, especially places near marshes that had an abundance of foul-smelling gases, and they blamed the spread of cholera on contact with those offensive gases.[5] This was

Lens	Sample Priority		Sample Priority	
Populations	Cardiovascular disease (CVD)	CVD is the leading cause of adult mortality worldwide.	Drinking water	Unsafe drinking water causes billions of cases of severe diarrhea annually.
Action	Hunger	There is enough food in the world to spare children from the lifelong consequences of not having access to adequate nutrition during their early years of development.	HIV	HIV medications can extend the lives of infected individuals by many years or even decades.
Cooperation	Air pollution	Air pollution generated by one country can cause adverse health effects for its neighbors.	Drug-resistant infections	One country with poor regulations for antibiotic use can put the whole world at risk.
Equity	Neglected tropical diseases	The world's poorest children are disabled and disfigured by parasitic diseases that do not affect children who happen to have been born in higher-income places.	Mental health	People with mental health disorders in every country face stigma that may exclude them from full participation in society.
Security	Violence	The violence in conflict areas can spill over into new locations and create refugee crises.	Emerging infectious diseases	Outbreaks of deadly infectious diseases threaten public safety and can cause social, economic, and political instability.

FIGURE 1–3 PACES: Examples of global health priorities.

a reasonable conclusion because the people who lived in the gassy, marshy areas were the same people who drank the bacterium-infected water that was the true cause of the outbreak. Public health efforts in the 19th century focused primarily on environmental sanitation, with special attention aimed at reducing epidemics thought to be associated with urban crowding and its associated grime.[6] Although outbreaks are no longer blamed on miasmas, good hygiene (like frequent handwashing) and the avoidance of known environmental hazards remain very important for preventing infections and injuries.

By the middle of the 20th century, most medical scientists had shifted their efforts from the identification of social and environmental risk factors for disease to the identification of specific infectious agents and genes.[7] But even with the emphasis on immunology and genetics, one of the biggest public health breakthroughs in the 20th century was a series of studies published in the 1950s that confirmed that cigarette smoking was a major cause of lung cancer, emphysema, and cardiovascular disease.[8] Later studies showed that exposure to secondhand smoke was an additional risk factor for lung disease.[9] Today, health scientists and clinicians agree that there are many social and behavioral, environmental, and biological contributors to disease. This means that there are diverse actions that can improve health status. The particular set of interventions recommended for global health concerns tends to reflect the disciplinary perspectives of the people designing and implementing the interventions.[10] Two of the most prominent voices in global health in the 21st century are medicine and public health.

Medicine focuses on preventing, diagnosing, and treating health problems in individuals and families. For thousands of years, various types of health practitioners in cultures across the globe have cared for people with health concerns, including herbalists adept at treating fevers, midwives skilled in delivering babies, and numerous other people equipped to provide physical and spiritual comfort to people with various ailments. As modern medical science has developed, clinical professionals like physicians, surgeons, nurses, dentists, psychologists, and physical therapists have developed highly specialized methods for caring for patients. Examples of common interventions in the medical field include antibiotics to treat infections, medications to manage chronic diseases (such as insulin for people with diabetes and inhaled bronchodilators for people with asthma), counseling to address mental health concerns, surgery to correct traumatic injuries, and physical therapy to restore function after an injury.

Public health focuses on promoting health and preventing illnesses, injuries, and early deaths at the population level by identifying and mitigating environmental hazards, promoting healthy behaviors, ensuring access to essential health services, and taking other actions to protect the health, safety, and well-being of groups of people (**FIGURE 1–4**).[11] Modern public health comprises a diversity of subdisciplines. **Environmental health** is the study of the connections between human

1	Monitor health status to identify community health problems.
2	Diagnose and investigate health problems and health hazards in the community.
3	Inform, educate, and empower people about health issues.
4	Mobilize community partnerships to identify and solve health problems.
5	Develop policies and plans that support individual and community health efforts.
6	Enforce laws and regulations that protect health and ensure safety.
7	Link people to needed personal health services and ensure the provision of health care when otherwise unavailable.
8	Ensure a competent public health and personal healthcare workforce.
9	Evaluate effectiveness, accessibility, and quality of personal and population-based health services.
10	Research for new insights and innovative solutions to health problems.

FIGURE 1–4 Essential public health services.

Reproduced from The public health system & the 10 essential public health services. Centers for Disease Control and Prevention website https://www.cdc.gov/stltpublichealth/publichealthservices/essentialhealthservices.html. Updated September 20, 2017.

health and environmental exposures, such as air quality, water quality, solid and hazardous waste, unsafe food, vermin and pathogen-transmitting insects, radiation, noise, and residential and industrial hazards. **Epidemiology** is the study of the distribution of health problems in populations, the risk factors for developing those conditions, and the effectiveness of interventions to address these concerns. **Biostatistics** is the science of analyzing health data and interpreting the results so that they can be applied to solving public health problems. **Health promotion** is an applied social science that encourages individuals and communities to take steps to improve their own health. The **Ottawa Charter** for Health Promotion was an international agreement sponsored by the WHO and approved at a conference in Canada in 1986 that identified the core health promotion actions as including healthy public policies, supportive environments, strong communities, skilled personnel, and expanded access to preventive health services.[12] There are also specialists in health policy and management, public health administration, health communication, maternal and child health, public health nutrition, health economics, and other public health fields. Examples of common public health interventions include policies that ensure that food and drinking water are safe, vaccination campaigns that prevent widespread outbreaks of infectious diseases, health education campaigns that promote active lifestyles for people of all ages, and school nutrition programs that ensure that children have access to the nutritious food they need to grow and learn.

The lines between medicine and public health are blurry (**FIGURE 1–5**). Medicine tends to focus on the clinical care of individuals, while public health has a focus on larger populations. Public health usually emphasizes the prevention of health problems while medicine has more of a focus on treating the existing problems. But many people trained in clinical fields work in population health and provide preventive services (including public health nurses, physicians specializing in community medicine and preventive medicine, and others), and many people trained in public health are dedicated to increasing access to treatment for individuals with critical health issues. Medical research informs the design of public health interventions, and the information generated from public health research helps clinicians to make differential diagnoses, prescribe appropriate therapies, and encourage healthy lifestyles for their patients in addition to helping communities set their own public health priorities and design and evaluate evidence-based programs to address these issues.

In global health, an **intervention** is a strategic action intended to improve individual and population health status. Interventions take many different forms: detection and treatment of physical and mental health

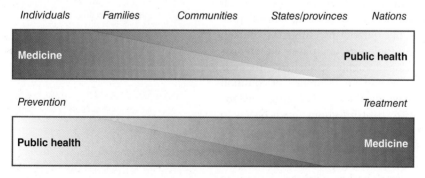

FIGURE 1–5 Comparing medicine and public health.

conditions, counseling and social marketing to promote healthier behaviors, development and enforcement of health policies, and numerous other actions.[13] Interventions targeted at any level from the individual to the community, the nation, and the world can be effective at improving personal and public health. For example, nutrition support programs for pregnant and breastfeeding women can reduce the risk of low birthweight and malnutrition in infants, the use of antibiotics to treat childhood pneumonia soon after the onset of a cough can prevent life-threatening illness, the availability of skilled birth attendants can prevent women from dying during childbirth, and numerous other interventions during adulthood, such as injury prevention activities, mental health care, and lifestyle changes that reduce the risk of heart attacks, can improve both quality of life and the number of years lived (**FIGURE 1–6**). Together, these interventions can have a strong positive impact on an individual's health, allowing a person who might otherwise have been in poor health in childhood and died young to instead have a healthy childhood and live to old age. When these interventions reach millions of people, they make a huge difference in population health, happiness, and productivity.

Because individual and community health status is the result of a complex mix of biological, socioeconomic, environmental, and other factors, the clinical disciplines and public health cannot on their own accomplish global health goals. People working in a diversity of fields make important contributions to the conditions that promote or inhibit the health of individuals and communities. Social workers, spiritual advisors, teachers, sanitation workers, farmers, scientists and engineers, policymakers and lawyers, a variety of government officials, and many others all have a role to play in the big-picture interventions that enable health.

▶ **1.3 Prevention Science**

The adage that prevention is better than a cure expresses one of the foundational principles of global health. It is usually cheaper to spend relatively small amounts of money on interventions that keep people healthy across the life span than it is to spend relatively large amounts of money helping people recover from serious health problems (**FIGURE 1–7**). Severe health problems, long-term disabilities, and untimely deaths are expensive for the affected individuals and for their families, who must pay the direct costs of medical care as well as bear the direct and indirect costs of caregiving. Health problems are also costly for the communities and nations that lose the economic and other contributions the affected individuals would have made through work productivity, tax revenue, and service if they had lived longer, healthier lives. **Prevention science** is the process of

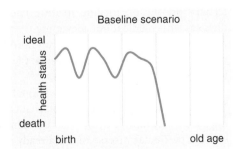

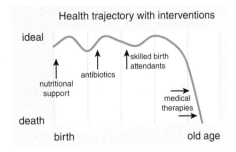

FIGURE 1–6 Examples of interventions that improve health trajectories across the life span.

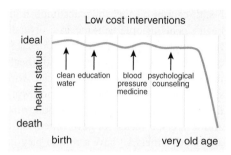
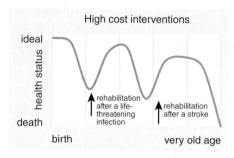

FIGURE 1-7 Maintaining good health status through preventive interventions is less costly than paying for rehabilitation after health crises.

determining which preventive health interventions are effective in various populations, how successful the interventions are, and how well they can be scaled up for widespread implementation.[14]

There are three levels of prevention (**FIGURE 1-8**). When an effective intervention for preventing disease or promoting health has been identified, **primary prevention** actions can keep an adverse health event from ever occurring. Numerous global health initiatives focus on primary prevention. Some promote health behaviors, such as vaccinating children to protect them from measles and polio infections, exercising to protect against heart disease, avoiding tobacco to reduce the risk of lung disease, and using a seatbelt to reduce the risk of serious injuries during a motor vehicle collision. Some programs work to modify the health environment by increasing access to improved sanitation facilities to prevent diarrhea, spraying insecticides to kill the mosquitoes that spread infections, implementing clean delivery room practices to prevent infections of newborns and their mothers, and building roads that are safe for bicyclists and pedestrians. Others use policy changes to improve access to healthcare services, essential medications, and nutritious foods.

The goal of **secondary prevention** is to detect health problems at an early stage when they have not yet caused significant damage to the body and can be treated more easily.

Secondary prevention interventions typically are targeted at people with early, asymptomatic (that is, not symptomatic) disease, so that health problems can be diagnosed before they become so severe that the affected individuals seek health services. There are numerous types of cancer screening tests that are forms of secondary prevention, such as mammography for breast cancer, Pap smears for cervical cancer, and colonoscopies that look for the polyps that are precursors to colorectal cancer. Other examples of screening tests include routine HIV tests, blood pressure checks in adults, and vision tests for children, all of which are intended to detect health issues in people who might otherwise remain unaware of the presence of these manageable health conditions for many years.

The aim of **tertiary prevention** is to reduce impairment, minimize pain and suffering, and prevent death in people with symptomatic health problems. Examples of tertiary prevention include treating chronic diseases with medication, alleviating the pain of people with advanced cancers, and providing physical therapy and occupational therapy to people recovering from strokes.

Given the three levels of prevention, there is almost always some intervention that could improve the health of those who are vulnerable to a particular disease or are already sick. Primary prevention is the preferred option when a cost-effective preventive intervention is available. When primary prevention is not

Level	Also Called...	Target Population	Goal	Examples
Primary prevention	Prevention	People without disease	Prevent disease from ever occurring	■ Vaccinating children to protect them from paralytic polio ■ Giving vitamin A capsules to at-risk children to prevent blindness
Secondary prevention	Early diagnosis	People with early, non-symptomatic disease	Reduce the severity of disease and prevent disability and death	■ Checking blood pressure routinely to detect the onset of hypertension ■ Screening with mammography to detect early-stage breast cancer
Tertiary prevention	Treatment and rehabilitation	People with symptomatic disease	Reduce impairment and minimize suffering	■ Extracting teeth with severe decay in order to alleviate pain ■ Providing physical therapy to people who have been injured in a vehicle collision in order to prevent long-term disability

FIGURE 1-8 Three levels of prevention: primary, secondary, and tertiary.

possible or health problems are already present, secondary prevention and tertiary prevention can improve longevity and quality of life.

▶ 1.4 Health Transitions

The changing health profiles observed in high-income countries over the last century are strong evidence that large-scale health interventions are effective at improving health throughout the life course. One hundred years ago, most populations across the globe had similar health profiles: high birth rates, high death rates, short life expectancies, and a considerable number of diseases and deaths due to infections and undernutrition. During the 20th century, most high-income nations made a transition to a lower birth rate, a lower death rate, longer life expectancies, and a higher burden from the chronic diseases often associated with overnutrition. For example, in the United States, the leading causes of death in 1800 and 1900 were pneumonia (including pneumonia caused by influenza), tuberculosis, and diarrhea, all of which are infectious diseases.[15] By 1950, the death rate had dropped significantly, life expectancy had increased, and the most common causes of death had shifted to heart disease, cancer, and stroke, the same noncommunicable diseases that remain the most frequent causes of death in the United States today.[16] These changes in population health status were due to a variety of factors, including new health technologies, such as new vaccines, new antibiotics, and new contraceptives, as well as improved sanitation, better nutrition, increased education, and economic growth.[17]

A **health transition** is a shift in the health status of a population that usually occurs in conjunction with socioeconomic development. Over the last century, high-income countries have experienced a diversity of health transitions: decreases in fertility rates, changes in population size and age structures, substantial reductions in the risk of death from pregnancy-related conditions, shifts from hunger to obesity as a dominant nutritional concern, increases in health problems associated with sedentary lifestyles, decreases in infectious diseases and corresponding increases in chronic diseases, reductions in infant and child mortality, and increases in life expectancy and the proportion of older adults in the population (**FIGURE 1–9**). Low-income countries have not experienced such dramatic changes.

Because some countries have gone through these health transitions and other countries have not, there are now significant differences in health status in the highest-income and lowest-income countries (**FIGURE 1–10**). A diversity of health statistics

Type of Transition	Pre-transition Populations	Post-transition Populations
Fertility transition	The typical woman gives birth to several children.	The typical woman gives birth to only one child or two children.
Demographic transition	The total population size may be increasing due to high birth rates.	The total population size may be shrinking because birth rates are so low.
Obstetric transition	Pregnancy-related conditions are a common cause of death in women of reproductive age.	The maternal mortality rate is very low.
Nutrition transition	Underweight is a major concern.	Obesity is a major concern.
Risk transition	Environmental exposures like unsafe drinking water and polluted indoor air are major contributors to disease.	Lifestyle factors like physical inactivity and tobacco use are major contributors to disease.
Epidemiologic transition	Infectious diseases in children are a significant burden to the population.	Chronic diseases in adults are the dominant health concern in the population.
Mortality transition	High death rates in children and reproductive-age adults mean that few people live to very old age.	Low mortality rates for children and reproductive-age adults allow many people to live to old age.
Aging transition	Children comprise the majority of the total population.	Older adults are a growing proportion of the population.

FIGURE 1–9 Examples of health transitions.

Today, in Very LOW-Income Populations...	Today, in Very HIGH-Income Populations...
■ There are high rates of poverty, illiteracy, and unemployment, which can have negative effects on personal, family, and community health.	■ Most people have access to the basic tools for health, although there are still health disparities based on socioeconomic status.
■ Many people do not have access to an outhouse or other type of toilet and many do not have reliable access to safe drinking water.	■ Almost everyone has indoor plumbing and safe drinking water.
■ Many infants and young children die from diarrhea, pneumonia, malaria, and other infections.	■ Almost every baby will survive to adulthood.
■ The typical woman gives birth to many children, and it is not uncommon for women to die in childbirth.	■ The typical woman gives birth to 1 or 2 children, and very few women die due to pregnancy-related conditions.
■ The median (average) age of the population is in childhood.	■ The median (average) age of the population is in adulthood.
■ A typical age at death for adults is 60 or 70 years old.	■ A typical age at death for adults is 80 or even 90 years old.
■ Visits to hospitals and clinics are usually because of infections (such as malaria or tuberculosis) or serious injuries.	■ Visits to hospitals and clinics are usually due to chronic noncommunicable diseases (such as arthritis, back pain, hypertension, and diabetes).
■ Access to effective management of chronic diseases (such as hypertension and diabetes) is very limited.	■ Screening tests (such as mammography for breast cancer) often detect emerging health problems early, when they are usually more treatable.
■ Undernutrition (including protein energy and micronutrient deficiencies) remains a significant public health concern.	■ Overweight and obesity are major public health concerns, and many people have diets that are excessively high in fat and calories.
■ Very few people with mental health disorders receive clinical care because there are so few psychiatrists and psychologists.	■ Clinical mental health services are usually available, but they are often underused.
■ Serious injuries often lead to death because no surgical services are available.	■ Serious injuries can often be treated with surgery and rehabilitation

FIGURE 1-10 Examples of significant differences in health status and access to the tools for health in low-income and high-income countries.

illustrate the wide gaps in health status.[18] A baby born in Japan in 2015 could expect to live to about 84 years old, but a newborn in Sierra Leone, in West Africa, could only expect to live to age 50. A woman giving birth in Sierra Leone in 2015 was about 450 times more likely to die of a pregnancy-related condition than a pregnant woman living in Finland, in northern Europe. A baby born in Angola, in southwestern Africa, was nearly 80 times more likely to die before his or her fifth birthday than a baby born in Iceland. A 30-year-old living in Mongolia, in central Asia, was 3.5 times more likely to die from heart disease, cancer, chronic respiratory diseases, or diabetes before age 70 than an adult of the same age living in Switzerland. Those multipliers would not have been as high 100 years ago when no one had access to neonatal intensive care units, advanced obstetric care, antibiotics, and medications for managing chronic diseases. As some populations have gained access to more tools for health, and others have not, the disparities in the health profiles of high- and low-income countries have become more extreme.

Middle-income countries tend to have intermediate health profiles with statistics somewhere between those of high-income and low-income countries. Many middle-income countries continue to have some populations burdened by undernutrition and infectious diseases while, at the same time, other populations within the same country experience the challenges associated with obesity and chronic noncommunicable conditions. This need for the health system in middle-income countries to address both "pre-transition" and "post-transition" health problems is sometimes called the "dual burden" of disease. Comparing high-, middle-, and low-income countries provides insights into how health transitions occur and insights into the types of interventions that are likely to be effective at achieving particular types of changes in population health status.

▶ 1.5 World Regions and Featured Countries

Throughout this book, data from eight large countries will be used to represent the diversity of the world's health profiles, including the three countries with the largest populations—China and India, which each have more than 1 billion residents, and the United States, which has more than 320 million inhabitants—as well as five other countries that are among the 19 countries that are each home to more than 1% of the world's population (that is, more than 75 million people).[19] Together, these eight countries are home to half of the world's people (**FIGURE 1–11**).

The featured countries represent a diversity of economic profiles (**FIGURE 1–12**). The World Bank divides countries into four categories based on the gross national income per person. Of the eight featured countries, two are classified as high income, three as upper-middle income, two as lower-middle income, and one as low income. This classification is

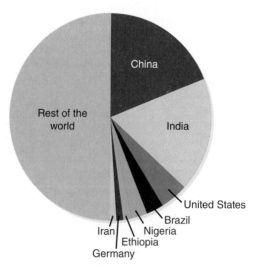

FIGURE 1–11 The eight featured countries represent nearly half of the world's population.

Data from *World development indicators 2016*. Washington DC: World Bank; 2016.

Country	World Bank Income Group	UNDP Human Development Level
United States	High	Very high
Germany	High	Very high
Iran	Upper middle	High
Brazil	Upper middle	High
China	Upper middle	High
India	Lower middle	Medium
Nigeria	Lower middle	Low
Ethiopia	Low	Low

FIGURE 1-12 Eight featured countries by income group.

The countries are listed in order from highest to lowest human development index.
Data from *World development indicators* 2016. Washington DC: World Bank; 2016. *Human development report 2016*. New York: UNDP; 2016.

similar to the distribution of the world's population by income level, since 70% of the world's people live in a country classified as middle income by the World Bank (**FIGURE 1-13**).[19] Many analyses of global health compare the health status in **low- and middle-income countries (LMICs)**, a category that includes all low-income, lower-middle-income, and upper-middle-income countries, to the health status in high-income countries (HICs). Some global health reports compare LMICs to countries that are members of the **Organisation for Economic Co-operation and Development (OECD)**, an intergovernmental organization that represents about three dozen of the world's richest countries. Six of the eight featured countries in this book are LMICs and two are OECD-member HICs.

The United Nations Development Programme (UNDP) divides countries into four groups (very high, high, medium, and low) based on a human development index calculated from income per person plus statistics about longevity and education.[20] These categories generally align with the World Bank group classifications, but one of the featured lower-middle-income countries (Nigeria) is classified as having a low rather than a medium human development level. The featured countries also represent geographic diversity (**FIGURE 1-14**), covering all seven World Bank analytical regions and all six of the WHO's regions (**FIGURE 1-15**).

There is often considerable diversity in the socioeconomic and health profiles of countries within the same world region. There is also considerable diversity among different states or provinces within countries and between urban and rural areas. These types of within-country differences can be observed in all eight of the featured countries. For example, parts of southern Nigeria have a middle-income economic profile while some of the northern areas of Nigeria have a very low-income profile and are at risk of famine.[21] National statistical reports present the average values for various metrics, and those averages do not

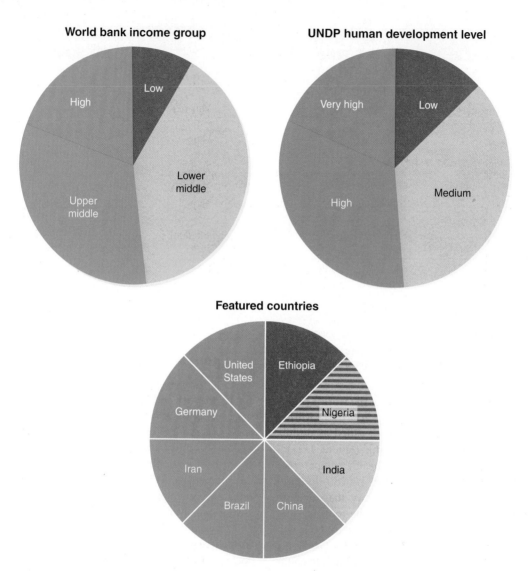

FIGURE 1–13 Most of the world's people live in a country classified as middle income by the World Bank.

Data from *World development indicators 2016*. Washington DC: World Bank; 2016; *Human development report 2016*. New York: UNDP; 2016.

express the wide range of values that may be present within diverse regions of the country. Despite that limitation, general patterns can be observed by comparing statistics from large countries. The differences between higher-income (high- and upper-middle-income) countries and lower-income (lower-middle and low-income) countries are often notable (**FIGURE 1–16**). For example, data from just the eight featured countries are sufficient to illustrate the patterns associated with the fertility transition (women in higher-income countries have fewer babies), the obstetric transition (higher-income countries have lower rates of maternal mortality), and the aging transition (higher-income countries have older populations) (**FIGURE 1–17**).[20] Similar trends can be observed for a great diversity of indicators.

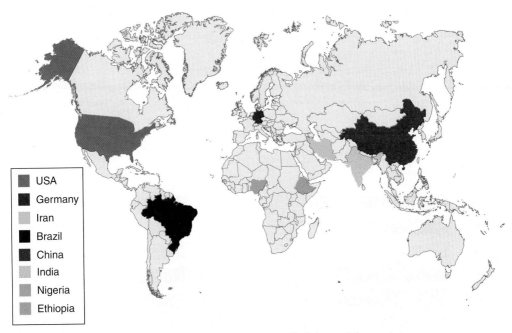

FIGURE 1–14 Eight featured countries representing nearly half of the world's population.

Data from *World development indicators 2016*. Washington DC: World Bank; 2016.

Country	Geographic Location	World Bank Region	WHO Region
United States	North America	North America	Americas
Germany	Europe	Europe and Central Asia	Europe
Iran	Middle East	Middle East and North Africa	Eastern Mediterranean
Brazil	South America	Latin America and the Caribbean	Americas
China	East Asia	East Asia and Pacific	Western Pacific
India	South Asia	South Asia	South-East Asia
Nigeria	West Africa	Sub-Saharan Africa	Africa
Ethiopia	East Africa	Sub-Saharan Africa	Africa

FIGURE 1–15 Eight featured countries by geographic location.

World development indicators 2016. Washington DC: World Bank; 2016; *World health statistics 2016: Monitoring health for the SDGs*. Geneva: WHO; 2016.

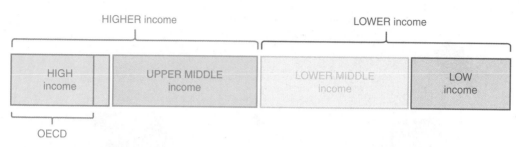

FIGURE 1–16 Income-level terminology.

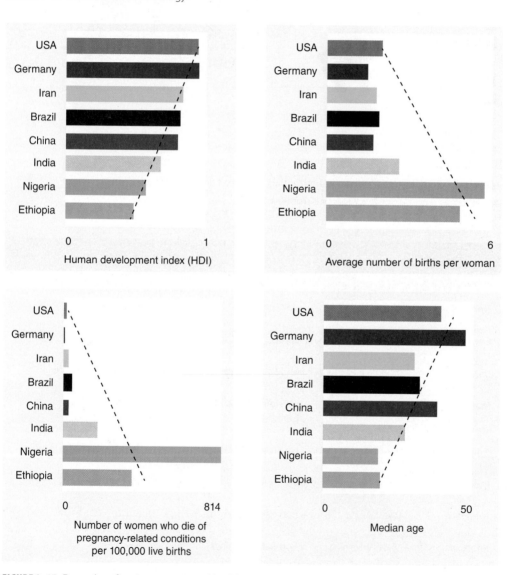

FIGURE 1–17 Examples of socioeconomic and health trends.

Data from *Human development report 2016*. New York: UNDP; 2016.

▶ 1.6 Global Health Security

The goal of the first international health initiatives was to prevent widespread outbreaks of infectious diseases. For example, a series of International Sanitary Conferences held in various European cities starting in 1851 assembled representatives from several countries to address concerns about travel and trade spreading cholera to new ports.[22] Signatories of the resulting agreements agreed to notify other countries about outbreaks of cholera, plague, yellow fever, and other epidemic diseases, and they pledged to monitor health at ports and impose quarantines on disease-carrying ships.[23] These treaties set the stage for the International Sanitary Regulations (later renamed the International Health Regulations) that were approved by the WHO 100 years later in 1951 and are still in force today. By the early 1900s, international regulations addressed several other cross-border health issues, including drugs and alcohol sales, occupational health and safety, and water pollution,[24] but the initial impetus for these deliberations was the recognition that countries had to collaborate with their neighbors to keep dangerous pathogens at bay.

A second set of early international health concerns focused on threats to economic and political interests. The field of tropical medicine blossomed in the late 1800s and early 1900s as more European (and American) military personnel, businessmen, and their families relocated to colonies in tropical climates.[25] Tropical medicine specialists aimed not only to protect settlers from parasitic and infectious diseases—a role similar to that of travel medicine specialists today—but also to ensure that the workforce in these areas could be productive.[26] Today, tropical medicine has expanded to become **international health**,[10] a term that now typically refers to initiatives targeted toward addressing poverty-related health conditions in lower-income areas, no matter which geographic region they happen to be located in.[27] While many international health programs are humanitarian, they also enable workers and consumers in the recipient countries to remain active participants in the global economy.

Human security was defined in the 1994 *Human Development Report* as the freedom from fear and want that results from having health security as well as food security (freedom from hunger), personal security (freedom from violence), environmental security (freedom from preventable environmental vulnerabilities), economic security (freedom from extreme poverty), community security (freedom from discrimination), and political security (freedom from human rights violations).[28] Human security focuses on individual and community well-being, while national security focuses on the protection of the collective interests of people living within a country's borders. For many countries, promoting health security and other aspects of human security in other countries is a core component of national security plans.[29] The investment in global health activities by high-income countries generates major returns through expanded markets for international trade, strengthened diplomatic relationships, and fortified homeland security.[30]

The nascent field of **global health security** seeks to protect populations from threats to health and safety by engaging a diversity of stakeholders, including governmental and military personnel, in public health interventions.[31] The current concept of global health security is an extension of the historic international health policies and practices that aimed to stem the spread of epidemics as international travel and trade became more common.[32] Communities and countries suffering from widespread health problems are more likely to have political and economic instability, and poverty and unrest can further exacerbate public health problems that might spill over into other parts of the world. International and global health initiatives can help to break this cycle, facilitating peace and productivity. Global health security recognizes that countries participating in global health activities reap the benefits of self-protection in addition to the humanitarian gains and goodwill that these actions may generate.[33]

▶ 1.7 Globalization and Health: Shared Futures

Globalization is the process of countries around the world becoming more integrated and interdependent across economic, political, cultural, and other domains. Globalization contributes to the health transitions that are occurring in many parts of the world by increasing access to health technologies, encouraging urbanization, changing social and cultural practices, and accelerating environmental changes.[34] Globalization can also be observed in the increasing number of global governmental and nongovernmental organizations, the proliferation of multilateral trade agreements, and increases in global supply chains, foreign direct investment, population mobility, communication, data sharing, and cultural diffusion.

The concept of globalization is not new to the field of public health. Infectious diseases like plague and smallpox spread across Asia and Europe more than a 1000 years ago, when sea and land trade routes like the Silk Road linked China, India, and the Mediterranean. The pathogens carried by the Europeans who explored the Americas in the 15th century caused the decimation of many indigenous American populations, while some infections indigenous to the Western hemisphere (such as syphilis) made their way back to Europe and sparked mass epidemics.[35] Pathogens have never stopped at national boundaries, and modern transportation allows for a new infectious disease that emerges in any part of the world to be transported by aircraft to any

other part of the world within hours rather than weeks or months. Concerns about globalization and health also encompass a diversity of other emerging health issues, like bioterrorism, drug resistance, food safety, and the health effects of climate change.

Globalization is not a uniformly good or bad process, but one that yields a mix of positive and negative outcomes.[36] For example, globalization has allowed more goods to be manufactured in middle-income countries and then sold in high-income countries where higher salaries for workers make manufacturing comparatively expensive. In middle-income countries, globalization often means more job opportunities, but there may also be pressures to increase productivity even if that causes environmental damage or creates unsafe working conditions. In high-income areas, international trade reduces the cost of consumer products but it also means that there are fewer local jobs in the manufacturing sector. Cheaper products created in middle-income countries also make it harder for the lowest-income countries to participate in the global economy because the poorest countries do not have educational systems geared toward producing a technologically skilled workforce. Globalization tends to create greater inequalities in income between countries and within countries.

Concerns about the adverse impacts of globalization have led in many countries to the rise of nationalistic political movements that call for greater self-reliance and less engagement with other nations. However, even if countries implement isolationist policies, it is not possible to eliminate the need for involvement in global health activities. The threat from emerging infectious diseases is an ancient one that will continue to exist for future generations, and environmental hazards can easily cross international borders when they are carried by air, water, or animals. Whether a country has pro- or anti-globalization policies, it is in every country's best interests to actively engage in communicating about transnational health concerns, sharing the scientific discoveries that enable populations to fortify themselves against threats to health, and collaborating on health interventions that promote peace, prosperity, and security.

Global health offers a proactive way to prevent outbreaks (and to respond to them when they happen), to protect economic and political interests at home and abroad, to promote goodwill and humanitarian values, and to achieve shared health and development goals.[37] Global health is a dynamic field. The health patterns that exist today are not the same as the patterns from 100 years ago, and new health transitions will occur in the coming decades. Global health provides an opportunity to use prevention strategies and other interventions to shape a healthier, safer future for the world's people.

▶ References

1. Huber M, Knottnerus JA, Green L, et al. How should we define health? *BMJ*. 2011;343:d4163.
2. Kuh D, Ben-Shlomo Y, Lynch J, Hallqvist J, Power C. Life course epidemiology. *J Epidemiol Community Health*. 2003;57:778–83.
3. Committee on Assuring the Health of the Public in the 21st Century. *The future of the public's health in the 21st century*. Washington DC: National Academies Press; 2002.
4. Susser M, Susser E. Choosing a future for epidemiology: I. Eras and paradigms. *Am J Public Health*. 1996;86:668–73.
5. Bingham P, Verlander NQ, Cheal MJ. John Snow, William Farr and the 1849 outbreak of cholera that affected London: A reworking of the data highlights the importance of the water supply. *Public Health*. 2004;118:387–94.
6. Shryock RH. The early American public health movement. *Am J Public Health*. 1937;27:965–71.
7. Pearce N. Traditional epidemiology, modern epidemiology, and public health. *Am J Public Health*. 1996;86:678–83.
8. Doll R, Hill AB. Lung cancer and other causes of death in relation to smoking. *Br Med J*. 1956;2:1071–81.
9. Hackshaw AK, Law MR, Wald NJ. The accumulated evidence on lung cancer and environmental tobacco smoke. *BMJ*. 1997;315:980–8.
10. Packard RM. *A history of global health: Interventions into the lives of other peoples*. Baltimore MD: Johns Hopkins University Press; 2016.
11. Harrell JA, Baker EL; Essential Services Work Group. The essential services of public health. *Leadersh Public Health*. 1994;3:27–30.
12. *The Ottawa Charter for Health Promotion*. Ottawa: 1st International Conference on Health Promotion; 1986.
13. Keller LO, Strohschein S, Lia-Hoagberg B, Schaffer MA. Population-based public health interventions: Practice-based and evidence-supported. *Public Health Nurs*. 2004;21:453–68.
14. Flay BR, Biglan A, Boruch RF, et al. Standards of evidence: Criteria for efficacy, effectiveness and dissemination. *Prev Sci*. 2005;6:151–75.
15. Jones DS, Podolsky SH, Greene JA. The burden of disease and the changing task of medicine. *New Engl J Med*. 2012;366:2333–8.
16. Guyer B, Freedman MA, Strobino DM, Sondik EJ. Annual summary of vital statistics: Trends in the health of Americans during the 20th century. *Pediatrics*. 2000;106:1307–17.
17. Martens P. Health transitions in a globalising world: Towards more disease or sustained health? *Futures*. 2002;34:635–48.
18. *World health statistics 2016: Monitoring health for the SDGs*. Geneva: WHO; 2016.
19. *World development indicators 2016*. Washington DC: World Bank; 2016.
20. *Human development report 2016*. New York: UNDP; 2016.
21. *National human development report 2015: Human security and human development in Nigeria*. Abuja: UNDP Nigeria; 2015.
22. Huber V. The unification of the globe by disease? The International Sanitary Conferences on cholera, 1951–1894. *Historical J*. 2006;49:453–76.
23. Fidler DP. From International Sanitary Conventions to global health security: The new International Health Regulations. *Chinese J Int Law*. 2005;4:325–92.
24. Fidler DP. The globalization of public health: The first 100 years of international health diplomacy. *Bull World Health Organ*. 2001;79:842–9.
25. Gibson AD. Miasma revisited: The intellectual history of tropical medicine. *Aust Fam Physician*. 2009;38:57–9.
26. Brown ER. Public health in imperialism: Early Rockefeller programs at home and abroad. *Am J Public Health*. 1976;66:897–903.
27. Koplan JP, Bond TC, Merson MH, et al. Consortium of Universities for Global Health Executive Board. Towards a common definition of global health. *Lancet*. 2009;373:1993–5.
28. *Human development report 1994*. New York: UNDP; 1994.

29. Oslo Ministerial Declaration: Global health: A pressing foreign policy issue of our time. *Lancet.* 2007;369:1373–8.

30. *The Case for U.S. Investment in the Global Fund and Global Health.* Washington DC: Friends of the Global Fight against AIDS, Tuberculosis and Malaria; 2017.

31. Aldis W. Health security as a public health concept: A critical analysis. *Health Policy Plan.* 2008;23:369–75.

32. Hoffman SJ. The evolution, etiology and eventualities of the global health security regime. *Health Policy Plan.* 2010;25:510–22.

33. Lakoff A. Two regimes of global health. *Humanity.* 2010;1:59–79.

34. McMichael AJ. Globalization, climate change, and human health. *N Engl J Med.* 2013;368:1335–43.

35. Morens DM, Folkers GK, Fauci AS. Emerging infections: A perpetual challenge. *Lancet Infect Dis.* 2008;8:710–19.

36. Osland JS. Broadening the debate: The pros and cons of globalization. *J Manage Inquiry.* 2003;12:137–54.

37. *Global health works: Maximizing U.S. investments for healthier and stronger communities.* Washington DC: Global Health Council; 2017.

CHAPTER 2

Global Health Priorities

Global health priorities are established based on population needs assessments, economic evaluations of the tools that are available to deploy as interventions, donor values, and security considerations. Health metrics provide valuable information for priority-setting, decision-making, and monitoring of progress toward achieving global health targets. Global partnerships for development like the Sustainable Development Goals also shape the global health agenda and encourage transnational cooperation to address shared priorities.

▶ 2.1 Global Health Achievements

Innovations in health technology during the last century have created an incredible set of tools for global health work. New antibiotics were discovered along with a host of medications for treating noncommunicable diseases (NCDs) like heart disease and cancer. Lifesaving vaccines were developed. Smallpox was eradicated. Oral contraceptives transformed family planning, and assisted reproductive technologies enabled many couples with infertility problems to have biological children. New diagnostic tools, such as electrocardiographs and MRIs, increased the quality of medical care, as did new therapies, like insulin for diabetes, dialysis for kidney disease, and contact lenses for vision impairments. Modern surgical techniques made joint replacements, open heart surgery, and organ transplants routine in some parts of the world. These technological advances enabled many of the top 10 public health achievements of the 20th century that were highlighted by the U.S. Centers for Disease Control and Prevention (CDC) at the start of the new millennium (FIGURE 2–1)[1] as well as many of the leading global health achievements during the first years of the 21st century (FIGURE 2–2).[2]

While these health technologies are indisputably beneficial, the uneven distribution of access to them has generated a massive intensification of health disparities. People living in the world's richest countries now have access to an array of tools for health that would have been unimaginable 100 years ago, while children living in the world's poorest areas continue to succumb to easily preventable conditions like starvation and vaccine-preventable and antibiotic-treatable infectious diseases. At the same time that the health profiles of populations worldwide were becoming more

1	Vaccination
2	Motor-vehicle safety
3	Safer workplaces
4	Control of infectious diseases
5	Decline in deaths from ischemic heart disease and stroke
6	Safer and healthier foods
7	Healthier mothers and babies
8	Family planning
9	Fluoridation of drinking water
10	Recognition of tobacco as a health hazard

FIGURE 2–1 The U.S. CDC's top 10 public health achievements of the 20th century (1900–1999).

Reproduced from Ten great public health achievements: United States, 1990–1999. *MMWR Morb Mort Wkly Rev* 1999;48:241–3.

1	Reductions in child mortality
2	Vaccine-preventable diseases
3	Access to safe water and sanitation
4	Malaria prevention and control
5	Prevention and control of HIV/AIDS
6	Tuberculosis control
7	Control of neglected tropical diseases
8	Tobacco control
9	Increased awareness and response for improving global road safety
10	Improved preparedness and response to global health threats

FIGURE 2–2 The U.S. CDC's top 10 global health achievements in the first decade of the 21st century (2001–2010).

Data from CDC, Ten great public health achievements: Worldwide, 2001–2010. *MMWR Morb Mort Wkly Rev* 2011; 60:814-8.

disparate, the 20th century brought potent reminders that all people around the world are at risk from a shared set of hazards. The emergence of HIV, virulent new strains of influenza, and drug-resistant pathogens prompted truly global research and response efforts. The goals of global health in the 21st century are to continue to create innovative solutions to public health problems; to increase access to health, healthcare services, and health technologies around the world; and to expand global communication and action about shared health concerns.

In an ideal world, there would be enough resources for all worthy global health goals to receive the funding they need to be achieved.

In the real world, the amount of funding available for health interventions is limited. Advocates for various health problems and solutions must compete for attention and support, and only the proposals that garner buy-in from well-resourced groups are able to move forward. The gap between commendable ideas and the resources to implement them has created a demand for prioritization strategies that allow funders to make informed decisions about where and how to invest in global health. When future generations compile lists celebrating the major global health accomplishments of the 21st century, those lists will reflect the decisions today's global health leaders make about which projects to prioritize.

▶ 2.2 Prioritization Strategies

Funding agencies and planning committees use a variety of strategies to prioritize the types of activities that they will support.[3] For example, some focus specifically on health and nutrition interventions, while others support broader education and economic development activities that enable healthier communities. Some give priority to prevention activities, and some prioritize treatment of existing health issues. Some prepare primary health facilities to address a diversity of health issues, and some focus on increasing access to advanced disease-specific care at tertiary hospitals. The priorities identified by groups viewing global health with different lenses provide insight into the common health challenges of nations and populations around the world, and they point toward solutions for shared concerns. The PACES definition of global health—one that considers populations, action, cooperation, equity, and security to be identifiers of global health issues—also provides a framework for prioritizing items for the global health agenda (**FIGURE 2–3**).

One approach is to establish priorities based on the health concerns that affect the most people. The term **burden of disease** (BOD) refers to the adverse impact of a particular health condition (or group of conditions) on a population. Disease burden can be measured using health metrics (like the number of deaths from a particular disease) and economic indicators (like the total direct costs of medical care for a disease plus the indirect costs of absences from work or school due to the condition). Groups that

Lens	Key Questions
Populations	What are the health issues that cause the greatest number of deaths, illnesses, and disability worldwide? Which populations have the greatest need?
Action	What are the "best buys" among the available interventions? How do we allocate resources to do the greatest good for the greatest number of people?
Cooperation	What are the goals of the partners? What problem is the partnership best equipped to solve?
Equity	What actions will do the most to improve the lives of children and other vulnerable populations? How will the intervention reduce health disparities?
Security	What are the greatest threats to peace? How will the intervention help to achieve the national interests of sponsoring governments?

FIGURE 2–3 PACES: strategies for prioritizing global health issues.

prioritize global health spending based on a population lens make their decisions after looking at statistics about the conditions that cause the greatest BOD. For example, the **Global Burden of Disease (GBD)** project, a massive collaborative effort to quantify the epidemiologic profiles of every country in the world that was initiated by the World Health Organization (WHO) in the 1990s and is now housed at the Institute for Health Metrics and Evaluation (IHME) in Seattle has identified unhealthy diets, child and maternal undernutrition, untreated high blood pressure, tobacco smoke, and indoor and outdoor air pollution as some of the most common modifiable exposures that cause poor health and early death globally.[4] The evidence that these risk factors cause a substantial BOD can be used to support proposals for interventions that will enable a large number of people to live longer, healthier lives. The GBD collaborators also release annual estimates of the causes of death, illness, and disability worldwide and for each country. These numbers inform the development of policy recommendations that can be acted on by governmental bodies and other public health funders and implementers.

Prioritization based on an action orientation often gives the highest ratings to the cost-effective interventions that have been identified as "best buys" because they help many people make meaningful gains in health status at a low cost per person (or at a low cost per adverse event averted by the intervention).[5] In general, low-cost primary prevention activities are the most cost-effective interventions.[6] The Disease Control Priorities (DCP) project has identified vaccinating children, preventing malaria and HIV infections, treating tuberculosis and common communicable childhood diseases to prevent them from spreading to other people, improving the basic care of newborns, distributing micronutrients to children and pregnant women, taxing tobacco products to reduce use, expanding the use of cardiovascular medications to prevent heart attacks and strokes, and enforcing traffic laws to reduce injuries as some of the highest-impact global health interventions (**FIGURE 2–4**).[7]

Some groups make decisions based on the special interests and capabilities of the collaborators. For example, the 14 Grand Challenges in Global Health identified by the Bill & Melinda Gates Foundation in 2003 highlighted critical needs for new health technologies (**FIGURE 2–5**),[8] and the Gates Foundation subsequently used that list as part of selecting proposals to fund. Because the Gates Foundation is led by people with expertise in computers and information technology, the foundation is uniquely prepared to support the development and dissemination of new tech products. When funding and implementation agencies have particular areas of expertise, they can maximize their impact by applying their existing knowledge and experience toward new projects that build on past successes.

Groups focused on equity prioritize projects that will address perceived injustices and reduce health disparities. Many equity-oriented programs focus on the health of infants and children because of the nearly universal belief that no child anywhere should suffer from abuse, hunger, or preventable diseases.[9] Equity-focused initiatives may also focus on the health of other vulnerable populations, like refugees and other migrants, people in prison, people with disabilities, and older adults, or they may advocate for human rights.

Another common approach is to make prioritization decisions based on the security interests of sponsoring governments, including direct and indirect threats to national, regional, and global peace and stability. For example, the top public health challenges that the U.S. CDC has identified for the United States

	Target	Action
1	Child health	Vaccinate children against major childhood killers, including measles, polio, tetanus, whooping cough, and diphtheria.
2	Child health	Monitor children's health to prevent or, if necessary, treat childhood pneumonia, diarrhea, and malaria.
3	Tobacco use	Tax tobacco products to increase consumers' costs by at least one-third to curb smoking and reduce the prevalence of cardiovascular disease, cancer, and respiratory disease.
4	HIV/AIDS	Attack the spread of HIV through a coordinated approach that includes promoting 100% condom use among populations at high risk; treating other sexually transmitted infections; providing antiretroviral medications, especially for pregnant women; and offering voluntary HIV counseling and testing.
5	Maternal and child health	Give children and pregnant women essential nutrients, including vitamin A, iron, and iodine, to prevent maternal anemia, infant deaths, and long-term health problems.
6	Malaria	Provide insecticide-treated bednets in malaria-endemic areas to drastically reduce malaria.
7	Injury prevention	Enforce traffic regulations and install speed bumps at dangerous intersections to reduce traffic-related injuries.
8	TB	Treat TB patients with short-course chemotherapy to cure infected people and prevent new infections.
9	Child health	Teach mothers and train birth attendants to keep newborns warm and clean to reduce illness and death.
10	Cardiovascular disease	Promote use of aspirin and other inexpensive medications to treat and prevent heart attack and stroke.

FIGURE 2–4 Ten "best buys" in global health from the Disease Control Priorities Project.

Reproduced from *Pathways to global health research: strategic plan 2008–2012*. Bethesda MD: The John E. Fogarty International Center, National Institutes of Health (NIH); 2008, p. 22.

	1	Create effective single-dose vaccines.
Improve childhood vaccines	2	Prepare vaccines that do not require refrigeration.
	3	Develop needle-free vaccine delivery systems.
	4	Devise testing systems for new vaccines.
Create new vaccines	5	Design antigens for protective immunity.
	6	Learn about immunological responses.
Control insects that transmit agents of disease	7	Develop genetic strategy to control insects.
	8	Develop chemical strategy to control insects.
Improve nutrition to promote health	9	Create a nutrient-rich staple plant species.
Improve drug treatment of infectious diseases	10	Find medications and delivery systems to limit drug resistance.
Cure latent and chronic infection	11	Create therapies that can cure latent infection.
	12	Create immunological methods to cure latent infection.
Measure health status accurately and economically in developing countries	13	Develop technologies to assess population health.
	14	Develop versatile diagnostic tools.

FIGURE 2–5 Grand Challenges in Global Health.

Data from Varmus H, Klausner R, Zerhouni E, Acharya T, Daar AS, Singer PA. Grand challenges in global health. *Science* 2003; 302:398-9.

include protecting the environment, responding to emerging infectious diseases (including pandemic influenza and drug-resistant pathogens), and reducing the burden from violence (including the physical and psychological traumas sustained by military personnel deployed to conflict areas) (**FIGURE 2–6**).[10] These types of threats to health and security cannot be alleviated by any one country working in isolation. Once a country has identified its own strategic global health priorities, that country is prepared to advocate for those priorities in conversations with potential partners. Working with partner nations on achieving shared aims will then advance health security at home and abroad.

1	Institute a rational healthcare system (balance equity, cost, and quality).
2	Eliminate health disparities.
3	Focus on children's emotional and intellectual development.
4	Achieve a longer "healthspan" (healthy aging).
5	Integrate physical activity and healthy eating into daily lives.
6	Clean up and protect the environment.
7	Prepare to respond to emerging infectious diseases.
8	Recognize and address the contributions of mental health to overall health and well-being.
9	Reduce the toll of violence in society.
10	Use new scientific knowledge and technological advances wisely.

FIGURE 2-6 The U.S. CDC's top public health challenges for the early 21st century.

Data from Koplan JP, Fleming DW. Current and future public health challenges. *JAMA* 2000; 284:1696-8.

▶ 2.3 Health Metrics

As more resources have been devoted to global health efforts, it has become increasingly important to quantify the health needs in various parts of the world, identify major modifiable risk factors for common diseases, assess the impact of new public health interventions, and monitor changes in the health status of populations over time. The key measures of health and disease in populations include information about population size, the birth rates and death rates, the causes of death, the frequency and causes of various illnesses and disabilities, and the rate at which members of the population engage in risky behaviors. All of these measures provide an evidence base for making policy and funding decisions.[11]

Health information comes from a wide variety of sources, including census data, registries, surveillance systems, household surveys, and health services records, such as hospital patient files and insurance claims.[12] Many types of health data are disseminated through the websites and annual reports of major governmental and nongovernmental health organizations and through academic journal articles. The websites of the WHO, the U.S. CDC, the U.S. National Institutes of Health (NIH), and other health agencies provide easy-to-read and regularly updated information about hundreds of diseases. For example, the WHO's *Weekly Epidemiological Record* and the CDC's *Morbidity and Mortality Weekly Report* (*MMWR*) provide timely information about emerging health issues, such as new outbreaks of serious infections.

For comparative global health statistics, the best sources are often the appendices of the annual reports of UN agencies, such as the WHO's annual *World Health Statistics* report and UNICEF's annual *State of the World's Children* report. For disease-specific statistics, the reports of specialty organizations can be helpful references. For example, some global cancer statistics are reported every year by the American Cancer Society and by the International Agency for Research on Cancer (IARC), which is part of the UN system.

For detailed information about particular research methods and findings, the best sources are academic and professional journals articles that have undergone **peer review**, which means that before the papers were published, the manuscripts were sent to experts in the field who scrutinized the methodology and evaluated the validity of the results. An **abstract** is a one-paragraph summary of the methods, results, and conclusions of a scientific investigation. Abstract databases like MEDLINE can be used to search for abstracts summarizing journal articles on selected topics. The full reports can then be found online or in a library. These various types of high-quality resources provide an evidence-based foundation for those who seek to create, implement, evaluate, or improve global public health policies and practices.

Most countries maintain **vital statistics** on their residents, population-level metrics about births, deaths, and other life events. Vital statistics are compiled from birth and death certificates, marriage and divorce certificates, census records, and other sources. Demographers use these statistics to understand the current population distribution and predict the size and characteristics of the population in future years. The **birth rate** is the annual number of births per 1000 people in the total population. The birth rate is usually highest in the lowest-income countries (**FIGURE 2–7**). The **death rate**, also called the **mortality rate**, is the annual number of deaths per 1000 people (or other units, such as per 100,000 people). Mortality rates can be presented for all-cause mortality and for specific causes of death. The all-cause death rate is usually higher in populations with a large percentage of older adults than in populations with an abundance of school-aged children because age-specific

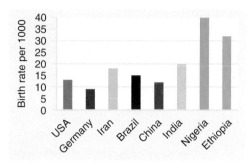

FIGURE 2–7 Birth rate per 1000 people in 2015 in featured countries.

Data from *World development indicators 2016*. Washington: World Bank; 2016.

mortality rates are higher for older adults than for younger people. Age-adjusted rates that account for differences in population age structures are usually used to compare mortality rates in two or more populations. While the crude (unadjusted) all-cause mortality rates are typically highest in high-income countries that have a large proportion of older adults, the age-standardized (adjusted) mortality rates are usually highest in low-income countries (**FIGURE 2–8**).

Measuring **mortality** (death) at the population level can be challenging for two principal reasons. The first is that in many parts of the world there is no system for reliably registering vital statistics. In places where most births and deaths occur in homes instead of in hospitals, few births and deaths are documented by government officials. The most disadvantaged populations—often the ones with the highest mortality rates—are the least likely to have their life events accurately counted. Thus, while very precise mortality statistics are available from high-income countries, death rates in low-income countries often must be estimated based on limited data. The second key challenge is assigning one cause of death to each deceased individual. Should a person with HIV/AIDS who dies of tuberculosis be recorded as an HIV death or a TB death? Should a person with advanced-stage

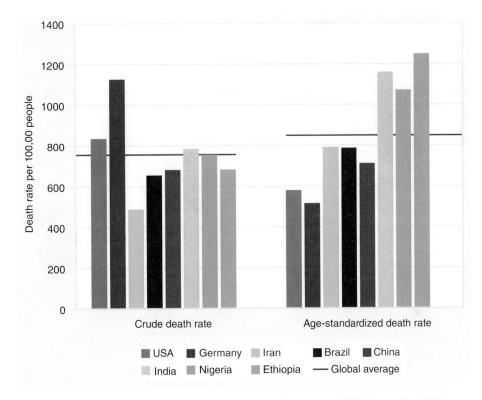

FIGURE 2-8 Crude and age-standardized all-cause mortality rates per 100,000 people in 2015 in featured countries.

Data from GBD Mortality and Causes of Death Collaborators. Global, regional, and national life expectancy, all-cause mortality, and cause-specific mortality for 249 causes of death, 1980–2015: a systematic analysis for the Global Burden of Disease Study 2015. *Lancet* 2016; 388:1459-544.

cancer who dies of pneumonia be counted as a cancer death or an infectious disease death? These decisions about how to assign causes of death can have a significant impact on which diseases appear to be the most common causes of mortality in a population. Even with these limitations, epidemiologists using standardized estimation methods and the best available data can make reasonably accurate assessments of the annual number and causes of death by age group and sex in every region of the world.

Another common way of examining mortality and survival at the population level is through the estimation of life expectancy (**FIGURE 2-9**). **Life expectancy** at birth is the

median expected age at death of all babies born alive. Life expectancy captures the burden from infant and child deaths in addition to the average age at death of adults. In places with high infant mortality rates, the median age at death is often in middle adulthood, which represents an age somewhere between a large number of child deaths and an even larger number of deaths in older adults. Life expectancies have increased over time in most countries, but they remain much higher in high-income countries than in low-income countries (**FIGURE 2-10**).[13] Some estimates of life expectancy instead focus on **healthy life expectancy (HALE)**, which is the number of years the average individual born into the

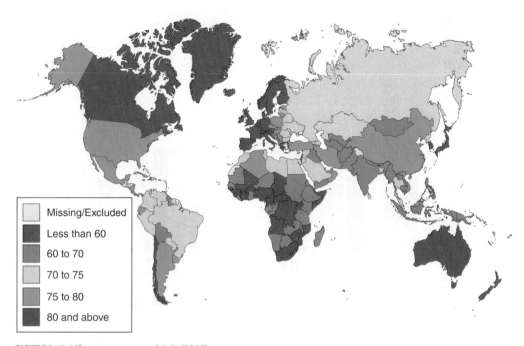

FIGURE 2–9 Life expectancy at birth (2015).

Data from *World development indicators 2016*. Washington: World Bank; 2016.

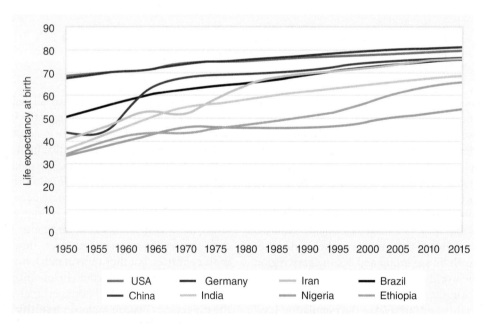

FIGURE 2–10 Life expectancy has increased over time.

Data from United Nations Department of Economic and Social Affairs. *World population prospects: the 2017 revision*. New York: UN; 2017.

population can expect to live without disability (**FIGURE 2–11**).[14] In most countries, adults experience about 10 years in poor health before dying. Global health aims to increase life expectancies and increase HALEs, so that people live to older ages without experiencing extended periods of disability prior to death.

Morbidity refers to the presence of illness or disease, whether that disease is relatively mild, like the common cold, or quite severe. The two most common terms used to describe the morbidity rate for a particular disease in a population are incidence and prevalence (**FIGURE 2–12**). **Incidence** is the number of new

cases of the disease occurring in a time period divided by the total number of people at risk for that disease in that time period. Incidence is usually used to study infectious diseases, acute diseases (diseases that occur suddenly), and outbreaks. **Prevalence** is the number of total existing cases, whether newly diagnosed or long-established, divided by the total number of people in the population at the time the prevalence is measured. Prevalence is usually used to describe the frequency of chronic (long-lasting) exposures and diseases in a population, such as the percentage of adults in a country who have diabetes or asthma or who smoke tobacco products.

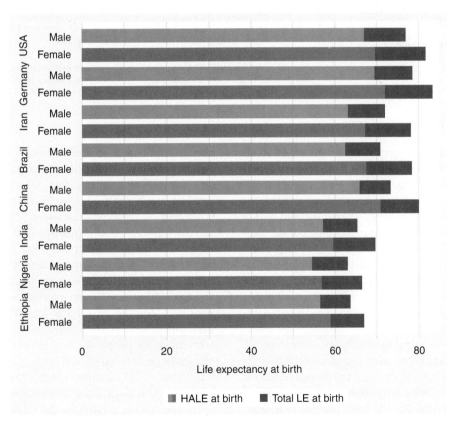

FIGURE 2–11 Life expectancy and healthy life expectancy (HALE) at birth.

Data from GBD 2015 DALYs and HALE Collaborators. Global, regional, and national disability-adjusted life years (DALYs) for 315 diseases and injuries and healthy life expectancy (HALE), 1990–2015: A systematic analysis for the Global Burden of Disease Study 2015. *Lancet* 2016; 388:1603-58.

December 31, 2017

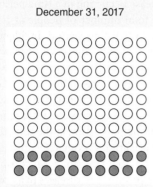

December 31, 2018

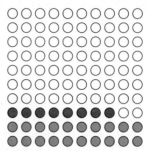

At the end of 2017, there were 100 adult residents of Villagetown and 20 of them had HIV infection.

The **prevalence** of HIV infection was 20/100 = 20%.

At the start of 2018, there were 80 susceptible adults in Villagetown. During 2018, 8 became newly infected with HIV.

The one-year **incidence rate** of HIV infection was 8/80 = 1/10. One in 10 susceptible adults became infected.

Assuming that all of the adults survived to the end of 2018, there were 100 adult residents of Villagetown and 28 of them had HIV infection.

The **prevalence** of HIV infection was 28/100 = 28%

FIGURE 2–12 An example of incidence and prevalence.

Epidemiologists measuring incidence and prevalence must establish a clear case definition that spells out exactly which characteristics indicate that a person has (or does not have) the conditions of interest. They must also have a system in place for ascertaining the total number of people in the population being studied, especially if changes in the health status of a population are being tracked over time and the population might be growing or shrinking or aging. Age-adjustment can be used to standardize two populations with different age structures before their morbidity rates are compared.

A variety of more complex health metrics also are used to examine the disease burden at the population level. **Years of life lost (YLLs)** quantify the burden from premature mortality in a population. Premature mortality is any death before a selected target survival age. For example, if the goal is for everyone in a population to live to age 70, someone who dies at 60 years of age would contribute 10 YLLs to the population total. If the target for survival

is age 80, someone who dies at 60 years of age would contribute 20 YLLs to the population total. Diseases that kill children, who would have had decades of productive life remaining if they had survived, generate more YLLs per case than diseases that primarily affect older adults. An intervention that keeps one 5-year-old from dying will prevent the loss of up to 75 YLLs in a population that has a target survival age of 80 years, while an intervention that keeps a 75-year-old alive for at least 5 more years will generate only 5 averted YLLs. An intervention for people who are already older than the target survival age will not help reduce the number of YLLs in the population because only premature deaths count toward the total.

In the models created for the GBD project, the term disability refers to any short- or long-term reduction in health status.[15] Weights are assigned to the level of disability caused by each type of physical or mental health condition. **Years lived with disability (YLDs)** quantify the burden to a population from nonfatal health conditions that cause significant impairment and distress (**FIGURE 2-13**). The total number of YLDs in a population is a function of how often a condition occurs, how much disability the condition causes (that is, the weight associated with the disability), and how long the condition typically persists.[16] A person who spends a year in a coma would

be considered fully disabled for that time period, contributing about one full YLD to the population total. Someone who is unable to work or go to school for 1 week due to a bout of influenza or a severely sprained ankle would contribute a tiny fraction of 1 YLD to the tally. The typical person contributes a small portion of one YLD to the population total each year. However, many small contributions from a particular cause can add up to a large number of YLDs across a population. Some of the most common causes of YLDs are back pain, depression, iron deficiency anemia, age-related hearing loss, diabetes, and migraine headaches.[17]

A **disability-adjusted life year (DALY)** is a measure of the total burden of disease in a population from both premature deaths and disability. The total number of DALYs in a population is the sum of YLLs and YLDs. One of the key benefits of using DALYs is that it highlights the high burden of disability caused by mental health disorders, pain, and other causes of reduced health status that are usually not fatal (**FIGURE 2-14**).[17] The main criticism of DALYs is the difficulty in assigning weights to the amount of disability caused by various illnesses and impairments. It will never be possible to assign an accurate weight to the decrease in quality of life caused by blindness, loss of a limb, depression, a brain tumor, or asthma, because the experience of disability varies so much based on the individual,

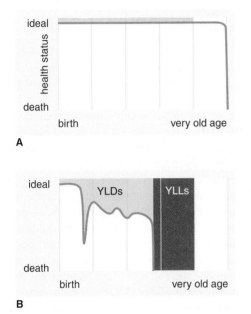

FIGURE 2-13 Examples of years lived with disability (YLDs) and years of life lost (YLLs) to premature mortality for different health trajectories.

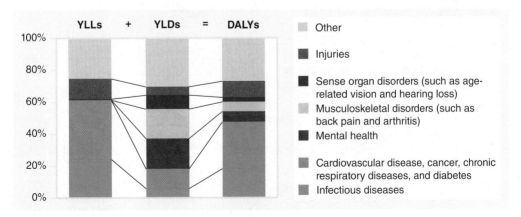

FIGURE 2-14 Global distribution of YLLs, YLDs, and DALYs in 2015.

Data from GBD 2015 Disease and Injury Incidence and Prevalence Collaborators. Global, regional, and national incidence, prevalence, and years lived with disability for 310 diseases and injuries, 1990–2015: A systematic analysis for the Global Burden of Disease Study 2015. *Lancet* 2016; 388:1545-602.

living conditions, the level of community support, access to health care, and other individual factors. For example, the amount of disability caused by an amputated foot would be much higher for a manual laborer in a low-resource setting where prosthetics are not available than it would be for an office worker in a place where high-tech prosthetics are common.

Economists frequently use health-adjusted life year estimates similar to the DALY as part of cost-effectiveness analyses. A **quality-adjusted life year (QALY)** quantifies the additional duration of life and quality of life conferred to populations by successful public health interventions.[18] A DALY is a bad thing to be avoided (the loss of a healthy year of life), while a QALY is a good thing to save.[19] While vital statistics and simple measures of morbidity (like incidence and prevalence) can be directly measured, more complicated health metrics like DALYs and QALYs are estimated using complex equations. The results of these types of computational models are dependent on the assumptions of the modelers, such as assumptions about the target survival age in a population and the disability weights assigned to various conditions. Health metrics from different populations should only be compared

when they were calculated based on similar methods and assumptions. Health metrics computed using the same methods allow different populations (or the same population at two points in time) to be compared.

▶ 2.4 Millennium Development Goals

The **Millennium Development Goals (MDGs)** that were adopted by the United Nations in 2000 and endorsed by nearly 200 countries worldwide were a major contributor to the global health successes thus far in the 21st century. The MDGs spelled out eight major goals for significantly reducing global poverty by 2015 (**FIGURE 2–15**).[20] While the MDGs overall were about general socioeconomic development, most of the goals had direct links to health: eradicating extreme poverty and hunger (MDG 1); reducing child mortality (MDG 4); improving maternal health (MDG 5); combatting HIV/AIDS, malaria, and other diseases (MDG 6); and ensuring environmental sustainability (MDG 7). Each signatory country was committed to working toward these

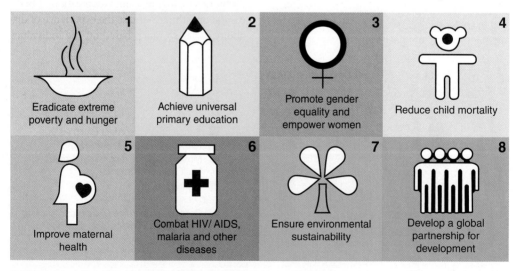

FIGURE 2–15 Millennium Development Goals (MDGs) (2000–2015).

goals, so the MDGs provided a blueprint for national- and international-level priority setting.

One of the main reasons the MDGs were so influential is that they provided a clear strategy for evaluation. When the eight MDGs were launched in 2000, they were accompanied by 18 targets that spelled out benchmarks for success (many of which used 1990 as the baseline year for comparison) and 48 specific indicators that were used to evaluate progress toward achieving those targets. These were later expanded to 21 targets and 60 indicators. Data about each of the 60 indicators were collected annually from most participating countries and were used to determine how much progress had been made toward reaching the goals at national, regional, and global levels. While some concerns were raised about how well the MDGs promoted equity, sustainability, local ownership of priorities, and holistic development (rather than relatively narrow, single-sector silos of focus), the general consensus was that the MDGs provided a helpful framework for global cooperation toward international development.[21]

The MDGs facilitated remarkable improvements in health status and quality of life for the world's lowest-income populations. Globally, there was a 44% reduction in hunger between 1990 and 2015, a 53% reduction in the mortality rate among children between birth and their fifth birthdays between 1990 and 2015, a 44% reduction in pregnancy-related deaths during that time period, a 45% reduction in new cases of HIV compared to the rate in 2000, and a 62% reduction in the percentage of people without reliable access to safe drinking water sources.[22] Although not all of the goals were achieved, most lower-income countries had healthier populations in 2015 than they had when the MDGs were launched in 2000.[20] The success of the MDGs was the impetus to create a follow-up set of goals, called the Sustainable Development Goals (SDGs). Many of the MDG targets that were not reached are now included among the SDG targets along with a host of new targets and indicators covering a broader diversity of socioeconomic, health, and environmental issues (**FIGURE 2–16**).

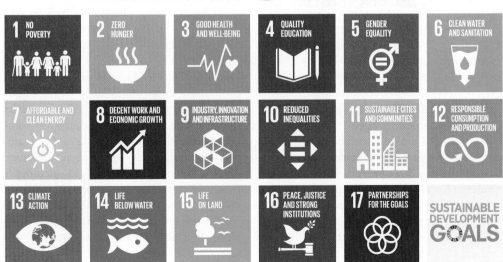

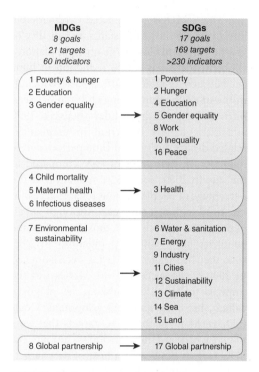

MDGs 8 goals 21 targets 60 indicators	SDGs 17 goals 169 targets >230 indicators
1 Poverty & hunger 2 Education 3 Gender equality	1 Poverty 2 Hunger 4 Education 5 Gender equality 8 Work 10 Inequality 16 Peace
4 Child mortality 5 Maternal health 6 Infectious diseases	3 Health
7 Environmental sustainability	6 Water & sanitation 7 Energy 9 Industry 11 Cities 12 Sustainability 13 Climate 14 Sea 15 Land
8 Global partnership	17 Global partnership

FIGURE 2–16 Transitioning from the MDGs to the SDGs.

▶ 2.5 Sustainable Development Goals

The **Sustainable Development Goals (SDGs)** are 17 goals established by the member countries of the United Nations at the end of 2015 that aim, by 2030, to end poverty, protect the planet, and promote prosperity and peace (**FIGURE 2–17**).[23] The 17 SDGs are operationalized through 169 targets and more than 230 indicators.[24] The preamble of the *2030 Agenda for Sustainable Development* that guides the SDG process states that the goals are "a plan of action for people, planet, and prosperity" that aim "to end poverty and hunger" in order to "ensure that all human beings can fulfill their potential in dignity and equality and in a healthy environment,"

"to protect the planet from degradation," "to ensure that all human beings can enjoy prosperous and fulfilling lives," and "to foster peaceful, just, and inclusive societies which are free from fear and violence."[23]

Like the MDGs, the SDGs consider health to be both a necessary prerequisite to and an outcome of economic growth. Two of the 17 SDGs focus specifically on health (SDG 3) and nutrition (SDG 2). Several of the SDGs address the socioeconomic determinants of health: poverty (SDG 1), education (SDG 4), gender equality (SDG 5), employment (SDG 8), equal opportunities for all people (SDG 10), peace (SDG 16), and good governance (SDG 17). The remaining SDGs address the environmental determinants of health: water and sanitation (SDG 6), affordable clean energy (SDG 7), safe work environments (SDG 9), healthy urban areas (SDG 11), sustainable consumption and production practices (SDG 12), and healthy climates (SDG 13), including healthy oceans (SDG 14) and land (SDG 15).

Unlike the MDGs, the SDGs are not singularly focused on the world's poorest billion people. While the SDGs remain "focused in particular on the needs of the poorest and most vulnerable," the SDGs mix goals for poverty reduction with a lengthy list of other targets that apply to countries across the economic spectrum, noting that "if we realize our ambitions across the full extent of the Agenda, the lives of all will be profoundly improved and our world will be transformed for the better."[23] The goal is to improve "the lives of all" and not just some countries and some stakeholders. For example, although there is only one SDG focused specifically on health, SDG 3 includes a much greater diversity of targets and indicators than were encompassed by the three MDGs that aimed to reduce the burden from child mortality, maternal mortality, and infectious diseases (primarily HIV, malaria,

SDG	Theme	Goal
1	No poverty	End poverty in all its forms everywhere
2	Zero hunger	End hunger, achieve food security and improved nutrition, and promote sustainable agriculture
3	Good health and well-being	Ensure healthy lives and promote well-being for all at all ages
4	Quality education	Ensure inclusive and equitable quality education and promote lifelong learning opportunities for all
5	Gender equality	Achieve gender equality and empower all women and girls
6	Clean water and sanitation	Ensure availability and sustainable management of water and sanitation for all
7	Affordable and clean energy	Ensure access to affordable, reliable, sustainable, and modern energy for all
8	Decent work and economic growth	Promote sustained, inclusive, and sustainable economic growth, full and productive employment, and decent work for all
9	Industry, innovation, and infrastructure	Build resilient infrastructure, promote inclusive and sustainable industrialization, and foster innovation
10	Reduced inequalities	Reduce inequality within and among countries
11	Sustainable cities and communities	Make cities and human settlements inclusive, safe, resilient, and sustainable
12	Responsible consumption and production	Ensure sustainable consumption and production practices
13	Climate action	Take urgent action to combat climate change and its impacts
14	Life below water	Conserve and sustainably use oceans, seas, and marine resources for sustainable development
15	Life on land	Protect, restore, and promote sustainable use of terrestrial ecosystems, sustainably manage forests, combat desertification, and halt and reverse land degradation and halt biodiversity loss
16	Peace, justice, and strong institutions	Promote peaceful and inclusive societies for sustainable development, provide access to justice for all, and build effective, accountable, and inclusive institutions at all levels
17	Partnership for the goals	Strengthen the means of implementation and revitalize the global partnership for sustainable development

FIGURE 2–17 Sustainable Development Goals (SDGs) (2016–2030).

Reproduced from United Nations. *Transforming our world: The 2030 agenda for sustainable development*. New York: UN; 2015, p. 14.

and tuberculosis). The health-focused SDG targets include ambitious aims for further reducing maternal and child mortality, alleviating the burden from a diversity of infectious diseases (including hepatitis B virus and neglected tropical diseases), reducing the number of adults who die before their 70th birthdays from common NCDs (cardiovascular disease, cancer, diabetes, and chronic respiratory diseases), improving treatment of substance use disorders and other mental health conditions, preventing transportation-related deaths, and increasing the accessibility of health services, medications, and vaccines (**FIGURE 2–18**).[25]

Because all of these health conditions and the socioeconomic and environmental conditions that influence them are now among the priorities for global action for the next decade, the SDGs are deployed as a framework for the outline of this book. The links between all of the SDGs and health are described in the next two chapters (**FIGURE 2–19**). The specific health topics and conditions included among the SDG targets are described in the remaining chapters (**FIGURE 2–20**).

Target	Theme	Target	Theme
2.2	Child nutrition	3.8	Universal health coverage
3.1	Maternal mortality	3.9	Mortality due to air pollution
3.2	Child mortality	3.9	Mortality due to unsafe water and sanitation
3.3	HIV		
3.3	Tuberculosis	3.9	Mortality due to unintentional poisoning
3.3	Malaria	3.a	Tobacco use
3.3	Hepatitis	3.b	Access to essential medicines and vaccines
3.3	Neglected tropical diseases		
3.4	Noncommunicable diseases	3.c	Health workers
3.4	Suicide	3.d	Emergency preparedness
3.5	Substance abuse	6.1	Drinking water
3.6	Road traffic injuries	6.2	Sanitation
3.7	Sexual and reproductive health	7.1	Clean household energy
16.1	Homicide	11.6	Air pollution
16.1	Conflicts	13.1	Natural disasters

FIGURE 2–18 Examples of Sustainable Development Goals targets related to health.

Data from *World health statistics 2016: monitoring health for the SDGs*. Geneva: WHO; 2016.

SDG	Theme	Section
1	No poverty	3.2
4	Quality education	3.3
5	Gender equality	3.4
8	Decent work	3.5
10	Reduced inequalities	3.6, 3.7
16	Peace and good governance	3.8
6	Clean water and sanitation	4.2
7	Affordable and clean energy	4.3
9	Industry and infrastructure	4.4
11	Sustainable cities	4.5
12	Responsible consumption and production	4.6
13	Climate action	4.7

FIGURE 2–19 Where in this book to find information about the Sustainable Development Goals as determinants of health.

SDG Target	Theme	Chapter
(Many)	Socioeconomic determinants of health	3
(Many)	Environmental determinants of health	4
3.c	Health workforce	5
3.b	Access to affordable medicines and vaccines	5
3.b	Official development assistance for health	6
3.d	Health emergency preparedness	7

(continues)

SDG Target	Theme	Chapter
3.3	HIV	8
3.3	Tuberculosis	8
3.2	Child mortality	9
3.3	Hepatitis	9
3.3	Malaria	10
3.3	Neglected tropical diseases	10
3.7	Sexual and reproductive health	11
3.1	Maternal mortality	11
2.1, 2.2	Nutrition	12
	Cancer	13
3.4	Cardiovascular disease	14
	Diabetes and chronic respiratory diseases	15
3.a	Tobacco use	15
3.5	Substance abuse	16
3.4	Suicide	16
3.6	Road traffic injuries	17
16.1	Violence	17
(Many)	Child health	18
(Many)	Adult health	19

FIGURE 2–20 Where in this book to find information about the health issues featured as Sustainable Development Goals targets.

▶ References

1. Ten great public health achievements: United States, 1990–1999. *MMWR Morb Mort Wkly Rev* 1999; 48:241–3.
2. Ten great public health achievements: worldwide, 2001–2010. *MMWR Morb Mort Wkly Rev* 2011; 60:814–8.
3. Yazbeck AS. *An idiot's guide to prioritization in the health sector.* Washington DC: World Bank; 2002.
4. GBD 2015 Risk Factors Collaborators. Global, regional, and national comparative risk assessment of 79 behavioural, environmental and occupational, and metabolic risks or clusters of risks, 1990–2015: A systematic analysis for the Global Burden of Disease Study 2015. *Lancet.* 2016;388:1649–724.
5. Glassman A, Chalkidou K, editors. *Priority-setting in health: Building institutions for smarter public spending.* Washington DC: Center for Global Development; 2012.
6. *The case for investing in public health: A public health summary report for EPHO 8.* Copenhagen: WHO Regional Office for Europe; 2014.
7. *Pathways to global health research: Strategic plan 2008–2012.* Bethesda MD: The John E. Fogarty International Center, National Institutes of Health (NIH); 2008.
8. Varmus H, Klausner R, Zerhouni E, Acharya T, Daar AS, Singer PA. Grand challenge in global health. *Science.* 2003;302:398–9.
9. *Convention on the Rights of the Child.* New York: United Nations; 1989.
10. Koplan JP, Fleming DW. Current and future public health challenges. *JAMA.* 2000;284:1696–8.
11. Murray CJ, Frenk J. Health metrics and evaluation: Strengthening the science. *Lancet.* 2008;371:1191–9.
12. AbouZahr C, Boerma T. Health information systems: The foundations of public health. *Bull World Health Organ.* 2005;83:578–83.
13. UN Department of Economic and Social Affairs. *World population prospects: The 2017 revision.* New York: UN; 2017.
14. GBD 2015 DALYs and HALE Collaborators. Global, regional, and national disability-adjusted life years (DALYs) for 315 diseases and injuries and healthy life expectancy (HALE), 1990–2015: A systematic analysis for the Global Burden of Disease Study 2015. *Lancet.* 2016;388:1603–58.
15. Chen A, Jacobsen KH, Deshmukh AA, Cantor SB. The evolution of the disability-adjusted life year (DALY). *Socioecon Plann Sci.* 2015;49:10–15.
16. Prüss-Üstün A, Mathers C, Corvalán C, Woodward A. *Assessing the environmental burden of disease at national and local levels: Introduction and methods.* Geneva: WHO; 2003.
17. GBD 2015 Disease and Injury Incidence and Prevalence Collaborators. Global, regional, and national incidence, prevalence, and years lived with disability for 310 diseases and injuries, 1990–2015: A systematic analysis for the Global Burden of Disease Study 2015. *Lancet.* 2016;388:1545–602.
18. Gold MR, Stevenson D, Fryback DG. HALYs and QALYs and DALYs, oh my: Similarities and differences in summary measures of population health. *Annu Rev Public Health.* 2002;23:115–34.
19. Sassi F. Calculating QALYs, comparing QALY and DALY calculations. *Health Policy Plan.* 2006;21;402–8.
20. *The Millennium Development Goals report 2015.* New York: United Nations; 2015.
21. Waage J, Banerji R, Campbell O, et al. The Millennium Development Goals: A cross-sectoral analysis and principles for goal setting after 2015. *Lancet.* 2010;376:991–1023.
22. *Health in 2015: From MDGs, Millennium Development Goals to SDGs, Sustainable Development Goals.* Geneva: WHO; 2015.
23. United Nations. *Transforming our world: The 2030 Agenda for Sustainable Development.* New York: UN; 2015.
24. *Tier classification for global SDG indicators (20 April 2017).* New York: Inter-agency Expert Group on SDG Indicators (IAEG-SDGs); 2017.
25. United Nations Economic and Social Council. *Report of the Inter-Agency and Expert Group on Sustainable Development Goal Indicators* (E/CN.3/2016/2 /Rev.1). New York: UN; 2016.

CHAPTER 3

Socioeconomic Determinants of Health

The disparities in health status between populations are largely due to gaps in economic development rather than differences in biology. People tend to have worse health profiles when they are poor, have low levels of education, are unemployed, experience discrimination, and have limited opportunities to participate in social and political processes. Increases in socioeconomic status are associated with improved health status, and better health enables further advancement in quality of life for individuals and communities.

▶ 3.1 Health Disparities and the SDGs

Socioeconomic status (SES), also called **socioeconomic position (SEP)**, describes an individual's standing in a society based on individual and household income, education, gender, occupation, ethnicity and race, and other characteristics that exist within a broader cultural, social, political, and policy environment.[1] There is no one measure of SES, but proxies, such as ownership of various assets (like a house, car, bicycle, television, radio, or livestock), amount and type of education, type of job, residential area, and other characteristics, can be used to evaluate a person's relative position in a community or larger population group. These socioeconomic characteristics have a significant impact on an individual's health status and ability to

access healthcare services. The personal factors and community conditions that enable or hinder access to health are collectively called the **social determinants of health**.[2] Many of these social determinants of health can be summarized using the acronym PROGRESS: place of residence, race and ethnicity, occupation and employment status, gender and sex, religion, education, social capital, and other socioeconomic indicators (**FIGURE 3–1**).[3]

Children and adults who have low SES, in terms of either absolute poverty or relative poverty compared to their neighbors, tend to have significantly reduced health status compared to people from wealthier socioeconomic groups.[4] The reduced health status in populations with lower SES is largely a function of economic, social, and political environments, and it is not caused by innate biological differences. An avoidable difference in health status between population groups is called a

P	Place of residence (rural/urban; particular state or province; housing characteristics)
R	Race, ethnicity, culture, and language
O	Occupation and employment status
G	Gender and sex
R	Religion
E	Education
S	Socioeconomic position (income, wealth, and other measures)
S	Social capital (neighborhood, community, and family support and other aspects of social relationships and networks)
Plus	Age, disability, sexual orientation, and other characteristics

FIGURE 3-1 The PROGRESS-Plus framework for the social determinants of health.

Data from Kavanagh J, Oliver S, Lorenc T. Reflections on developing and using PROGRESS-Plus. *Equity Update* 2008;2:1–3.

health disparity or an **inequality**.[5] When a health inequality is considered to be unfair and unjust, the difference is classified as an **inequity**.[6] **Social justice** is the principle that moving toward greater equality in the distribution of income and wealth, opportunities for education and employment, access to health and security, and involvement in civic and political activities is valuable for human flourishing.[7] One of the key goals of global public health is to reduce health disparities by increasing the health status of disadvantaged populations.[8] (Reducing health disparities by reducing the health status of the advantaged population would not be a global health gain.)

SES usually refers to individual characteristics. A related set of metrics can be used to compare the development status of different countries. The **Human Development Index (HDI)** is an estimate of national development calculated from composite data on longevity (life expectancy at birth), knowledge (such as the mean and expected years of schooling), and income (gross national income per capita in purchasing power parity dollars).[9] The HDI has increased in most countries over the past 25 years as life expectancies, school enrollment, and incomes have risen (**FIGURE 3-2**), but there are still significant gaps between the richest countries and the poorest countries (**FIGURE 3-3**).[9] These disparities are evident in the health metrics from high-income and low-income countries. Objective measures of socioeconomic development in a country, such as the components of the HDI, generally align with subjective measures of quality of life reported by the country's residents. A higher HDI is correlated with better health status and also with greater levels of happiness (**FIGURE 3-4**).[10] Making progress toward achieving the socioeconomic Sustainable Development Goals (SDGs) of ending poverty (SDG 1), ensuring quality education for all (SDG 4), achieving gender equality (SDG 5), promoting employment and decent work for all (SDG 8), reducing inequalities within and among countries (SDG 10), and promoting peaceful societies and good governance

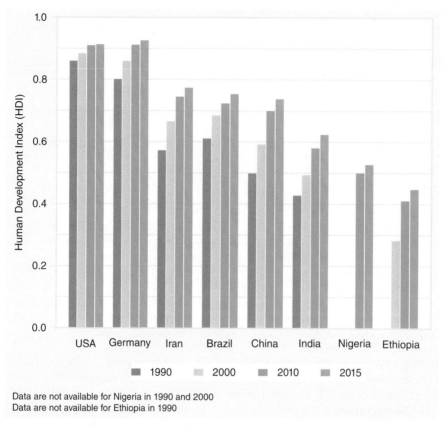

Data are not available for Nigeria in 1990 and 2000
Data are not available for Ethiopia in 1990

FIGURE 3–2 The Human Development Index (HDI) is increasing as people live longer, spend more years in school, and earn more.

Data from *Human development report 2016*. New York: UNDP; 2015.

(SDG 16) will improve the quality of life and the quality of health for billions of people.

▶ 3.2 Economics

SDG 1 sets an ambitious goal of "ending poverty in all its forms everywhere."[11] **Extreme poverty** is defined as surviving on less income than an international poverty line, typically set at an income of less than $1 or $2 per person per day.[12]

Many of the world's poorest people live in remote rural areas, where they try to grow enough as subsistence farmers with a small plot of land to feed all household members. Others are the urban poor, who often live in informal settlements that have no trash

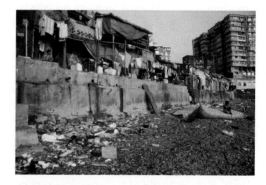

© Sam DCruz/Shutterstock

removal, running water, electricity, or other utilities. The percentage of the world's people living in extreme poverty decreased from approximately 35% in 1990 to 10% in 2015,

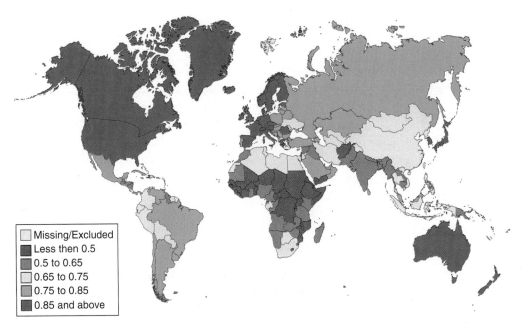

FIGURE 3–3 Human Development Index (2015).

Data from *Human development report 2016*. New York: UNDP; 2015.

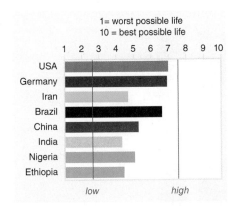

FIGURE 3–4 A higher proportion of people in countries with higher HDIs report being happy.

Data from Helliwell J, Layard R, Sachs J, editors. *World happiness report 2017*. New York: Sustainable Development Solutions Network; 2017.

and the SDGs aim to further reduce that percentage to 0% by 2030 (**FIGURE 3–5**).[12] As of 2015, however, the majority of people in many low-income countries (the lowest of the four country income level groupings) were living below international thresholds for poverty (**FIGURE 3–6**). An even higher percentage of people are considered to live in **relative poverty**, living on less than the nationally defined poverty line in their own countries.

Poverty is about more than income and consumption. Economic factors are intertwined with a variety of sociocultural, political, and environmental conditions that enable some people to thrive and cause others to struggle. The United Nations Development Programme (UNDP) calculates a Multidimensional Poverty Index (MPI) that combines data regarding health (including hunger and child mortality), education (including total years of school for adults and enrollment of children in school), and standard of living (including access to electricity, drinking water, and toilets, whether the floors in the home are dirt or some other material, the type of cooking fuel used, and the presence of economic assets). When the MPI is used as a measure of poverty rather than income alone, a large proportion of people living in lower-income countries are classified as living in poverty (**FIGURE 3–7**).[9] Poverty is not uniformly distributed within low-income countries, and there are often substantial variations in the poverty rate within

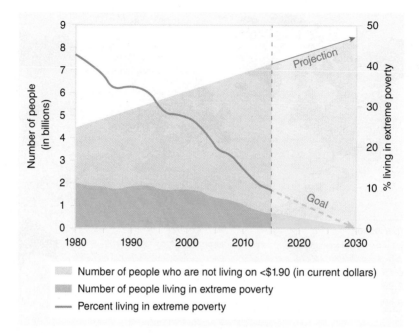

Number of people who are not living on <$1.90 (in current dollars)

Number of people living in extreme poverty

Percent living in extreme poverty

FIGURE 3–5 The percentage of the world's population living in poverty has decreased significantly.
Data from *World development indicators 2016* (Table 2.8.2). Washington: World Bank; 2016.

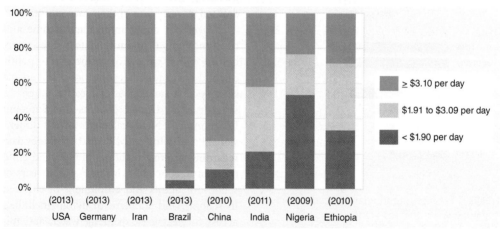

FIGURE 3–6 A large proportion of residents of lower-income countries live in poverty.
Data from *World development indicators 2016*. Washington: World Bank; 2016.

national borders. For example, in Nigeria the proportion of people with an MPI indicating poverty or severe poverty is higher in rural areas than in cities and is much higher in the north than in the south.[13] No matter where they are located, people living in poverty may have limited opportunities for education and employment, limited participation in social and cultural activities, and limited engagement in civic and political processes.[14] Poverty is also inextricably tied to health: living in poverty causes ill health, and ill health can cause poverty. Similarly, economic growth facilitates improvements in population health status, and investments in public health stimulate economic growth.[15]

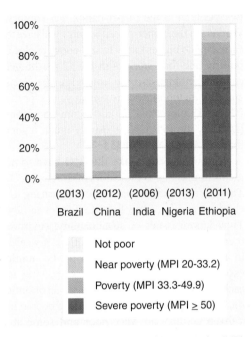

Not poor

Near poverty (MPI 20-33.2)

Poverty (MPI 33.3-49.9)

Severe poverty (MPI ≥ 50)

FIGURE 3-7 The Multidimensional Poverty Index (MPI). Data from *Human development report 2016: Work for human development.* New York: UNDP; 2016.

The economic status of a household is a function of both income and wealth. **Income** is the amount of take-home pay earned by household members in a week, year, or other time period. **Wealth** is the accumulated worth of the household's resources and can include a house, car, television or radio, livestock, and other consumer goods. When someone in a high-income or wealthy household has a health concern, that person usually has the resources to immediately access high-quality medical care, accurate diagnostic tests, and effective therapies. Attending to health issues early usually prevents mild issues from becoming severe problems. By contrast, low-income households generally have very little wealth, so they have few resources to draw on when someone in the household develops a severe illness or is seriously injured. People living in low-resource households may not be able to afford to seek care for health problems that are not immediately life-threatening or disabling. The direct costs of medical care add up quickly when they include transportation to a healthcare facility, fees for clinical consultations,

and payment for medications and supplies like bandages (which often are not provided by healthcare facilities and must be purchased by the patient). There are also indirect costs associated with lost wages for patients and caregivers, especially when outpatients must sit in a waiting area for a full day before seeing a clinician and when families of hospitalized patients must provide all food and most personal care for inpatients. The facilities where poor people can access health services are often underfunded, understaffed, and understocked, and they rarely have the clinical specialists, support staff, and equipment necessary to be able to offer advanced care.[16] These disparities in access to health services contribute to the significant gaps in health status between the average person from a high-income household and the average person living in a low-income household.

Just as the health status of individuals and families is related to their SES, the health status of communities and nations is linked to their economic status. Health economists use a variety of macroeconomic indicators to measure the amount of economic activity in a country. To distinguish between these measures, consider the way the GNI, GDP, and GNP of Germany would be calculated. The **gross national income (GNI)** is the total income from the selling of goods and services produced in Germany, including consumer spending, government spending, investments, and exports. The **gross domestic product (GDP)** is the total amount of goods and services produced in Germany by both German and foreign companies. The **gross national product (GNP)** is the total amount of goods and services produced by German companies in Germany and by German companies operating in other countries. All three of these metrics can be recorded in per capita (per person) terms by dividing the total monetary value by the population of the country.

It is impossible to accurately measure all economic transactions in a country, so macroeconomic metrics are estimated using the best available data. There are a variety of methods that can be used for the estimation process. The World Bank often uses an "Atlas method" to estimate the GNI. The Atlas method calculates the GNI by adding together the value of product sales and taxes (minus subsidies) within the country plus salaries and property income from abroad and then adjusting the total to account for inflation.[12] Because the amount of goods and services that can be purchased with a given amount of money varies from place to place—for example, it costs less to rent an apartment in Addis Ababa than to rent an apartment in New York City—it can be helpful for economic indicators to account for cost of living differences. GNI can be estimated in terms of **purchasing power parity (PPP)**, which adjusts the economic metric based on how many goods, services, and other products can be purchased in each country with a fixed amount of money, such as $1000 U.S. dollars. A clever example of PPP is the "Big Mac Index" that determines the relative price of a McDonald's hamburger in different countries and uses that exchange rate to determine the relative value of other items.[17] If a Big Mac costs $4 in one country and $2 in another, it is likely that the cost of living is about

twice as high in the $4-per-hamburger country. Workers in the higher-priced country will have to earn a much higher salary to stay above the local poverty line than workers in the $2-per-burger country. In high-income countries, the Atlas and PPP methods generate similar values for the GNI, but in low- and middle-income countries (LMICs), the PPP GNI is usually much higher than the Atlas GNI (**FIGURE 3–8**).[18]

Summary values like the GNI have some major limitations as indicators of development. They do not count unpaid labor like caring for children and growing food to feed a family. They ignore issues of sustainability, environmental damage, and the distribution of wealth in a country. These values show the economic experience of the "average" person living in each country, but the "average" economic measure may be misleading if most people in a given country are very poor and some are extremely rich and there is almost no middle class. Even when a large proportion of the population experiences something near the average

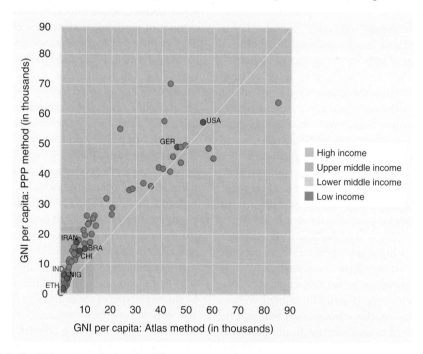

FIGURE 3–8 The GNI can be calculated in different ways, such as using an Atlas method or purchasing power parity (PPP). (The dots represent the 100 most populous countries.)

Data from *World development indicators 2016* (Table 2.1). Washington: World Bank; 2016.

reported for the country, there will still be variability in the experiences of individuals. There are millionaires in every country, even the countries with the poorest "average" person, and there are people in every country, even the wealthiest ones, who live on almost nothing.

However, at the population level, these metrics reveal important trends. For example, even small increases in the GNI per capita are associated with significant decreases in child mortality rates (**FIGURE 3–9**) and significant increases in life expectancy at birth (**FIGURE 3–10**).[19]

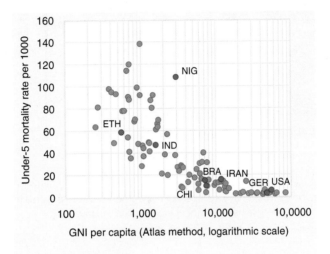

FIGURE 3–9 Small increases in GNI per capita in lower-income countries are associated with significant decreases in the rate of death for children between birth and their fifth birthdays. (The dots represent the 100 most populous countries. Note the use of the logarithmic scale on the *x*-axis.)

Data from *World development indicators 2016* (Table 2.21). Washington: World Bank; 2016.

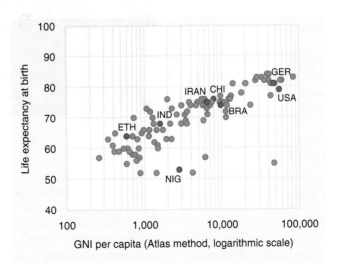

FIGURE 3–10 Small increases in GNI per capita in lower-income countries are associated with significant increases in life expectancy at birth. (The dots represent the 100 most populous countries. Note the use of the logarithmic scale on the *x*-axis.)

Data from *World development indicators 2016* (Table 2.21). Washington DC: World Bank; 2016.

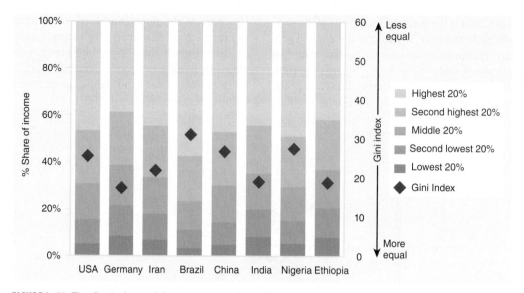

FIGURE 3–11 The Gini Index and the percentage share of income by income quintile. In a completely equal country, each of the quintiles would have a 20% share of income. In countries with a higher Gini Index (more inequality), the richest people have a higher percentage of income.

Data from *World development indicators 2016* (Table 2.9). Washington: World Bank; 2016.

The **Gini Index** is a measure of the inequality in the distribution of incomes within a particular country. A country in which everyone has exactly the same income has an index of 0 (perfect equality) and a country in which one person has all the income and everyone else has zero income has an index of 100 (perfect inequality). Brazil has a Gini Index of about 40, and the richest 10% earn more than forty times more than the poorest 10%. Germany has a Gini Index of about 30, and the richest 10% earn about seven times more than the poorest 10%.[20] However, the income level of a country is not a good predictor of Gini Index values (**FIGURE 3–11**).[21] Some high-income countries have relatively unequal income distributions, and some low-income countries have relatively equal income distributions. When two countries have similar economic profiles, the country with greater income inequality tends to have a less favorable health profile.[22]

Because economic status is so strongly tied to health status, progress toward achieving

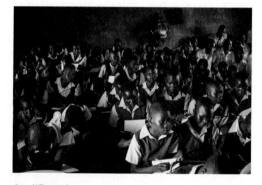

© punghi/Shutterstock

SDG 1 is necessary for sustained progress toward achieving the health-specific SDGs. The specific targets for ending poverty include eradicating extreme poverty, defined as living on less than $1.25 per day (SDG 1.1); reducing by half the proportion of people living in poverty according to national definitions (SDG 1.2); and implementing social protections for vulnerable populations, such as children, older adults, and people with disabilities (SDG 1.3).[23]

▶ 3.3 Education

Both the ability to read and a higher number of years of formal education are correlated with higher health status for adults and their children.[24] SDG 4 aims to "ensure inclusive and equitable quality education and promote lifelong learning opportunities for all," starting with access to early childhood education (SDG 4.2), and continuing with access for all girls and boys to primary and secondary education (SDG 4.1) and then to technical, vocational, or university education (SDG 4.3).[11] Most high- and upper-middle-income countries have strong enrollment in early childhood education and primary education, but in most lower-income countries, there is limited access to preschool education, and many school-aged children do not attend primary or secondary school (**FIGURE 3–12**).[25] Since many schools in lower-income countries have school health programs that provide hygiene and health education, nutritional support, treatment for common intestinal worm infections, and other health services, children who are not in school miss critical opportunities for both learning and healthy development.[26]

Literacy is the ability to read and write and apply those communication skills. Literacy exists along a spectrum from minimal recognition of written words to the advanced fluency gained through higher education. **Functional literacy** is the ability to understand written words well enough to complete normal daily tasks.[27] Functional literacy allows readers to acquire health information, navigate health systems, and attain other benefits associated with **health literacy**, the ability to access, understand, and apply health information.[28] Readers can learn about food preparation and exercise programs in newspapers and magazines, comprehend health and safety warnings on consumer products, access air and water quality reports, read posters advertising immunization and screening campaigns, follow directions on medicine containers and hospital discharge orders, understand the health benefits packages

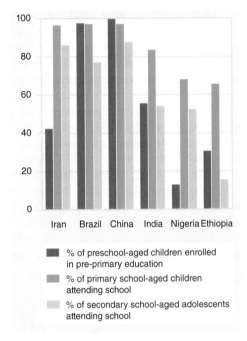

% of preschool-aged children enrolled in pre-primary education

% of primary school-aged children attending school

% of secondary school-aged adolescents attending school

FIGURE 3–12 Many children and adolescents in low- and middle-income countries are not enrolled in early childhood, primary, or secondary education (2014).

Data from *The state of the world's children 2016: A fair chance for every child.* New York: UNICEF; 2016.

offered by employers and the government, apply for aid and benefits, read brochures about their health conditions, use signs to navigate hospitals, and seek out additional information online or at libraries. People who cannot read will have difficulty with all of these health-related activities. They may delay seeking care for a health problem because they worry about being unable to complete paperwork at a doctor's office or being ridiculed for not knowing how to read or write. They may have difficulty taking their prescribed medications properly if their healthcare providers have not fully explained dosage and timing and they cannot read the instructions on the label. They may not be able to read the safety information provided by a pharmacist or know when to return for a follow-up examination.

Adult literacy in most LMICs increased between 2000 and 2015, but literacy rates among men and women remain low in many lower-income countries (**FIGURE 3–13**).[29] Female literacy and education are especially important for family and child health.[30] Women with more formal schooling are more likely to give birth at a healthcare facility (**FIGURE 3–14A**), which means that both mothers and newborns have an improved likelihood of survival if there are complications during or after delivery. The children of women with more education are also more likely to receive preventive medical services, such as vaccines (**FIGURE 3–14B**), and to receive professional clinical care for illnesses. Because women who have several years

of formal education are equipped to access the information they need to keep their children healthy and nourished, their children are more likely to survive past their fifth birthdays (**FIGURE 3–14C**). Increasing the proportion of girls and boys worldwide who complete at least a basic education (typically about seven years of primary school) will generate significant long-term benefits for the economic status and quality of life of those individuals and their families and communities. Reaching the target that "all youth and a substantial proportion of adults, both men and women, achieve both literacy and numeracy" by 2030 (SDG 4.6)[11] will also yield major benefits for the health and well-being of those individuals' future children.

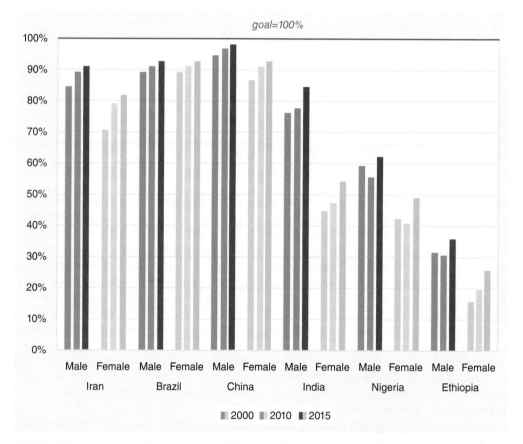

FIGURE 3–13 Literacy rates among adults (aged 15+ years) have increased in LMICs, but in many countries women lag behind men.

Data from *Education for all 2000–2015: Achievements and challenges.* Paris: United Nations Educational, Scientific and Cultural Organization (UNESCO); 2015.

A

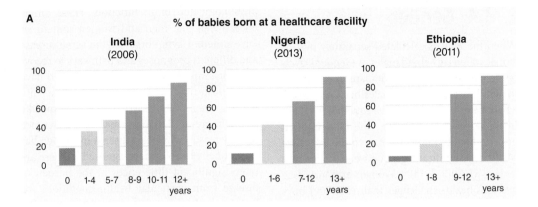

B

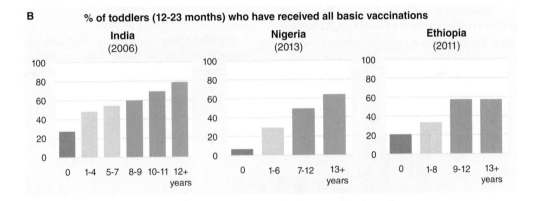

C

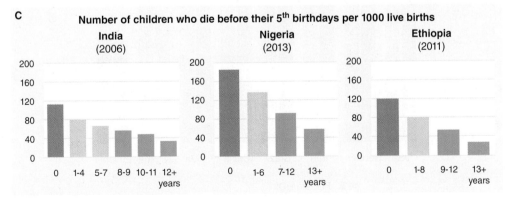

FIGURE 3–14 Women with more years of education (*x*-axis) have more interactions with the healthcare system, and their children are more likely to survive.

Data from *National Family Health Survey (NFHS-3) 2005–2006*. Mumbai: International Institute for Population Sciences (IIPS)/Macro International; 2007; *Demographic and Health Survey 2013*. Abuja: National Population Commission/ICF International; 2014; *Demographic and Health Survey 2011*. Addis Ababa: Central Statistical Agency/ICF International; 2012.

▶ 3.4 Gender

When the HDI is calculated separately by sex, females often lag behind males. A Gender Development Index (GDI) that compares the values of the HDI for females and males has a value of 1 when males and females have equal HDI values. In higher-income countries, the GDI is often near 1, but in lower-income countries, there is often a significant gap between males and females (**FIGURE 3–15**).[31] Women and girls face different health challenges than men and boys because of both biological characteristics related to sex and social structures related to gender.[32]

Sex refers to the biological classification of people as male or female based on genetics (such as the presence of XX or XY sex chromosomes) and reproductive anatomy. Males and females also have different body chemistry, hormones,

physiology, and brain function. These differences mean that men and women sometimes have different symptoms for the same disease and different prognoses and pathways to recovery. For example, men are more likely to have dramatic heart attacks with crushing chest pain, while women often have subtle symptoms like feeling more tired than normal. This difference is a key reason why heart disease in women has traditionally been underdiagnosed.[33] There are many significant differences in the burden of disease from particular health conditions for females and males that must be considered when planning for and implementing health education and preventive, diagnostic, and therapeutic health services (**FIGURE 3–16**).[34]

Gender refers to social, cultural, and psychological aspects of being male or female, and gender is shaped by the sociocultural

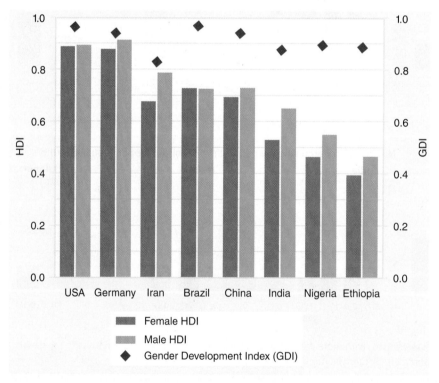

FIGURE 3–15 The Human Development Index (HDI) for females lags behind the HDI for males in many lower-income countries (2015).

Data from *Human development report 2015: Work for human development*. New York: UNDP; 2015.

FEMALES have a higher proportion of DALYs than males from...	MALES have a higher proportion of DALYs than females from...
■ Iron-deficiency anemia ■ Cancers of the reproductive system (such as breast cancer) ■ Depressive disorders, anxiety disorders, and migraine headaches ■ Musculoskeletal disorders (such as osteoarthritis and rheumatoid arthritis) ■ Alzheimer's disease and other dementias	■ Tuberculosis ■ Cancers of the lung, liver, stomach, and esophagus ■ Cirrhosis and other chronic liver diseases ■ Alcohol and drug use disorders ■ Autism spectrum disorders ■ Unintentional injuries (such as road traffic injuries and drowning) ■ Intentional injuries (such as violence and self-harm)

FIGURE 3–16 Examples of differences in the disability-adjusted life years (DALYs) attributed to various health risks for females and males.

Data from GBD Disease and Injury Incidence and Prevalence Collaborators. Global, regional, and national incidence, prevalence, and years lived with disability for 310 diseases and injuries, 1980–2015: A systematic analysis for the Global Burden of Disease Study 2015. *Lancet.* 2016;388:1545–602.

environment and experience in addition to biology. There is tremendous variability in the ways that individuals express their gender and in the ways that cultures define gender roles. **Gender roles** describe how a culture believes men and women should behave. For example, gender roles may indicate what tasks women are expected to do, such as cooking, cleaning, and taking care of children. They may also define what tasks women should not do, which might include working with heavy machinery or serving as religious leaders. Some cultures consider women to be under the authority of their fathers or other male relatives until marriage and under the authority of their husbands after marriage. In these places, laws may restrict women's ability to own property or manage their own finances. Some cultures have strict rules about what women can wear in public and whether they can be in public spaces unaccompanied by a male. This can limit the ability of women to participate in the marketplace and government, attend school and religious meetings, and acquire medical attention and information. Gender roles also define the social and behavioral norms for men. For example, young men may feel pressure to engage in risky behaviors like reckless driving or tobacco use in order to demonstrate their masculinity. Men may also be expected to take on hazardous jobs.[35]

SDG 5 aims to "achieve gender equality and empower all women and girls." The particular targets include eliminating "all forms of violence against all women and girls in the public and private spheres, including trafficking and sexual and other types of exploitation" (SDG 5.2) and ending harmful practices "such as child, early, and forced marriage and female genital mutilation" (SGD 5.3).[11] Achieving gender equity will require identifying and addressing the numerous preventable health issues that disproportionately affect women and girls and, at the same time, addressing the avoidable health conditions that disproportionately burden men and boys. Ideally, integrating gender-equity perspectives into new health policies, strategies, and plans will reduce within-country health disparities and improve overall population health status.[36]

▶ 3.5 Employment

Employment of at least one wage earner per household is generally critical for keeping a household out of poverty. In addition to the monetary income from working, employment often provides healthcare coverage, compensation for on-the-job injuries, and sometimes housing, food allowances, and schooling for employees and their children. These benefits can have a significant, positive impact on the health of workers and their families. SDG 8 aims to "promote sustained, inclusive, and sustainable economic growth, full and productive employment, and decent work for all."[11] Decent work for all means eradicating forced labor and ending child labor (SDG 8.7) as well as protecting labor rights and promoting safe working environments (SDG 8.8).

Unemployment occurs when a person who is not working for pay is unable to secure a position despite actively seeking a paid job. People who are retired, have opted not to work outside the home, or are not seeking employment for other reasons are not considered to be unemployed. **Underemployment** occurs when a person is involuntarily working part-time rather than full-time or is a low-wage worker whose earnings are below the local poverty level even after working long hours.[37] (In this usage, underemployment does not refer to people who are employed full-time and earning a living wage but who are underutilizing their education and training in their current positions.) Being unemployed or underemployed can be detrimental to mental and physical health status,[38] and so can precarious employment conditions.[39] People who have lost their jobs are more likely than working peers to develop depression and other mental health disorders.[40] Suicide rates are higher among people who are unemployed.[41] Unemployed people are more like to adopt unhealthy behaviors like smoking and harmful use of alcohol.[42] All-cause mortality rates are higher among unemployed men and women than employed people of the same age.[43]

Not all jobs are equally beneficial for health. People working as manual laborers have higher all-cause mortality rates, cardiovascular mortality rates, and cancer mortality rates than people of the same age who are working in nonmanual professional jobs.[44] Men and women who work in manual jobs also report lower self-rated health than same-age peers who work as managers or in other professional positions.[45] Among people doing manual labor, unskilled workers have higher mortality rates and lower self-rated health than skilled workers. People with limited job skills often have the most dangerous jobs, receive little compensation for their labor, and have little or no job security. Low-skilled workers who are injured or ill may not receive adequate treatment for their health problems when they cannot afford to take time off to consult with a medical professional and recuperate at home or they cannot afford to pay for health care.

Three of the key components that contribute to the SES of an individual or household—employment and occupational category, economic security, and educational level—are inextricably linked to each other and to health status (**FIGURE 3–17**). Any

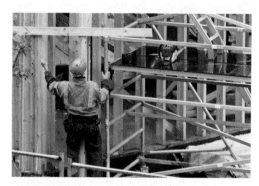

© Ari N/Shutterstock

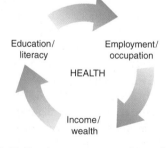

FIGURE 3–17 Employment, economics, and education are interrelated.

intervention aimed at one of these three categories may positively impact the others. For example, new reading skills may lead to a better job, increased job skills may lead to a higher hourly wage, and extra income may be used to pay for additional training. An improvement in any one of these dimensions of SES can lead to increased health.

▶ 3.6 Minority Populations

Major differences in health status exist between countries and also between different population groups within countries.[5] Some of these health disparities are a product of differences in SES, and some are a function of prejudice and discrimination against people from particular groups.[46] **Prejudice** is a perception about an individual based solely on preconceived notions about a sociocultural group to which that person belongs. Common forms of prejudice include racism, sexism, classism, ageism, and ableism (prejudice against people with disabilities). **Discrimination** encompasses the actions taken against an individual because of that person's membership in a sociocultural group. Unfair hiring and pay practices, restrictions on access to housing, and harassing jokes and insults are examples of discriminatory practices. Prejudice is a set of beliefs and attitudes. Discrimination is a set of practices and behaviors. Prejudiced thoughts lead to discrimination, but not all people who hold prejudicial beliefs act on them.

Culture is a way of living, believing, behaving, communicating, and understanding the world that is shared by members of a social unit. Culture encompasses a group's norms, values, morals, rules, and customs as well as the foods people eat, the clothes they wear, the language they use, the ways they interact with those inside and outside the cultural group, and how they describe and experience **illness** (how a person perceives his or her own experience of having an adverse health condition) and **sickness** (how a person with poor physical or mental health relates to and is regarded by the community).[47] Culture plays a role in how health and disease are experienced across the life span, from the way childbirth is approached to decisions about end-of-life care. Culture influences health beliefs, affects health behaviors, and shapes decisions about when and where to seek healthcare services. Different cultures may have distinct explanations about what causes disease. A mechanistic approach views disease as a dysfunction or breakdown of the human body, which is expected to function like a well-oiled machine. A moralistic perspective considers health to be the result of clean living and disease to be a type of punishment for wrongdoing. A supernatural viewpoint blames illness on demonic possession, evil eye, or the anger of God or the gods or ancestors. A disequilibrium approach considers disease to be caused by imbalances within the body, such as an imbalance between hot and cold, yin and yang, or the four humors. Disease may also be attributed to energy or qi imbalances; to emotions like fright or grief or jealously; or to stress, weather, food, germs, sex, genes, or age. These beliefs about health and illness may influence the way people interpret symptoms and diagnoses, the timeline for seeking treatment, the type of healer who is consulted (such as a physician or nurse, a counselor, a religious advisor, a massage therapist, or an acupuncturist), and the type of therapy that will be effective.

Celebrations of the various cultural traditions that exist within a nation or community can bring together people with diverse backgrounds. However, these differences can also be used to divide people. At worst, these divisions can lead to abuse, violence, hate crimes, war, and genocide. On a day-to-day basis, people who belong to minority racial, ethnic, tribal, or religious groups may encounter prejudice and discrimination along with language, cultural, and belief barriers. These obstacles may exist in the workplace and marketplace, and they may also be present within the healthcare system. Medical practitioners may be unfamiliar with the special health needs of patients from other backgrounds, in part because many population groups remain understudied by health researchers. Patients may be uncomfortable discussing health concerns and being examined by a medical professional who is not a member of their group or who is not sensitive to their cultural beliefs and practices. For example, women from some cultural and religious groups may be unwilling to be examined by a male clinician. Some barriers to healthcare access are legally sanctioned, such as when proof of legal residency is required before health care can be offered. Because of these obstacles to accessing health care, the health status of minority populations tends to be worse than that of majority populations.

Prejudice and discrimination are often related to race and ethnicity. **Ethnicity** is a social grouping based on many dimensions of cultural heritage, nationality, language, religion, tribal affiliation, and other factors. **Race** refers to superficial categories that group individuals based primarily on physical attributes like skin color. Significant cultural and genetic diversity is present within most racial groups. For example, the U.S. government typically collects and reports data for five racial categories and one ethnic category.[48] The five racial categories are American Indian or Alaskan Native, Asian, Black or African American, Native Hawaiian or other Pacific Islander, and White. The "Asian" category groups people with ancestors from countries as diverse as China, India, the Philippines, and Thailand. The "White" category includes most people whose ancestors were Europeans, North Africans, or Middle Easterners, and many with ancestors from other countries in the Americas. The only ethnic category classifies people as "Hispanic or Latino" versus "Not Hispanic or Latino." People who identify as "Hispanic or Latino" might have ancestry in places as diverse as Cuba, Ecuador, Mexico, and Spain.

Significant differences in health status often exist between different racial and ethnic groups. An assortment of explanations each partly explains the reasons for these health disparities.[49] Racial and ethnic categories may capture some genetic differences between population groups, including some differential risks for heritable genetic disorders. Ethnicity may be a marker for some health-related behaviors. If members of a population group tend to have similar dietary preferences and favorite foods, alcohol and tobacco use habits, and physical activity routines, these practices may account for some of the health differences observed between populations. Race and ethnicity may also be associated with socioeconomic factors. Members of marginalized population groups may have lower SES than other people in their town or city, and poverty is known to be associated with reduced health status. Additionally, discrimination because of race or ethnicity (or other characteristics) may cause chronic psychosocial stress that contributes to poor health outcomes.[50]

Members of indigenous communities tend to have especially low health status compared to other residents of their countries. About 370 million people worldwide identify as members of **indigenous population** groups that have maintained unique cultural traditions (and often also languages) for many generations after the colonization or domination of their traditional homeland by another group.[51] These populations include, among many others, the Cherokee and Navajo (and many other groups) of the United States, the Sami of Scandinavia, the Torres Strait Islanders of Australia, the Tangata Whenua (Māori) of New Zealand, the Quichua of Ecuador, the Maasai of Kenya, and the Hmong of Southeast Asia.[52] Members of indigenous people groups are more likely to be poor than their nonindigenous neighbors, and they usually have higher rates of morbidity and premature mortality.[53]

SDG 10 aims to "reduce inequality within and among countries" by taking steps to reduce poverty (SDG 10.1), ensure equal opportunities

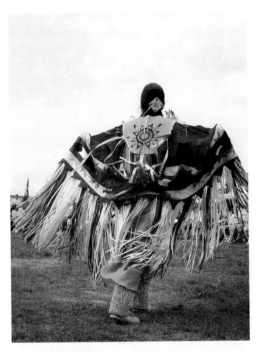

through the elimination of discriminatory laws (SDG 10.3), and "empower and promote the social, economic, and political inclusion of all, irrespective of age, sex, disability, race, ethnicity, origin, religion, or economic or other status" (SDG 10.2).[11] Actions to increase equity across these domains are expected to reduce health disparities by increasing the health status of currently disadvantaged groups.

▶ 3.7 Migrant and Refugee Health

A **migrant** is a person who has moved across an international border and has taken up residence in the new country.[54] By 2015, there were nearly 250 million people worldwide who were living in a country that was not their original homeland.[55] Some migrants intend to settle permanently in their new host country, while others are temporary residents or guest workers. An **immigrant** is a person who has

settled in a new country and intends to stay there permanently. A person who is temporarily living in another country and intends to return to his or her home country is called an **expatriate**. For example, people working in a foreign country for their home government, a business, the press corps, a nongovernmental organization, or another entity are usually considered to be "expats" rather than immigrants. Most migrants voluntarily move from one country to another to be closer to family, start a new job, or pursue educational opportunities. The majority of international migrants have moved from middle-income countries to high-income destination countries where their prospects for economic prosperity are greater (**FIGURE 3–18**).[55]

However, not all migration is voluntary. Some migrants are forced to move because of violence, persecution, or natural disasters. Some are involved in **trafficking**, which occurs when a migrant is forced into sex work, debt bondage, slavery, or other types of forced labor by the people who arranged the relocation. The experience of being an involuntary migrant is often accompanied by adverse health effects.[56] Smuggled migrants, victims of trafficking, and people fleeing conflict and persecution may experience violence and nutritional deprivation as well as other traumas during their travels. While some migrants gain greater access to healthcare services when they move from a country with poor health infrastructure to a country with an easily accessible healthcare system, many migrants encounter new health challenges as they settle into their new places of residence.[57]

A **refugee** is a person who has been forced to move across an international border because of security concerns like war, civil conflict, political strife, or persecution based on race, tribe, religion, political affiliation, or membership in some other group. Refugees typically secure permission to move to a new country prior to arriving in that country. An **asylum seeker** is an involuntary migrant who asks for protection from a host country after arriving in that country rather than waiting for a refugee application to be processed prior to traveling. Asylum seekers are often included in the refugee category in reports about involuntary international migration because the lived experiences of refugees and asylum seekers are similar. The primary difference between the groups is the status of their legal documents.

To be classified as a refugee or asylum seeker, an involuntary migrant must cross an international border. Nearly all refugees and asylum seekers originate in LMICs, and most move to middle-income countries (**FIGURE 3–19**).[58] An **internally displaced person (IDP)** is a person who fled his or her home community because of civil war, famine, natural disaster, or another crisis, but did not cross into another country and is, therefore, not afforded the same protection and assistance as a refugee.

In 2015, there were more than 21 million refugees and more than 3 million asylum seekers worldwide.[58] Half of all refugees were less than 18 years old.[58] The Office of the United Nations High Commissioner for Refugees (UNHCR) and other humanitarian

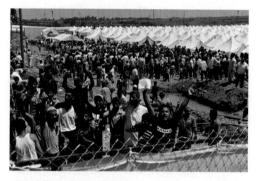

© Thomas Koch/Shutterstock

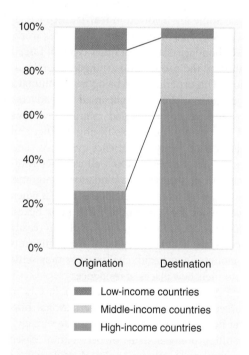

FIGURE 3–18 Most migrants were born in middle-income countries and most move to high-income countries (2015).

Data from *International migration report 2015*. New York: UN Department of Economic and Social Affairs; 2016.

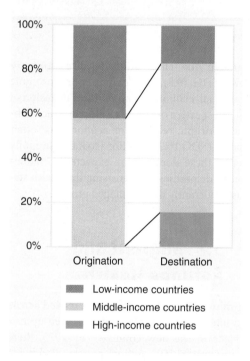

FIGURE 3–19 Most refugees and asylum seekers were born in low- and middle-income countries and relocate to middle-income countries (2015).

Data from *Global trends: Forced displacement in 2015*. Geneva: UNHCR; 2016.

organizations, both governmental and private, help provide for the basic needs of refugees, including water, food, sanitation, shelter, fuel, and health care for sick, pregnant, and vulnerable individuals. When possible, these organizations also offer treatment for malnutrition, address violence and security issues, and provide therapy for mental health problems, such as posttraumatic stress disorder. Fewer than half of refugees access these services in "camps" that provide long-term shelter. Most refugee camp residents are children, women, and the elderly. The rest are displaced to cities or rural areas, where they live alongside local residents (and other types of migrants) and rely on local social services for health care and other types of assistance.[59]

There were estimated to be about 28 million new IDPs worldwide in 2015, including about 8.6 million people displaced by conflict and violence and 19.2 million displaced by disasters.[60] More than 40 million people worldwide had IDP status after adding new IDPs to those who had been displaced in previous years and had not yet found a permanent residence.[60] IDPs and refugees share the experience of having lost their homes, jobs, social support networks, and some of their independence and sense of security. However, because IDPs have remained in their home countries, they are often not eligible for assistance from UNHCR and other international groups. IDPs usually do not live in camps. Most move to new rural areas or cities.

The services provided to involuntary migrants early in the cycle of displacement are not intended to be long-term solutions. The ultimate goal is for involuntary migrants (and IDPs) to secure permanent living situations and become self-sufficient by integrating into their host countries, resettling in a new host country, or returning to their home communities. Refugees and IDPs who return to their home communities after a period of displacement may face challenges related to the destruction of homes, healthcare facilities, schools, and other community buildings; the loss of farmland to environmental damage

and to hazards like unexploded ordnance; and the displacement of their family members, neighbors, and other members of their community. Those who settle in new areas often face challenges associated with learning new cultural practices and adapting to them, overcoming language and communication barriers, having limited occupational options, and potentially having limited access to health care. **Acculturation** is the complex process of adopting the practices, traditions, values, and identity of a new community after migrating.[61] Acculturation may be correlated with improved ability to navigate healthcare systems and access the tools for health.

Several of the SDGs specifically address the well-being of migrants. One of the SDG targets for reducing inequality is to "facilitate the orderly, safe, regular, and responsible migration and mobility of people, including through the implementation of planned and well-managed migration policies" (SDG 10.7).[11] Other SDG targets aim to protect migrants from being trafficked (SDG 5.2), forced into slavery (SDG 8.7), and working in unsafe environments (SDG 8.8). Policies and practices that address these issues and the other aspects of inequality covered by SDG 10 will improve the health of refugees and other migrants as well as the health of their neighbors.

▶ 3.8 Governance and Politics

SDG 16 focuses on peace, justice, and strong institutions, and aims to "promote peaceful and inclusive societies for sustainable development, provide access to justice for all, and build effective, accountable, and inclusive institutions at all levels."[11] The core of this goal is the need for good **governance**, the processes and structures that enable governments to set policies, provide services, and protect human rights. Good governance provides the policies, strategies, and resources that enable public agencies and other organizations to be well managed, and sound management ensures that health and social services are reliably delivered to the people who need them. Countries with good governance have low rates of violence (SDG 16.1), child abuse and human trafficking (SDG 16.2), organized crime (SDG 16.3), corruption and bribery (SDG 16.4), and discrimination (SDG 16.b); they have freedom of the press (SDG 16.10); they have justice systems that quickly and fairly enforce laws (SDG 16.3); and they are transparent (SDG 16.6) and allow diverse representatives to participate in decision-making (SDG 16.7). None of the other SDGs can be achieved when functioning governance systems are not in place to ensure that everyone has access to health services, education, clean drinking water, and other tools for health.

Access to health care and other services is associated with wealth, education, and employment, and it is also related to power. **Power** is the authority to control or influence the actions of others. Power can be conferred by political position and by socioeconomic advantages. Government officials may have the authority to demand certain services for themselves. Business leaders may have the money and connections to access care that is denied to others. Power can also be conferred by cultural systems. A tribal or religious leader may have the power to mobilize people and resources at will. A husband may have the power to control his wife's movements and activities. Powerful people can choose to limit or grant access to goods and resources like property, technology, social networks, and health care. **Corruption** occurs when politically powerful people abuse their positions for personal gain. LMICs tend to have less functional governance structures and more fraud, theft, bribery, kickbacks, and other types of corruption than high-income countries (**FIGURE 3–20**).[62]

In many countries, some people have the power to secure health for themselves and their families while others without power have limited or no access to the resources they need to be safe and healthy. Ethnic, racial, religious, and tribal minorities; immigrants, refugees, and internally displaced people; prisoners; people with mental health disorders or physical impairments; older persons; and members of other potentially vulnerable groups may not have the power to demand access to an equitable level of health care. An inclusive society is one in which all people have equitable access to governmental institutions and services, including health-related services.

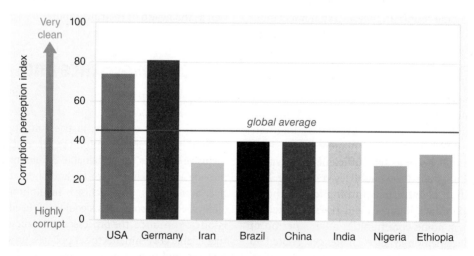

FIGURE 3–20 Low- and middle-income countries tend to have more corruption than high-income countries (2016).

Data from *Corruption perceptions index 2016*. Berlin: Transparency International; 2017.

▶ References

1. WHO Commission on Social Determinants of Health. *Health equity through action on the social determinants of health.* Geneva: WHO; 2008.

2. Marmot M. Social determinants of health. *Lancet.* 2005;365:1099–104.

3. Kavanagh J, Oliver S, Lorenc T. Reflections on developing and using PROGRESS-Plus. *Equity Update.* 2008;2:1–3.

4. Wilkinson R, Marmot M. *Social determinants of health: The solid facts.* Copenhagen: WHO; 2003.

5. Braveman P, Tarimo E. Social inequalities in health within countries: Not only an issue for affluent nations. *Soc Sci Med.* 2002;54:1621–35.

6. Gwatkin DR. Health inequalities and the health of the poor: What do we know? What can we do? *Bull World Health Organ.* 2000;78:3–18.

7. *Social justice in an open world: The role of the United Nations.* New York: UN Department of Economic and Social Affairs; 2006.

8. *Innov8 approach for reviewing national health programmes to leave no one behind: Technical handbook.* Geneva: WHO; 2016.

9. *Human development report 2015: Work for human development.* New York: UNDP; 2015.

10. Helliwell J, Layard R, Sachs J, editors. *World happiness report 2017.* New York: Sustainable Development Solutions Network; 2017.

11. United Nations. *Transforming Our World: The 2030 Agenda for Sustainable Development.* New York: UN; 2015.

12. *World development indicators 2016.* Washington DC: World Bank; 2016.

13. *National human development report 2015: Human security and human development in Nigeria.* Abuja: UNDP Nigeria; 2015.

14. *Report on the world social situation 2016: Leaving no one behind: The imperative of inclusive development.* New York: UN Department of Economic and Social Affairs; 2016.

15. Jamison DT, Summers LH, Alleyne G, et al. Global health 2035: A world converging within a generation. *Lancet.* 2013;382:1898–955.

16. Berendes S, Heywood P, Oliver S, Garner P. Quality of private and public ambulatory health care in low and middle income countries: Systematic review of comparative studies. *PLoS Med.* 2011;8:e1000433.

17. Ong LL. Burgernomics: The economics of the Big Mac standard. *J Int Money Finance.* 1997;16:865–78.

18. *World development indicators 2016 (Table 2.1).* Washington DC: World Bank; 2016.

19. *World development indicators 2016 (Table 2.21).* Washington DC: World Bank; 2016.

20. *World development indicators 2016 (Table 2.9).* Washington DC: World Bank; 2016.

21. *World development indicators 2016 (Table 2.9).* Washington DC: World Bank; 2016.

22. Wilkinson RG, Pickett KE. Income inequality and population health: A review and explanation of the evidence. *Soc Sci Med.* 2006;62:1768–84.

23. United Nations Economic and Social Council. *Report of the Inter-Agency and Expert Group on Sustainable Development Goal Indicators* (E/CN.3/2016/2/Rev.1). New York: UN; 2016.

24. Kickbusch IS. Health literacy: Addressing the health and education divide. *Health Promot Int.* 2001;16:289–97.

25. *The state of the world's children 2016: A fair chance for every child.* New York: UNICEF; 2016.

26. Bundy D, Schultz L, Sarr B. Platforms to reach school-age children (Chapter 20). *Disease control priorities.* 3rd ed. *Child and adolescent health and development (Volume 8).* Washington DC: IBRD/World Bank; 2017.

27. *Education for All (EFA) global monitoring report 2006: Literacy for life.* Paris: United Nations Educational, Scientific and Cultural Organization (UNESCO); 2005.

28. Nutbeam D. Health literacy as a public health goal: A challenge for contemporary health education and communication strategies into the 21st century. *Health Promot Int.* 2000;15:259–67.

29. *Education for All 2000–2015: Achievements and challenges.* Paris: UNESCO; 2015.

30. King EH, Hill MA. *Women's education in developing countries: Barriers, benefits, and policies.* Baltimore MD: Johns Hopkins University Press; 1993.

31. *Human development report 2016.* New York: UNDP; 2016.

32. Johnson JL, Greaves L, Repta R. Better science with sex and gender: Facilitating the use of a sex and gender-based analysis in health research. *Int J Equity Health.* 2009;8:14.

33. Arslanian-Engoren C, Engoren M. Physiological and anatomical bases for sex differences in pain and nausea as presenting symptoms of acute coronary syndromes. *Heart Lung.* 2010;39:386–93.

34. GBD 2015 Disease and Injury Incidence and Prevalence Collaborators. Global, regional, and national incidence, prevalence, and years lived with disability for 310 diseases and injuries, 1980–2015: A systematic analysis for the Global Burden of Disease Study 2015. *Lancet.* 2016;388:1545–602.

35. *Gender equality, work and health: A review of the evidence.* Geneva: WHO; 2006.

36. *Integrating equity, gender, humans rights and social determinants into the work of WHO: Roadmap for action (2014–2019).* Geneva: WHO; 2015.

37. Dooley D. Unemployment, underemployment, and mental health: Conceptualizing employment status as a continuum. *Am J Community Psychol.* 2003;32:9–20.

38. Wilson SH, Walker GM. Unemployment and health: A review. *Public Health.* 1993;107:153–62.

39. Benach J, Vives A, Amable M, Vanroelen C, Tarafa G, Muntaner C. Precarious employment: Understanding an emerging social determinant of health. *Annu Rev Public Health.* 2014;35:229–53.

40. Paul KI, Moser K. Unemployment impairs mental health: Meta-analyses. *J Vocational Behav.* 2019; 74:264–82.

41. Wanberg CR. The individual experience of unemployment. *Annu Rev Psychol.* 2012;63:369–96.

42. Dooley D, Fielding J, Levi L. Health and unemployment. *Annu Rev Public Health.* 1996;17:449–65.

43. Roelfs DJ, Shor E, Davidson KW, Schwartz JE. Losing life and livelihood: A systematic review and meta-analysis of unemployment and all-cause mortality. *Soc Sci Med.* 2011;72:840–54.

44. Toch-Marquardt M, Menvielle G, Eikemo TA, et al. Occupational class inequalities in all-cause and cause-specific mortality among middle-aged men in 14 European populations during the early 2000s. *PLoS One.* 2014;9:e108072.

45. Aldabe B, Anderson R, Lyly-Yrjänäinen M, et al. Contribution of material, occupational, and psychosocial factors in the explanation of social inequalities in health in 28 countries in Europe. *J Epidemiol Community Health.* 2011;65:1123–31.

46. Stuber J, Meyer I, Link B. Stigma, prejudice, discrimination and health. *Soc Sci Med.* 2008;67:315–7.

47. Boyd KM. Disease, illness, sickness, health, healing and wholeness: Exploring some elusive concepts. *Med Humanities.* 2000;26:9–17.

48. *Revisions to the standards for the classification of federal data on race and ethnicity.* Washington DC: Office of Management and Budget (OMB); 1997.

49. Dressler WW, Oths KS, Gravlee CC. Race and ethnicity in public health research: Models to explain health disparities. *Ann Rev Anthropol.* 2005;34:231–52.

50. Pascoe EA, Smart Richman L. Perceived discrimination and health: A meta-analytic review. *Psychol Bull.* 2009;135:531–54.

51. Gracey M, King M. Indigenous health part 1: Determinants and disease patterns. *Lancet.* 2009;374:65–75.

52. Bartlett JG, Madariaga-Vignudo L, O'Neil JD, Kuhnlein HV. Identifying indigenous peoples for health research in a global context: A review of perspectives and challenges. *Int J Circumpolar Health.* 2007;66:287–307.

53. King M, Smith A, Gracey M. Indigenous health part 2: The underlying causes of the health gap. *Lancet.* 2009;374:76–85.

54. *World migration report 2015.* Geneva: International Organization for Migration (IOM); 2015.

55. *International migration report 2015.* New York: UN Department of Economic and Social Affairs; 2016.

56. *International migration, health and human rights.* Geneva: IOM; 2013.

57. Gushulak BD, MacPherson DW. The basic principles of migration health: Population mobility and gaps in disease prevalence. *Emerg Themes Epidemiol.* 2006;3:3.

58. *Global trends: Forced displacement in 2015.* Geneva: UNHCR; 2016.

59. Spiegel PB, Checchi F, Colombo S, Paik E. Health-care needs of people affected by conflict: Future trends and changing frameworks. *Lancet.* 2010;375:341–5.

60. *Global report on internal displacement 2016.* Geneva: Internal Displacement Monitoring Centre (IDMC), Norwegian Refugee Council; 2016.

61. Fox M, Thayer Z, Wadhwa PD. Assessment of acculturation in minority health research. *Soc Sci Med.* 2017;176:123–32.

62. *Corruption perceptions index 2016.* Berlin: Transparency International; 2017.

CHAPTER 4

Environmental Determinants of Health

Human health is dependent on clean water, clean air, and other features of a healthy environment. Households, workplaces, communities, and cities can take steps to promote sustainable access to utilities, prevent hazardous exposures to toxins, support ecosystem vitality, and build resilience to withstand natural disasters. Combatting climate change and other large-scale threats to planetary health requires global cooperation.

▶ 4.1 Environmental Health and the SDGs

The most fundamental necessities for life are water, food, shelter, and fuel for heat and cooking. Where people live and work, the materials used to construct these buildings, what people eat and where that food comes from, the source and quality of drinking water, the quality of the air that is breathed, whether hazardous substances like cleaning agents, fertilizers, and motor oil are stored in or near the home, and numerous other components of the home environment play a role in health status. A broader set of environmental factors outside the home and workplace also contribute to health status, including geography, geology (such as the presence of earthquake fault lines or volcanoes), and climate (including whether the location is desert, tropical, arctic, or something more moderate, the types of vegetation and animals that are native to the location, and the usual weather and temperature patterns in the area).

Approximately 23% of deaths worldwide and 22% of disability-adjusted life years (DALYs) lost each year are attributable to water pollution, air pollution, occupational hazards, unsafe buildings and roads, and other modifiable environmental and occupational exposures (**FIGURE 4–1**).[1] These burdens fall on both adults and children.[2] Lack of access to safe drinking water, sanitation, and hygiene causes many cases of diarrheal diseases. Air pollution contributes to asthma, strokes, heart disease, respiratory infections, chronic obstructive pulmonary disease (COPD), and lung cancer. Failure to control insects and other pests enables the spread of malaria. The built environment contributes to the burden from drowning, road traffic accidents, falls, and other injuries. Occupational hazards cause low back pain and hearing loss. Numerous other factors contribute to other types of infections, noncommunicable diseases, and injuries (**FIGURE 4–2**).[1]

65

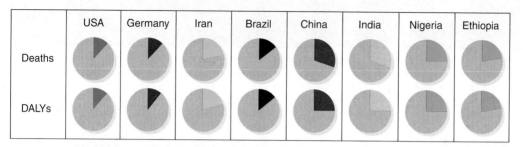

FIGURE 4–1 About one in four deaths and one in five disability-adjusted life years (DALYs) lost worldwide are attributable to environmental exposures.

Data from Prüss-Ustün A, Wolf J, Corvalán C, Bos, R, Neira M. *Preventing disease through healthy environments: A global assessment of the burden of disease from environmental risks.* Geneva: WHO; 2016.

Disease	Population Attributable Fraction (%)	Major Environmental Contributor(s)
Drowning	73	Safety of home and community environments, occupational risks
Diarrheal diseases	57	Water, sanitation, and hygiene
Asthma	44	Air pollution and occupational risks
Stroke	42	Air pollution
Malaria	42	Environmental vector management
Road traffic accidents	40	Occupational risks, built environment, traffic regulation, and land use
Ischemic heart disease	35	Air pollution
Acute lower respiratory infections	35	Air pollution
Chronic obstructive pulmonary disease	35	Air pollution and occupational risks
Falls	30	Built environment and occupational risks
Low back pain	26	Occupational risks
Hearing loss	22	Occupational noise
Self-harm	21	Chemicals, built environment, gun control, home and community safety
Cancers	20	Air pollution and many other factors

FIGURE 4–2 Percentage of disability-adjusted life years from selected conditions attributable to environmental risk factors.

Data from Prüss-Ustün A, Wolf J Corvalán C, Bos, R, Neira M. *Preventing disease through healthy environments: A global assessment of the burden of disease from environmental risks.* Geneva: WHO; 2016.

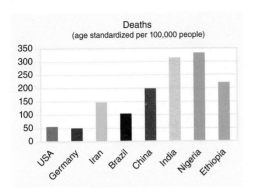
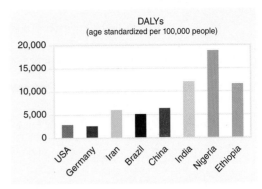

FIGURE 4–3 The age-standardized rates of deaths and DALYs attributable to environmental risk factors are highest in lower-income countries.

Data from Prüss-Ustün A, Wolf J, Corvalán C, Bos, R, Neira M. *Preventing disease through healthy environments: A global assessment of the burden of disease from environmental risks*. Geneva: WHO; 2016.

Public health requires safe home, work, and community environments. Public health is also dependent on healthy ecosystems at grander national, regional, and global scales.

Poverty is often linked to unhealthy living and occupational environments. Poverty impacts the type of dwelling a household lives in (which can be unstable, unventilated, and built with harmful materials), how crowded the home is (which can facilitate the spread of infectious diseases like tuberculosis), and whether it is in proximity to schools, healthcare facilities, public transportation, and waste dumps. Many poor communities do not have consistently safe drinking water, toilets, or enough water to practice good hygiene, so the risk of contracting an infection is greatly increased. In some places, the dwindling availability of wood for fuel limits the ability of households to boil water and cook food. Without electricity for refrigeration, it is difficult to store food safely. In rural areas, the lack of infrastructure for communication and transportation makes it difficult to access health education and healthcare services. Furthermore, low-income households may not have the money to purchase tools for disease prevention, because they must dedicate all income to immediate survival needs like food, housing, clothing, and emergency medical care. As a result of these challenges, environmental hazards place a particularly high burden on residents of low- and middle-income countries (**FIGURE 4–3**).[3]

One of the health-specific Sustainable Development Goals (SDGs) targets focuses specifically on environmental health, aiming to "substantially reduce the number of deaths and illnesses from hazardous chemicals and air, water and soil pollution, and contamination" (SDG 3.9).[4] Numerous additional SDG targets are related to environmental health (**FIGURE 4–4**), and making progress toward the environmental SDGs of ensuring drinking water and sanitation for all (SDG 6), ensuring modern energy for all (SDG 7), building resilient infrastructure (SDG 9), making cities safe and sustainable (SDG 11), ensuring responsible consumption and production patterns (SDG 12), and taking action to combat climate change and its impacts (SDG 12), along with the related goals of ocean conservation (SDG 14) and ecosystem restoration (SDG 15), will be necessary for achieving and maintaining poverty reductions and improvements in global health status.[5]

▸ 4.2 Water, Sanitation, and Hygiene

Everyone needs access to an adequate daily supply of water for drinking, cooking, hygiene,

1.5.3	Number of countries with national and local disaster risk reduction strategies
2.4.1	Proportion of agricultural area under productive and sustainable agriculture
3.9.1	Mortality rate attributable to household (indoor) and ambient (outdoor) air pollution
3.9.2	Mortality rate attributed to unsafe water, unsafe sanitation, and lack of hygiene
6.1.1	Percentage of the population using safely managed drinking water sources
6.2.1	Percentage of the population using safely managed sanitation services, including a handwashing facility with soap and water
6.3.1	Percentage of wastewater safely treated
6.b.1	Percentage of local administrative units with established and operational policies and procedures for participation of local communities in water and sanitation management
7.1.1	Percentage of the population with access to electricity
7.1.2	Percentage of the population with primary reliance on clean fuels and technology
7.2.1	Renewable energy share in the total final energy consumption
8.4.1 12.2.1	Material footprint, material footprint per capita, and material footprint per GDP
11.6.1	Proportion of urban solid waste regularly collected and with adequate final discharge out of total urban solid waste generated by cities
11.6.2	Annual mean levels of fine particulate matter in cities
12.4.1	Number of parties to international multilateral environmental agreements on hazardous and other chemicals and waste that meet their commitments and obligations
12.4.2	Hazardous waste generated per capita and proportion of hazardous waste treated
12.5.1	National recycling rate, tons of material recycled
12.7.1	Number of countries implementing sustainable public procurement policies and action plans
13.2.1	Number of countries that have communicated the establishment or operationalization of an integrated policy/strategy/plan that increases their ability to adapt to the adverse impacts of climate change

FIGURE 4–4 Examples of sustainable development goals targets related to environmental health.

Data from United Nations Economic and Social Council. *Report of the Inter-Agency and Expert Group on Sustainable Development Goal Indicators* (E/CN.3/2016/2 /Rev.1). New York: UN; 2016.

and cleaning tasks, such as washing clothes, scrubbing cooking pots, and cleaning homes. Water access is a function of water quality, reliability, quantity, proximity, and cost.[6] A household has access to **safe drinking water** when there is an adequate supply of affordable clean drinking water in or near the home (**FIGURE 4–5**).[6] The water needs to be free of bacteria, viruses, and parasites that can cause diarrhea and other infectious diseases, and it must also be free of harmful chemicals and sediments. The water should not appear cloudy, dirty, or strangely colored, so that it does not cause problems with cooking (such as giving food a strange flavor, color, or texture) or washing.[7] To be classified as an improved water source, the water must be protected, which means that people should not wash clothes or bathe in the vicinity where drinking water is collected, and animals, sewage, and garbage should be kept away from the water source. The water source must be available and functioning all the time, or the household must have access to adequate water storage and water treatment methods, such as filtering, boiling, and using chemicals like chlorine.

Hygiene is the practice of maintaining cleanliness in order to prevent disease. Personal hygiene behaviors include handwashing (hand hygiene), tooth brushing (oral hygiene), and bathing (body hygiene). Enough water must be available each day so people can stay hydrated

Service Level	Quality and Reliability	Quantity per Person per Day	Proximity	Hygiene Needs Met?	Level of Health Concern
No access	Neither quantity nor quality ensured	May be less than 5 liters	More than 1 kilometer or 30 minutes round trip	No because only available at source	Very high
Basic access	Quantity ensured but quality not ensured	About 20 liters	Between 100 and 1000 meters or 5–30 minutes round trip	Yes for handwashing and food hygiene; no for laundry and bathing	High
Intermediate access	Quantity and quality usually assured	About 50 liters	Water delivered through one tap that is within 100 meters or 5 minutes round trip	Yes	Low
Optimal access	Quantity and quality ensured	About 100 liters	Continuous supply through multiple taps	Yes	Very low

FIGURE 4–5 Water service level (quality, reliability, quantity, and proximity) and health effects.
Data from Howard G, Bartram J. *Domestic water quantity, service level and health.* Geneva: WHO; 2003.

and clean. The average minimum amount of water needed by one person each day just in order to survive is about 15–20 liters (about 4–5 gallons): about 1–3 liters for drinking, 2–3 liters for food preparation and cleanup, 6–7 liters for personal cleanliness, and 4–6 liters for laundry.[8] For healthy living, rather than mere survival, a minimum of about 50 liters (13 gallons) of water per person per day is recommended.[6] (As a comparison, the typical American uses about 90 gallons daily at his or her residence for indoor and outdoor purposes.[9])

To be considered accessible, the water source must be close enough to the home so that distance does not prevent people from using the water they need for health. At best, water is piped directly into an individual house. Public water taps, boreholes, and protected (and lined) dug wells that bring water near to homes, but not inside them, are also considered to be improved water sources (**FIGURE 4–6**).[10] Ideally, every person should live within 1 kilometer (about 0.6 miles) of a safe drinking water source.[6] When water sources are farther from the home, women and children may have to spend several hours each day walking to a water source, waiting for their turn to fill a container, and walking

home. In some places, it is possible for households to supplement their water access by collecting and storing rainwater for drinking and domestic use.

Water must be affordable enough that people have access to at least the minimum amount of water necessary for healthy living. This does not mean that water must be free. Households using a community water system may be asked to pay a reasonable fee so that the system can be maintained. These fees also promote water conservation if they are tied to the amount of water drawn from the pump by a household. However, it is problematic for public health when public water supplies are

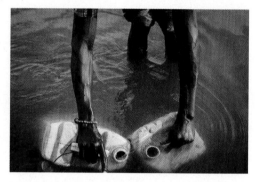

© punghi/Shutterstock

Unimproved		Improved	
• Surface water from a river, dam, lake, pond, stream, canal, irrigation channel, or other water body	• Unprotected dug well • Unprotected spring • Water from mobile vendors, such as tanker trucks or carts with a small tank or drum • Bottled water (when used as a primary source of water)	• Public tap or standpipe • Tube well or borehole • Protected dug well • Protected spring • Rainwater collection	• Piped water into the user's home or yard

FIGURE 4–6 Examples of improved and unimproved drinking water sources.

Data from *Progress on sanitation and drinking water: 2015 update and MDG assessment*. New York: UNICEF/WHO Joint Monitoring Programme for Water Supply and Sanitation; 2015.

not available and the prices charged for water are exorbitant.

Water used for drinking, hygiene, and other purposes must be free of toxins like arsenic, which can leak into wells when groundwater flows through fluvial deposits that contain arsenopyrites.[11] Arsenic in the water has long been a problem in Bangladesh,[12] where millions of residents remain at risk of **arsenicosis**, chronic arsenic poisoning from being exposed to contaminated water over a long period of time. The most visible symptoms are a change in skin color (hyperpigmentation) and the formation of hard skin patches (keratosis). Arsenicosis can also cause skin cancer and cancers of the lung, kidney, and bladder as well as liver damage and peripheral vascular disease. Low-cost filter systems can remove arsenic from drinking water, but even a very low-cost filter is more expensive than many Bangladeshi families can afford. Because the filters produce toxic waste, they are at best only a temporary solution. Deeper wells that bypass the geologic formations that contain arsenic might solve the problem, but digging a deeper well is an expensive solution in low-income communities.[13]

Sanitation is the safe disposal of human excreta (feces). A household has access to sanitation when there is a toilet in the home or a latrine near the home that can be used without a per-use payment (**FIGURE 4–7**).[10] One of the most basic sanitation systems is a simple pit latrine, which is a hole in the ground covered by an outhouse or encircled by a privacy blind. An improved toilet facility provides greater comfort, privacy, cleanliness, safety, and protection from dangers at night and from snakes and pests. For example, a ventilation-improved pit (VIP) latrine vents fumes away from the outhouse and keeps flies out of it. Pour-flush systems require some water for washing away the waste. Septic tanks and sewer connections are more advanced sanitation technologies that use water to remove waste from indoor toilets.

Open defecation occurs when people defecate in a field, a street, or another place that is not a toilet facility. Rural residents without access to sanitation systems may be able to go to an outdoor defecation site away from their living areas. Urban residents without access to a latrine often have no choice but to defecate at the side of a road or into a bag that is thrown outside, a waste disposal method that is sometimes called a "flying toilet." A desire for privacy means that many people without an improved

Unimproved			Improved
• Open defecation (using a field, forest, bush, open body of water, beach, or other open space as a toilet)	• Pit latrine without a slab or platform • Hanging latrine • Bucket (or bag) latrine • Flush or pour toilet that drains into a street, yard, open sewer, ditch, or drainage way	• Shared or public sanitation facilities	• Flush or pour toilet that diverts waste to a piped sewer system, a septic tank, or a pit latrine • Ventilated improved pit (VIP) latrine • Pit latrine with slab • Composting toilet

FIGURE 4–7 Examples of improved and unimproved sanitation facilities.

Data from *Progress on sanitation and drinking water: 2015 update and MDG assessment*. New York: UNICEF/WHO Joint Monitoring Programme for Water Supply and Sanitation; 2015.

sanitation facility, especially women, wait until dark to defecate, even though it is often dangerous for them to be out at night. A community is **open defecation free (ODF)** when all members are using designated toilet facilities and no one is defecating outside. Becoming an ODF community requires toilets to be present and used consistently by all community members. **Community-led total sanitation** (CLTS) programs are often implemented to encourage toilet use in places where residents are accustomed to open defecation and have not yet adopted new sanitation behaviors.[14]

The percentage of the world's people with an improved water source increased from 76% in 1990 to 91% in 2015 (**FIGURE 4–8**).[10] While nearly everyone in high-income countries has access to water, more than 1 in 10 people living in low- and middle-income countries—more than 650 million people—still did not have access to a reliable source of safe drinking water in 2015 (**FIGURE 4–9**). Access to an improved sanitation facility increased from 54% of the world's people in 1990 to 68% in 2015 (**FIGURE 4–10**).[10] However, in 2015 about 1 in 3 people worldwide—2.4 billion people— still did not have access to an improved toilet (**FIGURE 4–11**). Even though the proportion of people worldwide who practice open defecation has decreased, about 950 million people still practiced open defecation in 2015 (**FIGURE 4–12**). Rates of water and sanitation access are often especially low in rural areas (**FIGURE 4–13**). In 2015, 96% of urban residents had an improved water source and 82% had an improved sanitation facility. In rural areas, the rates were 84% for water and only 51% for sanitation.[10]

People who do not have access to improved water and sanitation are at increased risk for infectious diseases that are spread through contact with fecal matter.[15] In lower-income countries where few people have reliable access to water and sanitation, there is a substantial mortality rate associated with lack of access to these tools for health (**FIGURE 4–14**).[16] The presence of feces in or near homes significantly increases the risk of bacterial, viral, and protozoal diarrheal diseases and helminthic (worm) infections. Intestinal worm infections can be treated through the periodic distribution of de-worming medicines to school-age children and other at-risk population groups, but improved sanitation is a necessity for preventing new infections and reinfections. The best interventions for reducing the public health burden from diarrheal diseases and intestinal parasites are **water, sanitation, and hygiene (WASH)** programs that combine improved water and sanitation systems with health education to promote frequent handwashing and consistent use of toilets.[17]

Millennium Development Goal 7 aimed to reduce the proportion of people without access to water and sanitation by half between 1990 and 2015. The target for water

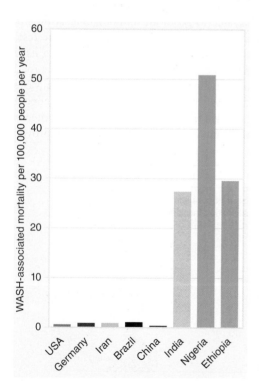

FIGURE 4–8 Mortality attributed to exposure to unsafe water, sanitation, and hygiene services per 100,000 people.

Data from *World health statistics 2016*. Geneva: WHO; 2016.

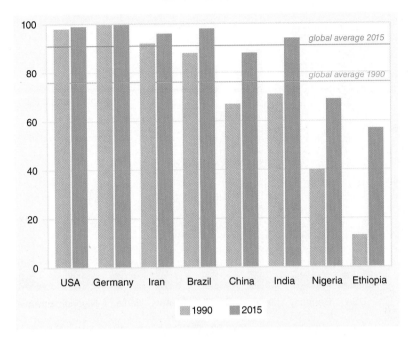

FIGURE 4–9 Improvement in access to improved drinking water sources, 1990–2015.

Data from *Progress on sanitation and drinking water: 2015 update and MDG assessment*. New York: UNICEF/WHO Joint Monitoring Programme for Water Supply and Sanitation; 2015.

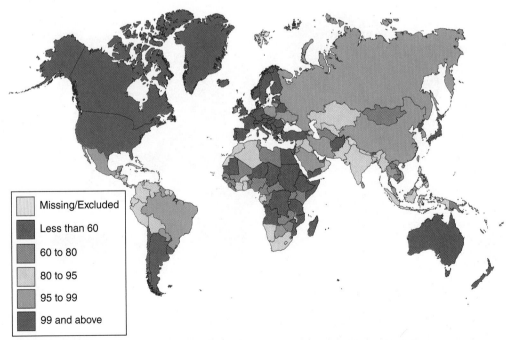

FIGURE 4–10 Proportion of the total population with access to an improved water source (2015).

Data from *Progress on sanitation and drinking water: 2015 update and MDG assessment*. New York: UNICEF/WHO Joint Monitoring Programme for Water Supply and Sanitation; 2015.

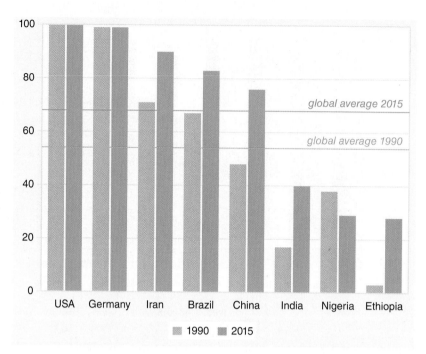

FIGURE 4–11 Improvement in access to improved sanitation facilities, 1990–2015.

Data from *Progress on sanitation and drinking water: 2015 update and MDG assessment.* New York: UNICEF/ World Health Organization; 2015.

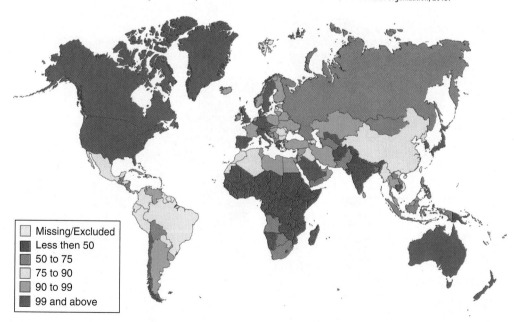

FIGURE 4–12 Proportion of the total population with access to an improved sanitation facility (2015).

Data from *Progress on sanitation and drinking water: 2015 update and MDG assessment.* New York: UNICEF/WHO Joint Monitoring Programme for Water Supply and Sanitation; 2015.

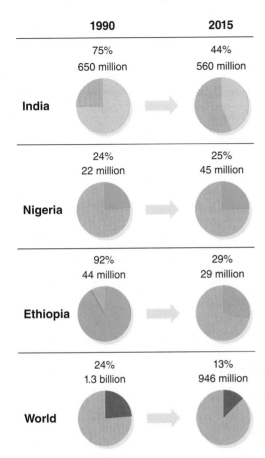

	1990	**2015**
India	75% 650 million	44% 560 million
Nigeria	24% 22 million	25% 45 million
Ethiopia	92% 44 million	29% 29 million
World	24% 1.3 billion	13% 946 million

FIGURE 4–13 Open defecation is still practiced by nearly 1 billion people worldwide.

Data from *Progress on sanitation and drinking water: 2015 update and MDG assessment.* New York: UNICEF/WHO Joint Monitoring Programme for Water Supply and Sanitation; 2015.

income per person in lower-income countries are associated with significantly greater levels of access to an improved drinking water source and sanitation (**FIGURE 4–17**).[18] Both economic growth and access to water and sanitation are associated with improvements in population health status.[19] WASH interventions are cost-effective means for reducing the preventable burden of water- and sanitation-related diseases in low- and middle-income countries.[20]

▶ 4.3 Energy and Air Quality

Energy is necessary for at least three important purposes: cooking food and boiling water for safe consumption, providing a source of heat when outdoor temperatures are low, and providing a source of light at night. The percentage of the world's people with electricity in their homes increased from about 75% in 1990 to about 85% by 2015 (**FIGURE 4–18**).[21] Nearly all of the 1.1 billion people without electricity at home live in lower-income countries.

Having electricity does not mean that electricity is the only source of household energy. About 40% of people worldwide—about 2.9 billion people who live in low- and middle-income countries—use solid fuels like wood, charcoal, coal, dung, and

was met, but the target for sanitation was not, despite good progress toward achieving it (**FIGURE 4–15**).[10] SDG 6 has the even more ambitious goal of "ensuring available and sustainable management of water and sanitation for all."[4] A series of targets spell out how universal access to WASH can be achieved (**FIGURE 4–16**). There is a synergy between economic growth, WASH, and health. Economic development improves access to utilities, and increased access to utilities enables economic growth. Even small increases in

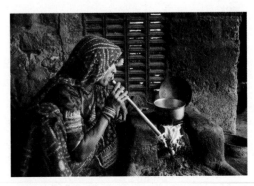

© Svetlana Eremina/Shutterstock

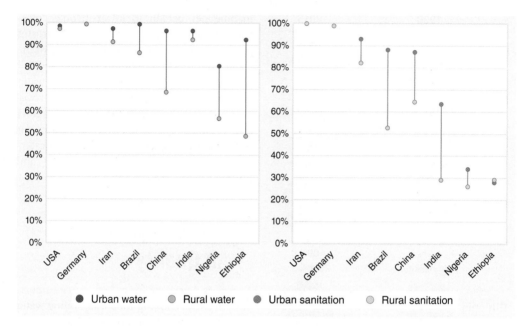

FIGURE 4–14 Rural areas often have less access to improved drinking water sources and sanitation facilities than urban areas.

Data from *Progress on sanitation and drinking water: 2015 update and MDG assessment*. New York: UNICEF/WHO Joint Monitoring Programme for Water Supply and Sanitation; 2015.

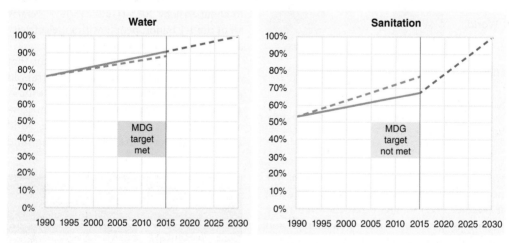

FIGURE 4–15 The Millennium Development Goal (MDG) target for water was met, but progress for sanitation was not met.

Data from *Progress on sanitation and drinking water: 2015 update and MDG assessment*. New York: UNICEF/WHO Joint Monitoring Programme for Water Supply and Sanitation; 2015.

crop waste as their primary source of energy for cooking (**FIGURE 4–19**).[21] **House-hold air pollution**, also called **indoor air pollution**, occurs when the air in or near

buildings is of poor quality. All fuels that are burned for energy release air pollutants, but **biomass** (fuel from organic materials like wood, vegetation, or animal waste) and

6.1	Achieve universal and equitable access to safe and affordable drinking water for all.
6.2	Achieve access to adequate and equitable sanitation and hygiene for all (including a handwashing facility with soap and water) and end open defecation, paying special attention to the needs of women and girls and those in vulnerable situations.
6.3	Improve water quality by reducing pollution, eliminating dumping and minimizing release of hazardous chemicals and materials, halving the proportion of untreated wastewater and substantially increasing recycling and safe reuse globally.
6.4	Substantially increase water-use efficiency across all sectors and ensure sustainable withdrawals and supply of freshwater to address water scarcity and substantially reduce the number of people suffering from water scarcity.
6.5	Implement integrated water resources management at all levels, including through transboundary cooperation as appropriate.
6.6	Protect and restore water-related ecosystems, including mountains, forests, wetlands, rivers, aquifers, and lakes.
6.a	Expand international cooperation and capacity-building support to developing countries in water- and sanitation-related activities and programs, including water harvesting, desalination, water efficiency, wastewater treatment, recycling, and reuse technologies.
6.b	Support and strengthen the participation of local communities in improving water and sanitation management.

FIGURE 4–16 Targets for Sustainable Development Goal 6, which focuses on water and sanitation.

Data from United Nations. *Transforming our world: The 2030 Agenda for Sustainable Development.* New York: UN; 2015.

other solid fuels are particularly unhealthy because they are usually burned in open fires or in simple stoves that release most of the smoke from burning into the home or cooking shelter.[22]

The health risks associated with indoor air pollution levels are particularly high for women and young children who spend several hours a day near fires while cooking.[23] Use of solid fuels for cooking and other energy needs can have adverse effects on respiratory health as well as other negative health outcomes.[24] Children are at risk of burns from falling into open fires or knocking over pots of boiling water. Women and children often spend hours each week collecting sticks and brush to use as fuel, and they are susceptible to injuries related to carrying heavy loads over uneven terrain. As sources of biomass close to the home are used up, fuel-gatherers must travel further distances to find fuel. There are also environmental consequences. Burning of solid fuels contributes to outdoor air pollution, and the demand for wood and charcoal contributes to deforestation.

Having electricity in the home and being able to cook without solid fuels has numerous benefits, including cleaner indoor air, safer food storage because of access to refrigeration, and greater access to health and safety messages delivered through radios or televisions. However, electricity is not a pollution-free form of energy when the energy is generated by burning coal or oil. Power plants, the exhaust from motor vehicles, and the wastes produced by industrial processes, forest fires, and the disposal of solid waste can all create **ambient air pollution**, also called **outdoor air pollution**, which is the presence of harmful chemicals or other substances in the air at concentrations above the thresholds established for human safety. People in higher-income countries use more energy than people in lower-income countries, and they also generate more emissions per person

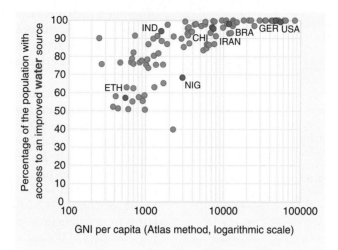

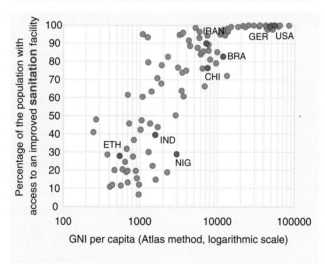

FIGURE 4–17 Small increases in income per person in low-income countries are associated with significant increases in access to an improved drinking water source and an improved sanitation facility. (The dots represent the 100 most populous countries. Note the use of the logarithmic scale on the *x*-axis.)

Data from *World development indicators 2016* (Table 2.9). Washington DC: World Bank; 2016.

than less-industrialized lower-income countries (**FIGURE 4–20**).[25]

Both indoor and outdoor air pollution are hazards to human health. The substances in polluted air include carbon monoxide (CO), nitrogen oxides (NOx), sulfur dioxide (SO_2), ozone (O_3), volatile organic compounds, and particulate matter. **Particulate matter** describes substances that are small enough to remain suspended in the air for long periods of time and can travel deep into the lungs.[26] Air pollutants can cause lung disease by triggering inflammation, damaging the cells that line the respiratory tract, and impairing immune response. They increase the risk of numerous respiratory diseases, including pneumonia, asthma, lung cancer, and other chronic respiratory diseases, and they exacerbate cardiovascular disorders.[27]

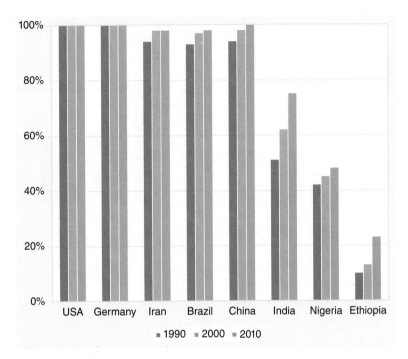

FIGURE 4–18 Many homes in lower-income countries do not have electricity.

Data from *Progress toward sustainable energy 2017: Global tracking framework report*. Washington DC: World Bank/IEA; 2017.

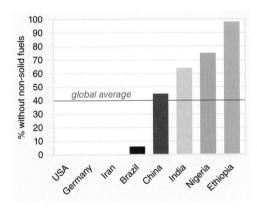

FIGURE 4–19 Most residents of low-income countries burn solid fuels to cook food rather than using clean fuels and technologies.

Data from *Progress toward sustainable energy 2017: Global tracking framework report*. Washington DC: World Bank/IEA; 2017.

In many low- and middle-income countries, a sizeable proportion of deaths are attributed to the combined effects of indoor and outdoor air pollution (**FIGURE 4–21**).[16]

SDG 7 is focused on "ensuring access to affordable, reliable, sustainable, and modern energy for all" (**FIGURE 4–22**).[4] In lower-income countries, progress toward this goal will be met by increasing the proportion of households with electricity, since indoor air pollution levels will be reduced when fewer people cook with solid fuels. There are also interventions that can reduce exposure to indoor air pollution among people without electricity.[28] Using a cook stove with a flue that diverts pollutants out of the home improves indoor air quality. When it is not possible to increase ventilation inside the home, moving the kitchen to the outside of the home reduces smoke inhalation (if the outside cooking area has a good ventilation system). Improved cooking devices such as those that use solar panels or other alternative energy sources generally create less smoke than biomass. It is also helpful to change behaviors to reduce the health risks associated with cooking, such as keeping children away

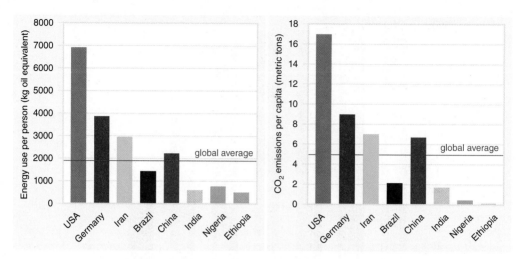

FIGURE 4–20 People in higher-income countries use more energy and generate more carbon dioxide emissions than people in low-income countries.

Data from *The little green data book 2016*. Washington DC: World Bank; 2016.

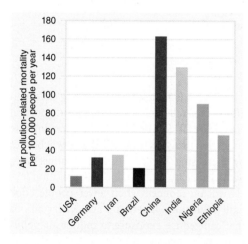

FIGURE 4–21 Mortality attributed to household and ambient air pollution per 100,000 people.

Data from *World health statistics 2016*. Geneva: WHO; 2016.

from smoke and using pot lids to conserve heat.

In higher-income countries, progress toward achieving SDG 7 will require generating a higher proportion of electricity from renewable sources that release fewer emissions into the air. **Renewable energy** is energy derived from a source like wind or solar power that is not depleted when it is used. Wind,

7.1	Ensure universal access to affordable, reliable, and modern energy services.
7.2	Increase substantially the share of renewable energy in the global energy mix.
7.3	Double the global rate of improvement in energy efficiency.
7.a	Enhance international cooperation to facilitate access to clean energy research and technology, including renewable energy, energy efficiency, and advanced and cleaner fossil-fuel technology, and promote investment in energy infrastructure and clean energy technology.
7.b	Expand infrastructure and upgrade technology for supplying modern and sustainable energy services for all in developing countries, in particular, least developed countries, small island developing states, and landlocked developing countries.

FIGURE 4–22 Targets for Sustainable Development Goal 7, which focuses on energy.

Data from United Nations. *Transforming our world: The 2030 agenda for sustainable development*. New York: UN; 2015.

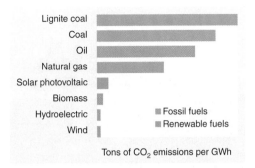

FIGURE 4-23 Renewable sources emit fewer greenhouse gases (CO_2 emissions per GWh) than nonrenewable energy sources.

Data from *Comparison of lifecycle greenhouse gas emissions of various electricity generation sources*. London: World Nuclear Association (WNA); 2011.

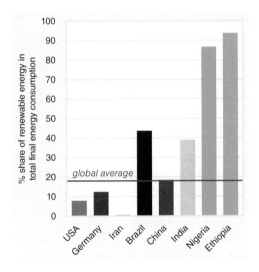

FIGURE 4-24 Countries with high rates of electrification generally have small shares of energy consumption from renewable energy sources (including biofuels, hydro, wind, solar, geothermal, and other renewable sources).

Data from *Progress toward sustainable energy 2017: Global tracking framework report*. Washington DC: World Bank/IEA; 2017.

solar, ocean, geothermal, and other renewable sources of energy produce less environmental damage than combustible fossil fuel sources like oil and coal (**FIGURE 4-23**).[29] Countries with high rates of electrification generally have small shares of energy consumption from renewable energy sources (**FIGURE 4-24**),[21] and

SDG 7 can only be met if the proportion of energy generated from renewable sources in those countries increases significantly.

▶ 4.4 Occupational and Industrial Health

The field of **occupational health**, also called occupational safety and health and workplace health and safety, focuses on primary prevention of injuries and other work-related health problems. Occupational health was one of the first public health specialty fields.[30] In 1713, Bernardino Ramazzini published *Diseases of Workers*, a book that detailed the environmental hazards encountered in 52 occupations, listing poisoning, respiratory diseases, problems related to prolonged postures and repetitive tasks, and psychological stress as some of many on-the-job threats to health. In 1753, James Lind published the results of an experiment that supported the hypothesis that sailors could prevent scurvy if they carried citrus fruit with them on long journeys.[31] (After this discovery, sailors were sometimes called "limeys" for the citrus fruit carried on ships.) In 1775, Percivall Pott identified chimney soot as the cause of elevated rates of scrotal cancer in chimney sweeps, which was the result of constant exposure to coal tar due to sweeps rarely bathing or changing their trousers.[32] New occupational risks continue to be identified today.

Many workers are exposed to a mix of biological, chemical, physical, mechanical, and psychosocial challenges at work.[33] Some occupations carry specific risks.[34] Workers exposed to loud noises are at risk of permanently impaired hearing. Office and factory workers have an increased risk of repetitive strain injuries, such as carpal tunnel syndrome, that can develop after repeatedly performing the same tasks. Some workers who have long-term exposure to industrial chemicals are at increased risk of developing certain types of cancers. Those who work in the manufacturing industry may be at risk of crush wounds from moving parts. Medical workers are at risk of contracting infectious diseases from needle sticks and contact with body fluids. All workers may be subject to stress that can impair mental health.[35] Specialists in **industrial hygiene** (also called occupational hygiene) assess and mitigate workplace hazards,[36] such as issuing ear protection to workers in factories with high noise levels, making sure that people who spend their days in front of a computer have ergonomically designed chairs and are taking steps to minimize repetitive motion injuries, providing education about proper use of heavy machinery and hazardous materials, equipping healthcare workers with personal protective equipment, and providing wellness coaching.

Each year, at least 1.1 million people die from on-the-job injuries and job-related diseases, including about 490,000 people who die from lung cancer, bladder cancer, and other cancers attributed to workplace exposure to harmful chemicals or radiation; 400,000 who die from work-related respiratory diseases, such as COPD, asthma, and pneumoconiosis, which is caused by inhalation of silica, asbestos, coal dust, and other substances; and 200,000 people who die from occupational injuries.[37] Occupational risks are estimated to be responsible for 31% of years of life lived with low back pain, 27% of hearing loss, 15% of COPD, 8% of asthma, 8% of injuries, and 2% of leukemia cases worldwide.[37] Every year there are more than 300 million occupational accidents that are severe enough to keep the injured person away from work for at least 4 days.[38] Most occupational injuries, diseases, and deaths could be prevented if worksite managers and government officials enforced compliance with safety regulations.[39]

Toxicology is the study of the harmful effects that chemicals and other environmental materials can have on living things. Chemicals and other substances produced, handled, stored, transported, or disposed of at work and chemicals released from work activities can pose both acute (immediate) and long-term

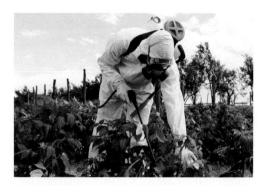
© hedgehog94/Shutterstock

health risks to people exposed to them.[40] Hazardous exposures in the workplace may include radiation, chemical pollutants, and toxic substances like polychlorinated biphenyls (PCBs), dioxins, asbestos, lead, mercury, cadmium, organic solvents, and pesticides. Many of these are released into the environment through industrial activities (**FIGURE 4–25**).[41] Toxicologists study the effect of exposure frequency (how often a person is exposed), duration (the length of exposure at a given time), and dose (the amount of hazardous substance contacted) on health. They also assess the various exposure routes (like inhalation, ingestion, and absorption through the skin) and pathways (through air, water, food, soil, or other mechanisms) related to hazardous exposures. **Carcinogens** (substances that can cause genetic mutations that lead to cancer), **teratogens** (substances that can cause birth defects), and other hazards can be regulated or banned.

Hazardous substances cause more than 500,000 deaths worldwide each year, including about 180,000 deaths attributable to asbestos, 120,000 attributable to diesel engine exhaust, 85,000 attributable to silica exposure, and several thousand deaths due to poisonings.[37] Although these hazardous substances are used and produced in industrial settings in countries across the income spectrum, workers in lower-income countries have greater risks from occupational exposure. Many highly toxic agents that are heavily

Substance	Uses
Arsenic	Used to make "pressure-treated" lumber, as a pesticide for cotton plants, and in copper and lead smelting
Lead	Used in the production of batteries, ammunition, metal products (solder and pipes), and devices to shield X-rays; released from the burning of fossil fuels and during mining and manufacturing; used in some gasoline, paints, caulks, and ceramic products
Mercury	Used in thermometers, dental fillings, batteries, and some antiseptic creams and ointments
Vinyl chloride	Used to make polyvinyl chloride (PVC), plastic products like pipes, wire and cable coatings, and packaging materials
Polychlorinated biphenyls (PCBs)	Used as coolants and lubricants in transformers, capacitors, and other electrical equipment
Benzene	Used to make other chemicals that form plastics, resins, nylon and synthetic fibers, rubbers, lubricants, dyes, detergents, drugs, and pesticides
Cadmium	Extracted during the production of metals like zinc, lead, and copper for use in batteries, pigments, metal coatings, and plastics
Polycyclic aromatic hydrocarbons (PAHs)	A group of more than 100 different chemicals that are formed during incomplete burning of coal, oil, gas, garbage, tobacco, charbroiled meat, and other organic substances; also found in coal tar, crude oil, creosote, roofing tar, some medicines and dyes, plastics, and pesticides

FIGURE 4–25 Harmful substances commonly found at worksites (ATSDR 2015 Substance Priority List).

Data from *2015 ATSDR Substance Priority List*. Atlanta GA: U.S. Agency for Toxic Substances and Disease Registry (ATSDR); 2015.

regulated or banned in high-income countries are still used in lower-income countries, and most workers in low-income countries where occupational regulations are rarely enforced do not have access to protective gear and safety training.[42] Furthermore, in some places where paid jobs are scarce, work that requires repeated exposure to dangerous chemicals may be seen as the only alternative to unemployment. The industries producing the most pollution-related health problems worldwide include used lead acid battery recycling, mining and ore processing, lead smelting, tannery operating, artisanal small-scale gold mining,

industrial and municipal dumping, chemical and product manufacturing, and the dye industry.[42]

Ecotoxicology examines the impact of toxic exposures on populations, communities, and ecosystems. When industrial accidents occur, they often affect people who do not work at the site of an incident. The pollutants, toxins, and other substances released into air or water as a result of an accident can affect the local community and may spread to a larger area. The radioactivity released during the meltdown of the nuclear reactor at Chernobyl in Ukraine (then part of the USSR) in

April 1986 spread a radioactive cloud across most of Europe. One health-related outcome of the meltdown was an increase in the incidence of thyroid cancer among children in the most contaminated regions.[43] An accident at a chemical plant in Bhopal, India, in December 1984 released liquid and vapor methyl isocyanate. Several thousand people died when they were exposed to the fumes, some in their beds and others in the street after they staggered out of their homes to try to escape from the chemical. Hundreds of thousands of people sustained lung injuries.[44] Routine industrial practices may also put entire communities at risk, especially in lower-income countries with few regulations to prevent environmental contamination.[42]

Chemical hazards in the home and community and at worksites can be especially dangerous for children who are still developing and growing. The risk of exposure to hazardous materials and other dangerous conditions is especially high for children who are sent to work at an early age. Some types of work, such as when rural children work alongside their parents on the family farm, can be a positive experience. But some children develop lasting physical and psychological scars from long hours doing domestic labor, agricultural work, or factory work. The International Labor Organization (ILO) makes a distinction between children participating in economic activity—working (whether for pay or not) for a few hours or full time doing activities other than household chores or schooling—and children who are involved in child labor.[45] It is permissible for children aged 12 years and older to spend a few hours a week doing light work that is not hazardous. It is a **child labor** violation when a child has an excessive workload, unsafe work conditions, or extreme work intensity. Any of these conditions may harm a child's physical health, mental health, or moral development. At worst, a child may be sold by his or her family into bonded labor, forced into sex work, or forced into armed conflict. In 2000, about 16% of all children between 5 and 17 years old were

engaged in child labor, about 245,000 children total. By 2012, the rate had dropped to about 10.6% of children, but there were still about 170,000 children engaged in child labor. That number included about 8.5% of children aged 5–11 years, 13.1% of children aged 12–14 years, and 13.0% of children aged 15–17 years.[46] The proportion of children between 5 and 17 years old who were engaged in hazardous work dropped by half between 2000 and 2012, from 11% to 5.4%, but in 2012 about 85,000 children were still doing hazardous work.[46]

Two of the SDGs have targets that focus on occupational health, aiming to end child labor (SDG 8.7), to "promote safe and secure working environments for all workers" (SDG 8.8), and to "build resilient infrastructure, promote inclusive and sustainable industrialization, and foster innovation" (SDG 9) with "increased resource-use efficiency and greater adoption of clean and environmentally sound technologies and industrial processes" (SDG 9.4).[4] Many countries from all income levels have passed occupational and environmental health and safety laws,[47] but meeting the SDG targets will require more attention on occupational health and safety, including protecting children from harmful labor, preventing workplace injuries and work-related diseases and disabilities, and safeguarding the health and safety of communities located near industrial sites.

▶ 4.5 Urbanization

Urbanicity is the degree to which a particular location is urban, and it is a function of total population size, population density, population diversity, and access to city services like retail facilities and public transportation (**FIGURE 4-26**).[48] Urbanicity is the opposite of **rurality**, the degree to which a particular location is rural. In 1950, about 30% of the world's people lived in urban areas. That percentage increased to more than 50% by 2010 and is projected to further rise to more than 65% by 2050 (**FIGURE 4-27**).[49] Most higher-income

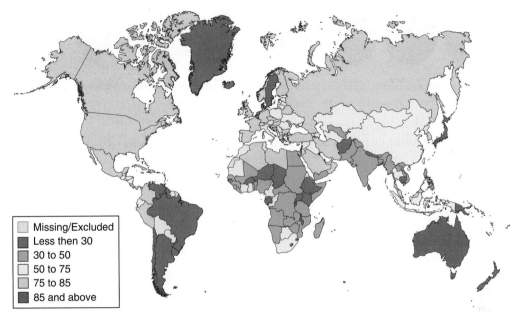

FIGURE 4–26 Proportion of people living in urban areas (2015).

Data from United Nations Department of Economic and Social Affairs. *World urbanization prospects: The 2014 revision.* New York: UN; 2014.

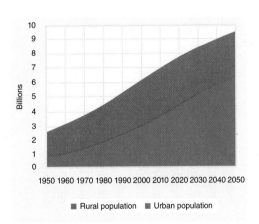

FIGURE 4–27 The global urban population will continue to grow.

Data from United Nations Department of Economic and Social Affairs. *World urbanization prospects: The 2014 revision.* New York: UN; 2014.

countries have highly urban populations, while most lower-income countries continue to have mostly rural populations (FIGURE 4–28). However, in nearly every country across the income spectrum, the proportion of the population

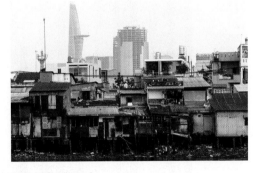

© Stephane Bidouze/Shutterstock

that lives in cities is increasing and is expected to continue to rise (FIGURE 4–29).[49] SDG 11 has an aim of "making cities and human settlements inclusive, safe, resilient, and sustainable" through targets related to housing (SDG 11.1), transportation (SDG 11.2), air quality and waste management (SDG 11.6), and open public spaces (SDG 11.7).[4] Because the majority of the world's people live in cities, urban health is a core component of global public health.[50]

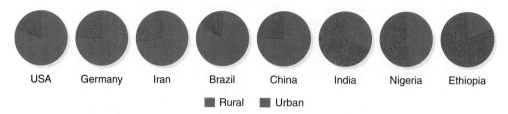

FIGURE 4–28 Percentage of each country living in an urban area (2015).

Data from United Nations Department of Economic and Social Affairs. *World urbanization prospects: The 2014 revision.* New York: UN; 2014.

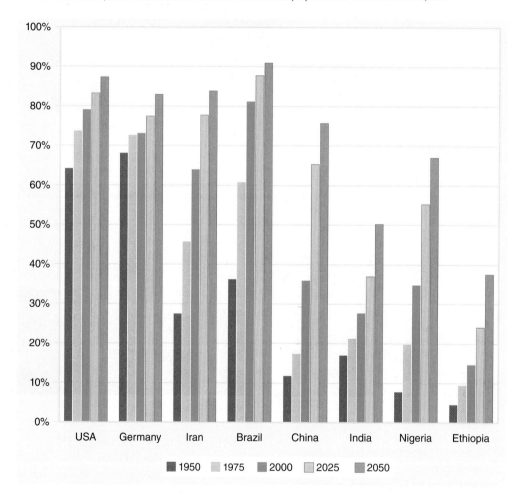

FIGURE 4–29 The proportion of the population living in an urban area is increasing in nearly every country and is projected to continue to increase.

Data from United Nations Department of Economic and Social Affairs. *World urbanization prospects: The 2014 revision.* New York: UN; 2014.

Urbanization is a shift toward more people living in cities and fewer people living in rural areas.[51] Each day, thousands of people move from rural areas to cities in search of better jobs, higher incomes, more social opportunities, and greater conveniences. Urbanization is occurring in nearly every part of the world, but this transition is happening

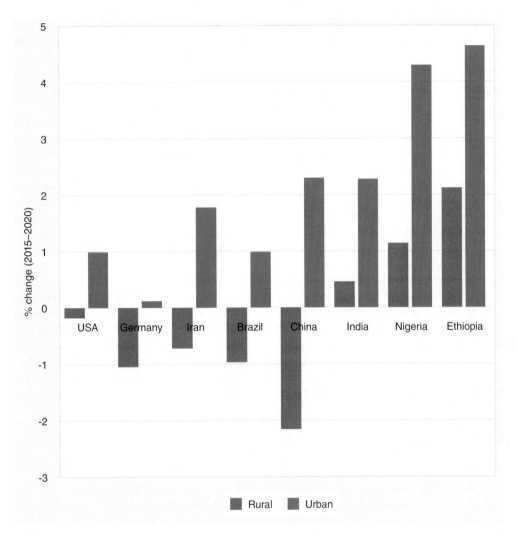

FIGURE 4–30 Urban areas are growing faster than rural areas (2015–2020).

Data from United Nations Department of Economic and Social Affairs. *World urbanization prospects: The 2014 revision.* New York: UN; 2014.

most dramatically in low- and middle-income countries (**FIGURE 4–30**).[49] In upper-middle-income countries, birth rates are relatively low and rapid rates of rural-to-urban migration are causing rural populations to shrink as cities grow. In lower-income countries, the birth rates remain high, but rural-to-urban migration is causing the urban population to grow much faster than the rural population. This process of urbanization affects both urban and rural residents. Rural women, for example, may bear a particularly heavy burden when their husbands move to cities to find wage employment, leaving the women with the responsibility of completing all household chores. Parents who move to a city may have to leave their children in the care of rural-dwelling grandparents, which puts a strain on three generations.

On average, urban residents have greater access than rural residents to water and sanitation, to a relatively reliable public transportation system, and to healthcare providers and health technologies. Electricity in cities reduces cooking time and makes it easier to store food safely. Communications systems broadcast news and entertainment shows as well as emergency warnings and health messages. Urban women have more opportunities to pursue additional education and find employment outside the home. Pregnancy in cities is safer because of greater access to antenatal care and assistance by medical professionals during delivery.

However, the benefits of urbanicity are not available to all urban residents (**FIGURE 4–31**). Many people who move to cities end up living in unplanned settlements (sometimes called shantytowns, slums, or squatter camps) where the quality of life is generally worse than rural life.[52] In low- and middle-income countries, clusters of temporary structures are often quickly erected at the outskirts of large cities to accommodate rural-to-urban migrants. The structures are often built with cardboard or scraps of metal, wood, or other found objects, and they may provide little comfort or privacy and only minimal protection from the sun, rain, wind, and other elements. These dwellings may eventually be replaced with shacks built from blocks or bricks with a tin or asbestos roof, or they may be replaced with sturdier houses constructed from cement. Many years may pass before these growing communities have access to critical utilities. Residents might not have access to toilets. Informal dwellings are often built in floodplains or on other vulnerable lands, and lack of drainage systems means that floods carry feces and other waste into homes. Trash and human waste might collect near the home and attract rodents and insects, increasing the risk of infectious diseases. Cooking indoors with solid fuels generates high levels of air pollution. Unplanned communities in urbanizing cities are often located in undesirable locations near noisy and polluted highways or industrial centers that exacerbate asthma and cardiovascular conditions. Urban workers may face new occupational hazards, and they might not have access to affordable emergency healthcare services.

Violence related to crowding and road-traffic accidents (often of the motor vehicle versus pedestrian variety) might be common. It might be difficult to grow or purchase nutritious foods, and there may be little time or space for exercising.

There are numerous public health responsibilities that are common to all large population centers globally, including maintaining a safe built environment, managing water and sanitation services, disposing of waste, minimizing pollutants, and addressing other infrastructure issues.[53] The similarities are especially prominent among megacities. A **megacity** is a metropolitan area with 10 million or more inhabitants. The number of megacities increased from 10 in 1990 to 29 in 2015, and that count is expected to rise to 41 by 2030 (**FIGURE 4–32**).[49] As the world urbanizes, the ability to achieve public health goals will depend on cities being safe, resilient, and sustainable. This will require cities in low- and middle-income countries to address the health-related challenges associated with poverty, socioeconomic inequalities, and environmental hazards.[54]

▶ 4.6 Sustainability

A sustainable system is one that is able to be maintained at a particular level. When the term is used as part of the SDGs, the word **sustainability** emphasizes the need to provide for current human needs without compromising the ability of future generations to meet their needs.[55] Sustainability has been described as a combination of "3 Es": ethics (or equity), environment, and economics.[56] These concepts have been expanded in the SDGs to include "5 Ps": people, planet, prosperity (or profit), peace, and partnership.[4] SDG 12 has an aim of "ensuring sustainable consumption and production patterns" through targets related to management of natural resources (SDG 12.2), reduction of food waste (SDG 12.3), management of hazardous waste (SDG 12.4), and improvements

Sector	Rural	Unplanned Urban	Planned Urban
Water	▪ May have minimal access to improved water sources ▪ Risk of microbial contamination	▪ May have minimal access to affordable clean water ▪ Risk of microbial exposure and industrial and agricultural chemical contamination	▪ Reliable access to safe, clean drinking water
Sanitation	▪ May have inadequate sanitation facilities ▪ Open defecation in a field away from the house may be common	▪ May have inadequate sanitation facilities ▪ Open defecation in the street may be common	▪ Sewage system
Trash disposal	▪ Solid waste is burned or buried	▪ No collection of solid waste ▪ Trash heaps create a habitat for insect and rodent vectors	▪ Solid waste is collected and removed
Chemical hazards	▪ Potential exposure to agrochemicals like fertilizer and pesticides	▪ Potential exposure to industrial waste	▪ Little exposure to industrial or agricultural hazards
Fuel	▪ Solid fuels, which may be able to be collected locally	▪ Solid fuels, which may be expensive	▪ Electricity
Air quality	▪ Indoor air pollution from burning biomass	▪ Both indoor and outdoor air pollution ▪ Noise pollution	▪ Some outdoor air pollution ▪ Some indoor air pollution from building materials
Nutrition	▪ May have limited ability to purchase food ▪ Can usually grow, gather, or hunt for food	▪ May have limited access to affordable, healthy foods ▪ May not have space for a garden	▪ Adequate access to healthy and safe dietary choices
Health facilities	▪ Facilities may be far from home and may provide only basic care	▪ Facilities may be crowded and understaffed	▪ Basic, emergency, and specialty healthcare (including mental health and rehabilitation) facilities are available

FIGURE 4–31 Comparison of health risks associated with living in rural, unplanned urban, and planned urban areas.

Rank	Metropolitan area	Country	Population (2015)
1	Tokyo	Japan	38.0 million
2	Delhi	India	25.7 million
3	Shanghai	China	23.7 million
4	São Paul	Brazil	21.1 million
5	Mumbai	India	21.0 million
6	Mexico city	Mexico	21.0 million
7	Beijing	China	20.4 million
8	Osaka	Japan	20.2 million
9	Cairo	Egypt	18.8 million
10	New York	USA	18.6 million
11	Dhaka	Bangladesh	17.6 million
12	Karachi	Pakistan	16.6 million
13	Buenos Aires	Argentina	15.2 million
14	Kolkata	India	14.9 million
15	Istanbul	Turkey	14.2 million
16	Chongqing	China	13.3 million
17	Lagos	Nigeria	13.1 million
18	Manila	Philippines	13.0 million
19	Rio de Janeiro	Brazil	19.9 million
20	Guangzhou	China	12.5 million
21	Los Angeles	USA	12.3 million
22	Moscow	Russia	12.2 million
23	Kinshasa	DR Congo	11.6 million
24	Tianjin	China	11.2 million
25	Paris	France	10.8 million
26	Shenzhen	China	10.8 million
27	Jakarta	Indonesia	10.3 million
28	London	UK	10.3 million
29	Bangalore	India	10.1 million

FIGURE 4–32 The world's megacities (urban areas of 10 million or more inhabitants).

Data from United Nations Department of Economic and Social Affairs. *World urbanization prospects: The 2014 revision.* New York: UN; 2014.

in recycling and reuse (SDG 12.5).[4] The concept of sustainability is also integrated into all of the other SDGs. The SDGs are intended to reduce poverty and disease for today's people while ensuring that future generations inherit a healthy planet that allows them to enjoy long, healthy lives.[57]

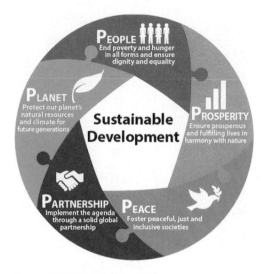

Courtesy of United Nations Information Centre

Sustainability has grown in prominence as a global priority in recent decades because of the rapid increase in the size of the human population. The dangers of overpopulation can be illustrated by comparing Earth to an island. Picture a small island in the middle of an ocean. It is arable (that is, it can grow food) and it has a variety of plant and animal species. At first, ten people settle on the island. They build homes, develop a system for collecting freshwater (because ocean water is too salty to drink or use for irrigation), and begin to farm the land. They also begin to have children, and eventually those children have children. Soon, the population has reached 100, and then it grows to 1000. The amount of land available for farming decreases as more homes are built, but the need for food is greater because there are more people to feed. Getting rid of waste products and finding energy sources are increasingly difficult. The limited amount of freshwater available is becoming a source of stress as the demand for water increases, but water quality is becoming poorer as waste pollutes water sources. Some plants and animals are threatened and at risk of extinction. Crime is increasing as resources become scarce. These challenges could be expected to become even worse as the population continues to grow.

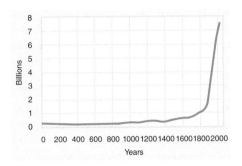

FIGURE 4–33 The "J-shaped curve" for world population growth.

Data from United Nations Department of Economic and Social Affairs. *World population to 2300*. New York: UN; 2004.

Overpopulation occurs when a population becomes so large that the amount of food and other environmental resources available are insufficient to support all members of the population. The size of the Earth's human population remained relatively steady for millennia, but recent growth has been exponential. A plot of the world's population shows a "J-shaped" growth pattern (**FIGURE 4–33**).[58] The doubling time, the number of years it takes for the world's population to double in number, is getting shorter. It took only 40 years—from 1950 until 1990—for the number of humans to double from 2.5 billion to 5 billion. The current world population is more than 7 billion, and demographers project that the global population may rise to 11 billion by 2100.[59] The population might stabilize after that time, but it might also grow or shrink depending on numerous socioeconomic and environmental factors that will unfold over the coming decades.

In 1798, Thomas Malthus hypothesized that overpopulation leads to catastrophes like famines, epidemics, and wars.[60] In the 21st century, this idea is expressed in terms of concerns about the unequal distribution of food and natural resources, the risks associated with the increased pollution and congestion that will occur with continued population growth, and the likelihood of increased crime and conflict as resources in some regions of the world become scarce. For example, many countries are already

facing water scarcity crises, especially small island nations and desert countries where internal freshwater resources are extremely limited, and water wars are seen as a possibility in the coming decades as more people compete for control over the world's finite supply of the freshwater that is essential for survival.[61]

Carrying capacity is the maximum human population the Earth can sustain. There is no easy way to calculate the carrying capacity, because it depends on the standard of living and cultural factors in addition to population density (measured as land area per person or as arable land area per person), climate, and the land and natural resources that are available. However, carrying capacity can be approximated based on estimations of the per capita area of land needed to meet a population's consumption patterns. The **ecological footprint** is a measure of how much burden human consumption places on the biosphere. People in high-income countries have large ecological footprints and use many more resources per person than people in low-income countries (**FIGURE 4–34**).[62] Earth likely could not support the current world population if everyone had the current ecological footprint of high-income countries, but most people in low- and middle-income countries aspire to the higher standards of living that come with larger ecological footprints. As countries' economies grow, their residents tend to use more resources per person. Sustainable development promotes economic growth while simultaneously protecting the environment from the adverse effects that typically accompany industrialization.[63]

Sustainable global health programs aim to generate long-term health benefits that endure even after specific projects end. A program that depletes natural resources and promotes overconsumption is not sustainable.[64] A program that is fully dependent on outside donors and does not involve recipients in planning, decision-making, and evaluation is not sustainable. Ideally, global health programs should foster capacity building and encourage the

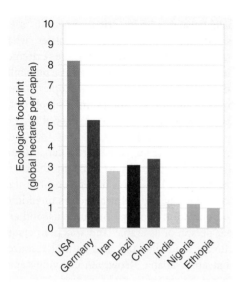

FIGURE 4–34 Ecological footprints are higher in high-income countries than in lower-income countries (2012).

Data from *National footprint accounts 2016*. Oakland CA: Global Footprint Network; 2016.

self-sufficiency of participating communities, such as by facilitating the integration of successful externally funded healthcare programs into the routine services offered by internally funded national healthcare systems.[65]

Sustainability applies to human behavior and also to larger ecological processes. **Biodiversity** is the presence of a wide variety of plant and animal species within a particular environment. An ecosystem is sustainable when it can maintain its biodiversity and level of productivity indefinitely. The **One Health** concept emphasizes the interconnectedness of human health, animal health, and ecological health.[66] Humans are dependent on plants and animals for food, and human lives are threatened when domestic animals, wildlife, agricultural crops, and other biological entities are harmed by environmental degradation and disease. The emerging field of **planetary health** emphasizes the dependence of human health on the Earth, and seeks to understand the damage that human actions can impose on ecosystem health.[67] Threats to the health of the planet

include habitat loss and degradation, species overexploitation, pollution, invasive plant and animal species that crowd out native species in a location, the dissemination of pathogens in new areas due to human transportation systems, and climate change.[68] Humans can promote planetary health by preserving and restoring natural resources, producing energy and goods more efficiently and less wastefully, and consuming resources more wisely.[68]

▶ 4.7 Climate Change and Health

Three of the SDGs address macro-level concerns about global environmental health. SDG 13 aims to "take urgent action to combat climate change and its impacts," with a focus on strengthening resilience to respond to "climate-related hazards and natural disasters" (SDG 13.1). SDG 14 aims to "conserve and sustainably use the oceans, seas, and marine resources." SDG 15 aims to "protect, restore, and promote sustainable use of terrestrial ecosystems, sustainably manage forests, combat desertification, and halt and reverse land degradation and halt biodiversity loss."[4]

At the local level, it can be easy to observe the health effects of human actions that alter the environment. Infrastructural development like building permanent structures, converting forests to farms, terracing slopes for agricultural use, paving streets, installing electrical lines and sewers, building dams, extracting fossil fuels to make oil and other petroleum products, and a host of other activities has increased the quality of life for billions of people. But any intentional change to the local environment may have some unintended side effects that adversely affect human health.[69] For example, building a dam may prevent flooding and improve agricultural productivity, but having a larger body of water nearby may increase the risk of some insect-transmitted infections and intestinal worm infestations.[70]

The immediate effects of most human activities are local, but the distinction between local and global environmental change is getting blurrier. In a globalized world, the choices any person makes about where to live, work, and travel and what to purchase can have an impact on people who live in distant lands. The air pollution created by millions of commuters driving to work each day in one city does not just damage their airspace, but that of their neighbors. When electronic waste (e-waste) and other types of garbage are discarded by people in high-income countries, the potentially toxic materials may be shipped to dumps in lower-income countries.[71] Deforestation and habitat destruction, soil erosion and salinization, water management problems, overhunting and overfishing, invasive species (which may crowd out local flora and fauna), human population growth, and increasing use of resources per capita all can have local and global impacts.[72]

Climate change is a long-term shift in weather patterns and average temperatures. One component of climate change is **global warming**, a gradual increase in the temperature of the Earth's atmosphere. The cumulative effect of the intensified use of natural resources across the planet appears to be contributing to global climate change. The **Intergovernmental Panel on Climate Change (IPCC)**, a scientific board that reviews and synthesizes scientific data about climate and weather under the auspices of the United Nations, has expressed certainty that global climate changes are occurring and will continue to occur for centuries to come.[73] The impacts of global climate change include land degradation, water and air quality issues, biodiversity loss, and temperature and precipitation extremes. The IPCC has also concluded that the observed changes are very likely due to human activity.[74] While cycles of climate change have occurred throughout history, there is growing concern about the pace of climate variability.[75] The IPCC predicts that climate change will mean more frequent hot days and nights, fewer cold days and nights, an increasing frequency of heat waves, an increase in the frequency of heavy precipitation events in some areas and an increase in droughts in others, an increase in tropical cyclone (hurricane) activity, and an increase in the incidence of extremely high sea levels.[76]

Many of these expected climate changes could have significant adverse impacts on human health (**FIGURE 4–35**).[77] Extreme heat increases the rate of cardiovascular disease

Climate Change	Health Impact
Hot days become hotter and more frequent	Increased rate of heat-related mortality from cardiovascular, respiratory, and kidney diseases exacerbated by heat
Precipitation events become more frequent and more intense, with more extreme floods in some places and more extreme droughts in others	Increased risks of undernutrition and of waterborne and vectorborne (insect-transmitted) infectious diseases
High sea levels become more extreme	Increased risk of drowning

FIGURE 4–35 Examples of observed climate change trends and their likely impacts on human health.

Data from Smith KR, Woodward A, Campbell-Lendrum D, et al. Human health: Impacts, adaptation, and co-benefits. In *Climate change 2014: Impacts, adaptation, and vulnerability. Contribution of Working Group II to the 5th Assessment Report of the Intergovernmental Panel on Climate Change.* Cambridge UK: Cambridge University Press; 2014.

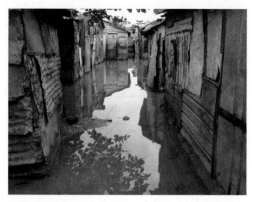

CDC/ Venecia Ramírez, Dominican Republic

mortality.[78] Extreme weather events decrease air quality by increasing particulates and pollen in the air, and poor air quality exacerbates illness and mortality from respiratory and cardiovascular diseases.[79] Floods, droughts, heat waves, and other weather extremes might reduce agricultural productivity, and ocean acidification might reduce aquacultural productivity, leading to greater levels of food insecurity.[80] Extreme weather events can also increase the risks of diarrheal diseases, insect-borne infectious like malaria and dengue fever, and drowning and other types of injuries.[81] The negative impacts of climate change are likely to be especially detrimental to the world's lowest-income people, who often live in places with greater environmental vulnerability and fewer resources to respond to threats.[82]

A series of international agreements have sought to combat climate change. The United Nations **Framework Convention on Climate Change (FCCC)** is an international environmental treaty that seeks to reduce greenhouse gas emissions.[83] A **greenhouse gas (GHG)** is a gas in the atmosphere that traps heat and causes surface temperatures to increase. The GHGs of greatest concern include carbon dioxide (CO_2), methane (CH_4), nitrous oxide (N_2O), and fluorinated gases such as sulfur hexafluoride (SF_6), hydrofluorocarbons, and perfluorocarbons. The FCCC was negotiated

in 1992 at the UN Conference on Environment and Development, colloquially called the Earth Summit, which was held in Rio de Janeiro, Brazil, and went into force in 1994. The 1997 Kyoto Protocol sought to toughen the FCCC commitments to reduce GHG emissions by the high-income signatory countries that generate the most emissions.[84] The 2015 Paris Agreement is a legally binding set of additional commitments from signatories across the income spectrum to reduce global warming and promote development that does not further exacerbate environmental damage.[85]

Regardless of arguments about the precise causes of global warming, the alarming trends documented by the IPCC support the value of humans treading more lightly on the Earth. For example, alternative energy sources that harness solar, wind, or wave power may be able to produce energy that creates less pollution and less environmental damage than carbon-based fuels, hydroelectric power (which requires the building of massive dams and flooding of large swaths of land), and nuclear power (which remains dangerous because of the risk of a meltdown). The short- and long-term risks and benefits of projects that alter the environment locally or more widely should be carefully considered before projects are initiated, and the assessments should include health and environmental evaluations as well as economic ones.[86] Strategic plans for public health initiatives should examine the links between human and environmental health in the targeted populations and then account for the possible impact of climate change on health risks.[87] In a globalized world, everyone has a stake in creating and sustaining a healthy environment.[88]

▶ References

1. Prüss-Ustün A, Wolf J, Corvalán C, Bos R, Neira M. *Preventing disease through healthy environments: A global assessment of the burden of disease from environmental risks.* Geneva: WHO; 2016.

2. *Don't pollute my future! The impact of the environment on children's health.* Geneva: WHO; 2017.

3. Landrigan PJ, Fuller R, Acosta NJR, et al. The *Lancet* Commission on pollution and health. *Lancet.* 2017. doi:10.1016/S0140-6736(17)32345-0

4. United Nations. *Transforming our world: The 2030 Agenda for Sustainable Development.* New York: UN; 2015.

5. UN Economic and Social Council. *Report of the Inter-Agency and Expert Group on Sustainable Development Goal Indicators* (E/CN.3/2016/2 /Rev.1). New York: UN; 2016.

6. Howard G, Bartram J. *Domestic water quantity, service level and health.* Geneva: WHO; 2003.

7. *Guidelines for drinking water quality: 4th edition incorporating the first addendum.* Geneva: WHO; 2017.

8. *Water for life: Community water security.* New York: Hesperian Foundation and UNDP; 2005.

9. Maupin MA, Kenney JF, Hutson SS, Lovelace JK, Barber NL, Linsey KS. *Estimated use of water in the United States in 2010.* Reston VA: U.S. Geological Survey; 2014.

10. *Progress on sanitation and drinking water: 2015 update and MDG assessment.* New York: UNICEF /WHO Joint Monitoring Programme for Water Supply and Sanitation; 2015.

11. Nordstrom DK. Worldwide occurrences of arsenic in ground water. *Science.* 2002;296:2143–4.

12. Smith AH, Lingas EO, Rahman M. Contamination of drinking-water by arsenic in Bangladesh: A public health emergency. *Bull World Health Organ.* 2000;78:1093–103.

13. Ahmed M, Jakariya M, Quaiyum M, Mahmud SN. *An implementation guide for the Arsenic Mitigation Program.* Dhaka: BRAC; 2002.

14. Kar K, Chambers R. *Handbook on community-led total sanitation.* London: Plan UK; 2008.

15. *Preventing diarrhoea through better water, sanitation and hygiene: Exposures and impacts in low- and middle-income countries.* Geneva: WHO; 2014.

16. *World health statistics 2016.* Geneva: WHO; 2016.

17. Mara D, Lane J, Scott B, Trouba D. Sanitation and health. *PLoS Med.* 2010; 7:e1000363.

18. *World development indicators 2016 (Table 2.9).* Washington: World Bank; 2016.

19. Hutton G, Chase C. Water supply, sanitation, and hygiene (Chapter 9). *Disease control priorities.* 3rd ed. *Injury prevention and environmental health (Volume 7).* Washington DC: IBRD/World Bank; 2017.

20. Watkins D, Dabestani N, Nugent R, Levin C. Interventions to prevent injuries and reduce environmental and occupational hazards: A review of economic evaluations from low- and middle-income countries (Chapter 10). *Disease control priorities.* 3rd ed. *Injury prevention and environmental health (Volume 7).* Washington DC: IBRD/World Bank; 2017.

21. *Progress toward sustainable energy 2017: Global tracking framework report.* Washington DC: World Bank/IEA; 2017.

22. *WHO guidelines for indoor air quality: Household fuel combustion.* Geneva: WHO; 2014.

23. Fullerton DG, Bruce N, Gordon SB. Indoor air pollution from biomass fuel smoke is a major health concern in the developing world. *Trans R Soc Trop Med Hyg.* 2008;102:843–51.

24. *Burning opportunity: Clean household energy for health, sustainable development, and wellbeing of women and children.* Geneva: WHO; 2016.

25. *The little green data book 2016.* Washington DC: World Bank; 2016.

26. Kampa M, Castanas E. Human health effects of air pollution. *Environ Pollut.* 2008;151:362–7.

27. Brunekreef B, Holgate ST. Air pollution and health. *Lancet.* 2002;360:1233–42.

28. Smith KR, Pillarisetti A. Household air pollution from solid cookfuels and health (Chapter 7). *Disease control priorities.* 3rd ed. *Injury prevention and environmental health (Volume 7).* Washington DC: IBRD/World Bank; 2017.

29. *Comparison of lifecycle greenhouse gas emissions of various electricity generation sources.* London: World Nuclear Association (WNA); 2011.

30. Abrams HK. A short history of occupational health. *J Public Health Policy.* 2001;22:34–80.

31. Hughes RE. James Lind and the cure of scurvy: An experimental approach. *Med Hist.* 1975;19:342–51.

32. Waldron HA. A brief history of scrotal cancer. *Br J Ind Med.* 1983;40:390–401.

33. Abdalla S, Apramian S, Cantley L, Cullen M. Occupation and risk for injuries (Chapter 6). *Disease control priorities.* 3rd ed. *Injury prevention and environmental health (Volume 7).* Washington DC: IBRD/World Bank; 2017.

34. *Encyclopedia of occupational health & safety.* Geneva: ILO; 2017.

35. Leka S, Jain A. *Health impact of the psychosocial hazards of work: An overview.* Geneva: WHO; 2010.

36. *A 5 step guide for employers, workers and their representatives on conducting workplace risk assessments.* Geneva: ILO; 2014.

37. *GBD 2015 Risk Factors Collaborators.* Global, regional, and national comparative risk assessment of 79 behavioural, environmental and occupational, and metabolic risks or clusters of risks, 1990–2015: A systematic analysis for the Global Burden of Disease Study 2015. *Lancet.* 2016;388:1545–602.

38. *Safety and health at work: A vision for sustainable prevention.* Geneva: ILO; 2014.

39. *The prevention of occupational diseases.* 4th ed. Geneva: ILO; 1998.

40. *Safety and health in the use of chemicals at work.* Geneva: ILO; 2013.

41. *2015 ATSDR Substance Priority List*. Atlanta, GA: U.S. Agency for Toxic Substances and Disease Registry (ATSDR); 2015.

42. *The world's worst pollution problems 2016: The toxins beneath our feet*. New York: Pure Earth; 2016.

43. Shibata Y, Yamashita S, Masyakin VB, Panasyuk GD, Nagataki S. 15 years after Chernobyl: New evidence of thyroid cancer. *Lancet*. 2001;358:1965–6.

44. Mehta PS, Mehta AS, Mehta SJ, Makhijani AB. Bhopal tragedy's health effects: A review of methyl isocyanate toxicity. *JAMA*. 1990;265:2781–7.

45. International Programme on the Elimination of Child Labour (IPEC). *Children in hazardous work: What we know, what we need to do*. Geneva: ILO; 2011.

46. *Making progress against child labour: Global estimates and trends 2000–2012*. Geneva: ILO; 2013.

47. *WHO Global Plan of Action on Workers' Health (2008–2017): Baseline for implementation*. Geneva: WHO; 2013.

48. Dahly DL, Adair LS. Quantifying the urban environment: A scale measure of urbanicity outperforms the urban-rural dichotomy. *Soc Sci Med*. 2007;64:1407–19.

49. UN Department of Economic and Social Affairs. *World urbanization prospects: The 2014 revision*. New York: UN; 2014.

50. *Health as the pulse of the new urban agenda: United Nations conference on housing and sustainable urban development, Quito, October 2016*. Geneva: WHO; 2016.

51. Vlahov D, Galea S. Urbanization, urbanicity, and health. *J Urban Health*. 2002;79(Suppl 4):S1–12.

52. Moore M, Gould P, Keary BS. Global urbanization and impact on health. *Int J Hyg Environ Health*. 2003;206:269–78.

53. Galea S, Vlahov D. Urban health: Evidence, challenges, and directions. *Annu Rev Public Health*. 2005;26:341–65.

54. McMichael AJ. The urban environment and health in a world of increasing globalization: Issues for developing countries. *Bull World Health Organ*. 2000;78:1117–26.

55. *Our common future*. Geneva: World Commission on Environment and Development (WCED); 1987.

56. Goodland R. The concept of environmental sustainability. *Annu Rev Ecol Systematics*. 1995;26:1–24.

57. *Inheriting a sustainable world? Atlas on children's health and the environment*. Geneva: WHO; 2017.

58. UN Department of Economic and Social Affairs. *World population to 2300*. New York: UN; 2004.

59. Gerland P, Raftery AE, Ševčíková H, et al. World population stabilization unlikely this century. *Science*. 2014;346:234–7.

60. Nekola JC, Allen CD, Brown JH, et al. The Malthusian–Darwinian dynamic and the trajectory of civilization. *Trends Ecol Evol*. 2013;28:127–30.

61. Shiva A. *Water wars: Privatization, pollution, and profit*. Cambridge MA: South End Press; 2002.

62. *National footprint accounts 2016*. Oakland CA: Global Footprint Network; 2016.

63. Lélé SM. Sustainable development: A critical review. *World Dev*. 1991;19:607–21.

64. Barbier EB. The concept of sustainable economic development. *Environ Conserv*. 1987;14:101–10.

65. Shediac-Rizkallah MC, Bone LR. Planning for the sustainability of community-based health programs: Conceptual frameworks and future directions for research, practice and policy. *Health Educ Res*. 1998;13:87–108.

66. Zinsstag J, Schelling E, Waltner-Toews D, Tanner M. From "one medicine" to "one health" and systematic approaches to health and well-being. *Prev Vet Med*. 2011;101:148–56.

67. Whitmee S, Haines A, Beyrer C, et al. Safeguarding human health in the Anthropocene epoch: Report of The Rockefeller Foundation–*Lancet* Commission on planetary health. *Lancet*. 2015;386:1973–2028.

68. *Living planet report 2016: Risk and resilience in a new era*. Geneva: WWW International; 2016.

69. McMichael AJ, Campbell-Lendrum DH, Corvalán CF, et al. *Climate change and human health: Risks and responses*. Geneva: WHO; 2003.

70. Morse SS. Factors in the emergence of infectious diseases. *Emerg Infect Dis*. 1995;1:7–15.

71. Heacock M, Kelly CB, Asante KA, Birnbaum LS, Bergman Å, Bruné MN. E-waste and harm to vulnerable populations. *Environ Health Perspect*. 2016;124:550–5.

72. Diamond J. *Collapse: How societies choose to fail or succeed*. New York: Viking; 2005.

73. Pachauri RK, Meyer LA, editors. *Climate change 2014: Synthesis report. Contribution of Working Groups I, II and III to the 5th Assessment Report of the Intergovernmental Panel on Climate Change*. Cambridge UK: Cambridge University Press; 2014.

74. Stocker TF, Qin D, Plattner GK, et al., editors. *Climate change 2013: The physical science basis. Contribution of Working Group I to the 5th Assessment Report of the Intergovernmental Panel on Climate Change*. Cambridge UK: Cambridge University Press; 2013.

75. *TBD*. Health risks and costs of climate variability and change (Chapter 8). *Disease control priorities*. 3rd ed. *Injury prevention and environmental health (Volume 7)*. Washington DC: IBRD/World Bank; 2017.

76. Field CB, Barros VR, Mastrandrea MD, et al., editors. *Climate change 2014: Impacts, adaptation, and vulnerability. Contribution of Working Group II to the 5th Assessment Report of the Intergovernmental Panel on Climate Change.* Cambridge UK: Cambridge University Press; 2014.

77. Costello A, Abbas M, Allen A, et al. Managing the health effects of climate change. *Lancet.* 2009;373:1693–733.

78. Luber G, McGeehin M. Climate change and extreme heat events. *Am J Prev Med.* 2008;35:429–35.

79. D'Amato G, Cecchi L, D'Amato M, Annesi-Maesano I. Climate change and respiratory diseases. *Eur Respir Rev.* 2014;23:161–9.

80. Watts N, Adger WN, Ayeb-Karlsson S, et al. The Lancet countdown: Tracking progress on health and climate change. *Lancet.* 2017;389:1151–64.

81. *Quantitative risk assessment of the effects of climate change on selected causes of death, 2030s and 2050s.* Geneva: WHO; 2014.

82. Watts N, Adger WN, Agnolucci P, et al. Health and climate change: Policy responses to protect public health. *Lancet.* 2015;386:1861–914.

83. *United Nations Framework Convention on Climate Change.* New York: UN; 1992.

84. *Kyoto Protocol to the United Nations Framework Convention on Climate Change.* New York: UN; 1998.

85. *Adoption of the Paris Agreement.* (FCCC /CP/2015/L.9/Rev.1). New York: UN; 2015.

86. *WHO guidance to protect health from climate change through health adaptation planning.* Geneva: WHO; 2014.

87. Frumkin H, Hess J, Luber G, Malilay J, McGeehin M. Climate change: The public health response. *Am J Public Health.* 2008;98:435–45.

88. McMichael AJ, Beaglehole R. The changing global context of public health. *Lancet.* 2000;356:495–9.

CHAPTER 5

Health and Humans Rights

Global health is founded on the principle that all people have the right to the highest attainable standard of health. By becoming signatories to the Universal Declaration of Human Rights, all of the world's countries have agreed that there are many human rights that every person is entitled to, including the right to medical care. Governments have an obligation to ensure that everyone has access to water, health services, essential medicines, and other basic human needs. Members of low-income households, victims of natural disasters and complex humanitarian emergencies, people in prison, and people with disabilities often have difficulty accessing health services and other human rights. One of the roles of global health is to advocate for the human rights of those vulnerable populations.

▶ 5.1 Health and Human Rights

The preamble to the Constitution of the World Health Organization (WHO), which has been affirmed by the nearly 200 countries that have membership in the United Nations (UN), lists nine principles that serve as the foundational values for the field of global health (FIGURE 5–1). The boldest claim is that "the enjoyment of the highest attainable standard of health is one of the fundamental rights of every human being" (principle 2).[1] This statement calls for quality health services to be accessible and affordable so that everyone has access to at least basic medical and psychological care (principle 7), especially children and people who are members of vulnerable population groups (principles 2 and 6). The preamble also notes that health is linked with peace

(principle 3) and security (principles 4 and 5), that everyone is at risk of outbreaks of infectious disease (principle 5), and that both the public (principle 8) and governments (principle 9) must take active responsibility for public health. Two key terms in the preamble require careful definition: human rights and standard of health.

Human rights are entitlements that are due to every person simply because that person is human. Human rights are considered to be universal, which means that they apply to every person of all ages in all circumstances. The **Universal Declaration of Human Rights (UDHR)**, which was unanimously adopted by the member states of the United Nations in 1948, spells out more than two dozen civil, political, economic, social, and cultural human rights (FIGURE 5–2).[2] Articles 3–21 define civil and political rights that protect the foundational freedoms of

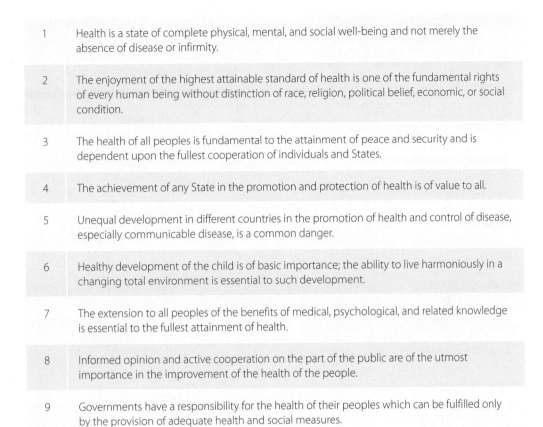

1	Health is a state of complete physical, mental, and social well-being and not merely the absence of disease or infirmity.
2	The enjoyment of the highest attainable standard of health is one of the fundamental rights of every human being without distinction of race, religion, political belief, economic, or social condition.
3	The health of all peoples is fundamental to the attainment of peace and security and is dependent upon the fullest cooperation of individuals and States.
4	The achievement of any State in the promotion and protection of health is of value to all.
5	Unequal development in different countries in the promotion of health and control of disease, especially communicable disease, is a common danger.
6	Healthy development of the child is of basic importance; the ability to live harmoniously in a changing total environment is essential to such development.
7	The extension to all peoples of the benefits of medical, psychological, and related knowledge is essential to the fullest attainment of health.
8	Informed opinion and active cooperation on the part of the public are of the utmost importance in the improvement of the health of the people.
9	Governments have a responsibility for the health of their peoples which can be fulfilled only by the provision of adequate health and social measures.

FIGURE 5-1 Health principles articulated in the Preamble to the Constitution of the World Health Organization.

Data from *Constitution of the World Health Organization*. New York: United Nations; 1946.

humans, such as the right to privacy and the right to freedom from torture. These rights are about protections rather than provisions, and they can be granted and upheld with limited financial costs to governments. Articles 22–28 outline economic, social, and cultural rights that, if realized, would contribute to human flourishing. These rights, such as the right to social security, the right to education, and the right to a standard of living adequate for health and well-being, obligate governments to provide certain services to their people.[3] Because these rights carry real monetary costs, they are somewhat aspirational. However, countries are called to make progress toward increasing the economic, social, and cultural rights of their populations.

The UDHR does not state that people have a right to be healthy. No government can guarantee health for anyone. For many diseases and disorders, there are currently no effective preventive methods or curative treatments, so there is no way for any entity to alleviate the burden from those health issues. But the UDHR does state that all people have the right to medical care and the underlying tools for health, such as safe drinking water and adequate nutrition, no matter where they live.[4]

Human Right	UDHR Articles
Right to equal dignity and human rights for all humans	1, 2
Right to life, liberty, and security of person	3
Freedom from slavery and servitude	4
Freedom from torture and cruel, inhuman, or degrading treatment or punishment	5
Right to recognition as a person	6
Freedom from discrimination	7
Right to legal protection of human rights	8
Freedom from arbitrary arrest, detention, or exile	9
Right to a fair trial	10
Right to be presumed innocent until proven guilty	11
Right to privacy	12
Freedom of movement	13
Right to asylum	14
Right to a nationality	15
Right to marry and found a family	16
Right to own property	17
Freedom of thought, conscience, and religion	18
Freedom of opinion and expression	19
Freedom of peaceful assembly and association	20
Right to participate in government	21
Right to social security	22
Right to work	23

(continues)

Human Right	UDHR Articles
Right to rest and leisure	24
Right to a standard of living adequate for the health and well-being of the individual and his/her family, including food, clothing, housing, medical care, and necessary social services, and the right to security in the event of unemployment, sickness, disability, widowhood, or old age	25
Right to education	26
Right to participate in the cultural life of a community	27

FIGURE 5–2 Key articles in the Universal Declaration of Human Rights.

Data from *The universal declaration of human rights*. New York: United Nations; 1948.

The term **standard of health** refers to targets that governments set for improving the health of the populations they govern. Achieving the "highest attainable standard of health" requires increasing access to healthcare services and to the tools for health. All governments can strive to increase access to preventive and therapeutic services, starting with a basic package of healthcare services (such as antenatal care, childhood vaccinations, treatment of common infectious diseases, and access to clean water) and then expanding the range of services that are available to the entire population.[5]

Health and human rights are intertwined. People who are denied their human rights are unable to advocate for their own health, and populations that are unhealthy are unable to advocate for their rights.[6] By adopting the UDHR, all UN member countries have affirmed their agreement that human rights are universal.[7] When people in one country are being denied their human rights, people in other countries have the obligation to call attention to those violations. The goals of the field of health and human rights include providing education about rights, exposing human rights violations, increasing accountability for governments and other organizations involved in health and human services, and improving access to health and related services.[8]

Before the concept of the "right to health" can be fully integrated into national health strategies and operationalized at the global level, four key questions will need to be answered[9]: (1) What are the services and goods guaranteed to every person under the human right to health? (2) What responsibilities do states have for the health of their own populations? (3) What duties do states owe to people beyond their borders in securing the right to health? (4) What kind of global governance for health is needed to ensure that all states live up to their mutual responsibilities? However, the shared commitment to ensuring that everyone has the basic tools for survival and health has already been recognized in numerous international agreements.

▶ 5.2 Access to Basic Human Needs

The most fundamental human right is the right to life. Human survival is dependent on having enough food, water, and air to support physiological processes and having sufficient shelter and clothing to protect the body from external exposures. These basic human needs are incorporated into the Sustainable Development Goals (SDGs) in targets that seek to "ensure that all men and women, in particular the poor and vulnerable, have equal rights to economic resources, as well as to basic services" (SDG 1.4) and to "ensure access for all to adequate, safe, and affordable housing and basic services" (SDG 11.1).[10] Additional aspects of meeting these basic human needs are included in targets specific to health and nutrition, education, water and sanitation, energy, housing, and other goals.

Because drinking water is something that everyone requires on a daily basis just to survive, access to water is considered to be a human right.[11] This does not mean that everyone has a right to an unlimited amount of free water, but it does mean that everyone has a right to an adequate quantity of clean water for consumption and hygiene at a reasonable cost.[12] Increasing access to water requires investments in water system infrastructure, which usually means digging new groundwater wells and protecting surface water sources, installing miles of pipelines and pumps to transport water from sources to consumers, and sometimes also constructing facilities to store and treat water. These improvements can be expensive, and the costs of building and maintaining the water system must usually be recouped through taxes or user fees. Additionally, user fees help promote conservation, which is important in places where freshwater resources are limited. Thus, freshwater is considered to be both an essential human need and a consumer good.[13]

Low-income households may struggle to access the water they need. For example, massive protests occurred in 2000 in Cochabamba, Bolivia's third largest city, after the government leased the city's water rights to a U.S.-based corporation in order to improve services and satisfy a condition of a World Bank loan.[14] To raise capital for modernizing the water system, the company significantly increased user fees. For many low-income households, the higher cost of water was a huge burden. There was no legal way to reduce the cost of the household's water. Residents were banned from using other water sources, such as personal wells and storage tanks, and they were even forbidden to collect rainwater without a paid permit.[15] After several months of escalating protests, the water system was re-nationalized. Water privatization schemes in countries in Latin America, Asia, Africa, and other parts of the world are generating similar concerns about how to guarantee that the poorest residents can access safe drinking water.[16]

Problems with ensuring equitable and affordable water access are not limited to low- and middle-income countries (LMICs). In 2015 alone, tens of thousands of households in both Detroit and Philadelphia, two large cities in the United States, had their water supplies shut off,[17] and the discovery of high levels of lead in the municipal water system in Flint, Michigan, triggered a state of emergency that forced tens of thousands of households to rely on bottled water for drinking, cooking, and hygiene.[18] In many western U.S. states, where a growing human population and agricultural intensification have placed extreme demands on the watershed, the ownership of various supplies of water is determined based on so-called water rights that were sold many decades ago to cities, farmers, ranchers, and miners. It is illegal for people who do not own rights to the local watershed to use river water or collect rainwater.[19] When large cities like Los Angeles and Las Vegas require additional water for their growing populations, they can buy water rights from distant sources. Then, large volumes of water from those source rivers are rerouted to the purchasing city. In some places, diversion of water or excessive use of water by upstream consumers has left downstream communities that have historically had adequate water supplies with an insufficient amount of water.[20] It can be difficult for those downstream populations to make a legal case for their right to the missing water, especially if the water crosses a state or national border (such as the U.S.–Mexican border). These sorts of ethical challenges will only become more acute as more people move to dry climates.

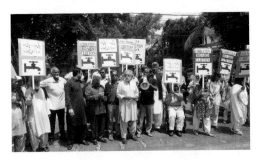

© Asianet-Pakistan/Shutterstock

Growing concerns about water scarcity in many countries and regions require conservation of precious freshwater resources (including the reduction of water loss during transport), clarification of the laws that govern water markets and water use, and a commitment to ensure adequate water access to vulnerable populations.

▶ 5.3 Access to Health Services

The right to health care is one of many human rights recognized in the Universal Declaration of Human Rights. Article 25 states that "everyone has the right to a standard of living adequate for the health and well-being of himself and of his family, including food, clothing, housing, and medical care and necessary social services."[1] Several key criteria are used to evaluate access to health care, including availability, accessibility, affordability, acceptability, and quality.[21] Health services are available when there are an adequate number of medical facilities that are functioning, staffed, and stocked with the necessary supplies. They are accessible when they are geographically and physically accessible to everyone, regardless of residential location and physical ability. Health services are affordable when they are economically accessible and payment for services is commensurate with ability to pay. They are acceptable when clinical care providers are respectful of patients from all ethnicities, sexes, ages, and other population groups. This may mean adapting to cultural expectations, such as ensuring that a female healthcare provider examines female patients in nonemergency situations if that is the cultural expectation of the patient. The quality of healthcare services is based on having well-maintained facilities that are stocked with appropriate supplies and staffed by appropriately skilled workers. These criteria set a minimum standard for access to health care. They do not specify what constitutes an acceptable level of access to health personnel, medical specialists, tests and procedures, medications, and health technology. Those details are expected to be defined by each country for its own people.

The right to health does not mean the right for everyone to have access to every health resource on demand. The economic reality is that most health systems cannot provide organ transplants to everyone who needs one to stay alive, expensive high-tech cancer treatments for everyone whose life could be extended by them, or years of intensive rehabilitation for everyone whose quality of life would improve with long-term care. Countries must make difficult decisions about which routine preventive health services and screenings will be covered by the national health plan, what types of emergency care will be provided to everyone with life-threatening injuries, which medications will be part of the health system's formulary, who will be eligible for particular surgical procedures, and countless other considerations. These selections should be made after evaluating the effectiveness and cost-effectiveness of various medications, devices, and procedures aimed at improving survival and quality of life.[22] The right to health requires equitable access to covered services, so the services included in a national health plan must be in alignment with the resources available, such as the number of medical specialists and support staff available to implement covered procedures.[23]

The level of access to quality health services is a major social, economic, and political concern in countries across the income spectrum. The United States has sought for decades to figure out how to increase the proportion of the population with health insurance, contain rising healthcare costs, and regulate private health insurance plans.[24] Brazil, India, and China are all committed to providing universal access to healthcare services, but they are struggling to fund their health systems, improve the quality of care, and ensure access in rural areas.[25] Every country has to make decisions about what healthcare services should be provided and who should pay for those services, and these decisions have human rights implications.

The SDGs aim to "substantially increase health financing and the recruitment, development, training, and retention of the health workforce in developing countries and small island developing states" (SDG 3.c).[10] At present, there is a very uneven distribution of healthcare workers across the globe. The WHO estimates that about 4.45 doctors, nurses, and nurse-midwives per 1000 people is the minimum ratio required for sustainable development. Higher ratios allow for higher-quality services to be provided. At present, there are about 14 skilled health professionals per 1000 people in high-income countries, 6 per 1000 in upper-middle-income countries, 4 per 1000 in lower-middle-income countries, and only 1.5 per 1000 in low-income countries (**FIGURE 5–3**).[26] This means that the number of people each clinician has to care for is higher in low-income countries than in high-income countries. For example, while there is about one physician, nurse, or nurse-midwife for every 75 residents of Germany, there is only one skilled health professional for every 3570 residents of Ethiopia (**FIGURE 5–4**).[27] Lower-income countries also have insufficient numbers of mental healthcare providers (**FIGURE 5–5**)[28] and an inadequate number of dentists (**FIGURE 5–6**).[29] Lower-income countries also have too few surgeons,[30] which means that the majority of residents in these areas do not have timely

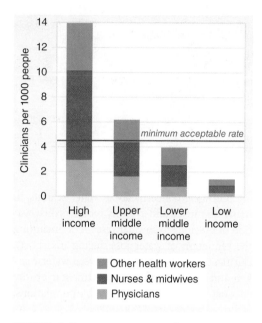

FIGURE 5–3 There are many more physicians, nurses and midwives, and other health workers per 1000 residents in high-income countries than in low-income countries.

Data from *Health workforce requirements for universal health coverage and the Sustainable Development Goals*. Geneva: WHO; 2016.

access to safe and affordable surgical services (**FIGURE 5–7**).[31]

One of the factors contributing to these inequalities in access to human resources for health is **brain drain**, the migration of healthcare professionals trained in LMICs to higher paying jobs in high-income countries.[32] In 2014, about 17% of physicians and 6% of nurses working in the 22 high-income countries that are members of the Organisation for Economic Co-operation and Development (OECD) had been trained in other countries.[33] In the United States, 25% of physicians and 6% of nurses were trained in other countries. In Germany, the percentages were 9% and 6%, respectively. Hundreds of thousands of physicians and nurses trained in India, China, Iran, Nigeria, and other LMICs work

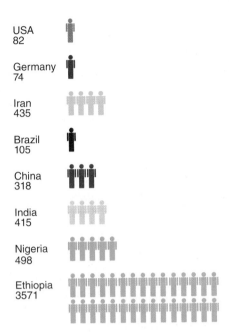

USA
82

Germany
74

Iran
435

Brazil
105

China
318

India
415

Nigeria
498

Ethiopia
3571

FIGURE 5–4 Skilled health professionals (physicians, nurses, and nurse-midwives) in low- and middle-income countries must serve many more people than clinicians in high-income countries.

Data from *World health statistics 2016*. Geneva: WHO; 2016.

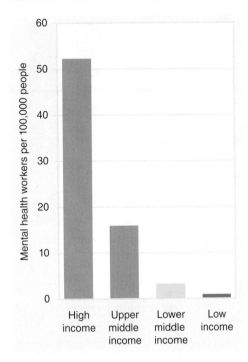

FIGURE 5–5 Mental health workers per 100,000 people.

Data from *Mental health atlas 2014*. Geneva: WHO; 2015.

in OECD countries.[33] This means that LMICs bear the cost of training these clinicians, and high-income countries reap the benefits of that investment in education. While it would be unethical to deny health professionals the opportunity to emigrate, it is problematic when skilled clinicians in countries with insufficient numbers of medical professionals are actively recruited by high-income countries.[34] The health SDGs will not be able to be met by 2030 if there is not a rapid expansion in the number of students enrolled in educational programs in medicine, nursing, and other health professions both in the lower-income countries that have the lowest clinician-per-population ratios as well as in the high-income countries that rely on foreign-born clinicians because they are not training enough clinicians within their own educational systems.[35]

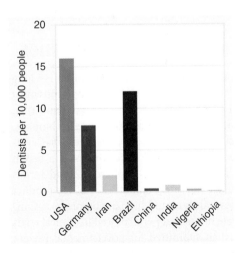

FIGURE 5–6 Dentists per 10,000 people.

Data from *The challenge of oral disease: A call for global action. The oral health atlas*. 2nd edition. Geneva: FDI World Dental Federation; 2015.

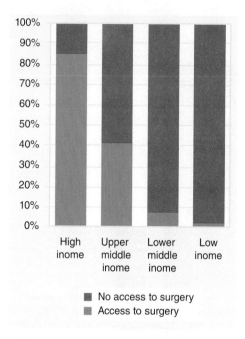

■ No access to surgery
■ Access to surgery

FIGURE 5–7 Most people in low- and middle-income countries do not have timely access to safe and affordable surgery.

Data from Alkire BC, Raykar NP, Shrime MG, Weiser TG, Bickler SW, Rose JA, et al. Global access to surgical care: A modelling study. *Lancet Glob Health* 2015;3:e316–23.

▶ 5.4 Access to Medicines

Creating and testing new medications is a long and expensive process.[36] New compounds must be created, tested in the laboratory, and then undergo several rounds of testing in humans. A **clinical trial** is a research study that evaluates the safety and effectiveness of a health intervention. A series of phase 1, 2, and 3 trials evaluate the safety and efficacy of the product in several thousand human volunteers.[37] Candidate drugs that perform well in clinical trials are then submitted for governmental review. In the United States, it takes about 15 years and costs about $1.4 billion in expenditures to move a new product through the process of development, testing, and review by the Food and Drug Administration (FDA).[38] It is similarly costly to move a new product from

discovery through the regulatory review process in Europe.[39] In exchange for their research and development (R&D) investments, pharmaceutical companies with a newly approved product are granted a **patent**, the exclusive rights to sell the new product for at least 20 years (or other periods of time negotiated with governmental and intergovernmental agencies).[40] This provides the company with a window of opportunity in which to recoup R&D costs and possibly make a profit.

The **World Trade Organization (WTO)** is a UN-related organization that negotiates and enforces trade agreements among UN member nations.[41] Three WTO-sponsored international agreements spell out the rules for trade in goods, services, and intellectual property: the General Agreement on Tariffs and Trade (GATT) that focuses on goods; the General Agreement on Trade in Services (GATS); and the **Trade-Related Aspects of Intellectual Property Rights (TRIPS)** Agreement, which protects patents, copyrights, registered trademarks, and industrial designs across national boundaries. Additional patent protections are provided to pharmaceutical and medical device companies through the World Intellectual Property Organization (WIPO) and some trade agreements between two or more countries. For example, trade agreements might extend the duration of a patent on a medication or device and enforce rules that prohibit generic versions of the products from being manufactured or imported.

Having a highly regulated international pharmaceutical industry protects public safety. Licensed brand-name and generic medications are subject to strict manufacturing and packaging regulations that ensure the quality and safety of the product. A **counterfeit** drug is an illegal product that is marketed deceptively. For example, counterfeiters may package sugar pills in boxes with the name of a brand-name medication on them or they may repackage legally produced medicines that are past their expiration dates in containers with new dates that make it look like the pills were just manufactured.

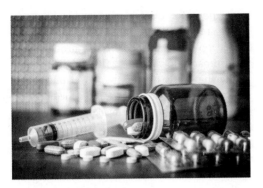

© Adul10/Shutterstock

Some counterfeit products are both ineffective and unsafe because they do not contain any active pharmaceutical agent but might contain dangerous contaminants. A rigorous approval process for medications and devices ensures the quality and safety of licensed products. However, trade agreements that regulate pharmaceutical products may restrict the ability of LMICs to legally produce or procure low-cost versions of medications. A **generic drug** is a medication with the same active ingredient as a brand-name medication that is produced after the patent for the brand-name medication expires. Generic medications usually cost less than brand-name ones, but generics cannot be sold legally until after the expiration of the exclusivity period granted to the patent recipient.

An **essential medication** is a drug that has been identified as a high priority for a country's health system to have in stock at all times because it is a cost-effective treatment for a common health issue.[42] Concerns about access to essential medications in LMICs became a prominent global health issue as the HIV/AIDS epidemic expanded in the 1990s. New antiretroviral medications (ARVs) that were saving lives in high-income countries were too expensive to be widely dispensed in LMICs. Countries like Brazil, India, and South Africa that tried to produce generic versions of patented ARVs or that imported generic medications produced elsewhere faced penalties for violating international intellectual property regulations.[43] In the early

2000s, pharmaceutical companies, governmental health agencies, and advocacy groups worked together to make patented medications available at lower prices in LMICs. The 2001 Doha Declaration clarified the relationship between TRIPS and public health, noting that the TRIPS Agreement "does not and should not prevent members from taking measures to protect public health," that "the Agreement can and should be interpreted and implemented in a manner supportive of WTO members' right to protect public health and, in particular, to promote access to medicines for all," and that countries facing a "national emergency or other circumstances of extreme urgency" could issue "compulsory licenses" for medications to be manufactured locally.[44] This has helped increase legal access to critical medications, but significant inequalities in access to medications remain.[45]

The WHO core list of essential medicines that healthcare systems should stock includes about 400 anti-infective, anti-allergic, analgesic, antipsychotic, and hormonal drugs along with medications for noncommunicable diseases such as epilepsy, migraines, heart disease, asthma, and gastrointestinal diseases.[42] In most low-income countries, the national formulary includes fewer than those 400 medications. In most high-income countries, more than 1000 additional products are on the list of approved and available medications.[46] People in high-income countries spend much more each year on medicines per person (public and private spending combined) than people in LMICs. The typical person in the United States (or his/her health insurance provider) spends about $1000 on pharmaceutical products each year. By contrast, annual spending on medication is only $12 per person in India, $6 in Nigeria, and $5 in Ethiopia (**FIGURE 5–8**).[47]

The ethical principle of **distributive justice** posits that needed resources in a population should be fairly allocated. The right to health in the Universal Declaration of Human Rights implies that signatories have an ethical responsibility to expand the availability of

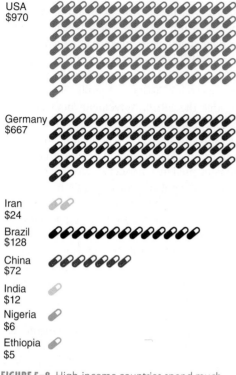

USA
$970

Germany
$667

Iran
$24

Brazil
$128

China
$72

India
$12

Nigeria
$6

Ethiopia
$5

FIGURE 5-8 High-income countries spend much more on pharmaceutical products per person each year than lower-income countries (2014).

Data from *The pharmaceutical industry and global health: Facts and figures 2017*. Geneva: International Federation of Pharmaceutical Manufacturers & Associations (IFPMA); 2017.

vaccines, diagnostic tests, and medicines that are free or affordable for people who live in low-income countries.[48] This value is expressed in the SDG target that aims to "support the research and development of vaccines and medicines for the communicable and non-communicable diseases that primarily affect developing countries, provide access to affordable essential medicines and vaccines, in accordance with the Doha Declaration on the TRIPS Agreement and Public Health, which affirms the right of developing countries to use the full provisions in the Agreement on Trade-Related Aspects of Intellectual Property Rights regarding flexibilities to protect public health, and, in particular, provide access to medicines for all" (SDG 3.b).[10] One model for achieving this goal is the creation of public–private partnerships that target development of

medications for diseases that for-profit companies are unlikely to invest in because of the limited revenue expected from a product created primarily for use in LMICs.[49] When these partnerships are funded by governments or philanthropic organizations, the medications they produce can be made available at an affordable price as soon as they are proven to be safe and effective. Other types of partnerships work to accelerate the time line for making existing vaccines, diagnostic tools, and medicines legally available at affordable prices in LMICs.[50]

▶ 5.5 Health and Natural Disasters

Both natural and human-generated disasters can lead to urgent humanitarian situations (**FIGURE 5-9**). The critical needs immediately after any humanitarian incident include (1) water, sanitation, and hygiene; (2) food; (3) shelter and essential nonfood items, such as personal care items, clothing, bedding, cooking and eating utensils, fuel, and lighting; and (4) essential health services for injuries, infections, sexual and reproductive health, mental health, and noncommunicable diseases.[51]

The players involved in a particular humanitarian response depend on the scale of the incident (**FIGURE 5-10**).[52] A **crisis** is a small-scale event that can easily be addressed locally, like when a tornado damages several homes in a small town and neighbors provide aid to the affected households. An **emergency** is a larger event that stresses local resources but can still be managed locally. A **disaster** occurs when the need for assistance exceeds local capacity. The type of response is also dependent on whether an incident affects just a small community or is an international event (**FIGURE 5-11**).[53] A **catastrophe** overwhelms the local response network and requires extensive outside assistance.[54]

A well-managed international response to a natural disaster or catastrophe begins when

Natural Disasters	Human-Generated Disasters
Weather-related disasters ■ Floods ■ Landslides/mudslides ■ Hurricanes/cyclones/typhoons ■ Tornadoes ■ Winter storms Geophysical disasters ■ Earthquakes ■ Tsunamis ■ Volcanic eruptions Climate-related disasters ■ Droughts ■ Extreme heat ■ Extreme cold ■ Wildfires and forest fires Biological disasters ■ Pandemic disease ■ Insect infestations	Intentional ■ War ■ Genocide/ethnic cleansing ■ Terrorism ■ Refugee crises ■ Internally displaced person crises Unintentional ■ Transportation accidents ■ Industrial accidents ■ Hazardous materials spills ■ Explosions/fires ■ Radiation ■ Structural collapses (buildings, bridges, dams, and tunnels)

FIGURE 5–9 Examples of types of disasters.

1	Crisis	Capacity > demand	Local response is sufficient
2	Emergency	Capacity = demand	Local response is sufficient
3	Disaster	Demand > capacity	Outside assistance is necessary
4	Catastrophe	Demand >> capacity	Extensive outside assistance is necessary

FIGURE 5–10 The scale of critical incidents depends on capacity and demand.

Data from Quarantelli E.L. Just as a disaster is not simply a big accident, so a catastrophe is not just a big disaster. *J Am Soc Prof Emerg Planners* 1996;3:68–71.

an affected country invites the United Nations and other organizations to assist. A lead agency, usually the UN Office for the Coordination of Humanitarian Affairs (OCHA), is designated to coordinate the response by other UN agencies, government agencies (including militaries), the national Red Cross or Red Crescent society, and nongovernmental organizations. These groups work together to meet essential needs that have been designated as humanitarian response "clusters" (**FIGURE 5–12**).[55] National and local responses

benefit from similar coordination strategies. In the United States, for example, the **National Incident Management System (NIMS)** specifies how different governmental agencies and nongovernmental organizations work together to respond to a disaster, and the **Incident Command System (ICS)** is an organizational structure used in the field to provide a clear chain of command for responders. The national response plan also identifies 15 **Essential Support Functions (ESFs)**, critical service areas that require immediate attention

PICE Stage	Potential for Additional Casualties	Effect on Local Resources	Extent of Geographic Involvement	Projected Need for Outside Assistance	Status of Outside Help
0	Static	Controlled	Local	Little to none	Inactive
1	Dynamic	Disruptive	Regional	Small	Alert
2	Dynamic	Paralytic	National	Moderate	Standby
3	Dynamic	Paralytic	International	Great	Dispatch

FIGURE 5–11 PICE (potential injury-creating event) nomenclature.

Data from Koenig KL, Dinerman N, Kuehl AE. Disaster nomenclature—a functional impact approach: The PICE system. *Acad Emerg Med* 1996;3:723–7.

Cluster		Lead UN Agency
Overall Coordination		OCHA
Technical Clusters	Camp coordination and management	IOM and UNHCR
	Early recovery	UNDP
	Education	UNICEF (and Save the Children)
	Food security	WFP and FAO
	Health	WHO
	Nutrition	UNICEF
	Protection	UNHCR
	Shelter	IFRC and UNHCR
	Water, sanitation, and hygiene	UNICEF
Support Clusters	Emergency telecommunications	WFP
	Logistics	WFP

FIGURE 5–12 Humanitarian response clusters.

Data from Stumpenhorst M, Stumpenhorst R, Razum O. The UN OCHA cluster approach: Gaps between theory and practice. *J Public Health* 2011;19:587–92.

after a disaster, and names a lead agency that is responsible for each ESF during a disaster response (**FIGURE 5–13**).[56] A coordinated response maximizes resources and saves lives.

Interagency coordination helps facilitate a timely and comprehensive response, especially when this process ensures that volunteers and their host organizations complete appropriate training before traveling to the disaster site and are prepared to fully provide for themselves in the field.[57] If the various responders do not coordinate their efforts, the result can be chaos. In the weeks after the massive earthquake in Haiti in 2010, thousands of well-intentioned volunteers flew to Port-au-Prince to assist. Many of these spontaneous volunteers were unaffiliated with a Haiti-based host organization and arrived without adequate personal supplies, so they ended up being a burden rather than a help.[58] Supplies remained stockpiled at the airport because the Haitian government, local institutions,

ESF #1	Transportation
ESF #2	Communications
ESF #3	Public works and engineering
ESF #4	Firefighting
ESF #5	Emergency management
ESF #6	Mass care, emergency assistance, housing, and human services
ESF #7	Logistics management and resource support
ESF #8	Public health and medical services
ESF #9	Search and rescue
ESF #10	Oil and hazardous materials response
ESF #11	Agriculture and natural resources
ESF #12	Energy
ESF #13	Public safety and security
ESF #14	Long-term community recovery
ESF #15	External affairs

FIGURE 5–13 Essential support functions (ESFs) in the National Incident Management System (NIMS) of the United States.

Data from *National incidence management system*. Washington U.S. Department of Homeland Security; 2008.

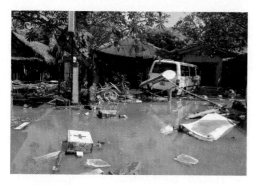

© Stefano Ember/Shutterstock

and various international governmental and nongovernmental organizations had difficulty communicating about on-the-ground needs, securing local transportation, and coordinating distribution efforts. Similar logistical issues have occurred after other large-scale natural disasters, including the devastating tsunami that hit Southeast Asia in 2004.[59]

The SDGs address disaster preparedness and response in several targets, including a recognition of the need to "strengthen the capacity of all countries, in particular developing countries, for early warning, risk reduction, and management of national and global health risks" (SDG 3.d) (**FIGURE 5–14**).[10] Mitigating risks and preparing for potential critical incidents before they happen are the best ways to enable a smooth response and recovery when a natural or human-generated disaster does occur. The **Sendai Framework** for Disaster Risk Reduction is a global agreement that aims to significantly diminish the number of deaths and the magnitude of destruction caused by natural disasters.[60] The priority areas with the Sendai Framework include increasing awareness of disaster risks, strengthening emergency management capacities in all countries, promoting investment in risk reduction, and enhancing the effectiveness of response and recovery efforts, including ensuring that the rebuilt structures are more resilient to future hazardous events.[61] The need for improved disaster preparedness is especially acute in lower-income countries.

Emergency management is about more than just responding to crises.[62] **Emergency management**, also called disaster management, oversees all resources and responsibilities related to emergencies and disasters, including prevention, preparedness, response, and recovery. The emergency management cycle includes four steps, sometimes called the "4 Rs" (**FIGURE 5–15**): (1) Reduction of risks, or **mitigation**, is the process of implementing preemptive measures to protect people and property from hazards, such as by enforcing building codes. These activities enhance **resilience**, the ability of a community or nation to resist, survive, adapt to, and recover from natural disasters and other adverse events. (2) Readiness, or preparedness, for responding to an emergency includes the creation and refinement of emergency operations plans, the establishment of emergency communication infrastructure, and the training of public employees and emergency response volunteers. (3) Response to an imminent, ongoing, or recent threat includes provision of emergency medical assistance, shelter, and other critical services. (4) Recovery is a phase in which continued efforts focus on rebuilding affected communities and attending to other aspects of reconstruction and rehabilitation.

▶ 5.6 Conflict and War

A **complex humanitarian emergency** occurs when civil conflict or war causes mass migration of civilian populations, food insecurity, and long-term public health concerns.[63] Natural disasters usually create an immediate period of acute need but quickly transition into recovery mode. By contrast, complex humanitarian emergencies may remain in an acute phase for years or even decades. Because natural disasters are generally seen as apolitical events, it is usually fairly easy for aid agencies to assist survivors. Responses to complex humanitarian emergencies are much more complicated because military commanders

1.5	Build the resilience of the poor and those in vulnerable situations and reduce their exposure and vulnerability to climate-related extreme events and other economic, social, and environmental shocks and disasters.
2.4	Ensure sustainable food production systems and implement resilient agricultural practices that … strengthen capacity for adaptation to climate change, extreme weather, drought, flooding, and other disasters.
9.1	Develop quality, reliable, sustainable, and resilient infrastructure.
11.5	Significantly reduce the number of deaths and the number of people affected and substantially decrease the direct economic losses relative to global gross domestic product caused by disasters, including water-related disasters, with a focus on protecting the poor and people in vulnerable situations.
11.b	Substantially increase the number of cities and human settlements adopting integrated policies and plans toward inclusion, resource, efficiency, mitigation and adaptation to climate change, resilience to disasters, and develop and implement, in line with the Sendai Framework for Disaster Risk Reduction 2015–2030, holistic disaster risk management at all levels.
13.1	Strengthen resilience and adaptive capacity to climate-related hazards and natural disasters in all countries.
16.1	Significantly reduce all forms of violence and related death rates everywhere.

FIGURE 5–14 SDG targets focused on disaster preparedness and response.

Data from United Nations. *Transforming our world: The 2030 agenda for sustainable development.* New York: UN; 2015.

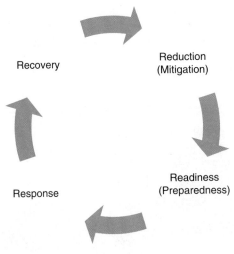

FIGURE 5–15 Four stages of the emergency management cycle.

and faction leaders engaged in armed conflicts are often disinclined to allow outsiders to assess and assist vulnerable populations.[64]

Numerous public health challenges arise during complex emergencies. The breakdown of water and sanitation systems and public health services may lead to frequent outbreaks of communicable diseases. Diarrheal diseases may become very common. Vaccine-preventable diseases such as measles and meningitis may resurge when routine childhood vaccination programs are interrupted. Respiratory infections like pneumonia and tuberculosis may become more prevalent due to inadequate shelter. Other infectious disease concerns include the intensification of malaria in endemic areas, outbreaks of viral hepatitis, and an increased incidence of sexually transmitted infections, which may be spread through gender-based violence and then remain untreated because of lack of access to health care.[65]

International humanitarian laws are supposed to protect civilians and combatants,[66] but these rules are not always enforced.[67] Rape and sexual violence have been used as military tactics in many conflicts.[68] Reproductive health services, including family planning and obstetric care, and psychiatric services tend to be severely inadequate during conflicts. Malnutrition is also a major concern during war and civil conflicts.[69] Food production tends to decrease as farms are abandoned, and it is more difficult to import affordable food during times of instability. Food supply chains that enable food products to be processed, transported, stored, and sold are often interrupted by conflict and uncertainty. Large numbers of people may be migrating and in need of a daily supply of nutrients. The combination of too few calories, vitamins, and minerals plus lack of care for other diseases often leads to severe undernutrition.

Two of the most prominent organizations involved in providing health services and other types of assistance during times of war are the Red Cross and Médecins Sans Frontières. The International Committee of the **Red Cross** (ICRC) is unique among private organizations because it is an independent organization guided by its own set of rules and principles—humanity, impartiality, neutrality, independence, voluntary service, unity, and universality—but it is officially sanctioned by the Geneva Convention and international law to provide specific humanitarian services.[70] The ICRC works with more than 185 national Red Cross and Red Crescent societies and the International Federation of Red Cross and Red Crescent Societies to provide humanitarian aid to both civilian and military victims of conflicts. Red Cross representatives visit prisoners of war, search for missing persons, transmit messages between separated family members, reunify dispersed families, monitor compliance with the international laws that pertain to armed

conflict, and provide basic services to civilians, such as food, water, and medical assistance. The ICRC is funded through governmental support, contributions from national Red Cross and Red Crescent societies, and private donations. National Red Cross and Red Crescent societies are autonomous from the ICRC, and they provide a variety of services that meet needs in their communities, such as maintaining blood banks, providing first aid training, and offering assistance to residents who have been affected by natural disasters. The ICRC and its affiliates generally attempt to maintain neutrality by carefully avoiding actions that could appear to take sides with any particular political party and by not releasing statements that could be construed as political.[71]

MSF plays a very different role in global health than the ICRC. **Médecins Sans Frontières (MSF)**, more often called **Doctors Without Borders** in the United States, provides medical care to people harmed by violence no matter what the victims' races, religions, and political affiliations are.[72] MSF often sets up clinics in places that are so unstable that other organizations refuse to deploy resources to them.[73] The core values of MSF include independence, impartiality, and bearing witness to violations of human rights.[72] To MSF, impartiality does not mean silence.[74] Impartiality means that all governmental agencies and other bodies are equally open to criticism from MSF when they engage in or allow injustices.[75]

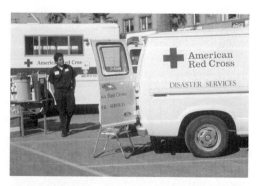

© Joseph Sohm/Shutterstock

In postconflict areas (and also in areas that have been devastated by natural disasters), a diversity of local, national, and international organizations typically help with reconstruction by responding to urgent needs, assisting with long-term recovery, and helping to prevent future crises. Political and economic systems need to be rebuilt, and educational and social services need to be restored after a civil conflict or war. Postconflict areas also need to repair health systems (because of lost infrastructure and personnel, among other issues), expand access to physical rehabilitation and mental healthcare services, and address environmental health concerns. Contaminated environments often take longer to renovate than hospitals and clinics.[76] For example, a **landmine** is a buried explosive device, and landmines and other unexploded ordnance buried during wartime remain hazards to workers, children, and communities long after the conflict is over. This means, among many other problems, that large tracts of potential farmland are unable to be cultivated because of the risk of encountering a mine while clearing a field. Most people who sustain landmine injuries are civilians. Children may have elevated risk of injuries because they do not know how to recognize explosive devices and may pick them up and even play with them. Landmines and other explosive remnants of war remain a concern in many parts of the world, killing thousands of civilians each year and seriously injuring thousands of others.[77] Although it only costs a few dollars to purchase and plant a mine, it can cost thousands of dollars to safely remove one.[78] The direct costs to injured individuals and their families can be very high when they must pay for surgery, a lengthy hospitalization, and a lifetime of assistive devices for people who survive with lost limbs, burn contractures, blindness, and other permanent disabilities. A **prosthetic** is a replacement body part, such an artificial leg or arm that might be used after a limb is lost in a landmine explosion. Even a low-tech prosthetic can be expensive, and children with amputated limbs need to be refitted with new devices as they grow.[79]

Access to basic health care is considered to be a fundamental human right, but wars and civil conflicts often restrict access to health services and the foundational tools for health.[80] International organizations can play a critical role in advocating for human rights, promoting health, and providing medical care during times of conflict and war. In postconflict areas, public health work can facilitate the transition back to peace by implementing initiatives that improve population health status and strengthen social connections across diverse populations.[81]

▶ 5.7 Bioterrorism

Bioterrorism is the deliberate release of pathogens, chemicals, or other agents that can cause illness and possibly death of people, animals, or plants. Chemical and biological warfare are not new.[82] During the Tartar siege of the city of Kaffa (now in the Ukraine) in the 14th century, the bodies of plague victims were catapulted over city walls to spark an epidemic. During the French and Indian War in the 1760s, the British army sent smallpox-infected blankets to American Indians who supported the French. During World War I, several European nations used biological agents against the livestock of enemies. What is new is that there are now more tools available for creating and spreading bioterror agents and the scale on which such acts can occur is much larger.

A bioweapon may be selected because it produces severe disease or death, the target population is susceptible to the agent, and the target population has limited or no access to immunization or treatment. Additionally, a particular agent may be selected for use because it can be produced relatively easily and rapidly, it is relatively inexpensive, it is environmentally stable, it has a low infectious dose, it has a simple delivery mechanism (such as through air, water, or food), it is highly infectious, it has a desirable incubation period (either short so immediate disease is produced or longer so that the asymptomatic contagious stage is lengthy), and it causes disease that is difficult to diagnose.[83] While the goal of some bioterrorists is to kill or seriously injure large numbers of people, the most common goal is to cause widespread fear, panic, and social disruption.

In the United States, potential bioterror agents are classified into three groups (**FIGURE 5–16**).[84] Category A represents high-priority agents that pose a significant risk because they can be easily transmitted from one person to another or have high mortality rates. Category A agents include anthrax, smallpox, plague, botulism, tularemia, and viral hemorrhagic fevers like Ebola and Marburg virus. **Anthrax** (*Bacillus anthracis*) is of particular

concern because the bacterium was used in a postal bioterrorism attack in the United States in 2001.[85] Naturally occurring cases of anthrax are diagnosed every year in people who work with sheep and livestock because anthrax spores (dormant bacteria) can survive in the environment for years. These cases are usually cutaneous (skin) infections. In the laboratory, anthrax can be made into a fine powder that can cause an inhalational anthrax that affects the lungs. Anthrax is not passed from person to person, but the weaponized form can be aerosolized and breathed in.[86] Anthrax disease can be cured with antibiotics if is detected early, but advanced cases are often fatal. Category B agents are moderately easy to spread but usually cause relatively few deaths. Examples of Category B agents include brucellosis, ricin (a toxin from the plant *Ricinus communis*, also known as castorbean or caster

Category	Agents
Category A	▪ Anthrax (*Bacillus anthracis*) ▪ Botulism (*Clostridium botulinum* toxin) ▪ Plague (*Yersinia pestis*) ▪ Smallpox (variola major) ▪ Tularemia (*Francisella tularensis*) ▪ Viral hemorrhagic fevers (such as Ebola, Marburg, Lassa, and Machupo viruses)
Category B	▪ Brucellosis (*Brucella* species) ▪ Glanders (*Burkholderia mallei*) ▪ Melioidosis (*Burkholderia pseudomallei*) ▪ Psittacosis (*Chlamydia psittaci*) ▪ Q fever (*Coxiella burnetii*) ▪ Toxins (such as ricin, *Staphylococcus* enterotoxin, and the epsilon toxin of *Clostridium perfringens*) ▪ Typhus fever (*Rickettsia prowazekii*) ▪ Food- and waterborne diseases (such as *Cryptosporidium parvum*, *Escherichia coli* O157:H7, hepatitis A virus, *Salmonella*, *Shigella*, and *Vibrio cholerae*) ▪ Mosquito-borne encephalitis viruses
Category C	▪ Emerging infectious diseases, including drug-resistant pathogens

FIGURE 5–16 U.S. classifications of potential bioterrorism agents.

Data from Rotz LD, Khan AS, Lillibridge SR, Ostroff SM, Hughes JM. Public health assessment of potential biological terrorism agents. *Emerg Infect Dis* 2002;8:225–30.

oil plants), Q fever, typhus fever, viral encephalitis infections, food safety threats, such as *Salmonella*, *Shigella*, and *E. coli* O157:H7, and water supply threats, such as cholera and cryptosporidiosis. Category C agents are emerging infectious diseases like hantaviruses that are potential threats in part because they are not well understood. Chemical agents may also pose a threat (**FIGURE 5–17**).[87]

The best defense against a bioterrorism attack is early detection so that an outbreak can be contained and exposed or at-risk people can receive immunization, post-exposure prophylaxis, and medical treatment. This requires a strong laboratory network, trained public health departments that are prepared to coordinate response activities, the cooperation of healthcare providers and emergency responders, and an adequate stockpile of essential vaccines and medications.[84] Strong communication systems are also necessary for keeping the public informed of developments and encouraging appropriate personal responses. Global communication may also play a role in preventing some acts of terrorism and responding to attacks that do occur.

In any response, careful attention must be paid to protecting the civil, political, economic,

Category	Examples
Nerve agents	Tabun, sarin, soman, GF, VX
Blood agents	Hydrogen cyanide, cyanogen chloride
Blister agents	Lewisite, nitrogen and sulfur mustards, phosgene oxime
Heavy metals	Arsenic, lead, mercury
Volatile toxins	Benzene, chloroform, trihalomethanes
Pulmonary agents	Phosgene, chlorine, vinyl chloride
Incapacitating agents	BZ
Explosive nitro compounds and oxidizers	Ammonium nitrate combined with fuel oil
Flammable industrial gases and liquids	Gasoline, propane
Poisonous industrial gases, liquids, and solids	Cyanides, nitriles
Corrosive industrial acids and bases	Nitric acid, sulfuric acid
Other agents	Esticides, dioxins, furans, polychlorinated biphenyls

FIGURE 5–17 Possible chemical bioweapons.

Data from Biological and chemical terrorism: Strategic plan for preparedness and response. Recommendations of the CDC Strategic Planning Workgroup. *MMWR Recomm Rep.* 2000;49(RR-1):1–14.

social, and cultural rights of affected persons. In some situations, individual and collective rights must be balanced. A **nonderogable right** is a human right that is irrevocable, such as the rights to freedom from slavery and freedom from torture. But some other rights may be temporarily suspended under special circumstances when restrictions on some individual rights protect the community as a whole. For example, freedom of movement for people with highly contagious infections may be temporarily limited during an outbreak so that the health rights of other people can be protected.[88] If rights are derogated during or immediately after a critical incident, the new rules must not be discriminatory, and full rights should be restored as soon as possible.

▶ 5.8 Health in Prisons

On any given day, nearly 10 million people across the globe are incarcerated, including more than 2.2 million people in the United States and 1.7 million in China (**FIGURE 5–18**).[89] The incarceration rate varies considerably between countries, but the country with the highest rate, by far, is the United States

(**FIGURE 5–19**).[89] Prisons, jails, and detention centers house convicted criminals and may also accommodate suspects waiting for trial, juvenile offenders, and undocumented immigrants.

Many people entering prison already have health problems related to mental illness, drug abuse, and poverty. Incarceration may exacerbate existing health conditions and create new health problems as a result of exposure to severe overcrowding, poor ventilation, poor nutrition, unhygienic conditions, lack of access to medical care, abuse by guards, and prisoner-on-prisoner violence, including beatings and sexual assault. Prison populations worldwide have higher rates of HIV, tuberculosis, and other infectious diseases than the general population.[90] Tuberculosis (TB) is of particular concern because it is an airborne infectious disease. TB spreads easily in crowded prison blocks, and late diagnosis and inadequate treatment may allow prisoners with TB to remain contagious for lengthy periods of time. Interruptions in treatment can facilitate the emergence and spread of drug-resistant strains that are not able to be cured by the standard antibiotics used

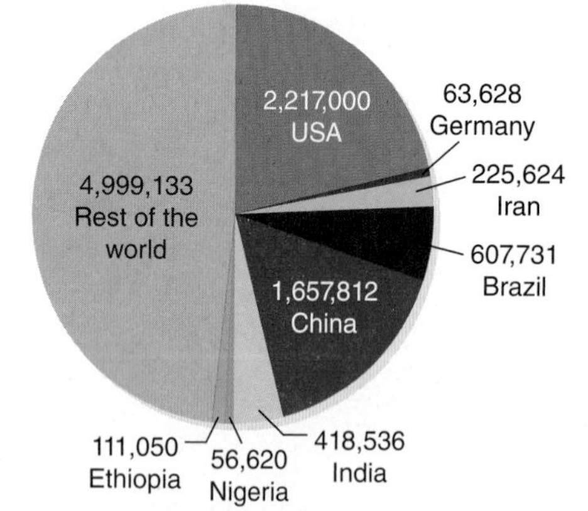

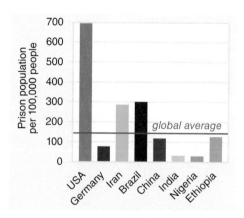

FIGURE 5–18 More than 10 million people worldwide are in prison each day.

Data from Walmsley R. *World prison population list*. 11th ed. London: International Centre for Prison Studies; 2016.

FIGURE 5–19 The United States has the world's highest incarceration rate.

Data from Walmsley R. *World prison population list*. 11th ed. London: International Centre for Prison Studies; 2016.

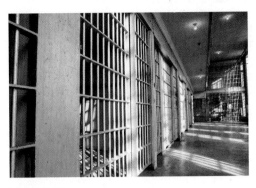

© txking/Shutterstock

to treat TB. Over time, an increase in TB in prisons will increase the amount of TB in the general population. When individuals infected with TB are released from prison, they may spread TB to their family and friends. To prevent further increases in the prevalence of TB in prisons, it is important for every case of TB in incarcerated people to be detected early and treated consistently with no interruptions in antibiotic therapy.[91]

Prisoners are entitled to all fundamental human rights, and they have a right to be protected from medical neglect, starvation, abuse, forced medical experimentation, and other civil rights violations.[92] Contracting potentially life-threatening infections is not part of any prisoner's sentence. It is considered unjust not to provide incarcerated people with medical and dental care, adequate nutrition, protection from infectious diseases, and safe conditions.[93]

▶ 5.9 People with Disabilities

An **impairment** is a difference or limitation in an anatomical structure, mental or sensory function, or physiological function that constrains the capacity of an individual to do a task or action. A **disability** occurs when an impairment leads to restrictions in activity and participation. Disability is the result of both an impairment and the social and environmental context in which a person with impairment interacts with other people and the world (**FIGURE 5–20**). About 15% of the world's people—more than 1 billion people total—have a moderate or severe disability.[94] People with disabilities are entitled to all of their human rights, including the right to be treated with dignity, to have the autonomy to make decisions for themselves (if they are cognitively capable of doing so), and to be active members of society.[95]

An impairment may affect numerous domains, such as self-care, mobility, communication, and learning (**FIGURE 5–21**).[96] Some people with impairments need assistance with **activities of daily living (ADLs)**, the routine daily self-care functions that are required for health and survival, such as dressing, eating, ambulating, using the toilet, and taking care of personal hygiene (**FIGURE 5–22**). Some people with impairments can manage the ADLs but require assistance with the **instrumental activities of daily living (IADLs)** required for independent living, such as shopping, housekeeping, managing personal finances, preparing foods, and navigating transportation. Some people with impairments manage their own ADLs and IADLs, but experience limitations in full participation in social events because of stigma and other barriers.

Rehabilitation is the process of restoring, improving, or maintaining the highest

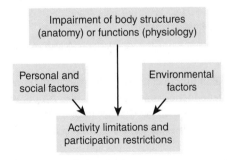

FIGURE 5–20 Disabilities are a function of biological, social, and environmental factors.

Domain	Activities
Learning and applying knowledge	Watching, listening, learning to read, learning to write, learning to calculate, solving problems
General tasks and demands	Undertaking a single task, undertaking multiple tasks
Communication	Receiving spoken messages, receiving nonverbal messages, speaking, producing nonverbal messages, conversation
Mobility	Lifting and carrying objects, fine hand use (such as picking up objects or grasping them), walking, moving around using equipment (such as a wheelchair), using transportation
Self-care	Washing oneself (such as washing hands, bathing, and using a towel), caring for body parts (by brushing teeth, shaving, and grooming), toileting, dressing, eating, drinking, looking after one's own health
Domestic life	Acquisition of goods and services (such as by shopping), preparation of meals (such as by cooking), doing housework (such as cleaning house, washing dishes, doing laundry, and ironing), assisting others
Interpersonal interactions and relationships	Basic interpersonal interactions, complex interpersonal interactions, relating to strangers, formal relationships, informal social relationships, family relationships, intimate relationships
Major life areas	Informal education, school education, higher education, remunerative employment, basic economic transactions, economic self-sufficiency
Community, social, and civic life	Community life, recreation and leisure, religion and spirituality, human rights, political life, and citizenship

FIGURE 5–21 Domains of activity and participation from the International Classification of Functioning, Disability, and Health.

Data from *International Classification of Functioning, Disability, and Health (ICF)*. Geneva: WHO; 2001.

level of function possible in order to maximize independence and quality of life. Adults and children of all ages who have impairments can benefit from timely access to appropriate physical therapy, occupational therapy, speech–language therapy, and other types of rehabilitation services.[97] A condition that might be preventable or treatable in a high-income country where rehabilitation facilities are routinely accessible might cause permanent disability in a low-income country where rehabilitation services are not available. People with physical and mental impairments and disabilities also benefit from being included to the fullest extent possible in the activities of their families and communities.

Activities of Daily Living (ADLs): Self-care	Instrumental Activities of Daily Living (IADLs): Independence
Dressing	Shopping
Eating	Housekeeping
Ambulating (mobility)	Accounting (personal finances)
Toileting	Food preparation
Hygiene	Transportation

FIGURE 5–22 Activities of daily living.

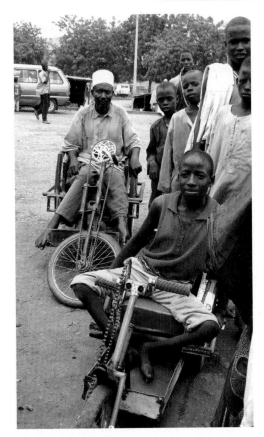

CDC/Molly Kurnit, M.P.H./Paul Chenoweth

People with impairments may have their activities facilitated or restricted by their environment and the resources available to them. An **assistive device**, also called assistive technology, is a tool that helps with the performance of a task. Assistive devices such as wheelchairs and canes, prosthetics for people with missing arms or legs, orthotics and braces for people with various types of musculoskeletal disorders, hearing aids, and glasses can enable independence and fuller participation in social activities. However, only about 10% of people worldwide who would benefit from medical assistive devices have them.[98] A person who uses a wheelchair may easily access public transportation, sidewalks, and public buildings in Germany, but might find it impossible to navigate the unpaved pathways of rural Ethiopia. An American with a visual impairment may have access to books through Braille editions, electronic magnifiers, and audio recordings, but a similarly impaired person in Nigeria might not have access to any of these tools.

The SDGs feature numerous targets geared toward increasing the ability of people with disabilities to access social protections (SDGs 1.3 and 10.2), education (SDGs 4.5 and 4.a), work (SDG 8.5), transportation (SDG 11.2), public spaces (SDG 11.7), and civic events (SDG 16.7).[99] People with disabilities have an increased risk of living in poverty. The direct costs associated with paying for medical care and assistance can be overwhelming. Health issues restrict the ability of some people with disabilities to work, and family caregivers may need to limit their paid employment and home productivity. These economic factors are exacerbated when people with disabilities have limited access to the public services, education, and employment opportunities that would enable a higher standard of living. A safe and accessible physical environment and a strong social network are critical for maximizing the activities and social participation of all people who have impairments and disabilities (**FIGURE 5–23**).[96]

Environment	Environmental Characteristics
Products and technology	Products for personal consumption (food, medicines), for personal use in daily living, for personal indoor and outdoor mobility and transportation, for communication; design, construction, and building materials of buildings for public use and buildings for private use
Natural environment and human-made changes to the environment	Climate, light, sound
Support and relationships	Support of and relationships with immediate family, friends, acquaintances, peers, colleagues, neighbors, community members, people in positions of authority, personal care providers and personal assistants, healthcare professionals
Attitudes	Individual attitudes of immediate family members, friends, personal care providers and personal assistants, healthcare professionals; societal attitudes; social norms, practices, and ideologies
Services, systems, and policies	Services, systems, and policies related to housing, communication, transportation, legal, social, health, education and training, labor and employment

FIGURE 5–23 Environmental characteristics that relate to activities and participation.

Data from *International Classification of Functioning, Disability, and Health (ICF)*. Geneva: WHO; 2001.

The WHO defines health as "a state of complete physical, mental, and social well-being."[1] By that definition, any action that improves social well-being will improve overall health status. Increasing the social inclusion of people with disabilities will yield health benefits for those individuals and their families, and also for their communities. Global health is founded on the principle that all people have the right to the highest attainable standard of health. Advocating for everyone's human rights is a core part of achieving that shared goal.

▶ References

1. *Constitution of the World Health Organization*. New York: United Nations; 1946.
2. *The Universal Declaration of Human Rights*. New York: United Nations; 1948.
3. Leckie S. Another step towards indivisibility: Identifying the key features of violations of economic, social and cultural rights. *Human Rights Q.* 1998;20:81–124.
4. Hunt P. The human right to the highest attainable standard of health: New opportunities and challenges. *Trans R Soc Trop Med Hyg.* 2006;100:603–7.
5. *International Covenant on Economic, Social and Cultural Rights (A/RES/21/2200)*. New York: UN; 1966.
6. Mann JM, Gostin LO, Gruskin S, Brennan T, Lazzarini Z, Fineberg HV. Health and human rights. *Health Hum Rights.* 1994;1:6–23.
7. *Global health ethics: Key issues*. Geneva: WHO; 2015.
8. Farmer P. Pathologies of power: Rethinking health and human rights. *Am J Public Health.* 1999;89:1486–96.
9. Gostin LO, Friedman EA, Ooms G, et al. The joint action and learning initiative: Towards a global agreement on national and global responsibilities for health. *PLoS Med.* 2011;8:e1001031.
10. United Nations. *Transforming Our World: The 2030 Agenda for Sustainable Development*. New York: UN; 2015.

11. Gliek PH. The human right to water. *Water Policy.* 1998;1:487–503.

12. Howard G, Bartram J. *Domestic water quantity, service level and health.* Geneva: WHO; 2003.

13. Bleumel EB. The implications of formulating a human right to water. *Ecol Law Q.* 2004;31:957–1006.

14. Nickson A, Vargas C. The limitations of water regulation: The failure of the Cochabamba concession in Bolivia. *Bull Latin Am Res.* 2002;21:99–120.

15. Morgan. Water: Frontier markets and cosmopolitan activism. *Soundings J Polit Nat.* 2004;28:10–24.

16. Mirosa O, Harris LM. Human right to water: Contemporary challenges and contours of a global debate. *Antipode.* 2012;44:932–49.

17. Jones PA, Moulton A. *The invisible crisis: Water unaffordability in the United States.* Cambridge MA: Unitarian Universalist Service Committee (UUSC); 2016.

18. Markel H. Remember flint. *Milbank Q.* 2016;94:229–36.

19. Hundley N Jr. *Water and the West: The Colorado River compact and the politics of water in the American West.* Los Angeles CA: University of California Press; 2009.

20. Glennon R. Water scarcity, marketing, and privatization. *Texas Law Rev.* 2005;83:1873–902.

21. United Nations Committee on Economic, Social and Cultural Rights. *General Comment 14: The right to the highest attainable standard of health (E/C 12/2000/4).* Geneva: UN Office for the High Commissioner for Human Rights; 2000.

22. Spiegelhalter DJ, Gore SM, Fitzpatrick R, Fletcher AE, Jones DR, Cox DR. Quality of life measurements in health care. III: Resource allocation. *BMJ.* 1992;305:1205–9.

23. *A universal truth: No health without a workforce.* Geneva: WHO/Global Health Workforce Alliance (GHWA); 2014.

24. Berwick DM, Nolan TW, Whittington J. The triple aim: Care, health, and cost. *Health Aff.* 2008; 27:759–69.

25. Marten R, McIntyre D, Travassos C, et al. An assessment of progress towards universal health coverage in Brazil, Russia, India, China, and South Africa (BRICS). *Lancet.* 2014;384:2164–71.

26. *Health workforce requirements for universal health coverage and the Sustainable Development Goals.* Geneva: WHO; 2016.

27. *World health statistics 2016.* Geneva: WHO; 2016.

28. *Mental health atlas 2014.* Geneva: WHO; 2015.

29. *The challenge of oral disease: A call for global action. The oral health atlas.* 2nd ed. Geneva: FDI World Dental Federation; 2015.

30. Meara JG, Leather AJM, Hagander L, et al. Global Surgery 2030: Evidence and solutions for achieving health, welfare, and economic development. *Lancet.* 2015;386:569–624.

31. Alkire BC, Raykar NP, Shrime MG, et al. Global access to surgical care: A modelling study. *Lancet Glob Health.* 2015;3:e316–23.

32. Taylor AL, Hwenda L, Larsen BI, Daulaire N. Stemming the brain drain: A WHO Global Code of Practice on International Recruitment of Health Personnel. *N Engl J Med.* 2011;365:2348–51.

33. Dumont J, Lafortune G. *International migration of doctors and nurses to OECD countries: Recent trends and policy implications.* Geneva: WHO High-Level Commission on Health Employment and Economic Growth; 2016.

34. *User's guide to the WHO Global Code of Practice on the International Recruitment of Health Personnel.* Geneva: WHO; 2010.

35. *Global strategy on human resources for health: Workforce 2030.* Geneva: WHO; 2016.

36. *The pharmaceutical industry and global health: Facts and figures 2017.* Geneva: International Federation of Pharmaceutical Manufacturers & Associations (IFPMA); 2017.

37. *Good review practice: Clinical review of investigational new drug applications.* Silver Spring MD: U.S. Food and Drug Administration (FDA); 2013.

38. DiMasi JA, Grabowski HG, Hansen RW. Innovation in the pharmaceutical industry: New estimates of R&D costs. *J Health Econ.* 2016;47:20–33.

39. Van Norman GA. Drugs and devices: Comparison of European and U.S. approval processes. *JACC Basic Transl Sci.* 2016;1:399–412.

40. *Managing access to medicines and health technologies (MDS-3).* Arlington VA: Management Sciences for Health (MSH); 2012.

41. Fidler DP, Drager N, Lee K. Managing the pursuit of health and wealth: The key challenges. *Lancet.* 2009;373:325–31.

42. *WHO model list of essential medicines (19th list).* Geneva: WHO; 2015.

43. 't Hoen E, Berger J, Calmy A, Moon S. Driving a decade of change: HIV/AIDS, patents and access to medicines for all. *J Int AIDS Soc.* 2011;14:15.

44. World Trade Organization (Doha WTO Ministerial 2001). Declaration on the TRIPS agreement and public health (WT/MIN(01)/DEC/2); 2001.

45. Smith RD, Correa C, Oh C. Trade, TRIPS, and pharmaceuticals. *Lancet.* 2009;373:684–91.

46. van den Ham R, Bero L, Laing R. Selection of essential medicines. In: *The world medicines situation 2011.* 3rd ed. Geneva: WHO; 2011.

47. *The pharmaceutical industry and global health: Facts and figures 2015.* Geneva: International Federation of Pharmaceutical Manufacturers & Associations (IFPMA); 2015.

48. Lee JY, Hunt P. Human rights responsibilities of pharmaceutical companies in relation to access to medicines. *J Law Med Ethics.* 2012;40:220–33.

49. Howitt P, Darzi A, Yang GZ, et al. Technologies for global health. *Lancet.* 2012;380:507–35.

50. *Access to medicine index 2016.* Haarlem, Netherlands: Access to Medicine Foundation; 2016.

51. The Sphere Project. *Humanitarian charter and minimum standards in humanitarian response.* 3rd ed. Rugby UK: Practical Action Publishing; 2011.

52. Quarantelli EL. Just as a disaster is not simply a big accident, so a catastrophe is not just a big disaster. *J Am Soc Prof Emerg Planners.* 1996;3:68–71.

53. Koenig KL, Dinerman N, Kuehl AE. Disaster nomenclature—A functional impact approach: The PICE system. *Acad Emerg Med.* 1996;3:723–7.

54. Holguín-Veras J, Jaller M, Van Wassenhove LN, et al. On the unique features of post-disaster humanitarian logistics. *J Oper Manag.* 2012;30:494–506.

55. Stumpenhorst M, Stumpenhorst R, Razum O. The UN OCHA cluster approach: Gaps between theory and practice. *J Public Health.* 2011;19:587–92.

56. *National Incident Management System.* Washington DC: U.S. Department of Homeland Security; 2008.

57. Krin CS, Giannou C, Seppelt IM, et al. Appropriate response to humanitarian crises. *BMJ.* 2010;340: c562.

58. Jobe K. Disaster relief in post-earthquake Haiti: Unintended consequences of humanitarian volunteerism. *Travel Med Infect Dis.* 2011;9:1–5.

59. VanRooyen M, Leaning J. After the tsunami: Facing the public health challenges. *N Engl J Med.* 2005;352:435–8.

60. Aitsi-Selmi A, Egawa S, Sasaki H, Wannous C, Murray V. The Sendai framework for disaster risk reduction: Renewing the global commitment to people's resilience, health, and well-being. *Int J Disaster Risk Sci.* 2015;6:164–76.

61. *Sendai Framework for Disaster Risk Reduction 2015–2030.* Geneva: United Nations Office for Disaster Risk Reduction (UNISDR); 2015.

62. McLoughlin D. A framework for integrated emergency management. *Public Admin Rev.* 1985;45(Special Issue):165–72.

63. Salama P, Spiegel P, Talley L, Waldman R. Lessons learned from complex emergencies over past decade. *Lancet.* 2004;364:1801–13.

64. Spiegel PB. Differences in world responses to natural disasters and complex emergencies. *JAMA.* 2005;293:1915–18.

65. Toole MJ, Waldman RJ. The public health aspects of complex emergencies and refugee situations. *Annu Rev Public Health.* 1997;18:283–312.

66. Melzer N. *International humanitarian law: A comprehensive introduction.* Geneva: ICRC; 2016.

67. Kalshoven F, Zegveld L. *Constraints on the waging of war.* 4th ed. Cambridge UK: Cambridge University Press; 2011.

68. Kivlahan C, Ewigman N. Rape as a weapon of war in modern conflicts. *BMJ.* 2010;340:c3270.

69. Young H, Borrel A, Holland D, Salama P. Public nutrition in complex emergencies. *Lancet.* 2004;364:1899–909.

70. *The fundamental principles of the Red Cross and Red Crescent.* Geneva: ICRC; 2016.

71. Minear L. The theory and practice of neutrality: Some thoughts on the tensions. *Int Rev Red Cross.* 1999;833.

72. *International activity report 2015.* 2nd ed. Geneva: MSF; 2016.

73. *Hope in hell: Inside the world of Doctors Without Borders.* 3rd rev. ed. Richmond Hill ON: Firefly Books; 2010.

74. Barnett M. Humanitarianism transformed. *Persp Politics.* 2005;3:723–40.

75. Redfield P. A less modest witness: Collective advocacy and motivated truth in a medical humanitarian movement. *Am Ethnologist.* 2006; 33:3–26.

76. Brown VJ. BattleScars: Global conflicts and environmental health. *Environ Health Perspect.* 2004;112:A994–1003.

77. *Landmine monitor 2016.* Geneva: International Campaign to Ban Landmines; 2016.

78. Machel G. *Impact of armed conflict on children* (report A/51/306). New York: United Nations; 1996.

79. *Assistance to victims of landmines and explosive remnants of war: Guidance on child-focused victim assistance.* New York: UNICEF; 2014.

80. *Protecting health care: Key recommendation.* Geneva: ICRC; 2016.

81. MacQueen G, Santa-Barbara J. Peace building through health initiatives. *BMJ.* 2000;321:293–6.

82. Noah DL, Huebner KD, Darling RG, Waeckerle JF. The history and threat of biological warfare and terrorism. *Emerg Med Clin N Am.* 2002;20:255–71.

83. Beeching NJ, Dance DAB, Miller ARO, Spencer RC. Biological warfare and bioterrorism. *BMJ.* 2002;324:336–9.

84. Rotz LD, Khan AS, Lillibridge SR, Ostroff SM, Hughes JM. Public health assessment of potential biological terrorism agents. *Emerg Infect Dis.* 2002;8:225–30.

85. Inglesby TV, O'Toole T, Henderson DA, et al. Anthrax as a biological weapon, 2002: Updated recommendations for management. *JAMA.* 2002;287:2236–52.

86. Jernigan DB, Raghunathan PL, Bell BP, et al. Investigation of bioterrorism-related anthrax, United States, 2001: Epidemiologic findings. *Emerg Infect Dis.* 2002;8:1019–28.

87. Biological and chemical terrorism: Strategic plan for preparedness and response. Recommendations of the CDC Strategic Planning Workgroup. *MMWR Recomm Rep.* 2000;49(RR-1):1–14.

88. Thompson AK, Faith K, Gibson JL, Upshur REG. Pandemic influenza preparedness: An ethical framework to guide decision-making. *BMC Med Ethics.* 2006;7:12.

89. Walmsley R. *World prison population list.* 11th ed. London UK: International Centre for Prison Studies; 2016.

90. Watson R, Stimpson A, Hostick T. Prison health care: A review of the literature. *Int J Nurs Stud.* 2004;41:199–28.

91. Dara M, Grzemska M, Kimerling ME, Reyes H, Zagorskiy A. *Guidelines for control of tuberculosis in prisons.* Washington DC: USAID; 2009.

92. Møller L, Stöver H, Jürgens R, Gatherer A, Nikogosian H, editors. *Health in prisons: A WHO guide to the essentials in prison health.* Copenhagen: WHO Europe; 2007.

93. *Standard minimum rules for the treatment of prisoners.* Geneva: Office of the United Nations High Commissioner for Human Rights; 1977.

94. *World report on disability 2011.* Geneva: WHO; 2011.

95. *Convention on the Rights of Persons with Disabilities and optional protocol.* New York: UN; 2006.

96. *International Classification of Functioning, Disability, and Health (ICF).* Geneva: WHO; 2001.

97. *WHO Global Disability Action Plan 2014–2021: Better health for all people with disability.* Geneva: WHO; 2014.

98. *Priority assistive products list.* Geneva: WHO; 2016.

99. United Nations Economic and Social Council. *Report of the Inter-Agency and Expert Group on Sustainable Development Goal Indicators* (E/CN.3/2016/2/Rev.1). New York: UN; 2016.

CHAPTER 6

Global Health Financing

Health is a big business, with trillions of dollars spent annually on health services worldwide. Most individual and public health expenses in high-income countries are paid for with tax revenue or mandatory insurance plans that enable universal access to critical health services. In lower-income countries, people who are unable to pay out-of-pocket for health services may be denied access to clinical care. Global health activities financed with government funds from host and donor countries as well as by charitable contributions from philanthropies, businesses, and private donors facilitate improvements in health promotion and disease prevention in vulnerable populations.

▶ 6.1 Personal and Public Health

Health expenditures are a significant component of the global economy, accounting for more than 8% of the world's total gross domestic product (GDP) (**FIGURE 6–1**).[1] The costs of health can be divided into two categories: (1) money spent on personal health and (2) money spent on public health. Personal health expenses relate to the health of one individual or family, such as the cost of purchasing antibiotics to treat a bacterial infection, paying for a midwife to help deliver a baby, or buying test strips for self-monitoring of blood glucose levels by people with diabetes. Public health expenses relate to shared activities that protect a community, a nation, or the global population at large, such as the costs associated with

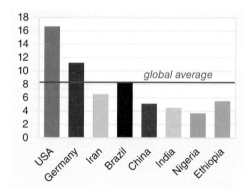

FIGURE 6–1 High-income countries spend a high percentage of their gross domestic product on health.

Data from Global Burden of Disease Health Financing Collaborator Network. Evolution and patterns of global health financing 1995–2014: development assistance for health, and government, prepaid private, and out-of-pocket health spending in 184 countries. *Lancet* 2017; 389:1981–2004.

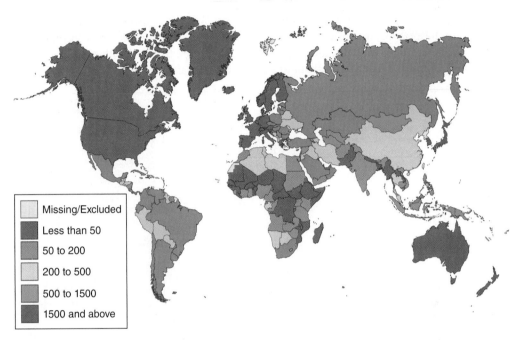

FIGURE 6–2 Health spending per capita (2014).

Data from Health system financing profile by country. Geneva: WHO Global Health Expenditure Database; 2017.

investigating and containing outbreaks of infectious diseases, marketing the mass polio vaccination days that are part of the global eradication campaign, using insecticides in outdoor areas to kill the mosquitoes that can transmit dangerous pathogens to humans, and developing evidence-based clinical guidelines for managing chronic diseases.

Worldwide, more than $9 trillion was spent on health care in 2015, and annual spending could increase to $16 trillion by 2030.[2] High-income countries spend much more per resident on healthcare services than low-income countries do (**FIGURE 6–2**). This difference remains significant even after adjusting for differences in the cost of living (**FIGURE 6–3**).[1] There are a diversity of mechanisms for paying for personal health expenses. Some countries have a publicly funded healthcare system that is paid for with tax revenue, some have a healthcare system in which the medical care of individuals is usually funded by private health insurance or the personal funds of the

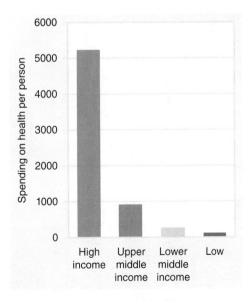

FIGURE 6–3 Total spending on health care per capita by country income level (2014).

Data from Global Burden of Disease Health Financing Collaborator Network. Evolution and patterns of global health financing 1995–2014: development assistance for health, and government, prepaid private, and out-of-pocket health spending in 184 countries. *Lancet* 2017; 389:1981–2004.

individual and his or her family, and some countries pay for personal health services with a combination of public and private sources (**FIGURE 6–4**).[3] Most public health activities in higher-income countries are funded by taxes. Public health initiatives in lower-income countries are often financed with a combination of governmental and external support.

		PERSONAL HEALTH	PUBLIC HEALTH
FUNDERS *Who pays?*	*Typical* **HIGH**-*income country*	Governments (via taxes)	Governments (via taxes)
	Typical **LOW**-*income country*	Households & others	Governments & donors

FIGURE 6–4 Governments in high-income countries use tax revenue to pay for most health services; in low-income countries, a more diverse set of funders pay for health activities.

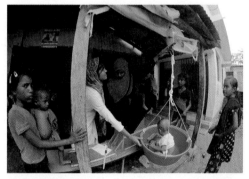

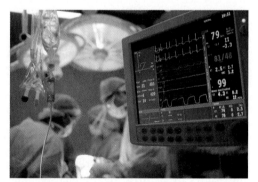

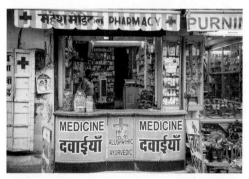

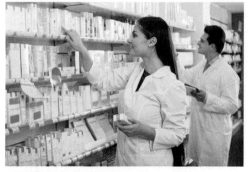

Financing is the provision of money for a particular activity and the management of that investment. Financing for global health is allocated to both personal and public functions. Some global health funding helps lower-income countries expand the personal healthcare services that they offer to residents. For example, some donors have provided financing that enables more women in low-income countries to give birth at hospitals at no cost to the family, more children to be treated for intestinal worm infections through school-based programs, and more people living with HIV to access free and low-cost antiretroviral medications. Some global health funding supports global health governance,[4] pandemic preparedness and response, the development and dissemination of new health technologies, and other public health functions.[5] There are also expenses that blend the personal and public health categories, like the costs associated with educating healthcare workers, ensuring that clinicians are licensed and staying up to date on best practices, and building and maintaining hospitals to ensure that everyone has access to essential health services. These activities are public health functions that enable individuals to have access to quality personal health care. All of these activities are part of functioning health systems.

▶ 6.2 Health Systems

A **health system** includes all of the people, facilities, products, resources, and organizational structures that deliver health services to a population. The World Health Organization (WHO) has identified six core building blocks of health systems: (1) the provision of effective personal and population-based healthcare services; (2) a well-trained and productive health workforce that is able to provide quality care to all population groups; (3) a strong **health information system** that collects, analyzes, and disseminates the

information about population health and health systems performance that is critical for health system decision-making;[6] (4) access to essential medicines, medical devices, vaccines, and other health technologies; (5) a health financing system that enables everyone to access affordable services when they are needed while providing incentives to limit overuse of services; and (6) effective oversight of the system to ensure safety, efficiency, and accountability.[7]

The Sustainable Development Goals (SDGs) aim by 2030 to "achieve universal health coverage, including financial risk protection, access to quality essential healthcare services, and access to safe, effective, quality, and affordable medicines and vaccines for all" (SDG 3.8).[8] **Universal health coverage (UHC)** is present when everyone in a country has access to high-quality health services (including preventive care, diagnosis, treatment, and rehabilitation) and everyone is protected from major health-associated financial shocks via a tax-based financing system or a health insurance plan.[9] In places where patients and their families pay out-of-pocket for most health services, the poorest households are often excluded from accessing quality care. By contrast, countries that spread the cost of health services across the entire population through tax revenue or mandatory participation in highly regulated insurance plans enable everyone to access the services that are included in the national health plan (**FIGURE 6–5**).[10] These services typically include family planning (contraception), obstetric and newborn care, child vaccines, medications for common infections and noncommunicable diseases (such as high blood pressure and diabetes), care for acute injuries, and other services that have been identified as population priorities.[11]

Every government has finite financial reserves, so it is not possible for national health systems to provide every procedure for every condition for every person. Government officials and other people with health leadership

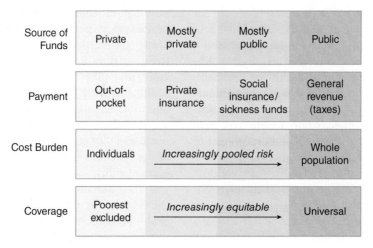

Source of Funds	Private	Mostly private	Mostly public	Public
Payment	Out-of-pocket	Private insurance	Social insurance/ sickness funds	General revenue (taxes)
Cost Burden	Individuals	*Increasingly pooled risk* →		Whole population
Coverage	Poorest excluded	*Increasingly equitable* →		Universal

FIGURE 6–5 Universal health coverage spreads the cost burden for health services across the entire population.

Data from *World health report 1999*. Geneva: WHO; 1999.

responsibilities in countries aiming to achieve UHC must make difficult decisions about which goods and services will be provided to everyone. For example, health system leaders must decide which procedures will and will not be available in public hospitals and which medications will and will not be included in the national formulary. Resource limitations may mean that only part of a comprehensive strategy for improving population health status can be publicly funded. For example, budgeting authorities might determine that it is possible to improve access to in-hospital trauma care for injured people but there is not sufficient funding to simultaneously support injury prevention activities, train and equip more emergency responders, and provide more physical therapy and rehabilitation services for survivors. The decision to increase coverage for one type of service sometimes requires decreases in support for other types of health services.

Government officials must also make critical determinations about how much funding can be allocated to the health system and how much must be dedicated to maintaining other necessary services. Increases in government spending on health often require decreases in funding for education and other social services. Funding decisions have a very tangible impact on the quality of services that are provided. The governments of high-income countries with aging populations usually allocate more of their budget to health than to education.[12] In these countries, surveys that ask residents about their perceptions of social services and their overall quality of life typically show that satisfaction with health services exceeds levels of satisfaction with the education system (**FIGURE 6–6**).[13] The governments of low- and middle-income countries with a large proportion of children in their populations usually allocate more funding to education than to health. Surveys in these countries usually show a higher level of satisfaction with schools than with the healthcare system. Health system strengthening requires a process of identifying priorities and resources, strategizing about the policies that will achieve key goals, transforming those ideas into operational action plans, and then implementing changes and tracking progress toward meeting the targets.[14]

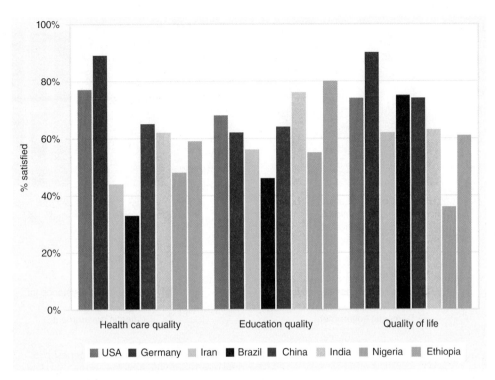

FIGURE 6–6 Satisfaction with healthcare quality is highest in high-income countries.
Data from *World health statistics 2016*. Geneva: WHO; 2016.

▶ 6.3 Paying for Personal Health

Each country has a unique mix of strategies for paying for personal health expenses, but there are some general patterns by country income level (**FIGURE 6–7**).[1] Most high-income countries have a government-sponsored healthcare system that is paid for through general tax revenue, mandatory payments into a government-run social security system, or other types of compulsory contributions. Health services are typically provided at government health facilities or at private facilities that receive most of their funds from the government. (The health financing and delivery system in the United States is a notable exception to the general global trend for high-income countries.)

In most middle-income countries, governments pay for a portion of health costs but the remaining money spent on health is expended in the form of **out-of-pocket (OOP) payments**, cash disbursements made by patients and their families in order to receive health services (**FIGURE 6–8**).[1] The range of services covered by government health plans vary widely. Some health systems pay for all the expenses of hospitalization for a range of causes, while others require the patient to pay part or most of the cost of a hospital stay. Some health systems require users to pay a fee at the time of service and pay OOP for prescription medications and therapy, while others do not. Only a few government health plans include dental care and vision care in their health packages. In places where private healthcare coverage is available to supplement government services, there are

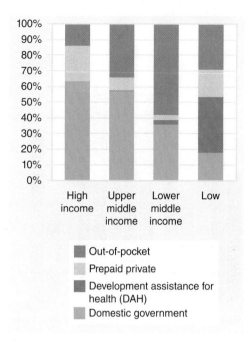

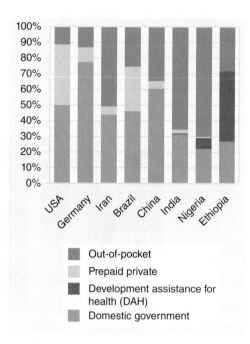

FIGURE 6-7 Total spending on health by payer and country income level.

Data from Global Burden of Disease Health Financing Collaborator Network. Evolution and patterns of global health financing 1995–2014: development assistance for health, and government, prepaid private, and out-of-pocket health spending in 184 countries. *Lancet* 2017; 389:1981–2004.

FIGURE 6-8 Sources of funding for health in featured countries. (Prepaid private spending includes private insurance and spending by nongovernmental organizations.)

Data from Global Burden of Disease Health Financing Collaborator Network. Evolution and patterns of global health financing 1995–2014: development assistance for health, and government, prepaid private, and out-of-pocket health spending in 184 countries. *Lancet* 2017; 389:1981–2004.

wide variations in the prices of private plans and differences in the quality of services covered by the plans.

In most low-income countries, some basic clinical services that have been deemed necessary for achieving high-priority global health goals are financed by domestic governments and international donors to ensure that these services are available to everyone who needs them. For other health conditions, both public and private healthcare facilities may charge user fees and require additional OOP payments for medications and supplies.[15] When subsidized healthcare services are unavailable or the quality of local health services is poor, families are often unable to access any type of skilled care. For example, in some low-income countries, all pregnant women can give birth for free at public hospitals (if they can afford transportation to a hospital, which is not always possible for women who live in rural areas). In other low-income countries, women must pay OOP to give birth at a hospital or must pay midwives OOP to help deliver their babies at home. When families cannot afford to hire help, women must deliver at home without a trained birth assistant. Similarly, in some low-income countries, everyone with HIV can access free or low-cost antiretroviral medications, with the price tied to income to ensure free access to low-income individuals. However, in other countries, people from higher-income households who can afford the medications take them and those from lower-income households who cannot afford the medications do not take them. Increasing access to affordable health services for the most vulnerable populations is one of the major goals for health system strengthening in most low-income countries.

▶ 6.4 Health Insurance

Insurance is a risk management strategy that protects purchasers against major financial losses. Health insurance is intended to protect insured people from incurring overwhelming expenses if they happen to develop an expensive health condition. Health insurance systems, whether private or public, are funded based on the principle of pooled risk. **Pooled risk** assumes that if many low-risk people and a few high-risk people all pay premiums to the insurance system over many years, there will be a pot of money that can be used to pay for major illnesses and injuries when they occur. Only a few people will

develop a very serious chronic condition or suffer a catastrophic injury. However, because everyone is at risk of unexpected health crises, most people are willing to pay additional taxes or purchase insurance that protects them against the small possibility of needing to forego essential medical care because they cannot afford it or acquiring a lifetime of unmanageable, impoverishing debt as a result of one medical incident.[16]

The country that spends the most on health each year, by far, is the United States (**FIGURE 6–9**),[1] which has a health system that is unique among high-income countries because it is not a universal health coverage system. Nearly all health services are provided in private facilities, and a mix of private insurance and government funding is used to pay for healthcare services. Pooled risk was at the core of the U.S. Patient Protection and Affordable Care Act (ACA) of 2010, which made participation in an insurance plan mandatory for those who could afford it and provided financial support for lower-income households to purchase private coverage or

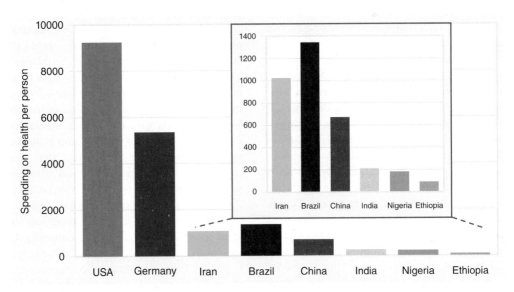

FIGURE 6–9 Total spending on health care per capita in featured countries (2014).

Data from Global Burden of Disease Health Financing Collaborator Network. Evolution and patterns of global health financing 1995–2014: development assistance for health, and government, prepaid private, and out-of-pocket health spending in 184 countries. *Lancet* 2017; 389:1981–2004.

gain access to government-sponsored health coverage plans. The proportion of Americans who were uninsured decreased after the ACA insurance mandate went into effect in 2014, but the percentage of uninsured people did not reach 0%.[17] In 2015, about 91% of Americans had health insurance coverage and 9% had no health insurance.[17] Of the insured individuals, about two-thirds had private health insurance and about one-third were on a government plan.[17]

Most working-aged Americans and their children have employment-based private health insurance. The majority of adults who are employed full-time (and some who are employed part-time) receive healthcare coverage for themselves, their spouses, and their minor children through an employer's plan. Most plans require the employee to pay for a portion of the coverage through monthly **premiums**. Most plans also have deductibles. A **deductible** is the amount that an insured person must spend OOP on health care each year, in addition to premiums, before the insurance company begins paying for health services. Insurance plans with lower premiums have higher deductibles, which means that patients are only reimbursed for expenses after they have paid thousands of dollars OOP. After meeting the deductible for a plan year, patients sometimes must continue to pay OOP copays or co-insurance payments until they reach the maximum OOP amount for the plan year. A **copay** is usually a fixed fee that is paid when receiving routine health services, such as a fee of $50 for each clinic visit or $25 for each prescription for a generic medication. **Co-insurance** requires patients to pay a percentage of the costs of care, such as 20% of the total cost. Copays and co-insurance are intended to discourage overuse of the health system. Insurance plans that cover the full spectrum of care, including medications, preventive care, clinic visits for minor conditions, hospitalizations for serious illnesses, and surgeries, are often expensive for businesses and employees.

The major governmental insurance plans provide healthcare coverage for older adults, low-income households, and military personnel. **Medicare** is the federal health funding system for people who are 65 years old and older, and it also provides coverage for some younger people with serious permanent disabilities. Medicare coverage is based on age and disability status, and it is not tied to income. **Medicaid** is a federal program that provides funding to states to support state-sponsored health coverage for very low-income citizens. The government also provides healthcare services to injured military veterans through the Veterans Administration hospital system and to some indigenous Americans through the Indian Health Services.

Health insurance in the United States was originally designed to cover only the catastrophic expenses that arise from serious illnesses or injuries. Today, many insurance plans also pay for preventive care and minor health problems. This is because health economists have determined that health systems save money when minor conditions are treated before they become major problems. For example, an insurance company may calculate that it is cheaper to pay for thousands of people to be screened for early-stage cancer, which can usually be treated at a relatively low cost, than it is to pay for expensive treatment for one person with advanced-stage cancer. If screening many people and treating several patients with early-stage cancer will prevent a few insured people from requiring expensive treatments for cancers that were not detected until they were at an advanced stage, the insurance company may conclude that encouraging all of its clients to participate in the cancer screening program will yield financial benefits for the company. Or the company may calculate that it is cheaper to pay for frequent routine checkups for people with chronic diseases like diabetes and asthma than it is to pay for emergencies that require hospitalization. The company may provide incentives for people with these chronic diseases to participate in disease management programs that catch emerging problems early and avert the need for expensive emergency care.

Some other high-income countries use health insurance as part of their strategies for UHC. For example, in Germany, every resident must belong to a highly regulated "sickness fund."[18] All sickness funds provide the same services to members at the same cost to users, and OOP payments for health services are minimal. Employers pay half of the sickness fund costs for employees, and the government covers the full cost for children and unemployed adults. Inpatient care is provided at both public and private hospitals, and most outpatient care is provided at private clinics. The payments that providers receive for their services are identical no matter where they work.

Health insurance is also being used by a growing number of residents of middle-income countries so they can access advanced care from high-quality private healthcare providers.[19] For example, lower-income households in Brazil usually receive healthcare services at public facilities that are funded by tax revenue, but a large proportion of higher-income households (or their employers) purchase private insurance plans and seek medical and surgical care at private facilities.[20] Everyone in Brazil can access free primary and emergency health care at public facilities—this is an important right guaranteed under Brazil's constitution—but the public health system offers a limited range of services and technologies.[21] Health insurance allows wealthier households to access a greater range of health services, procedures, medications, and equipment from their preferred providers, and having those individuals use the private health system allows the public health system to allocate more of its resources to care for the lowest-income residents.

▶ 6.5 Paying for Global Health Interventions

The money spent on global public health initiatives comes from a different set of sources than the money that pays for individual health care. In addition to the local and national governmental spending that pays for most of the public health interventions around the world, global health activities are funded by a combination of grants from one country to another, grants and loans from intergovernmental agencies, and gifts from private-sector foundations, businesses, and individuals (**FIGURE 6–10**).[22] The best financing mechanisms for new global health initiatives are sources that are stable and sustainable over time, that are new funding lines rather than money redirected from other health programs, and that are managed efficiently without demanding heavy administrative costs or burdening recipient populations.[23]

Donors have a variety of motivations for giving.[24] For the governments of high-income countries, health funding for lower-income countries is part of foreign policy strategies for building trade alliances and protecting homeland security.[25] Multilateral lending groups may consider global health projects to be good financial investments, especially when aid is provided in the form of loans that will be repaid with interest. Philanthropic organizations focused on reducing poverty and promoting human flourishing may view global health as a tool for achieving their missions. Disease-specific charities may be able to multiply their impact by addressing concerns worldwide rather than limiting their work to a single country or region. Expanding their project portfolios may also attract new donors and volunteers. Large corporations may use global health work to cultivate customer

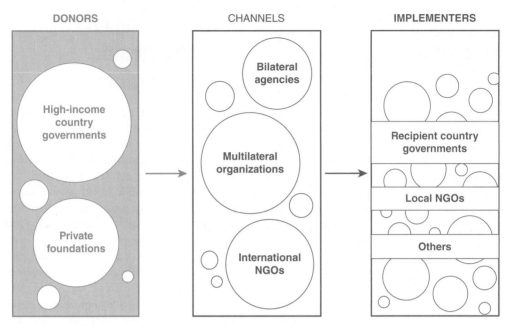

DONORS   CHANNELS   IMPLEMENTERS

High-income country governments

Private foundations

Bilateral agencies

Multilateral organizations

International NGOs

Recipient country governments

Local NGOs

Others

FIGURE 6–10 Typical pathway from global health funders to implementers.

loyalty in new markets, take advantage of tax breaks, and foster a shared sense of purpose among employees. Most of these rationales for funding global health involve benefits for both the recipients and the donors, and the best global health projects achieve goals that are beneficial to all involved parties.

▶ 6.6 Official Development Assistance

Official development assistance (ODA) is money given by the government of a high-income country to the government of a low-income country to support socioeconomic development. Although some aid is given simply to fight poverty, aid is often tied to the political and economic interests of the donor country. For example, bilateral food aid agreements may require food to be purchased in the donor country and shipped by donor-country carriers to the recipient (as is the case for most U.S. food assistance[26]).

Most ODA is donated to low- and middle-income countries (LMICs) by high-income countries that are members of the Development Assistance Committee (DAC) of the Organisation for Economic Co-operation and Development (OECD), but a growing number of upper middle-income countries are including small amounts of ODA in their annual budgets. The SDGs call for "developed countries to implement fully their official development assistance commitments, including the commitment by many developed countries to achieve the target of 0.7% of gross national income (GNI) for ODA to developing countries and 0.15%–0.20% of GNI to least developed countries" (SDG 17.2).[8] In 2015, the five donor nations that provided the greatest amount of ODA in total dollars were the United States, the United Kingdom, Germany, Japan, and France.[27] As a percentage of their GNI, the largest donors were Sweden, Norway, Luxembourg, Denmark, the Netherlands, and the United Kingdom, which all spent at least 0.7% of their GNI on ODA. Germany invested about 0.52% of GNI on ODA in 2015 and the United States spent 0.17% of its GNI on ODA, a rate far below the 0.7% target in the SDGs even though the United States had the world's largest ODA budget.

The foreign aid spending by the United States in 2015 provides an illustration of an annual foreign aid budget. In 2015, the United States spent about $32 billion on humanitarian and other foreign aid, which was about 0.9% of the total national government spending. When the $17 billion spent on foreign military and security assistance (which is only a small portion of the military budget used for international humanitarian operations and other joint responses with allies) is combined with non-military/security foreign aid, the total spending on foreign assistance was about 1.3% of the national governmental spending

(**FIGURE 6–11**).[26] Aid may be given in the form of cash transfers, equipment and commodities (such as food and computers), training and expert advice, or infrastructure development (such as building schools and health clinics in post-conflict areas). Most non-military/security ODA flows through the U.S. Agency for International Development (USAID). Most military aid flows through the Department of Defense (DOD). The U.S. Government considers foreign aid to be a critical contributor to national security because aid supports economic growth, promotes stability, and combats illegal activities.[26] The top recipients of non-military/ security ODA from the United States in 2015 were Afghanistan, Jordan, Pakistan, Kenya, Ethiopia, South Sudan, Syria, and the Democratic Republic of the Congo.[28] All of these countries were engaged in civil conflicts or were located adjacent to conflict areas and were housing large refugee populations.

The amount spent on foreign aid by donor countries and the various types of projects that are supported by ODA can vary considerably from year to year, but global health has become a prominent ODA priority.

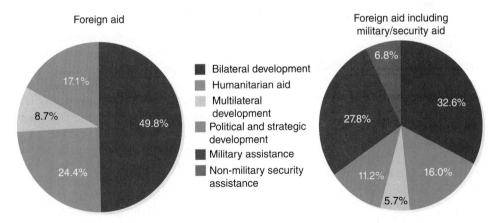

FIGURE 6–11 Foreign aid expenditures by the United States in 2015 by spending category, with and without military/security assistance.

Data from Tarnoff C, Lawson ML. Foreign aid: an introduction to U.S. programs and policy. Washington: Congressional Research Service (CRS); 2016.

Development assistance for health (DAH), sometimes called donor aid for health, is ODA designated for health activities. DAH is an important component of the health budget in low-income countries (**FIGURE 6–12**),[29] and it is a large portion of current foreign aid budgets. Globally, more than $20 billion of ODA was spent on global health in 2015.[30] The United States allocated nearly $10 billion of its foreign aid budget to global health activities in 2015,[30] making the United States the largest contributor of DAH worldwide both in terms of the percentage of its foreign aid budget assigned to DAH and the total budget for DAH (**FIGURE 6–13**).[31] About 70% of those funds were dedicated to HIV/AIDS, tuberculosis, and malaria programs.[32] Other supported activities were in the areas of neglected tropical diseases, reproductive health, child health, nutrition, water and sanitation, and global health security.

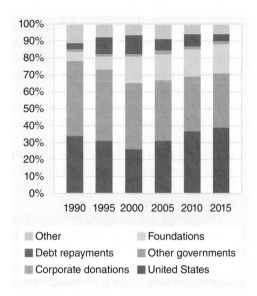

FIGURE 6–13 The United States is a large donor of development assistance for health (DAH).

Data from Financing global health 2015: development assistance steady on the path to new Global Goals. Seattle: Institute for Health Metrics and Evaluation (IHME); 2016.

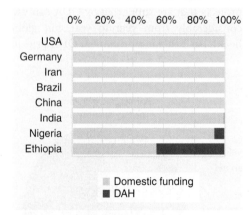

FIGURE 6–12 Development assistance for health (DAH) is an important component of total spending on health in low-income countries.

Data from Global Burden of Disease Health Financing Collaborator Network. Evolution and patterns of global health financing 1995–2014: development assistance for health, and government, prepaid private, and out-of-pocket health spending in 184 countries. *Lancet* 2017; 389:1981–2004.

The SDGs emphasize that ODA is only part of the plan for funding development activities, and they call for action to "strengthen domestic resource mobilization, including through international support to developing countries, to improve domestic capacity for tax and other revenue collection" (SDG 17.1) and to "mobilize additional financial resources for developing countries from multiple sources," including foreign direct investments and remittances (SDG 17.3).[8] **Foreign direct investment (FDI)** is a business investment made by a corporation or an individual in another country. **Remittances** are funds transferred by international workers back to family members in their home communities. The total amount of ODA globally in 2015 neared $150 billion (about 0.3% of GNI in DAC countries).[27] That was a lower amount than the money distributed to lower-income countries through FDI and remittances.[33] In 2015, about $765 billion in FDI was invested in LMICs[34] and about $430 billion in remittances were sent to LMICs.[35]

▶ 6.7 Multilateral Aid

There are two main types of ODA: bilateral aid and multilateral aid. **Bilateral aid** is money given directly from one country (usually a high-income country) to another country (usually a lower-income country). **Multilateral aid** is funding pooled from many donor countries. The largest multilateral organizations include the United Nations, the World Bank and other development banks, and the European Union.

Multilateral organizations, sometimes called intergovernmental organizations, receive two types of funds from member nations. Assessed contributions are mandatory dues calculated from each country's economic and population statistics. Voluntary contributions are extra funds a country opts to donate. Mandatory funds go to the general budget of the multilateral organizations. Voluntary contributions can be designated as core (unrestricted) or noncore (restricted) funding. Core funding can be used by the recipient multilateral organization on any projects the organization deems to be priorities. Some of these projects address the specific needs of particular low-income countries, but many of them are global initiatives that are of value to all countries (such as support for outbreak prevention and control). Noncore funding is given for a specific purpose by the donor and must be spent on that particular activity. In 2013, about 59% of ODA was bilateral ODA distributed by bilateral agencies, about 28% was core multilateral ODA from assessed and voluntary contributions, and about 13% was noncore bilateral aid that was distributed through multilateral organizations to designated recipient countries.[33]

Two multilateral institutions have played a unique role in financing economic development projects because they offer both **loans** (borrowed money that must be repaid with interest) and **grants** (money that does not have to be repaid): the World Bank and the International Monetary Fund (IMF). Both institutions were founded in 1944 during a summit held at Bretton Woods, New Hampshire, in the United States. Both are headquartered in Washington, DC. Both are owned by their nearly 180 member nations. Both the World Bank and the IMF may require recipient countries to implement economic policy reforms as a condition of receiving loans, such as raising taxes, reducing government spending, devaluing the country's currency, eliminating price controls and subsidies, and increasing the production of exports. However, the two institutions have distinct functions and modes of operating.[36]

The **World Bank** is an investment bank that makes loans to developing countries. Its board of governors is composed of representatives from each member country, who are usually member countries' ministers of finance (or the equivalent, such as the Secretary of the Treasury of the United States). Its president has always been a U.S. citizen. World Bank loans must be repaid with interest. Debt repayments are usually used to make new loans for development projects in other countries, including projects focused on health.

The World Bank's primary lending institute is the International Bank for Reconstruction and Development (IBRD), which issues bonds in order to be able to make loans to middle-income member countries. These loans carry an interest rate that is slightly above the market rate, and they are usually supposed to be repaid within 15 years. Most IBRD loans are for specific infrastructure projects, although funds can also be used for other economic development purposes. The International Development Association (IDA) makes interest-free loans to low-income member nations using money that has been donated from high-income countries. IDA loans are usually supposed to be paid back over a 40-year period. The World Bank Group is also home to the International Finance Corporation, which supports private sector development; the Multilateral Investment Guarantee Agency, which supports FDI in low- and middle-income countries; and the International Centre for Settlement of Investment Disputes.

The **International Monetary Fund (IMF)** provides a structure for international monetary policy and currency exchanges, and it also makes loans to countries of any income level that have a balance of payment need and would otherwise not be able to make payments on their other international loans. The IMF's managing director has always been a European. The IMF is funded by membership fees (called quotas) paid by its member countries, and it operates like a credit union. The goal of IMF loans is to allow countries to rebuild their monetary reserves, stabilize their currencies, continue paying for imports, and create conditions for economic growth and high employment rates. The interest rates for IMF funds are usually slightly below market rates, and loans from the IMF are usually supposed to be paid back within a few years.

A major criticism of the international loan system is that interest payments divert money away from education, health, clean water, and other essential human services in lower-income countries. When interest rates are high, countries that are allocating large portions of their annual budgets to interest payments may still not be making good progress toward lowering the amount of principal that must be repaid in the future. The SDGs acknowledge the significant problems associated with overwhelming debt in low-income countries, and they aim to "assist developing countries in attaining long-term debt sustainability through coordinated policies aimed at fostering debt financing, debt relief, and debt restructuring, as appropriate, and address the external debt of highly indebted poor countries to reduce debt distress" (SDG 17.4).[8] The World Bank and the IMF have established plans for debt forgiveness in the poorest, most indebted countries, so that those countries can devote more of their resources to their own health and educational systems rather than requiring those countries to prioritize debt repayment. However, concerns about debt burden are one of the reasons that development banks are now playing less of a role in global health funding than they did in the past. In 2000, more than 20% of DAH came from development banks. By 2015, less than 10% of DAH was disbursed through development banks.[31]

▶ 6.8 Foundations and Corporate Donations

A **foundation** is a charitable trust that gives grants to other nonprofit organizations. A private foundation is one that is established and funded by an individual, family, or corporation as a mechanism for making tax-deductible donations to entities that align with values of the funders. The word foundation is also often used to describe public charities that solicit financial support from other individuals, foundations, and government agencies in order to engage in nonprofit activities. The particular regulations that apply to various types of foundations are specific to each country, but tax laws typically require public charities to have a diverse board of directors and disburse a set percentage of their assets each year in order to maintain their tax-exempt status.

An **endowment** is a large donation made to a nonprofit organization so that the funds can be invested and the interest from the investments can be used to support the operation of the charity. The **Bill & Melinda Gates Foundation** is the largest private foundation in the world. It had $40.4 billion in assets at the end of 2015. Other foundations with large endowments include the Ford Foundation ($12.2 billion in assets in 2015), the Robert Wood Johnson Foundation (RWJF) ($10.3 billion), the W. K. Kellogg Foundation ($8.4 billion), and the Bloomberg Family Foundation ($7.2 billion).[37] These endowments are so large that they enable the foundations to give away large sums of money each year. The Gates Foundation distributed nearly $4 billion in 2015, with about $2.9 billion of that total allocated to health projects.[31] The recipients of Gates Foundation funding included, among others, the Global Alliance for TB Drug Development, the International AIDS Vaccine Initiative, CARE, Family Health International, PATH, UNICEF, the World Health Organization, other organizations that do applied global health work, and a diversity of universities and other research institutes working on agricultural and health technologies.[38] The Ford Foundation gave away $512 million in 2015, RWJF gave $348 million, the Kellogg Foundation gave $322 million, and Bloomberg Philanthropies gave $280 million.[37]

Many large companies have established corporate foundations to do charitable work related to their areas of expertise, and many also support other forms of benevolent engagement.[39] A **corporate social responsibility (CSR)** plan spells out the positive social and environmental actions a company voluntarily supports. For example, a company may choose to build its facilities with sustainable materials and implement a recycling program, even when these actions are not legally required, or it may sponsor local charities

that are important to employees. The major multinational companies that manufacture food and beverage products and produce personal care items are among the many corporations with CSR strategies that support global health. For example, Unilever, Nestlé, Danone, Mondelēz (formerly Kraft Foods), Mars, PepsiCo, the Kellogg Company, General Mills, and Coca-Cola have made commitments to improve access to nutritious food products,[40] and all of them are taking action to improve their social and environmental practices.[41]

In-kind donations of goods or services related to the corporation's core business are often part of CSR programs. Pharmaceutical companies are some of the largest donors to global health initiatives. Each year, GlaxoSmithKline (GSK), Merck, Johnson & Johnson, Eisai, Novartis, Pfizer, and other drug companies donate millions of doses of medications to disease control programs.[42] For example, many millions of people have been treated through Merck's Mectizan® (ivermectin) donation program that targets onchocerciasis (river blindness) and lymphatic filariasis, Pfizer's Zithromax® (azithromycin) program for trachoma, and GSK's Zentel® (albendazole) program for lymphatic filariasis and soil-transmitted helminths.

In addition to being an expression of humanitarian values, and often a tax deduction, corporate donations help develop international markets and increase brand recognition among potential customers. Populations with increased incomes and decreased health expenditures as a result of successful charitable health initiatives have more money to spend on other goods and services. By investing in helping potential and current consumers become healthy and maintain their health, companies are doing good work while expanding their markets and gaining brand loyalty.

▶ 6.9 Personal Donations

Charitable donations are crucial sources of funding for a diversity of health-related projects, and many people all over the world have been and continue to be generous in their support of nonprofit entities. For example, people in the United States donated nearly $375 billion to charity in 2015, with 71% of this total given by individuals, 16% by foundations, 9% from bequests (donations released to a charity from the estate of a deceased person who named the charity in her or her will), and 5% by corporations.[43] In total, those donations represent about 2.1% of the country's total GDP, and individual donations account for 2% of all disposable income in the United States. The major recipients of funding were religious groups (32% of donations), educational institutions (15%), human services organizations (12%), and health charities (8%).[43] Because many of the non-profit organizations within all of these categories provide services that support health and the tools for health, a large proportion of all donations went toward activities related to health promotion.

The generosity of individual donors is especially visible after major natural disasters, when charities may receive millions of dollars of donations in the days immediately after the event.[22] The American Red Cross received $488 million in designated donations after the massive earthquake in Haiti in 2010,[44] $581 million in designated donations after the devastating Indian Ocean tsunami in 2004,[45] and $2.1 billion after Hurricane Katrina hit the Gulf Coast of the United States in 2005.[46] These amounts represent only a fraction of all donated funds, since the Red Cross was just one of numerous organizations receiving humanitarian donations after these catastrophes. Americans gave billions of dollars to charities providing humanitarian services in the affected areas, and individuals from other countries were also generous with their donations.

Another popular giving option for individual donors is **child sponsorship**, a charitable donation model in which a donor selects a child to sponsor and then receives regular updates about that particular child (often including an annual photograph and a thank-you letter written by the child) in exchange for continued monthly contributions to the host organization. Some child sponsorship programs make direct cash transfers to the families of sponsored children, but many use the funds to support community development projects (like clean water and sanitation projects and school improvement projects) that benefit both sponsored and non-sponsored children in a community. Well-run child sponsorship programs are effective at increasing the educational attainment of participating children and improving their employment opportunities in adulthood.[47]

While many of the recipients of individual donations are charities that work on a small scale, some have large budgets and are prominent players in global health initiatives. More than twenty nonprofit organizations in the United States that work in the international arena generated revenue exceeding $250 million in the 2015 fiscal year (including funds from charitable donations and from governmental contracts for implementing international development projects) (**FIGURE 6–14**), as did a variety of nonprofit health and social service charities focused primarily on work within the United States (**FIGURE 6–15**).[48] The best-rated charities spend a relatively small proportion of their budgets on administration and fund-raising, and they apply most of their income to direct program expenses. The annual reports of registered charities allow potential donors to evaluate the financial performance of organizations before making a contribution, and the organizations' websites and other online tools allow potential donors to assess the importance and effectiveness of the organizations' work.[49]

Name	Location	Total Revenue	Contributions from Government Grants (%)	Total Expenses	Admin. Expenses (%)	Fund-Raising Expenses (%)	Amount Spent to Raise $1
Food for the Poor	Coconut Creek, FL	$1158 million	0.1	$1158 million	0.7	3.4	$0.03
World Vision	Federal Way, WA	$1005 million	17.2	$993 million	5.3	10.6	$0.10
Direct Relief	Goleta, CA	$889 million	0	$717 million	0.4	0.2	<$0.01
Compassion International	Colorado Springs, CO	$768 million	0	$776 million	6.8	10.0	$0.10
Americares	Stamford, CT	$752 million	0.2	$641 million	0.6	1.4	<$0.01
Catholic Relief Services	Baltimore, MD	$731 million	46.9	$733 million	3.3	4.2	$0.04
International Rescue Committee	New York, NY	$689 million	66.5	$674 million	4.9	2.6	$0.02
Save the Children	Fairfield, CT	$641 million	41.5	$636 million	4.9	5.3	$0.05
Samaritan's Purse	Boone, NC	$594 million	5.8	$505 million	4.6	7.5	$0.06
MAP International	Brunswick, GA	$547 million	0	$487 million	0.1	0.5	<$0.01
CARE	Atlanta, GA	$530 million	26.1	$528 million	5.7	4.6	$0.04
U.S. Fund for UNICEF	New York, NY	$515 million	0	$541 million	2.6	7.0	$0.06

(continues)

Name	Location	Total Revenue	Contributions from Government Grants (%)	Total Expenses	Admin. Expenses (%)	Fund-Raising Expenses (%)	Amount Spent to Raise $1
Feed the Children	Oklahoma, OK	$451 million	0.4	$449 million	3.0	6.6	$0.06
Doctors Without Borders, USA	New York, NY	$351 million	0	$296 million	1.1	10.4	$0.09
Mercy Corps	Portland, OR	$329 million	70.8	$326 million	11.3	4.8	$0.04
The Rotary Foundation of Rotary International	Evanston, IL	$318 million	0	$274 million	3.3	6.5	$0.06
Catholic Medical Mission Board	New York, NY	$311 million	3.1	$314 million	1.4	1.1	<$0.01
PATH	Seattle, WA	$289 million	27.8	$277 million	15.4	0.9	<$0.01
Operation Blessing International	Virginia Beach, VA	$256 million	0.8	$258 million	0.3	0.6	<$0.01
Project HOPE	Millwood, VA	$254 million	4.3	$272 million	1.6	2.9	$0.02

FIGURE 6–14 Major nonprofit organizations based in the United States and working internationally.

Data are for the 2015 fiscal year.
Data from *Charity Navigator*. Glen Rock NJ: Charity Navigator; 2017.

Name	Location	Total Contributions	Contributions from Government Grants (%)	Total Expenses	Admin. Expenses (%)	Fund-Raising Expenses (%)	Amount Spent to Raise $1
American Red Cross	Washington, DC	$2727 million	7.0	$2886 million	3.8	5.9	$0.21
Feeding America	Chicago, IL	$2201 million	0	$2185 million	0.3	1.1	<$0.01
ALSAC St. Jude Children's Research Hospital	Memphis, TN	$1388 million	6.6	$1095 million	10.8	16.1	$0.15
American Cancer Society	Atlanta, GA	$862 million	0.6	$840 million	5.8	34.2	$0.36
American Heart Association	Dallas, TX	$780 million	0.8	$744 million	8.8	12.3	$0.14
Alzheimer's Association	Chicago, IL	$314 million	4.4	$279 million	7.4	19.5	$0.19
The Leukemia & Lymphoma Society	Rye Brook, NY	$282 million	0	$277 million	8.8	17.9	$0.18
American Kidney Fund	Rockville, MD	$265 million	0	$266 million	0.7	1.8	<$0.01

FIGURE 6–15 Major multipurpose human services and disease-specific charities based in the United States.

Data for the 2015 fiscal year.
Data from *Charity Navigator*. Glen Rock NJ: Charity Navigator; 2017.

▶ References

1. Global Burden of Disease Health Financing Collaborator Network. Evolution and patterns of global health financing 1995–2014: Development assistance for health, and government, prepaid private, and out-of-pocket health spending in 184 countries. *Lancet.* 2017;389:1981–2004.

2. Global Burden of Disease Health Financing Collaborator Network. Future and potential spending on health 2015–40: Development assistance for health, and government, prepaid private, and out-of-pocket health spending in 184 countries. *Lancet.* 2017;389:2005–30.

3. Kutzin J, Witter S, Jowett M, Bayarsaikhan D. *Developing a national health financing strategy: A reference guide.* Geneva: WHO; 2017.

4. Frenk J, Moon S. Governance challenges in global health. *N Engl J Med* 2013;368:936–42.

5. Schäferhoff M, Fewer S, Kraus J, et al. How much donor financing for health is channeled to global versus country-specific aid functions? *Lancet.* 2015;386:2436–41.

6. *Monitoring the building blocks of health systems: A handbook of indicators and their measurement strategies.* Geneva: WHO; 2010.

7. *Everybody's business: Strengthening health systems to improve health outcomes: WHO's framework for action.* Geneva: WHO; 2007.

8. United Nations. *Transforming Our World: The 2030 Agenda for Sustainable Development.* New York: UN; 2015.

9. *The world health report 2013: Research for universal health coverage.* Geneva: WHO; 2013.

10. *World health report 1999.* Geneva: WHO; 1999.

11. *Tracking universal health coverage: First global monitoring report.* Geneva: WHO/World Bank; 2015.

12. *Human development report 2016.* New York: UNDP; 2016.

13. *World health statistics 2016.* Geneva: WHO; 2016.

14. Schmets G, Rajan D, Kadandale S, editors. *Strategizing national health in the 21st century: A handbook.* Geneva: WHO; 2016.

15. Basu S, Andrews J, Kishore S, Panjabi R, Stuckler D. Comparative performance of private and public healthcare systems in low- and middle-income countries. *PLoS Med.* 2012;9:e1001244.

16. Gottret P, Schieber G. *Health financing revisited: A practitioner's guide.* Washington DC: World Bank; 2006.

17. Barnett JC, Vornovitsky MS. *Health insurance coverage in the United States: 2015.* Washington DC: U.S. Census Bureau; 2016.

18. Busse R, Blümel M. Germany: Health system review. *Health Syst Transit.* 2014;16:2.

19. Mills A. Health care systems in low- and middle-income countries. *N Engl J Med.* 2014;370:552–7.

20. Paim J, Travassos C, Almeida C, Bahia L, Macinko J. The Brazilian health system: History, advances, and challenges. *Lancet.* 2011;377:1778–97.

21. Macinko J, Harris MJ. Brazil's family health strategy: Delivering community-based primary care in a universal health system. *N Engl J Med.* 2015;372:2177–81.

22. *Global humanitarian assistance report 2016.* Bristol UK: Development Initiatives Ltd; 2016.

23. *Fast-track: Ending the AIDS epidemic by 2030.* Geneva: UNAIDS; 2014.

24. Stuckler D, McKee M. Five metaphors about global-health policy. *Lancet.* 2008;372:95–7.

25. Yach D, Bettcher D. The globalization of public health, II: The convergence of self-interest and altruism. *Am J Public Health.* 1998;88:738–41.

26. Tarnoff C, Lawson ML. *Foreign aid: An introduction to U.S. programs and policy.* Washington DC: Congressional Research Service (CRS); 2016.

27. *Development co-operation report 2016.* Paris: OECD; 2016.

28. *Aid at a glance.* Paris: OECD; 2016.

29. Bendavid E, Ottersen T, Schaferhoff M, Padian N, Nugent R, Rottingen JA. Donor assistance for health (Chapter 15). *Disease control priorities.* 3rd ed. *Disease control priorities (Volume 9).* Washington DC: IBRD/World Bank; 2017.

30. *The U.S. Government engagement in global health: A primer.* Menlo Park CA: The Henry J. Kaiser Family Foundation; 2017.

31. *Financing global health 2015: Development assistance steady on the path to new Global Goals.* Seattle WA: Institute for Health Metrics and Evaluation (IHME); 2016.

32. Salaam-Blyther T. *U.S. global health assistance: FY2001-FY2016.* Washington DC: Congressional Research Service (CRS); 2015.

33. *Multilateral aid 2015: Better partnerships for a post-2015 world.* Paris: OECD Publishing; 2015.

34. *World investment report 2016.* Geneva: United Nations Conference on Trade and Development (UNCTAD); 2016.

35. *Migration and remittances: Recent developments and outlook.* Washington DC: World Bank; 2016.

36. Driscoll DD. *The IMF and the World Bank: How do they differ?* Washington DC: IMF; 1996.

37. *Foundations: Top 50 by assets.* New York: Foundation Center; 2017.

38. *2015 Annual tax return (Form 990-PF).* Seattle WA: Gates Foundation; 2016.

39. *Giving in numbers: 2016 edition.* New York: The Committee Encouraging Corporate Philanthropy (CECP); 2016.

40. *Access to Nutrition Index: Global index 2016.* Utrecht: Access to Nutrition Foundation; 2016.

41. *The journey to sustainable food: A three-year update on the Behind the Brands campaign.* Oxford: Oxfam; 2016.

42. *Access to medicine index 2016.* Haarlem, Netherlands: Access to Medicine Foundation; 2016.

43. *Giving USA 2015: Highlights.* Chicago IL: The Giving Institute; 2016.

44. *Haiti earthquake response: Five-year update (January 2015).* Washington DC: American Red Cross; 2015.

45. *Tsunami recovery program: Five-year report.* Washington DC: American Red Cross; 2009.

46. *The face of recovery: The American Red Cross response to Hurricanes Katrina, Rita, and Wilma.* Washington DC: American Red Cross; 2007.

47. Wydick B, Glewwe P, Rutledge L. Does international child sponsorship work? A six-country study of impacts on adult life outcomes. *J Political Econ.* 2013;121:393–436.

48. *Charity Navigator.* Glen Rock NJ: Charity Navigator; 2017.

49. MacAskill W. *Doing good better: How effective altruism can help you help others, do work that matters, and make smarter choices about giving back.* New York: Gotham Books; 2015.

CHAPTER 7

Global Health Implementation

Global health interventions are implemented in countries and communities by national and local governments as well as by international cooperation agencies, United Nations organizations, public–private partnerships, nonprofit organizations, and corporate contractors. Monitoring and evaluation processes help ensure that initiatives aiming to expand access to clinical services, distribute relief aid, promote community development, disseminate new health products, and support other health-related activities are achieving their stated goals.

▶ 7.1 Global Health Interventions

The groups that set global health priorities and fund global health activities usually are distinct from the entities that implement health projects at the national and community levels.[1] The typical funding pathway for a global health initiative is for a donor (usually a high-income country government or a large foundation) to give money to a first-level recipient (such as an international cooperation agency, a United Nations agency, or a global partnership), which then passes funding along to numerous second-level recipients (such as government agencies, nongovernmental organizations, and private-sector contractors) that implement the projects (**FIGURE 7–1**).

Funders often use terms like strategy and policy to describe the outputs they generate. A **strategy** is a big picture plan for how to achieve a major goal. A **policy** is a set of principles and procedures that guide decision-making and resource allocation. An action **plan** describes all of the steps that will be taken to achieve strategic goals and implement approved policies. A scheme is an operationalized plan that spells out the desired outcomes and completion timelines for an action plan.

By contrast, implementers more often use terms like program and project to describe their work. A **program** is a portfolio of related projects that together achieve part of an action plan. A **project** is a series of coordinated tasks that are completed within a limited time period in order to achieve a specific target. A **deliverable** is a product, service, or other result of a project. **Project management** is the process of initiating, planning, executing, monitoring and controlling, and closing out projects.[2] Most funded projects have stated outcomes that must be achieved by the project implementation team to meet the terms of the contract between the funder and the recipient. A project manager is responsible for ensuring that deliverables are completed on time and within budget. The same series of steps are implemented for nearly all global health projects, even when they have very different objectives.

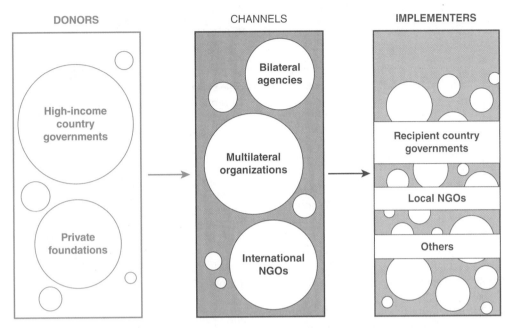

DONORS   **CHANNELS**   **IMPLEMENTERS**

High-income country governments

Private foundations

Bilateral agencies

Multilateral organizations

International NGOs

Recipient country governments

Local NGOs

Others

FIGURE 7–1 Typical pathway from global health funders to implementers.

Global health implementers provide services in a diversity of specialty areas. Many implementation groups provide clinical care at hospitals and clinics or through community-based healthcare providers. Clinical initiatives are often described as being horizontal or vertical.[3] A **horizontal program** strengthens an existing health system so that it can deliver additional health services. Horizontal programs are often described as integrating newly funded packages of health services into existing primary care delivery systems. A **vertical program** delivers disease-specific services that are not fully integrated into the health system. Vertical programs are often used to address global health priorities like disease eradication efforts that demand an intensive but time-limited series of coordinated efforts.

Some agencies and organizations have expertise in responding quickly to emergencies, and others have experience in working alongside communities to promote lasting economic growth. **Relief** is aid that meets the immediate needs of people who might otherwise not have access to water, food, shelter, emergency medical care, and other urgent necessities after major natural disasters and during wars and other types of humanitarian crises. **Development** is a long-term process of improving the socioeconomic and environmental conditions that are associated with poor population health status. Some development programs are designed centrally by professionals and disseminated to participating localities. Some use a slower **community development** process in which community members identify their own priorities and take action to achieve them with the support of partner organizations. Relief groups quickly deliver the material goods needed for survival, while community development groups make long-term investments in capacity building and sustainable change.

Some global health groups have strengths in **advocacy**, the process of increasing awareness of a specific cause in order to influence policy and resource allocation decisions related to that issue. A variety of communication tactics are used for advocacy. For example, **social media**, electronic communication tools that allow users to generate and

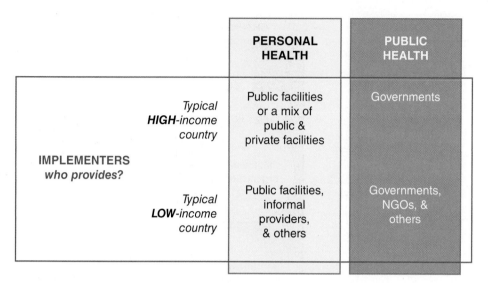

		PERSONAL HEALTH	PUBLIC HEALTH
	Typical **HIGH**-*income country*	Public facilities or a mix of public & private facilities	Governments
IMPLEMENTERS *who provides?*	*Typical* **LOW**-*income country*	Public facilities, informal providers, & others	Governments, NGOs, & others

FIGURE 7–2 Governments are responsible for implementing most public health activities.

share content, are often used to disseminate news about emerging public health problems to large audiences in live time. Some global health implementers have expertise in **logistics**, the process of coordinating complex operations, especially the movement of supplies and equipment. Logistics specialists are able to efficiently procure or produce, package, transport, store, and deliver food, medications, medical devices, and other goods to people and communities in need. Advocacy calls for an action to be taken, and logistics makes that action happen after funding for the activity has been secured.

Many of the most prominent global health implementers are governmental and intergovernmental agencies, large nonprofit organizations, and businesses that work in several functional areas in multiple world regions. Smaller implementing entities may focus on one area of expertise and work within a limited geographic zone.

▶ 7.2 Local and National Governments

In most countries, the majority of clinical health services are provided at government-owned

and operated health facilities or at private non-profit or for-profit health facilities that are regulated by governments. Governments decide, at least in part, the list of services that are covered by public funds, social security, or health insurance schemes and the choices (if any) that people have about which healthcare facilities and clinicians provide their care. Governments are also responsible for the public health system (**FIGURE 7–2**).[4] Government public health agencies protect residents from unsafe foods, medications, medical products, and environmental hazards; provide recommendations and regulations about nutrition, vaccination, screening tests, worker safety, and other actions that promote health and prevent disease; and respond to outbreaks and other threats to public health.[5]

The lead governmental health agency in a country is often called the **Ministry of Health**. In most countries, the majority of clinical health services and public health programs are implemented by national ministries of health and their state or provincial and district health offices or with the approval of these agencies.[6] The national health agency also typically takes the lead on communicating about health-related issues with intergovernmental agencies (such as the World Health Organization), global partnerships, and other external groups. For example, international laws require a country's lead health agency to submit timely reports about outbreaks of dangerous infectious diseases and make formal requests for assistance before international teams can be deployed to support epidemic containment efforts. Ministries of health also oversee the training and licensure of all clinicians working within their borders, including ensuring that visiting clinicians providing patient care are qualified practitioners.

Even when formal approval prior to the implementation of a new health initiative is not mandated, projects often benefit from the advice and support of governmental officials. For example, suppose that a nonprofit organization based in the United States wants to distribute free insecticide-treated bednets (ITNs) in rural communities in Nigeria. A typical first step toward implementation would be for representatives from the nonprofit organization and their Nigerian partner organization(s) to meet with leaders from the local government and other community organizations, including religious groups, to ask for their support. If the project is deemed to be one that will benefit the targeted communities, these local leaders and other community representatives will be able to help the nonprofit group design an appropriate distribution system and spread the word about the free ITNs to the participating communities. The local leaders will also be able to tell American visitors if their community members do not need or do not want ITNs, if the visitors are scheduled to come at a bad time (such as arriving during harvest time or on the day of a special event), or if hosting the visitors, who might need meals and places to sleep, will place an undue burden on some communities. Without doing these sorts of pre-implementation checks, well-intentioned groups might unintentionally inconvenience recipient communities, violate laws about taxation of imported products, duplicate existing malaria control programs, undermine the community health outreach programs of local hospitals and clinics, financially harm local vendors who sell ITNs, or encounter other preventable problems.

In the United States, the Department of Health and Human Services (HHS) performs the functions of a health ministry plus additional tasks. HHS's lead health protection agency is the **Centers for Disease Control and Prevention (CDC)**. One of the many roles of CDC is responding to outbreaks and other public health emergencies, including participating in international responses when foreign governments invite CDC to collaborate.[7] The CDC also works with partners in other countries to conduct field research, set up monitoring and surveillance systems, and train public health workers. The **National Institutes of Health (NIH)** is HHS's division that conducts health research. Although most NIH research is conducted at study sites within the United States, NIH research may be conducted internationally when the research protocol meets the rigorous standards for ethical research established by NIH and by host country governments. Other operating divisions of HHS include the Agency for Healthcare Research and Quality (AHRQ), the Agency for Toxic Substances and Disease Registry (ATSDR), the Centers for Medicare & Medicaid Services, the Food and Drug Administration (FDA), the Health Resources and Services Administration (HRSA), the Indian Health Service, and the Substance Abuse and Mental Health Services Administration (SAMHSA), among others. Other countries have similarly complex organizational structures within their health ministries.

▶ 7.3 International Cooperation

Foreign policy describes the strategies and approaches a country uses to engage with other nations and protect its own interests as they pertain to security, trade, and other critical functions.[8] The "3 Ds" of foreign policy have been described as diplomacy, defense, and development.[9] **Diplomacy** is the process of negotiating agreements between countries, resolving disputes peacefully, and navigating other aspects of international relations.[10] **Health diplomacy**

Country	Abbreviation	Agency
Austria	ADA	Austrian Development Agency
Belgium	BTC	Belgian Development Agency
Czech Republic	CzDA	Czech Development Agency
France	AFD	Agence Française de Développement
Germany	GIZ	Deutsche Gesellschaft für Internationale Zusammenarbeit
Iceland	ICEIDA	Icelandic International Development Agency
Ireland	Irish Aid	Irish Aid
Japan	JICA	Japan International Cooperation Agency
Republic of Korea	KOICA	Korean International Cooperation Agency
Luxembourg	LuxDev	Lux-Development
Norway	Norad	Norwegian Agency for Development Cooperation
Spain	AECID	Agencia Española de Cooperación Internacional para el Desarrollo (Spanish Agency for International Development Cooperation)
Sweden	Sida	Swedish International Development Cooperation Agency
Switzerland	SDC	Swiss Agency for Development and Cooperation
United Kingdom	DFID	Department for International Development
United States	USAID	United States Agency for International Development

FIGURE 7-3 Examples of international development and cooperation agencies.

uses health projects as part of meeting foreign policy goals.[11] Defense is carried out by militaries. Development in the foreign policy context is often called **international cooperation** or development cooperation, and it includes financial assistance, capacity building, and other actions that improve the economic situation in lower-income countries, promote stability, and foster future opportunities for expanded trade. Many donor countries have a specialized agency that leads bilateral cooperation efforts (**FIGURE 7-3**). Other countries implement international cooperation initiatives through a Ministry of Foreign Affairs (or an equivalent agency). International cooperation agencies typically send representatives to recipient countries to oversee projects and provide technical and logistical support.

International cooperation is about more than high-income countries (and a growing number of upper-middle-income countries) sending money to a low- or middle-income partner country to alleviate poverty and improve health. Sponsored projects are integral parts of donor countries' foreign policy strategies. The targeted recipient countries, goals, and methods are selected based on the political situations and historic connections of the donor

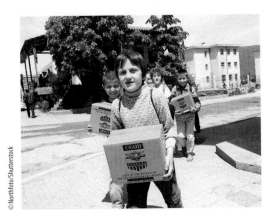

nation. For example, the United Kingdom's Department for International Development (DFID) tends to work especially closely with members of the Commonwealth of Nations (formerly the British Commonwealth), which are almost exclusively former British colonies or protectorates,[12] and the Japan International Cooperation Agency (JICA) works worldwide but is especially active in the Asian countries with which it has strong economic ties.[13]

USAID, the United States Agency for International Development, is a major donor to global health activities and also operates global health programs, partners with other groups to implement global health activities, engages in global health diplomacy, supports research and development, and provides technical assistance related to global health.[14] USAID has been active for several decades in supporting maternal and child health programs, infection control efforts, and health systems strengthening, as well as other aspects of global health.[15] The State Department and the Millennium Challenge Corporation also engage in health diplomacy on behalf of the United States.

▶ ## 7.4 The World Health Organization and the United Nations

The **United Nations** (UN) is the world's largest intergovernmental organization. The UN was founded by 51 member states in 1945, at the end of World War II. The membership list has expanded to include more than 190 member nations. The goals of the UN are "to maintain international peace and security," "to develop friendly relations among nations," and "to achieve international cooperation in solving international problems of an economic, social, cultural, or humanitarian character."[16] The UN is governed by its main bodies: the UN General Assembly, which is the chief policy-setting group for the UN and is composed of one voting representative from each member state; the 15-member UN Security Council, which is responsible for peace-building, mediation, and security operations; the Economic and Social Council; the International Court of Justice, which provides legal judgments and advisory opinions; and the UN Secretariat, which is run by the Secretary-General of the UN and manages numerous departments and offices, including the Department of Economic and Social Affairs, the Office of the UN High Commissioner for Human Rights (OHCHR), and the UN Office on Drugs and Crime (UNODC). The UN also hosts programs and funds, specialized agencies, and several UN-related organizations, including the International Atomic Energy Agency (IAEA), the International Organization for Migration (IOM), and the World Trade Organization (WTO).

The programs and funds of the UN are overseen by the General Assembly and financed through voluntary contributions from member nations (**FIGURE 7-4**). The **UN Development Programme (UNDP)** focuses on poverty reduction. The **UN Environment Programme (UNEP)** promotes healthy ecosystems and sustainable use of natural resources.[17] The **UN Population Fund (UNFPA)**, formerly the UN Fund for Population Activities, supports reproductive health programs. The **United Nations Children's Fund (UNICEF)**, formerly the UN International Children's Emergency Fund, advocates for children's rights and

Program or Fund		Primary Work Area
UNCTAD	United Nations Conference on Trade and Development	International trade
UNDP	United Nations Development Programme	Poverty reduction and resilience
UNEP	United Nations Environment Programme	Environment
UNFPA	United Nations Population Fund	Reproductive health
UN-HABITAT	United Nations Human Settlements Programme	Urban development
UNHCR	Office of the United Nations High Commissioner for Refugees	Refugees
UNICEF	United Nations Children's Fund	Children and mothers
UNODC	United Nations Office on Drugs and Crime	Drugs
UNRWA	United Nations Relief and Works Agency for Palestinian Refugees	Palestinian refugees
UN Women	UN Women	Women
WFP	World Food Program	Hunger and malnutrition

FIGURE 7-4 United Nations programs and funds.

provides humanitarian assistance for children. UNICEF aims to end preventable deaths of children, newborns, and their mothers and to promote the healthy development of all children from birth through adulthood.[18] UN-Habitat, the United Nations Human Settlements Programme, advises on sustainable urban development. The Office of the UN High Commissioner for Refugees (UNHCR) is the UN Refugee Agency. UN Women is the UN Entity for Gender Equality and the Empowerment of Women. The World Food Programme (WFP) aims to eradicate hunger and malnutrition.

The specialized agencies of the UN are autonomous international organizations that

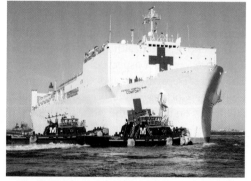

work with the UN and are funded through both assessed contributions and voluntary donations (FIGURE 7-5). The Food and

Agriculture Organization (FAO), the World Bank, and many of the other agencies work on sociopolitical, economic, and environmental issues that are related to health. The **Joint United Nations Programme on HIV/AIDS (UNAIDS)** is an entity co-sponsored by 10 UN system agencies—UNHCR, UNICEF, WFP, UNDP, UNFPA, UNODC, the International Labour Organization (ILO), UNESCO, WHO, and the World Bank—to advance HIV/AIDS prevention and control. Other UN entities that are not specialized agencies but work with them include the UN Office for Disaster Reduction (UNISDR) and the UN Office for Project Services (UNOPS).

Agency		Primary Work Area
FAO	Food and Agriculture Organization	Hunger
ICAO	International Civilian Aviation Organization	Aviation
IFAD	International Fund for Agricultural Development	Rural development
ILO	International Labour Organization	Labor rights
IMF	International Monetary Fund	Economic growth
IMO	International Maritime Organization	Shipping
ITU	International Telecommunication Union	Information and communication technologies
UNESCO	United Nations Educational, Scientific and Cultural Organization	Culture
UNIDO	United Nations Industrial Development Organization	Industrial development
UNWTO	World Tourism Organization	Tourism
UPU	Universal Postal Union	Postal services
WHO	World Health Organization	Health
WIPO	World Intellectual Property Organization	Intellectual property
WMO	World Meteorological Organization	Meteorology
World Bank Group	World Bank	Poverty reduction

FIGURE 7–5 United Nations agencies.

The **World Organisation for Animal Health** (known as **OIE**, the acronym for the Office International des Epizooties, the organization's original name in French) is an intergovernmental group that is not part of the UN system but works closely with FAO and World Health Organization to control the spread of zoonotic infectious diseases and to promote food safety.

The **World Health Organization (WHO)**, launched in 1948, is a specialized agency of the UN that serves as its primary health agency.[19] The WHO is governed by the World Health Assembly (WHA), composed of one representative from each UN member state. The WHA convenes every May to approve a budget, make policy decisions, and approve conventions, agreements, and regulations. The core functions of the WHO are to provide leadership for the health work being done across the UN; identify global health research priorities; develop standards of practice, such as child growth charts and recommendations for laboratory and diagnostic procedures; formulate evidence-based policy recommendations; provide technical support to UN member nations; and monitor disease epidemics and compile health statistics.[20] Current priority areas include health systems strengthening, health promotion across the life span, and emergency preparedness and response.[20]

▶ 7.5 International Health Regulations

Globalization means that humans are tied together more tightly than ever before, and a problem in one part of the world can quickly become a global issue.[21] One of the roles of global health agencies is to prevent dangerous outbreaks from spreading across national borders and causing widespread morbidity and mortality. The **International Health Regulations (IHR)** are a global health security agreement between all of the member countries of the UN. Under the IHR, all countries agree to notify the WHO immediately about situations that might become public health emergencies and to share critical information with all member nations when outbreaks are occurring.[22] The member nations also agree to develop and maintain public health systems that are able to monitor population health status, identify emerging problems, and respond to health crises, and they pledge to engage in travel and transportation practices that protect global public health.

The IHR are derived from agreements negotiated in the mid-1800s by several European countries that worked together to prevent the spread of cholera outbreaks without stifling international shipping and trade.[23] The WHO was established in 1948. In 1951, the member nations adopted a set of International Sanitary Regulations that were based on the existing cholera control frameworks. These international laws governing global health security were renamed the International Health Regulations in 1969 and were updated to focus on controlling six infectious diseases: cholera, plague, relapsing fever, smallpox, typhus, and yellow fever. Modifications made in 1973 and 1981 reduced the number of reportable diseases to just three: cholera, plague, and yellow fever. A major overhaul of the IHR adopted in 2005 increased requirements for shared communication about and coordinated responses to influenza, viral hemorrhagic fevers, and other emerging infectious diseases and events of potential international public health concern.[24]

The 2005 updates were a response to the emergence of **SARS (severe acute respiratory syndrome)**, a coronavirus infection that caused its victims to become critically ill with pneumonia.[25] The first cases of SARS were identified in Guangdong, in southern China, in November 2002. In March 2003, SARS spread to Hong Kong, and a secondary outbreak occurred in Toronto, Canada. Cases were diagnosed in more than two dozen countries across five continents.[26] The SARS pandemic was contained by isolating patients and carefully observing the people they had contact with, so that anyone who developed symptoms could be isolated immediately and treated under strict infection control protocols.[27] However, the outbreak raised alarms about gaps in global health communication, surveillance, and response capacity.[28] The 2005 IHR address all types of risks, mandating more communication about health events from member nations and obligating countries to strengthen their surveillance and response activities.[29]

Health **surveillance** is the process of continually monitoring health events in a population so that emerging problems can be detected and appropriate control measures can be implemented quickly. Surveillance is the first step in a public health approach to responding to threats (**FIGURE 7–6**).[30] Surveillance systems, which are usually run by governments, track infectious disease reports from hospitals and other information sources to look for possible outbreaks or clusters of disease, which occur when there is an unusually high incidence of disease in a particular place (spatial clustering) or time (temporal clustering). The health statistics collected as part of surveillance allow communities, states and provinces, and nations to know what diseases are common in their populations and to recognize when an unusual health situation is emerging. Baseline data about incidence and prevalence from routine surveillance allow epidemiologists to identify when an atypically large number of cases are being diagnosed.

It is not necessary for surveillance systems to track an entire population. **Sentinel surveillance** is the continuous collection and analysis of high-quality data from a limited number of clinics or hospitals so that public health officials will be able to detect changes in health status in the larger population from which the sentinel sites were sampled. If an outbreak is suspected based on data from sentinel sites, a more rigorous investigation involving additional clinics, hospitals, and laboratories can be conducted. **Passive surveillance** collects mandatory reports of notifiable disease diagnoses from medical laboratories. **Active surveillance** involves public health officials contacting healthcare providers to ask about how often they are diagnosing particular types of diseases. **Syndromic surveillance** tracks potential outbreaks or other disease events based on reports of symptoms, school absentee reports, spikes in Internet searches for particular diseases, and other types of data rather than relying solely on counts of laboratory-confirmed diagnoses.

Several epidemiological terms are used to describe how often diseases occur in a population. An **endemic** disease is an adverse health condition that is always present in a particular population. For example, malaria and dengue are constant threats to health in many parts of the world and are considered to be endemic in those places. An **outbreak** is characterized by at least several people becoming ill from a disease that is not usually present in a population, as happens when dozens of people contract a foodborne illness by eating at the same restaurant. An **epidemic** occurs when a disease is occurring more often than usual and there are more than a few sporadic occurrences of disease. A **pandemic** is a worldwide epidemic. The term pandemic describes the distribution of disease

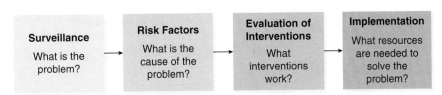

FIGURE 7–6 Surveillance is the first step in a public health approach to responding to threats to health.

Adapted from Holder Y, Peden M, Krug E, Lund J, Gururaj G, Kobusingye O, editors. *Injury surveillance guidelines*. Geneva: WHO; 2001.

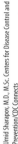

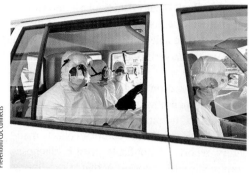

events across the globe, and it is not necessarily an indicator of the severity of the disease. Pandemics of highly pathogenic infectious diseases are global health priorities because they have the potential to wreak havoc on global travel and trade in addition to causing widespread illness and death. Historic pandemics of influenza, cholera, and other severe infectious diseases have shaped international health agreements and global preparedness and response plans.[31]

Under the 2005 IHR, a **public health emergency of international concern (PHEIC)** can be declared when an infectious disease outbreak is causing serious illnesses, is likely to spread to other countries, and requires a coordinated global response. Several events have been declared to meet the PHEIC criteria, including the 2009 H1N1 influenza pandemic; a resurgence of polio that occurred in 2014; the 2014 West African outbreak of **Ebola** virus disease, a hemorrhagic fever transmitted via contact with the body fluids of infected individuals; and the spread of Zika virus in the Americas in 2016.[32] PHEIC status enables international resources to be released to support the response to the disease event, and it also obligates the affected countries to act on the disease control recommendations issued by the WHO.

▶ 7.6 Global Partnerships

A **public–private partnership (PPP)** is a long-term collaboration in which the costs, risks, and benefits are shared by governmental

and nongovernmental entities. For global health PPPs, the public partners are the national governments of countries from across the income spectrum. Since 2000, PPPs have been increasing in popularity as channels for dispersing development assistance for health (DAH) (**FIGURE 7–7**).[33] The private partners in global health PPPs include nonprofit foundations and for-profit corporations. Global health PPPs are developing new products (such as new medications, vaccines, and diagnostic tools), improving the quality and regulation of products, distributing donated and subsidized health products, educating the public about particular health issues, strengthening health services and health informatics systems, and coordinating complex global health efforts.[34]

Dozens of PPPs are currently working to set and accomplish goals for selected global health issues. The two largest global health

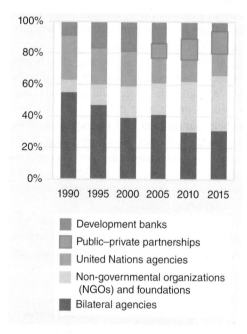

FIGURE 7–7 The channels involved in disbursing development assistance for health (DAH) are shifting in prominence.

Data from *Financing global health 2015: Development assistance steady on the path to new global goals*. Seattle: Institute for Health Metrics and Evaluation (IHME); 2016.

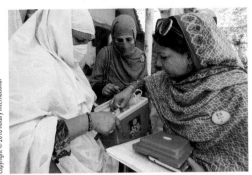

partnerships are The Global Fund to Fight AIDS, Malaria and Tuberculosis and Gavi, the Vaccine Alliance.[33] The Global Fund finances infection control and prevention initiatives in low- and middle-income countries. Applicant countries propose their own sets of projects, and they manage the implementation of funded programs. The Global Fund provides technical support and negotiates with pharmaceutical companies and other manufacturers to procure medications and other health products at low costs. The Global Fund is able to make these tools for health affordable by signing contracts to purchase massive quantities of commonly desired products—enough to meet the demand in many countries— and guaranteeing that the manufacturer will receive payment for its products.[35] Gavi works with low- and middle-income countries to identify priority vaccines and negotiates with manufacturing companies to increase the production of desired vaccines. Gavi and the recipient countries share the costs of the vaccines. Countries pay larger shares of the costs as their economies grow, until they are fully sustaining their own vaccination programs.[36]

One of the goals of many PPPs is to increase access to new technologies and other tools for health. A health product is only valuable for global health when the intended users can afford the product and when they choose to use the product for its intended purposes. Increasing the number of users requires the product to gain local acceptance and be adopted by end users, and that process requires

product advocacy and buy-in from a variety of stakeholders, including donors, policymakers, and end users.[37] **Social marketing** is the use of marketing strategies to change behaviors in targeted populations. Partners with expertise in social marketing can increase demand for products, and partners with expertise in manufacturing can ensure that there are enough supplies to meet demand.

Successful global health partnerships yield benefits for all of the partners who contribute to research, production, and distribution activities. Corporate partners are able to make a profit on reduced-price products by selling a larger volume of products than they would sell if they were not part of the partnership. They also benefit when subsidized health products open up new markets to the company and enhance their reputations. The governments of high-income countries attain an effective mechanism for achieving their foreign policy, scientific, and humanitarian goals. Most importantly, the health of the world's people is advanced when partnerships increase the visibility of specific health issues, raise funds to address those issues, stimulate research and development, implement new treatment protocols and technical standards, and improve access to health care and the tools for health.[38]

▶ 7.7 The Nonprofit Sector

A **nonprofit organization** (NPO) is a mission-driven group that reinvests surplus revenue in the organization rather than distributing extra income to owners or shareholders. Some NPOs are led by unpaid volunteers, but many have paid staff. A **nongovernmental organization (NGO)**, sometime called a private voluntary organization, is a nonprofit organization that is privately managed and receives at least some of its funding from private sources. NGOs from countries across the income spectrum are involved in providing clinical care and public health services, disseminating relief aid, leading community development work, engaging in advocacy, and managing logistics for health programs and projects. NGOs with global health portfolios may focus on one key health issue (such as specializing in raising awareness about HIV prevention or providing surgical services) or they may address multiple issues in a particular location (such as delivering a comprehensive set of socioeconomic development, environmental sustainability, and health interventions in one country or a smaller geographic area). Some large **international NGOs (INGOs)** have diverse portfolios of projects that they implement in numerous countries. Some NGOs are **faith-based organizations (FBOs)** sponsored by a religious or religiously affiliated entity. FBOs rarely require that aid recipients adhere to a particular faith or listen to an evangelistic message, but they openly represent a particular religious tradition. Examples of FBOs include the American Jewish World Service, Catholic Relief Services, Church World Service, Islamic Relief, and World Vision.

Most large global health NGOs raise funds from individuals, private foundations, and governmental sources. One challenge for many NGOs is balancing the goals of donors and the desires and needs of recipients.[39] Directed donations are ones in which the donor stipulates that the contributed funds or supplies must be used in a particular way. Sometimes this works well, but when donors are not aware of conditions in the recipient community, the donation may not generate the intended outcome. A community that wants to upgrade its local health clinic by adding a solar panel to provide electricity to the building may instead receive a microscope that cannot be used without electricity. A nursing school may receive a donation of textbooks written in a language not spoken by any of the students or containing obsolete content. Or a donor may send used medical equipment that cannot be maintained by the community, expired medications that

have to be discarded immediately, or a water pump that cannot be locally repaired. (**Appropriate technology** is affordable and environmentally sustainable technology that can be locally operated and maintained.) Donors may also demand input into operational decisions. They may insist that expatriates, rather than host-country staff, manage projects and oversee budgets. This may inhibit capacity building in host communities.

NGOs working in global health aim to improve the well-being of individuals, communities, and nations, but well-intentioned efforts can sometimes have harmful side effects. The actions of an NGO may have unintended social and political consequences.[40] For example, the presence of a relief NGO may exacerbate conflicts by providing supplies that allow violence and instability to continue or by encouraging displaced people to congregate in one area that could be targeted for attack. The long-term presence of a community development NGO may promote a "culture of dependency" and prevent the development of governmental or commercial service providers.

Skills in effective cross-cultural communication are a requirement for everyone working in global health, especially for INGO leaders who have to navigate complex political terrains. For example, some of the largest U.S.-based INGOs receive a substantial portion of their budgets from the U.S. government. Their workers may be seen by host communities as agents of a foreign government. Other challenges arise from the political landscapes in host countries. INGOs must decide how closely they will work with officials from host countries and how to address potential problems with corruption and mismanagement. Some humanitarian groups feel that it is important to remain publicly neutral about political matters, while others feel compelled to speak openly about any injustices they witness.

NGOs that successfully maneuver through these complex situations play a very important role in global health. Since NGOs often work for decades in the same communities, their employees and volunteers build relationships and trust with community members. NGOs can then serve as points of connection between communities and donors (and other funding channels), with NGOs using their networks to help new projects and programs quickly reach their target audiences. NGOs are often the organizations that actually deliver global health interventions to the people who will most benefit from them. For example, Rotary International members worldwide have worked together on the global polio eradication campaign, with local Rotary clubs in endemic areas facilitating vaccination campaigns in their own communities.[41]

▶ 7.8 The Corporate Sector

A variety of businesses play a role in global health. Some companies specialize in project implementation, and they receive contracts from funding agencies and other global health financing channels to manage the delivery of global health services. Some companies are the private partners in PPPs, and they are paid to manufacture the medications, vaccines, and other products that are distributed as part of global health initiatives. (These companies might also donate some of their products as part of their corporate social responsibility plans, but that is a separate function from participation in contracted manufacturing of health products.) Some companies involved in global health excel at **supply chain management**, the process of coordinating all the steps from selecting and procuring products through the logistics of transporting, storing, and delivering them.[42] Many companies that are not primarily focused on global health play a role in influencing health behaviors and health status, whether they are multinational corporations or smaller businesses.

USAID is one of the major channels for disbursing global health funding to companies. USAID does not have the staff to implement all of its own projects, so many of its projects are managed by outside groups. Several of the leading USAID contractors are for-profit companies, including Chemonics, John Snow Inc., DAI, Abt Associates, and Tetra Tech (**FIGURE 7-8**).[43] Most of the other leading USAID contractors are nonprofit organizations that receive nearly all of their funds from government contracts and are not dependent on fund-raising from private donors. These groups include FHI 360, Management Sciences for Health (MSH), Jhpiego, and RTI. Only a few of the major recipients of USAID funding are charities that manage large government contracts but still rely heavily on private donations for a large portion of their portfolio of projects, such as Catholic Relief Services and Mercy Corps.

Among the global health implementing groups that have annual budgets of millions of dollars, the functional differences between for-profits and nonprofits are often minimal. For example, both for-profit and nonprofit contractors typically offer their professional staff from high-income countries professional-level salaries and compensation packages, no matter what setting they are working in. For both, professional staff from low- and middle-income countries who are working in their home countries—"host-country nationals," in international development lingo—typically earn salaries that are locally competitive but lower than their peers from high-income countries,[44] even though these pay differentials can become a source of workplace tension.[45] Charities that primarily remain dependent on private donors tend to offer smaller compensation packages to employees.

Food and beverage companies, pharmaceutical companies, manufacturers of medical devices, manufacturers of hygiene supplies and personal care products, and other corporations that produce health-related goods and provide health-related services play an important role in facilitating

Name	Headquarters	Type
Chemonics International, Inc.	Washington, DC	For-profit
Partnership for Supply Chain Management (a collaboration founded by JSI and MSH)	Arlington, VA	Nonprofit
FHI 360 (formerly Family Health International)	Durham, NC	Nonprofit
John Snow Incorporated (JSI)	Boston, MA	For-profit
DAI	Bethesda, MD	For-profit
Management Sciences for Health (MSH)	Medford, MA	Nonprofit
Jhpiego	Baltimore, MD	Nonprofit
Abt Associates	Cambridge, MA	For-profit
RTI International	Research Triangle Park, NC	Nonprofit
Catholic Relief Services	Baltimore, MD	Charity
Mercy Corps	Portland, OR	Charity
Tetra Tech, Inc.	Pasadena, CA	For-profit

FIGURE 7–8 Many of the groups with the largest USAID contracts in 2015 were for-profit corporations.
This list excludes multilateral organizations, such as the World Bank, the World Food Program, UNICEF, Gavi, and WHO.
Data from *Top 40 vendors*. Washington DC: USAID; 2015.

health for populations around the world. These businesses are typically not part of the funder–channel–implementer pathway for large-scale global health initiatives, but they are key contributors to achieving global health goals via market-based strategies. Any company may play a role in influencing health via marketing (especially if its products are ones that promote or inhibit health), lobbying, and corporate social responsibility activities.[46] Corporations can also play a role in health promotion by protecting the health and safety of their employees and the communities where they work, producing and selling healthy products, and participating in public health alliances.[47]

▶ 7.9 Research and the Academic Sector

Universities in countries across the income spectrum play several roles in global health. The most important role is education. Universities provide training in medicine, nursing, dentistry, physiotherapy, counseling, other clinical disciplines, public health, pharmacology, engineering, statistics, informatics, business, marketing, public policy, public administration, law, international relations, education, the biomedical sciences, and all the other fields that contribute to global health.

Universities also conduct research. **Research** is the process of systematically investigating a topic in order to discover new insights about the world. Researchers conduct epidemiological studies that quantify the burden of various health conditions; identify the socioeconomic, behavioral, environmental, and other risk factors for diseases and the protective factors that can keep people healthy; and carry out experimental trials to determine which interventions are the safest and most effective. Research at universities contributes to the development of new medications, vaccines, diagnostic tools, and medical devices.[48] The journal articles and other publications written by researchers in the academic sector and by people who work at research institutes, think tanks, and other organizations provide a critical foundation of scientific evidence that is used to develop global health strategies and design intervention plans. Researchers also contribute to needs assessments, prioritization exercises, and evaluations of the outcomes of global health initiatives.

While most of the global health funding that flows through universities is for educational and research activities, some universities also accept contracts to implement global health programs and subcontracts from other implementers to participate in some aspects of program implementation. Many students, trainees, professors, staff, and other members of university communities are also active in voluntary service that contributes to global health. The traditional functions of universities are teaching, research, and service, and all three of these areas are being used to advance global health.

▶ 7.10 Measuring Impact

Many public health intervention packages would increase the quality of life of millions of people at a relatively low cost per person. However, all of these interventions together add up to a lot of money, especially for low-income countries where the total amount spent on health per person per year is significantly less than $100. Trillions of dollars each year would be required to implement global health strategies for all of the various causes of disease, disability, and death. Difficult decisions have to be made about how to allocate limited resources. Because resources for global health are scarce, funding recipients are expected to demonstrate to global health financers that their resources are being well used.

A typical project passes through planning, implementation, and evaluation stages, with assessment strategies applied throughout the project cycle. **Monitoring** is a process of ongoing assessment of a project or program to track progress toward achieving predefined targets. If the monitoring process reveals that a project or program is not fulfilling its mandate, adjustments can be made to increase the impact of the intervention. **Evaluation** is an assessment of how well a project, program, or policy has met its goals. Together, **monitoring and evaluation (M&E)** is the systematic collection of information about an ongoing intervention (process evaluation) and the determination of whether the intervention achieved its objectives (impact evaluation). Most contracts for global health implementation work mandate that the recipient group have a robust M&E plan that examines the inputs into a program, the processes used during the intervention period, the outputs generated during the implementation process, and the short-term outcomes and longer-term impacts that can be attributed to the program.

M&E uses quantitative indicators (numeric metrics) and qualitative indicators (descriptive observations) as measures of the success of a program. In addition to measuring population health outcomes like mortality and disability, M&E can be used to track the performance of health systems by quantifying the coverage rates for various interventions, tallying the financial, human, and material resources invested in health systems, evaluating the satisfaction of clients with health service providers and public health programs, determining which interventions are cost-effective, and tracking the inequalities that may remain within a health system.[49] M&E can also examine whether progress is being made toward a program becoming locally sustainable.

Effectiveness is a measure of the success of an intervention under real-world conditions (as opposed to efficacy, which measures success in ideal, laboratory-controlled conditions). **Efficiency** is an evaluation of the cost-effectiveness of an intervention that is based on both its effectiveness and resource considerations. **Cost-effectiveness analysis** (CEA) is a type of economic analysis that compares the health gains from an intervention to the financial costs of that intervention. The goal of CEA is to confirm that the funds spent on a health initiative are achieving the planned outcomes and are making efficient use of financial and other resources. CEA works best when the goals of a project are specific and measurable.

The most cost-effective global health interventions tend to be relatively inexpensive, can be easily distributed to many people, focus on prevention rather than treatment, and are targeted toward children and young adults so that they can avert many potential years of life lost to long-term disability or premature death. Some of the most cost-effective interventions include hygiene promotion for the prevention of diarrheal diseases, deworming medications to reduce the prevalence of soil-transmitted helminths in endemic areas, first-aid training for emergency care, intermittent preventive treatment of malaria in pregnant women in endemic areas, and bednets for malaria prevention.[50] Expensive, high-tech solutions, such as coronary artery bypass surgery for treatment of ischemic heart disease, tend to be among the least cost-effective interventions.

CEA is not by itself sufficient for making decisions about health financing priorities and evaluating the value of global health programs. One limitation is that cost-benefit analyses tend to promote interventions that have already proven to be successful, and they tend to undervalue pioneering interventions that have not yet been proven to reliably achieve results. New innovations are necessary for moving global health forward, but creative ideas are sometimes considered to be risky uses of resources. For example, successful vaccine programs are very cost-effective, but the upfront cost of research and development for a new vaccine is high and there is no guarantee that a safe, effective, licensed vaccine will be produced. It is important for some funding agencies and research organizations to be willing to risk failure so that new technologies and innovative approaches to solving global health problems can be developed.

Some cost-effectiveness analyses compare the cost of action to the cost of inaction. The costs of inaction include lost lives, lost productivity due to disease and disability, and the direct and indirect costs of medical care that are incurred when an intervention is not implemented to reduce the incidence and prevalence of preventable and treatable health conditions. When it is expensive not to address public health problems, cost-effectiveness analyses can demonstrate that disease prevention and control initiatives will yield long-term savings. However, this reveals another shortcoming of cost–benefit analysis: CEA often requires analysts to make judgments about what a healthy life is worth. The calculations may require an estimate of how much it costs a disabled person to be unable to work, or they may demand an approximation of how much an additional year of life is worth for a

70-year-old compared to a 7-year-old. While these sorts of estimates may be helpful at the population planning level, they break down at the individual level. Estimates of lost wages do not capture the burden of lost self-sufficiency that may accompany a disability, and few families would put a price tag on grandpa and deem his year of life to be worth less than that of his grandchild.

Global health statistics, budget spreadsheets, and numbers-heavy progress reports sometimes seem to reduce real people to nameless, faceless masses: a few million children dying from preventable diseases like diarrhea and malaria, a few million people with treatable mental health disorders lacking access to therapy, a few million young adults with HIV infection gaining access to lifesaving antiretroviral medications, and a few million households gaining access to a reliable source of clean drinking water. But statistics cannot capture the profound grief experienced by families who lose a child, just as they cannot fully express how life-changing a new water well can be. Many groups include photographs of people in their annual reports and other publications as a reminder that their work is about real people whose lives are being affected in very real ways by health problems and health interventions. Even when monitoring and evaluation activities appear to be coldly quantitative, empathy and shared humanity are central to the process.

▶ References

1. McCoy D, Chand S, Sridhar D. Global health funding: How much, where it comes from and where it goes. *Health Policy Plann.* 2009;24:407–17.
2. *A guide to the project management body of knowledge (PMBOK® guide).* 5th ed. Newtown Square PA: Project Management Institute (PMI); 2013.
3. Oliveira-Cruz V, Kurowski C, Mills A. Delivery of priority health services: Serving for synergies within the vertical versus horizontal debate. *J Int Dev.* 2003;15:67–86.
4. Szlezák NA, Bloom BR, Jamison JT, et al. The global health system: Actors, norms, and expectations in transition. *PLoS Med.* 2010;7:e1000183.
5. Frieden TR. Government's role in protecting health and safety. *N Engl J Med.* 2013;368:1857–9.
6. Macfarlane S, Racelis M, Muli-Musiime F. Public health in developing countries. *Lancet.* 2000;356:841–6.
7. *Centers for Disease Control and Prevention's Strategic Framework FY 2016–FY 2020.* Atlanta GA: CDC; 2016.
8. Feldbaum H, Lee K, Michaud J. Global health and foreign policy. *Epidemiol Rev.* 2010;32:82–92.
9. *3D planning guide: Diplomacy, development, defense.* Washington DC: USAID; 2012.
10. Katz R, Kornblet S, Arnold G, Lief E, Fischer JE. Defining health diplomacy: Changing demands in the era of globalization. *Milbank Q.* 2011;89:503–23.
11. Feldbaum H, Michaud J. Health diplomacy and the enduring relevance of foreign policy interests. *PLoS Med.* 2010;7:e1000226.
12. *Annual Report and Accounts 2015–16.* London: DFID; 2016.
13. *Japan International Cooperation Agency Annual Report 2016.* Tokyo: JICA; 2016.
14. *Shared progress, shared future: Agency financial report fiscal year 2016.* Washington DC: USAID; 2016.
15. Himelfarb T. *50 years of global health: Saving lives and building futures.* Washington DC: USAID; 2013.
16. *Charter of the United Nations.* San Francisco CA: UN; 1945.
17. *Global environmental outlook 5 (GEO5): Environment for the future we want.* Nairobi: UNEP; 2012.
18. *UNICEF's strategy for health (2016–2030).* New York: UNICEF; 2015.
19. Brown TM, Cueto M, Fee E. The World Health Organization and the transition from "international" to "global" public health. *Am J Public Health.* 2006;96:62–72.
20. *WHO 12th General Programme of Work 2014–2019: Not merely the absence of disease.* Geneva: WHO; 2014.
21. Bettcher D, Lee K. Globalisation and public health. *J Epidemiol Commun Health.* 2002;56:8–17.
22. *International Health Regulations (2005): Areas of work for implementation.* Geneva: WHO; 2007.
23. Lee K, Dodgson R. Globalization and cholera: Implications for global governance. *Glob Gov.* 2000; 6:213–36.
24. *International Health Regulations (2005).* 3rd ed. Geneva: WHO; 2016.
25. Peiris JSM, Yuen KY, Osterhaus ADME, Stöhr K. The severe acute respiratory syndrome. *N Engl J Med.* 2003;349:2431–41.
26. Cherry JD. The chronology of the 2002–2003 SARS mini pandemic. *Pediatr Respir Rev.* 2004;5:262–69.

27. Lipsitch M, Cohen T, Cooper B, et al. Transmission dynamics and control of severe acute respiratory syndrome. *Science.* 2003;300:1966–70.

28. Heymann DL. The international response to the outbreak of SARS in 2003. *Philos Trans R Soc Lond B Biol Sci.* 2004;359:1227–9.

29. Fidler DP, Gostin LO. The new International Health Regulations: An historic development for international law and public health. *J Law Med Ethics.* 2006;34:85–94.

30. Mercy JA, Rosenberg ML, Powell KE, Broome CV, Roper WL. Public health policy for preventing violence. *Health Aff.* 1993;12:7–29.

31. Madhav N, Opopenheim B, Gallivan M, Mulembakani P, Rubin E, Wolfe N. Pandemics: Risks, impacts, and mitigation (Chapter 17). *Disease control priorities*, 3rd ed. *Disease control priorities (Volume 9)*. Washington DC: IBRD/World Bank; 2017.

32. Bennett B, Carney T. Public health emergencies of international concern: Global, regional, and local responses to risk. *Med Law Rev.* 2017;25:223–39.

33. *Financing global health 2015: Development assistance steady on the path to new Global Goals.* Seattle: Institute for Health Metrics and Evaluation; 2016.

34. Widdus R. Public–private partnerships for health: Their main targets, their diversity and their future directions. *Bull World Health Organ.* 2001;79:713–20.

35. *Results Report 2016.* Geneva: The Global Fund; 2016.

36. *Keeping children healthy: The vaccine alliance progress report 2015.* Washington DC: Gavi; 2015.

37. Frost LJ, Reich MR. *Access: How do good health technologies get to poor people in poor countries?* Cambridge MA: Harvard Center for Population and Development Studies; 2008.

38. Buse K, Harmer AM. Seven habits of highly effective global public-private health partnerships: Practice and potential. *Soc Sci Med.* 2007;64:259–71.

39. Antrobus P. Funding for NGOs: Issues and options. *World Dev.* 1987;15(Suppl 1):95–102.

40. Stein JG. In the eye of the storm: Humanitarian NGOs, complex emergencies, and conflict resolution. *Peace Conflict Stud.* 2001;8:2.

41. Majiyagbe J. The volunteers' contribution to polio eradication. *Bull World Health Organ.* 2004;82:2.

42. *The logistics handbook: A practical guide for the supply chain management of health commodities.* 2nd ed. Arlington VA: USAID; 2011.

43. *Top 40 vendors.* Washington DC: USAID; 2015.

44. Carr SC, McWha I, MacLachlan M, Furnham A. International–local remuneration differences across six countries: Do they undermine poverty reduction work? *Int J Psychol.* 45:321–40.

45. Bonache J, Sanchez JI, Zárraga-Oberty C. The interaction of expatriate pay differential and expatriate inputs on host country nationals' pay unfairness. *Int J Hum Resour Manage.* 2009;20:2135–49.

46. Kickbusch I, Allen L, Franz C. The commercial determinants of health. *Lancet Global Health.* 2016;4:e895–6.

47. *The Bangkok Charter for Health Promotion in a Globalized World.* Geneva: WHO; 2005.

48. Moran M. The grand convergence: Closing the divide between public health funding and global health needs. *PLoS Biol.* 2016;14:e1002363.

49. Murray CJ, Frenk J. Health metrics and evaluation: Strengthening the science. *Lancet.* 2008;371:1191–9.

50. Laxminarayan R, Mills AJ, Breman JG, et al. Advancement of global health: Key messages from the disease control priorities project. *Lancet.* 2006;367:1193–208.

CHAPTER 8

HIV/AIDS and Tuberculosis

The coordinated global efforts to respond to the HIV pandemic in the 1990s and 2000s transformed global health, significantly expanding the financial resources available for combatting infectious diseases and bringing together public- and private-sector partners from countries across the income spectrum. Collaborative approaches for financing and implementing global health activities are also being used to address shared concerns about tuberculosis, drug-resistant infections, and other dangerous infectious diseases.

▶ 8.1 HIV/AIDS, TB, and Global Health

HIV/AIDS, tuberculosis (TB), and malaria are among the infections that cause the most deaths worldwide each year. These "big three" infectious diseases have been the target of numerous initiatives that aim to prevent, diagnose, and treat as many cases as possible. The rapid expansion of the global HIV epidemic during the 1980s and 1990s, in particular, was the primary driver of the shift from traditional international health practices to modern global health approaches.[1] Together, the three diseases are the focus of the Global Fund to Fight AIDS, TB and Malaria (usually just called the **Global Fund**), which was founded in 2002 and has used more than $30 billion donated by the governments of high-income countries and other partner organizations to provide antiretroviral medications to millions of people with HIV, distribute billions of condoms, dispense antibiotics to millions of people with TB, distribute hundreds of

millions of bednets to people living in malaria-endemic areas, treat millions of cases of malaria, and strengthen health systems in low- and middle-income countries, among other achievements.[2] These diseases are also the focus of specialized multilateral organizations and agencies, like the Joint United Nations Programme on HIV/AIDS (UNAIDS); global partnerships and alliances, like the Stop TB Partnership; diplomatic efforts, such as the President's Emergency Plan for AIDS Relief (PEPFAR) and the President's Malaria Initiative (PMI) in the United States; scientific collaborations like the International AIDS Vaccine Initiative (IAVI) and the TB Drug Accelerator program; and countless charitable organizations. These investments are made for a diversity of overlapping reasons: the humanitarian impulse to save lives, the recognition that contagious diseases can easily spread across national borders, and the observation that healthier countries and communities promote global security because they tend to have stronger economies and more stable political systems.[3]

Disease	HIV/AIDS	TB	Malaria
Type of infectious agent	Virus	Bacterium	Protozoan
Infectious agent	Human immunodeficiency virus (HIV)	Mycobacterium tuberculosis	Several types of *Plasmodium*
Primary mode(s) of transmission	Sexual contact and injecting drug use	Airborne by droplet spread	Mosquito bites
Can it be cured with medication?	No	Yes	Yes
Estimated number of deaths in 2015	1,100,000	1,769,000 (including 389,000 people with HIV)	438,000
Estimated number of deaths of children in 2015	Aged 0–14 years 110,000	Aged 0–14 years 210,000 (including 41,000 children with HIV)	Aged 0–5 years 306,000
% of deaths from the disease that occur in children	Aged 0–14 years 10%	Aged 0–14 years 12%	Aged 0–5 years 70%

FIGURE 8–1 Comparison of HIV/AIDS, TB, and malaria.

Data from *AIDS by the numbers 2016*. Geneva: UNAIDS; 2016. *Global tuberculosis report 2016*. Geneva: WHO; 2016. *World malaria report 2015*. Geneva: WHO; 2015.

Most large-scale HIV, TB, and malaria programs have targeted just one of the diseases, and a comparison of the three conditions shows why integrated programs have not been the norm (**FIGURE 8–1**). Each of the three infections is caused by a different type of agent, and they require different types of clinical care. Each has a distinct primary mode of transmission, which means that different prevention strategies are required. Each causes hundreds of thousands of deaths each year, so each demands a large-scale response. Each affects people of all ages, but children bear a greater burden from malaria than from HIV and TB. However, there are similarities across the disease control strategies, too, with all requiring the financial, technical, and operational support of dozens of different players,

including international and national governmental agencies, a variety of nongovernmental organizations, businesses, charitable foundations, scientists and other researchers, health professionals, and local volunteers.

▶ 8.2 Viruses, Bacteria, and Fungi

There are many different types of pathogens that can cause infection, including viruses, bacteria, fungi, and parasites (**FIGURE 8–2**). Different infectious agents require different methods of prevention and treatment. Approaches for the prevention and control of HIV, TB, and other infections must be tailored to the type of

Type of Agent	Viruses	Bacteria	Fungi
Relative size	Small	Medium	Large
Number of cells	Acellular (non-cellular)	Single-celled prokaryote	Single-celled or multi-cellular eukaryote
Nucleic acids	DNA or RNA (1 nucleocapsid)	DNA and RNA (1 chromosome)	DNA and RNA (2+ chromosomes)
Cell nucleus	None	Nucleoid region	True nucleus
Nuclear membrane	No	No	Yes
Cell organelles	No	No	Yes
Cellular membrane	No	Yes	Yes
Cell wall	No	Yes (peptidoglycan)	Yes (chitin)

FIGURE 8–2 Comparison of viruses, bacteria, and fungi.

infection, the usual mode of transmission, and the technologies and other resources that are available to prevent and treat the infection.

A **virus** is a piece of nucleic acid (DNA or RNA) encased in a shell made of proteins and sometimes also fatty acids. Viruses are extremely tiny, and because they are acellular (not cells), they are generally not considered to be alive. They can only replicate by invading the cells of a living host and taking control of the cells' nuclei. When a virus enters the body, spikes on the outer part of the virus, called a capsid, attach to the surface of a human cell. The outside of the virus is shed and the genetic material from inside the virus penetrates the cell and travels to the nucleus, where the virus takes command and directs the infected cell to make many new copies of the virus. The newly formed copies of the virus travel to the edge of the cell and enter new capsids. When released from the cell, the new virus particles travel to other parts of the body, infecting other cells, or they are shed from the body to infect other people.

The human body will clear most acute viral infections on its own, but some viruses become chronic infections, such as HIV and hepatitis C virus. For some types of viral infections, it is possible to take medications that reduce the number of virus particles present in the body and help mitigate the symptoms of infection. For example, antiviral medications can slow the progression of HIV infection, suppress the lesions caused by the herpes virus, and make influenza infections less severe. However, the better option is to take steps to prevent contracting a virus. Some viral infections can be prevented by vaccines, including chickenpox, hepatitis B, human papillomavirus (HPV), measles, polio, and rotavirus. Personal hygiene and health practices, such as handwashing and covering one's mouth when sneezing or coughing, can limit the transmission of many other viruses. Viral infections cannot be cured by antibiotics designed to kill bacteria and parasites. Treating viral infections inappropriately by prescribing antibiotics poses a serious threat to global health by contributing to the development of antimicrobial resistance.

A **bacterium** is a microscopic single-celled prokaryotic organism. Bacteria can be differentiated based on their shapes, such as rods (bacilli), spheres (cocci), and spirals (spirochetes, vibrios, and spirilla); by relative size (although all are very small); and by the amount of a substance called peptidoglycan in their cell walls. The peptidoglycan on the surface of Gram-positive bacteria will bond to a special dye. Gram-negative bacteria have an outer membrane over the peptidoglycan layer, so the dye will not stain them. Bacteria are found nearly everywhere on the planet, from the arctic tundra to hot springs deep in the ocean. They play an important role in decomposition and chemical cycling, in the fixation of nitrogen into plants, and in the production of alcohol and foods like cheese and yogurt. Millions of helpful bacteria line the digestive tracts and other surfaces of humans, crowding out harmful bacteria. However, some types of bacteria can cause disease. For example, some strains of *Escherichia coli* can cause diarrhea, and some strains of *Staphylococcus* can cause skin disease.

Bacteria cause illness in a variety of ways. Many symptoms of gastrointestinal bacterial infections are the result of endotoxins being released from Gram-negative bacteria when the bacteria die and disintegrate. Some bacteria produce exotoxins, like the ones that cause botulism and tetanus. Tetanus and several other bacterial diseases are vaccine-preventable, including whooping cough, pneumococcal pneumonia, and bacterial meningitis. Most bacterial infections can be cured with antibiotics, although a growing number of pathogenic (disease-causing) bacteria are becoming resistant to common antibiotics.

A **fungus** is a eukaryotic organism. Fungi come in many forms, including molds (multicellular threads or filaments called hyphae) and yeasts (single-celled fungi that reproduce by budding). Fungi are important decomposers used to make bread, wine, and cheese, but some are pathogenic. Fungal diseases frequently occur after the bacteria that normally live in or on the body are disturbed by antibiotic use or immunosuppression. For example, the fungus *Candida albicans* is normally found on human skin, especially around moist areas like the mouth, groin, and underarms. Sometimes an overgrowth of *Candida*, called

candidiasis, occurs and presents as thrush (a white coating on the tongue), a vaginal yeast infection, or diaper rash. Other examples of fungal infections include histoplasmosis, which is spread through animal droppings, and dermatomycoses (fungal diseases of the skin) like ringworm and athlete's foot. Fungi thrive in moist, dark places, and are especially common in the tropics. Antifungal medications can treat some fungal diseases.

▶ 8.3 HIV and AIDS

Human immunodeficiency virus (HIV) is a viral infection spread when body fluids like blood, semen, vaginal fluid, or breastmilk are exchanged during sexual contact, the sharing of needles used to inject drugs, or by mother-to-child transmission during childbirth or breastfeeding. HIV is not transmitted through casual contact like shaking hands, sharing eating utensils, or using the same toilet. Transmission of HIV through blood transfusions is rare now that donated blood and blood products can be tested for HIV. The virus destroys specialized white blood cells that are needed by the immune system to fight infection, especially **CD4 cells**, also called T cells or CD4+ T-helper cells, which are lymphocytes that have a CD4 glycoprotein on their surfaces. Most HIV infections are caused by HIV virus type 1, or HIV-1. There is also an HIV-2 virus that accounts for a small fraction of the HIV cases, primarily in West Africa. HIV-2 progresses more slowly and causes milder symptoms than HIV-1.[4]

Acquired immunodeficiency syndrome (AIDS) is characterized by the onset of illnesses occurring as a result of the destruction of immune system cells by the HIV virus. A **sign** is an objective indicator of disease that can be clinically observed, such as a rash, cough, fever, or elevated blood pressure. A **symptom** is a subjective indication of illness that is experienced by an individual but cannot be observed by others, such as a headache, stomachache, pain, or fatigue. A **syndrome** is a collection of signs and symptoms that occur together. HIV is contagious, because it is a transmissible virus; AIDS is not contagious, because it is a syndrome related to HIV infection and it is not an infectious agent. The secondary infections associated with AIDS are called **opportunistic infections (OIs)** because they only occur when the body's immune system is weakened enough to give the infectious agents an opportunity to invade. The

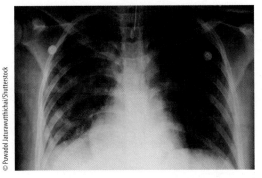

X-ray showing signs of pulmonary tuberculosis.

most common OIs include TB, bacterial pneumonia, chronic diarrhea, and fungal infections, such as *Cryptococcus*.[5]

A person newly infected with HIV may experience flu-like symptoms for a few days or weeks, but is often asymptomatic (**FIGURE 8-3**). During this stage, the newly infected individual still has a normal number of CD4 cells, but there is a high viral load in the blood (with many virus particles per cubic millimeter) and it is possible to transmit the virus. The World Health Organization (WHO) identifies four clinical stages of HIV infection and AIDS disease that follow primary infection (**FIGURE 8-4**).[5] In stages 1 and 2, which can last from a few weeks to more than 20 years, the infected person is asymptomatic or has only minor symptoms like skin infections and recurrent respiratory infections. Stage 3 is marked by more severe symptoms like recurrent respiratory infections, persistent fevers, TB, mouth ulcers, and the loss of more than 10% of body weight

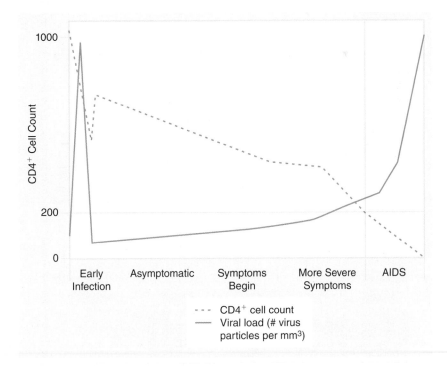

FIGURE 8-3 CD4+ cell count and viral load following HIV infection.

Stage	Primary HIV Infection	Clinical Stage 1	Clinical Stage 2	Clinical Stage 3	Clinical Stage 4 (AIDS)
HIV-associated symptoms	Mild	Asymptomatic	Mild	Advanced	Severe
Weight	Normal	Normal	Loss of less than 10% of body weight	Loss of more than 10% of body weight	HIV wasting syndrome
Activity level	Asymptomatic	Asymptomatic, normal activity	Symptomatic, normal activity	Bedridden less than 50% of the day in the last month	Bedridden more than 50% of the day during the last month
Examples of common clinical conditions	Acute retroviral syndrome: flu-like symptoms about 2–4 weeks after initial infection that resolve within a few weeks	Persistent enlargement of lymph nodes in several parts of body	Minor skin problems (like fungal infections and mouth ulcers) and upper respiratory infections	Chronic diarrhea, chronic fevers, thrush, pulmonary TB, and severe bacterial infections like pneumonia and meningitis	Chronic diarrhea, chronic fevers, complex infections, and HIV-associated cancers

FIGURE 8–4 Clinical staging system for HIV/AIDS.

Data from *WHO case definitions of HIV for surveillance and revised clinical staging and immunological classification of HIV-related disease in adults and children. Geneva: WHO; 2007.*

due to chronic diarrhea. The CD4 count begins to fall and the viral load in the blood begins to increase. In stage 4, serious OIs mark the onset of AIDS, and the CD4 count becomes very low (below 200 particles per mm³) and may fall to undetectable levels.

There is currently no HIV vaccine and no medication that can cure HIV infection.[6] However, people who have contracted the virus can take **antiretroviral (ARV)** medications to keep the viral count low and slow the progression of symptoms. **Antiretroviral therapy (ART)**, also called **highly active antiretroviral therapy (HAART)**, uses combinations (sometimes called "cocktails") of three or more different medicines to combat HIV, including nucleoside reverse transcriptase inhibitors (NRTIs), such as tenofovir, lamivudine, abacavir, emtricitabine, and zidovudine (AZT); non-nucleoside reverse transcriptase inhibitors (NNRTIs), such as efavirenz and nevirapine; protease inhibitors, such as lopinavir, ritonavir, and darunavir; and integrase inhibitors. ART does not work for all people with HIV: some cannot tolerate the side effects, some do not adhere to the treatment regimen and skip too many doses for the medicines to be effective, and some have a drug-resistant strain of HIV.[7] Even if the medications reduce the viral load, they do not cure the HIV infection or alleviate all of the symptoms. However, for most people with HIV, ART is effective at managing HIV as a chronic condition and enabling many years of healthy life that would be impossible without the medicines. Even if one of the many HIV candidate vaccines under development proves to be highly effective and is added to the tools available for HIV prevention,[8] there will still be a continued need for HIV treatment services for individuals who already have HIV infections.[9]

The **natural history of disease** describes the typical timeline from initial infection with a particular agent to either recovery or death. The median survival time after infection with HIV if a person does not take ART is about 10 years, including an average of 2 years from onset of clinical AIDS to death.[10] ART prolongs both the duration of time between infection and the onset of clinical AIDS and the time between onset of AIDS and death, extending the lives of people with HIV infection by years or even decades.[11] The current WHO recommendation is for treatment with ARVs to begin immediately after diagnosis, since earlier use of ARVs is associated with better outcomes than delayed treatment.[12] Use of prophylactic doses of co-trimoxazole (a combination of two antibiotics, sulfamethoxazole and trimethoprim) is recommended for people with advanced HIV to reduce the risk of bacterial, fungal, and protozoal OIs, and isoniazid can be used as preventive treatment in people with HIV who are at risk of TB disease.[12]

▶ 8.4 HIV/AIDS Epidemiology

Phylogenetic analysis of stored serological specimens suggest that the first cases of HIV infection in humans probably occurred in the 1920s in Central Africa in what is now the Democratic Republic of the Congo.[13] The first cases of AIDS were not diagnosed until 1981, when clusters of homosexual men in the United States were diagnosed with fungal *Pneumocystis carinii* pneumonia (PCP)[14] and with Kaposi's sarcoma, which until then had been a very infrequently observed type of cancer.[15] The HIV-1 virus was not identified by virologists until several years later.[16] Over the subsequent years, the epidemic spread across the globe and the prevalence of HIV infection increased dramatically.[17] By 1990, there were nearly 10 million people living with HIV. That number increased to 20 million by the mid-1990s, more than 30 million by 2005, and about 37 million by 2015 (**FIGURE 8–5**).[18] Sub-Saharan Africa was hit the hardest. In the 1990s and early 2000s, AIDS caused life expectancies to plummet in many countries, and it dramatically altered the social structure in many communities.[19]

Because nearly all infections and deaths were occurring in young- and middle-aged adults, many older adults had to become caregivers for both their sick adult children and their young grandchildren. Orphans and vulnerable children (OVCs) without family caregivers often ended up homeless and living in extreme poverty.[20]

UNAIDS estimates that about 2 million people contract HIV each year. This is an improvement from the more than 3 million cases per year that were occurring at the turn of the century.[21] However, it is concerning that the incidence plateaued after the year 2010 rather than continuing to decrease. UNAIDS and its many collaborators aim to dramatically reduce both the number of new HIV infections and the number of AIDS-related deaths between 2010 and 2030.[22] The ultimate target is to shrink the incidence to zero. As of 2015, little progress had been made toward reducing the annual number of incident cases to below 500,000 by 2020 and being on track to reduce the number of new cases to below 200,000 by 2030 (**FIGURE 8–6**).[21]

By contrast, the increasing number of people living with HIV is seen as a public health success, because it is the result of people with

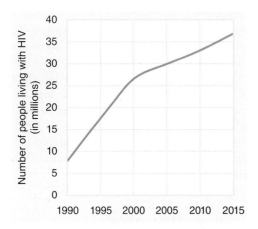

FIGURE 8–5 HIV prevalence: The number of people living with HIV worldwide has increased.

Data from GBD 2015 HIV Collaborators. Estimates of global, regional, and national incidence, prevalence, and mortality of HIV, 1980–2015: The Global Burden of Disease Study 2015. *Lancet. HIV* 2016;3:e361–87.

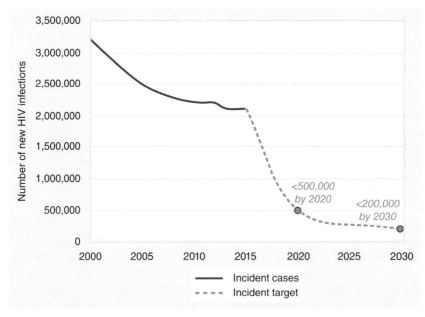

FIGURE 8–6 HIV incidence: The number of new HIV infections each year has stabilized rather than continuing to decrease.

Data from *AIDS by the numbers 2016*. Geneva: UNAIDS; 2016.

HIV living longer. There were about 1.1 million HIV/AIDS deaths in 2015, which was much lower than the 2 million deaths that occurred during the peak of the epidemic in 2005.[21] This represents good progress toward reducing HIV mortality to below 500,000 deaths in 2020 and 200,000 deaths in 2030 (**FIGURE 8–7**). In the absence of a cure for HIV, the long-term goal is to stabilize the prevalence of HIV by reducing the incidence to zero and lowering the mortality rate from AIDS to zero, and then for the prevalence of HIV to slowly decrease to zero as people with HIV die in older adulthood of diseases not related to HIV infection.

One of the challenges in tracking progress toward achieving these epidemiological goals is that many countries do not compile and disseminate reliable statistics about HIV incidence, prevalence, and mortality. However, model-based estimates, such as those from the Global Burden of Disease collaboration, allow for a comparison of the epidemiological situations in each nation.[18] About 1 in 200 people worldwide (across all ages) has HIV infection

(**FIGURE 8–8**). Some countries (such as Iran) have a rate close to 0%, while some countries in sub-Saharan Africa (such as Nigeria) have a prevalence considerably higher than the global average (**FIGURE 8–9**). The **proportionate mortality rate** is the percentage of all deceased people who succumbed to a particular cause. About 1 in 50 people worldwide who died in 2015 died from HIV/AIDS, but the proportionate mortality rates for HIV/AIDS by country are heterogeneous (**FIGURE 8–10**). There are also significant differences by country in the HIV mortality rate per 100,000 residents (**FIGURE 8–11**).

More than half of the people living with HIV worldwide in 2015 were females (**FIGURE 8–12**), and half of new cases of HIV worldwide occurred in females (**FIGURE 8–13**), with significant variations between countries in the distribution of cases by age and sex.[18] Hormones and vaginal anatomy, physiology, and microbiology make females more susceptible than males to HIV and other sexually transmitted infections.[23] Women are at least twice as likely as men to acquire HIV from an

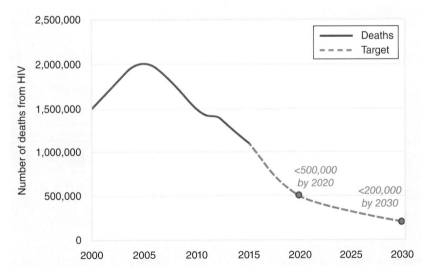

FIGURE 8–7 HIV mortality: The number of deaths from HIV each year has decreased as more people gain access to ART.

Data from *AIDS by the numbers 2016*. Geneva: UNAIDS; 2016.

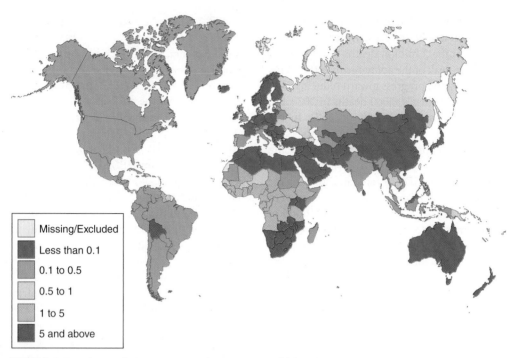

FIGURE 8–8 Prevalence of HIV among people 15–49 years old (2015).

Data from GBD 2015 HIV Collaborators. Estimates of global, regional, and national incidence, prevalence, and mortality of HIV, 1980–2015: The Global Burden of Disease Study 2015. *Lancet. HIV* 2016;3:e361–87.

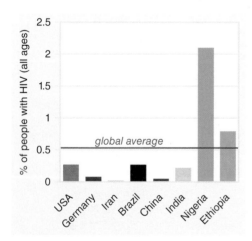

FIGURE 8–9 HIV prevalence: Percentage of people (all ages) living with HIV in featured countries in 2015.

Data from GBD 2015 HIV Collaborators. Estimates of global, regional, and national incidence, prevalence, and mortality of HIV, 1980–2015: The Global Burden of Disease Study 2015. *Lancet. HIV* 2016;3:e361–87.

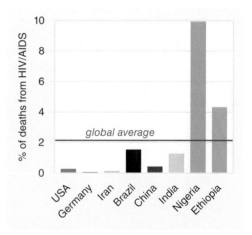

FIGURE 8–10 HIV mortality: Percentage of total deaths (all ages) due to HIV/AIDS in featured countries in 2015.

Data from GBD 2015 HIV Collaborators. Estimates of global, regional, and national incidence, prevalence, and mortality of HIV, 1980–2015: The Global Burden of Disease Study 2015. *Lancet. HIV* 2016;3:e361–87.

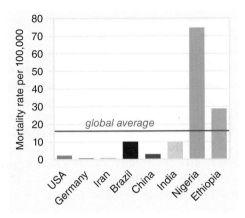

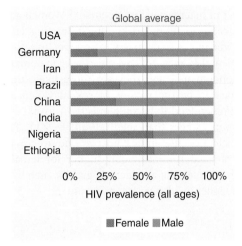

FIGURE 8–11 HIV mortality: HIV death rates per 100,000 people (all ages) in featured countries in 2015.

Data from GBD 2015 HIV Collaborators. Estimates of global, regional, and national incidence, prevalence, and mortality of HIV, 1980–2015: The Global Burden of Disease Study 2015. *Lancet. HIV* 2016;3:e361–87.

FIGURE 8–12 HIV prevalence: Percentage of people living with HIV in featured countries in 2015 who were female.

Data from GBD 2015 HIV Collaborators. Estimates of global, regional, and national incidence, prevalence, and mortality of HIV, 1980–2015: The Global Burden of Disease Study 2015. *Lancet. HIV* 2016;3:e361–87.

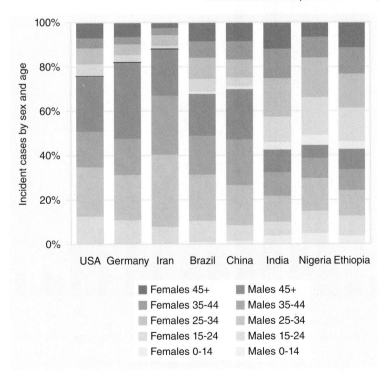

FIGURE 8–13 HIV incidence: Percentage of new cases by age and sex in featured countries in 2015.

Data from GBD 2015 HIV Collaborators. Estimates of global, regional, and national incidence, prevalence, and mortality of HIV, 1980–2015: The Global Burden of Disease Study 2015. *Lancet. HIV* 2016;3:e361–87.

act of heterosexual intercourse.[24] Women also face sociocultural risks for contracting HIV. Women generally marry at younger ages than men, they may not have the power to demand condom use, and they are more likely than men to be the victims of sexual violence.[25] Women tend to become infected with HIV at younger ages than men (**FIGURE 8–14**).[18] The incidence rate among people who are 15–29 years old is considerably higher for females than males. For all older age groups, men have a higher incidence rate than women.

Some populations have an elevated rate of HIV infection because they engage in behaviors that increase the likelihood of contact with blood and other body fluids or because discrimination may limit their access to health care. Key populations known to have special vulnerability to HIV infection include men who have sex with men (MSM), people who inject drugs (PWID), people in prison or other criminal justice detention centers, sex workers, and transgender people.[26] In most high-income countries, MSM, PWID, and their partners account for the

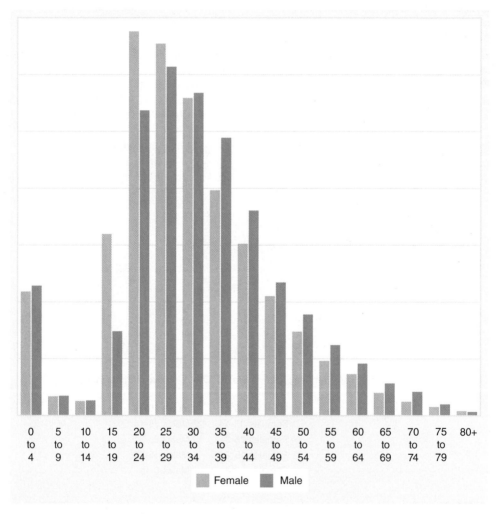

FIGURE 8–14 HIV incidence: The peak incidence rate occurs at younger ages for females than for males.

Data from GBD 2015 HIV Collaborators. Estimates of global, regional, and national incidence, prevalence, and mortality of HIV, 1980–2015: The Global Burden of Disease Study 2015. *Lancet. HIV* 2016;3:e361–87.

majority of new infections, and most incident cases occur in men; in the sub-Saharan African countries with the highest incidence rates, the majority of incident cases occur in women and members of these key populations account for only a minority of cases.[21]

▶ 8.5 HIV Interventions

The ultimate goal for control of the global HIV epidemic is to reduce the incidence of new viral infections to zero cases while simultaneously allowing all people who already have HIV infection to live long, healthy lives.[27] The reduction in the HIV mortality rate in recent years is a direct function of increased access to ART. Treating people with HIV is also a critical component of HIV prevention strategies because people who are taking ARVs often reduce their viral counts to such low levels that there is almost no risk of them passing the virus on to a sexual partner, even though the use of condoms is still recommended.

Testing for HIV enables people who have HIV infection to be diagnosed so that they can access treatment. **Voluntary counseling and testing (VCT)**, also called HIV testing and counseling (HTC), is a process of pre-test counseling about risk assessment, the testing process, and planned prevention and coping strategies; performance of an HIV test, typically using a rapid diagnostic test of blood or oral fluids; receipt of test results; and posttest counseling about risk reduction and disclosure of HIV status.[28] Testing is recommended for a diversity of individuals, including everyone with known exposure to HIV, everyone who is a member of a high-risk population, everyone with symptoms consistent with HIV infection, everyone diagnosed with a sexually transmitted infection, everyone diagnosed with TB, all pregnant women, and all blood donors.[29] All HIV testing services should ensure that the "5Cs" are present: consent, confidentiality, counseling before and after the test, correct (valid) test results, and connection through referral to prevention and treatment services.[29]

There has been a rapid increase in the percentage of people with HIV who are receiving ARVs (**FIGURE 8–15**).[21] The "15 by 15" goal of

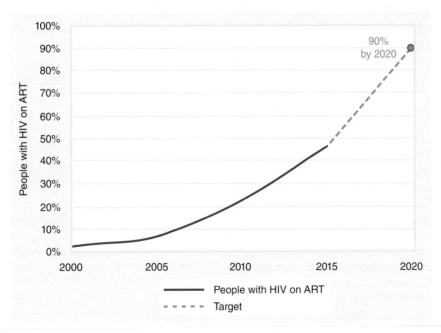

FIGURE 8–15 HIV treatment: The percentage of people with HIV who are taking ART has increased rapidly.

Data from *AIDS by the numbers 2016*. Geneva: UNAIDS; 2016.

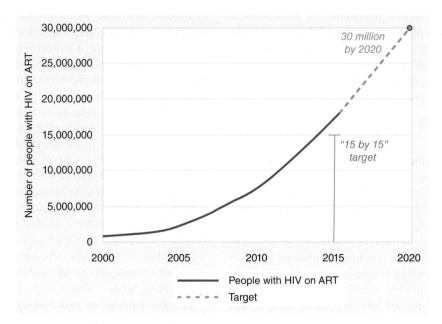

FIGURE 8–16 HIV treatment: The number of people with HIV who are taking ART has increased rapidly. Data from *AIDS by the numbers 2016*. Geneva: UNAIDS; 2016.

15 million people taking ART daily by 2015 was achieved (**FIGURE 8–16**).[30] However, an acceleration in the scale-up of ART programs will be necessary to meet the Fast-Track "90–90–90" goal of having at least 90% of people with HIV infection know their status, at least 90% of people with diagnosed HIV taking ART, and at least 90% of people on ART achieving viral suppression by 2020 (and then raising all three values to 95% by 2030).[31] Projections suggest that the target of having 30 million people with HIV on ART by 2020 is achievable, but many low- and middle-income countries are not on track to reach 90% ART use by 2020 (**FIGURE 8–17**). There are still millions of people with HIV infection who would benefit from access to HAART but do not have access to it because they cannot afford the treatment.

Mother-to-child transmission (MTCT), also called **vertical transmission**, is a mode of HIV transmission in which a pregnant woman passes a pathogen on to her offspring during pregnancy, delivery, or breastfeeding.[32] ARV use by pregnant women is a form of prevention of MTCT (PMTCT). In the absence

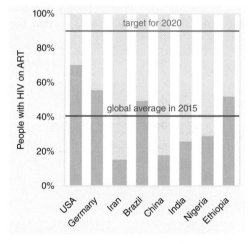

FIGURE 8–17 HIV treatment: ART use in featured countries in 2015.

Data from GBD 2015 HIV Collaborators. Estimates of global, regional, and national incidence, prevalence, and mortality of HIV, 1980–2015: The Global Burden of Disease Study 2015. *Lancet. HIV* 2016;3:e361–87.

of any ARV interventions, a baby born to an HIV-infected mother has about a 15%–30% risk of contracting HIV during delivery.[33] If the infant is breastfed for several months, the cumulative risk can be as high as 25%–45%.[33] If the mother takes ARVs during pregnancy and delivery—and in the weeks after delivery, if she is breastfeeding—the likelihood of transmission is much lower, only about 1% or 2%.[34] New mothers taking ARVs who have undetectable HIV viral counts are encouraged to breastfeed.[35] Some mothers with HIV infection who are not taking ARVs are encouraged to use formula instead of breastmilk when replacement feeding is acceptable, feasible, affordable, sustainable, and safe (AFASS).[35] When women cannot reliably afford formula or do not have consistent access to clean water, the risk of infant death due to diarrhea from unsafe water used to mix the formula may be greater than the risk of contracting HIV through breastmilk.

An increase in access to ARVs for pregnant women has helped to significantly decrease the number of new cases of HIV in children occurring each year (**FIGURE 8–18**).[21] Unfortunately, the tens of thousands of infants who are still acquiring HIV infection each year are evidence that too many pregnant and breastfeeding women with HIV are not taking ARV, because most incident cases of HIV in children are due to MTCT. Some of these women are not able to access the formal health system or prefer not to take medications. Some cannot afford ARVs or would be at risk of violence if they were found to be taking HIV medications. Some do not know their infection status, so they do not take steps to prevent vertical transmission.

ARVs are also used for **post-exposure prophylaxis (PEP)**, the process of taking medications after exposure to a pathogen in order to reduce the likelihood of contracting an infection. People with occupational exposures to HIV, such as a healthcare workers who have sustained a needle stick injury while treating a patient with HIV, and those with other unexpected potential exposures to HIV, such as the victims of sexual assaults, can take ARVs for a month as PEP to reduce the likelihood of infection.[36]

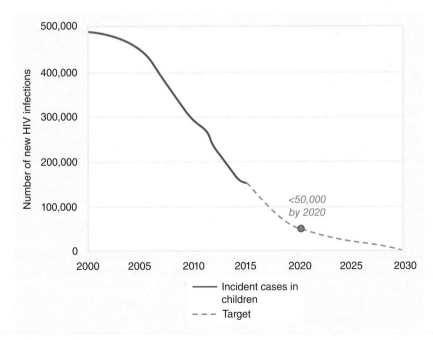

FIGURE 8–18 HIV incidence: The number of new HIV infections each year among children has decreased.
Data from *AIDS by the numbers 2016*. Geneva: UNAIDS; 2016.

Pre-exposure prophylaxis (PrEP) is the process of taking medications prior to a likely exposure to a pathogen in order to reduce the risk of contracting an infection. When both partners in a relationship undergo HIV testing and they are found to be discordant, with one member HIV-positive and the other HIV-negative, the HIV-negative partner can opt to take PrEP to reduce the risk of infection.[37]

There are also behavioral prevention methods that are recommended for all people to reduce the risk of contracting HIV. One is **universal precautions**, the use of barriers like gloves to prevent contact with blood or body fluids when caring for a sick person or cleaning up a spill or soiled laundry. Another is following the ABCs of HIV prevention: abstinence, being faithful to a partner if sexually active, and consistently and correctly using a condom during all sexual acts.[38] Although the risk of HIV per sexual act is usually low—less than 1 in 250 heterosexual contacts with a person who has HIV infection—the cumulative risk can be high, so consistent condom use is necessary.[39] Routine use of health services is also beneficial, since detection and treatment of other sexually transmitted infections reduce biological vulnerability to HIV.[40] Health workers in all regions of the world must continue HIV/AIDS education efforts because the incidence of new cases tends to increase when people stop worrying about their risk.

Several other harm reduction strategies are also being used for HIV prevention. Male **circumcision** is the surgical removal of the foreskin of the penis. Voluntary male medical circumcision (VMMC) in countries with high levels of HIV transmission where circumcision of male infants has not been the traditional practice has been shown to reduce incidence of HIV infection in men who undergo the procedure.[41] VMMC reduces the risk of HIV infection, but it does not negate the need to use condoms as protection against HIV and other sexually transmitted infections.[42] In some places, needle exchanges for injecting drug users have successfully helped reduce incidence.[43] Using a combination of approaches is often the best option to ensure protection of individuals and communities.[44] However, limited budgets for disease prevention and control mean that in most places only a few types of HIV services can be offered.[45]

Low- and middle-income countries (LMICs) are paying an increasing share of the costs of HIV prevention and treatment programs within their own borders—reaching nearly $11 billion by 2015—but international assistance for ARV programs and other services remains critical to the success of global control efforts.[22] In 2015, the governments of high-income countries invested about $7.5 billion in HIV/AIDS programs in LMICs.[46] About three-quarters of this spending was bilateral, with funding from the donor country being directly transferred to the recipient country. The remaining governmental funds were multilateral spending distributed through the Global Fund, Unitaid, and other partnerships. Private-sector donations to HIV/AIDS programs in LMICs from foundations, corporations, and individuals were estimated to exceed $600 million in 2015, with the Bill & Melinda Gates Foundation being the largest donor.[46]

The United States is the largest funder of HIV programs in LMICs in terms of dollars spent each year. The U.S. President's Emergency Plan for AIDS Relief (**PEPFAR**) was launched in 2003 when few people living with HIV in sub-Saharan Africa had access to ART. PEPFAR funding has enabled millions of people in LMICs to gain access to life-extending medications, and it has allowed millions of babies to be born HIV-free to mothers with HIV infection. In 2015 alone, nearly 6 million people in partner LMICs were receiving ARVs as a result of direct support from PEPFAR and nearly 4 million more were benefiting from technical support for ART programs.[47] PEPFAR also supports VCT programs that test tens of millions of people annually, sponsors VMMC programs in targeted regions, and funds programs that care for OVCs.[47]

▶ 8.6 Other Sexually Transmitted Infections

Besides HIV, several other pathogens can be transmitted through sexual contact (**FIGURE 8–19**). A **sexually transmitted infection (STI)** is an infection spread through sexual intercourse or other types of sexual contact.[48] STIs are often asymptomatic. When symptoms of an STI are present, the affected individual is considered to have a sexually transmitted disease (STD), also called a venereal disease.

Some of the most frequently occurring bacterial STIs worldwide are chlamydia, gonorrhea, and syphilis. About 130 million people each year contract **chlamydia**, an infection with *Chlamydia trachomatis*.[49] About 80 million people each year contract **gonorrhea**, an infection with *Neisseria gonorrhoeae*.[50] Gonorrhea and chlamydia are both often asymptomatic, especially in women,[51] but they may cause reproductive tract discharge and a burning sensation when urinating. If left undiagnosed and untreated, both infections can cause chronic health problems, such as **pelvic inflammatory disease (PID)**, an infection in the upper reproductive system (the uterus, ovaries, and other structures) that can cause pain and lead to scarring and infertility. Cases of drug-resistant gonorrhea that do not respond to standard therapies are a growing global health concern.[52] **Syphilis** is an infection with *Treponema pallidum*. About 5.6 million people contract syphilis each year, and the global prevalence is about 18 million because many people with syphilis have not been treated for it.[53] Untreated syphilis progresses through three clinical stages. Primary syphilis presents as a painless skin lesion called a chancre. The second stage is characterized by a rash on the palms of the hands and the soles of the feet as well as other symptoms, such as swollen lymph nodes and fatigue. Late stage syphilis may persist for years and cause weakened arterial walls and nervous system impairment.[54] When pregnant women have syphilis, there is a high rate of stillbirth, neonatal mortality, and birth defects associated with congenital syphilis.[55]

Disease	Agent Name	Type of Agent
Chlamydia	*Chlamydia trachomatis*	Bacterium
Gonorrhea	*Neisseria gonorrhoeae*	Bacterium
Syphilis	*Treponema pallidum*	Bacterium
HIV	Human immunodeficiency virus (HIV, retrovirus family)	Virus
Herpes	Herpes simplex virus (HSV-2, herpesvirus family)	Virus
HPV	Human papillomavirus (HPV, papillomavirus family)	Virus
Trichomoniasis	*Trichomonas vaginalis*	Protozoan
Crabs	*Pthirus pubis* (crab louse)	Insect

FIGURE 8–19 Examples of sexually transmitted infections (STIs).

Several STIs are caused by viruses, including herpes and HPV. Genital **herpes** is an infection with herpes simplex virus type 2 (HSV-2) that can cause painful genital ulcers.[56] More than 400 million people worldwide have HSV-2 infections, with an annual incidence of about 20 million cases.[57] (A related virus, HSV-1, causes lesions on the mouth that are often called "cold sores."[58]) Human papillomavirus (HPV) causes genital warts and significantly increases the risk of cervical cancer and cancers of the oropharynx, especially the throat.[59] A vaccine for HPV is now available in some countries,[60] but no successful vaccine has been developed for HIV or herpes. Although some medications, such as interferon, can help suppress some viral infections, no cures for these viral infections have been discovered.

A few parasites are also transmitted through sexual contact. **Trichomoniasis** is a protozoal infection with *Trichomonas vaginalis* that affects about 140 million people each year.[61] Pubic lice (*Phthirus pubis*), also called crabs or pediculosis pubis, are ectoparasites that cling to human hair, feed on human blood, and cause intense itching.[62]

STIs can be prevented by abstinence from sexual activity, the use of barriers such as condoms that limit direct contact with body fluids (although some infections may occur even with condom use), and treatment of infected individuals so that they do not transmit the infection to sexual partners.[63] Public health interventions to reduce the population-level burden from STIs include sex education, risk reduction counseling, condom distribution, HPV vaccination, screening for asymptomatic infections, treatment or management of diagnosed cases, and offering testing and treatment to sexual partners of known cases.[64] **Partner notification** is the process of a patient diagnosed with an STI communicating with his or her sexual partners (or a public health official communicating with the partners of the diagnosed individual) about their need to be tested so that they can receive appropriate treatment, if necessary, and they can take steps to protect the health of future partners.[65]

▶ 8.7 Tuberculosis

Tuberculosis (TB) is caused by the bacterium *Mycobacterium tuberculosis*, which is spread through airborne droplets.[66] TB can affect any part of the body, but it usually occurs in the lungs. TB affecting the lungs is called pulmonary TB. TB outside of the lungs is called extrapulmonary TB. Pulmonary TB used to be called consumption because people with the disease were "consumed" by it and developed a bloody cough, persistent fever, wasting, and pale skin. Anyone can become infected with TB, but the rate of infection is higher among low-income individuals and those who are undernourished, have underlying medical conditions, smoke tobacco, and live or work in crowded facilities that have poor ventilation and high levels of indoor air pollution.[67]

A distinction is made between having TB infection (latent TB) and having TB disease (active TB). An **infection** occurs when an infectious agent begins to reproduce inside a person. This usually causes an immunologic response specific to the agent, and that response can often be detected through laboratory testing. Many infections have a latent phase (also called an incubation period) when the infectious agent multiplies in the host but the infected individual does not feel sick. For TB, this stage is called **latent TB infection (LTBI)**. LTBI may persist for decades. **Disease** occurs when an infected person develops symptoms and becomes ill. When LTBI converts into a symptomatic, contagious form, it is called **TB disease** (or **active TB**). The symptoms of TB disease include fevers, weight loss, night sweats, and a cough that may produce bloody sputum (phlegm from the lungs). People with active TB are contagious, and if untreated they may infect several other people each year, especially if they have frequent and prolonged interactions with susceptible individuals.[68] About one in three people worldwide has been infected with the TB bacillus, but only about 5%–15% of people with LTBI who do not have HIV infection will develop TB disease during their lifetimes.[69] **Bacillus Calmette-Guérin (BCG)** is a TB vaccine used in many countries to confer some childhood protection against TB disease (and related complications, such as disseminated TB disease, which is the spread of TB bacteria from the lungs into other parts of the body), but BCG is not effective at preventing TB infection.[70]

The standard test for TB is the purified protein derivative (PPD) test, also called the Mantoux tuberculin skin test (TST), in which a small amount of TB bacterial protein is injected under the skin and the reaction is monitored. A person with TB infection will have an immune response and develop a rash at the injection site. (One of the disadvantages of BCG is that people who have received BCG usually test positive on PPD tests. Some workplaces and schools require employees and students to prove that they do not have TB, and people who have received BCG may require extra testing to show that they do not actually have TB.) An interferon-gamma release assay (IGRA) blood test is also available. If a person has a positive skin or blood test, a chest X-ray will be taken to look for lesions that might be pockets of TB infection. If pulmonary TB is suspected, a sputum smear test is conducted on the phlegm produced by deep coughs. A microscope is used to check the stained specimen for the presence of acid-fast bacilli (AFB). The diagnosis can be confirmed with a positive culture grown in a laboratory for several days. Laboratory tests for TB are used for clinically diagnosing people with symptoms of TB disease; as part of routine screening for people who have elevated risk for TB, such as people with HIV infection and those who have occupational exposure to silica;[71] and as part of outbreak responses that test contacts of TB cases so that treatment can be initiated before infected contacts develop TB disease.[72]

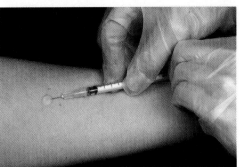

Tuberculin skin test (TST).

CDC/Gabrielle Benenson/Greg Knobloch

▶ 8.8 TB Interventions

The standard treatment regimen for TB involves taking a combination of up to five different medications (isoniazid, rifampicin, pyrazinamide, ethambutol, and streptomycin) every day for 6 months or longer.[73] The first 2 months are the most crucial, but following through with the full course of treatment is essential so that all of the bacteria are killed, including the hardiest organisms. The WHO-recommended treatment protocol is called **DOTS**, which is an acronym for directly observed therapy, short-course. DOTS is sometimes shortened to just DOT to emphasize that the key part of DOTS is the directly observed component. TB patients receiving DOTS are required to have a trained observer watch them take their pills every day. If the patient is hospitalized or reports to a clinic for his or her daily treatment, the observer might be a physician or nurse. If the treatment is community-based, the observer might be a shopkeeper or other community leader, or a family member who is supervised by another community member. If the patient misses a dose, a public health worker will track the patient down and try to ensure compliance. (Some countries have public health laws stipulating that people who are not compliant with TB treatment can be hospitalized under guard or imprisoned for the duration of their treatment, but most do not enforce these regulations.) However, the **case detection rate**

(CDR), the proportion of people with TB disease who are diagnosed, is low in many places. This means that many people who should take DOTS for TB are not undergoing treatment. A higher CDR would increase the treatment rate and decrease the TB mortality rate.

The Stop TB Strategy (2006–2015) led by the WHO spelled out a plan for achieving the Millennium Development Goals (MDGs) plans to reduce the prevalence of TB disease, reduce the number of deaths each year from TB, and increase the proportion of TB disease cases that are diagnosed and treated using a DOTS protocol.[74] The TB prevalence, which is the total number of people with active TB at any point in time, is reduced by lowering the incidence of TB and by curing active TB cases more quickly. The incidence of TB disease can be reduced by decreasing the incidence of LTBI and treating LTBI before it advances to TB disease. (Several new TB vaccines are being developed and tested, but they are not yet ready for widespread use.[75]) People with a high likelihood of developing active TB, such

as those with HIV, are a priority for LTBI treatment programs.[76] Strategies to reduce TB prevalence also reduce TB mortality.

Good progress toward reducing the global burden from TB was made under the Stop TB Strategy, with the incidence of TB disease decreasing gradually but steadily after 2000.[77] Between 2000 and 2015, there was a 42% reduction in overall prevalence of TB disease and a 47% reduction in mortality among people without HIV infection.[77] The Stop TB strategy has been replaced by a new End TB plan. The End TB Strategy (2016–2035) supports the achievement of the Sustainable Development Goals that aim to reduce TB incidence by 80% and TB deaths by 90% between 2015 and 2030. By 2035, the End TB Strategy aims to reduce TB incidence by 90% and TB deaths by 95% compared to 2015 levels.[78]

In 2015, there were an estimated 10.4 million new cases of TB disease worldwide, which is equivalent to an incidence rate of 142 per 100,000 people (**FIGURE 8–20**).[69] However, there is considerable uncertainty

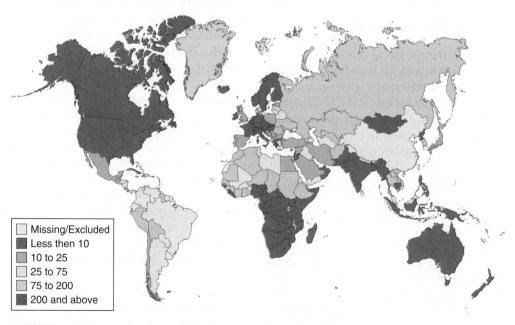

Missing/Excluded
Less then 10
10 to 25
25 to 75
75 to 200
200 and above

FIGURE 8-20 Incidence of new cases of TB disease per 100,000 people (2015).

Data from *Global tuberculosis report 2016*. Geneva: WHO; 2016.

about this number because of underdiagnosis and underreporting.[79] The actual incidence might be higher. The End TB Strategy aims to reduce the global incidence rate to 10 new cases per 100,000 people per year by 2035 (**FIGURE 8–21**). There is a special emphasis on the countries that have the highest TB rates and those with the highest number of cases. In 2015, six countries were home to 60% of the world's TB cases: India, Indonesia, China, Nigeria, Pakistan, and South Africa. That year, 1.4 million people died from TB, for a global mortality rate of 24 per 100,000 people.[69] The End TB Strategy aims to reduce the global TB mortality rate by 95% between 2015 and 2035 (**FIGURE 8–22**).

HIV treatment programs are an important contributor to TB control. People with HIV infection are about 30 times more likely to develop active TB disease than people without HIV infection, and TB is the leading cause of death for people with HIV.[80] In 2015, about one in three people who died from HIV/AIDS

died as a result of TB infection.[69] HIV-negative people who develop TB disease and are not treated for it have about a 43% case fatality rate; HIV-positive people who develop TB disease and are not taking ARVs or receiving TB treatment have about a 78% case fatality rate.[77] However, people with HIV infection can be successfully treated for TB if they are strong enough to survive several months of antibiotic treatment.[81] Treatment of LTBI, early diagnosis and initiation of treatment of TB disease, and early initiation of ART after HIV diagnosis all contribute to improved survival rates for people with HIV/TB coinfection.[82]

HIV/TB coinfections occur in every country, but the countries with the highest HIV prevalence rates have the highest burden from HIV-associated TB. In 2015, 1.2 million (11%) of the 10.4 million incident cases of TB disease worldwide occurred in people with HIV infection (**FIGURE 8–23**).[69] TB fatalities among people with HIV are classified as HIV deaths rather than as TB deaths, and in 2015, there

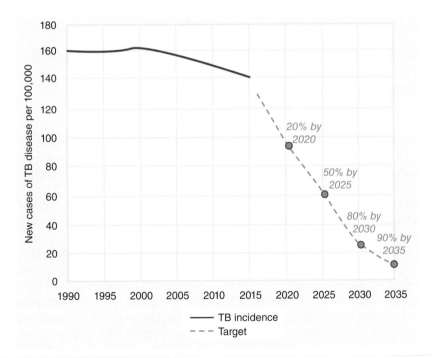

FIGURE 8–21 TB incidence: Approximate targets for reduction of the TB incidence rate.

Data from *Global tuberculosis report 2016*. Geneva: WHO; 2016.

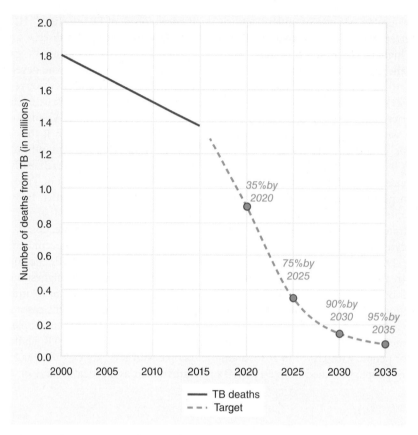

FIGURE 8-22 TB mortality: Approximate targets for reduction in the number of TB deaths (not including death from TB/HIV coinfection).

Data from *Global tuberculosis report 2016*. Geneva: WHO; 2016.

were about 390,000 people with HIV who died from TB in addition to the 1.4 million TB deaths in people without HIV (**FIGURE 8-24**). With access to treatment for HIV and TB, the TB survival rate for people with HIV infection is only slightly lower than the survival rate for people without HIV.[69]

Control of the spread of TB requires structures to be in place to support diagnosis and treatment, including a supply chain that provides consistent access to all essential TB medications in every country and a reporting system that allows governments to track their progress toward improved prevention, diagnosis, and treatment. Clinicians, public health workers, and members of communities with a high prevalence of TB play critical roles in local and national TB control by diagnosing, treating, and supporting individuals with TB disease. At the global level, TB control efforts are being led by the **Stop TB Partnership**, founded in 2000, which brings together representatives from hundreds of organizations— including WHO and other UN agencies, national and subnational governmental organizations, foundations, charities (including patient support networks), private-sector entities (including pharmaceutical and diagnostic companies), and universities and research institutions—to develop and operationalize action plans for reducing the global burden from TB.

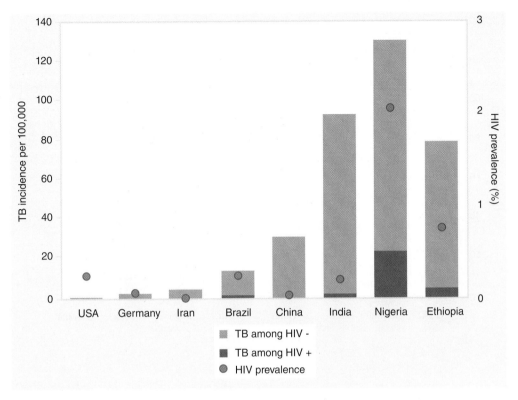

FIGURE 8–23 TB incidence: New cases of TB disease per 100,000 residents in 2015.

Data from *Global tuberculosis report 2016*. Geneva: WHO; 2016.

The Stop TB partners aim to eliminate TB as a public health problem by reducing the incidence of TB to less than 1 case per 1 million people by 2050.[83] This will be impossible to achieve without increased funding from domestic and international sources. In 2016, about $6.6 billion was spent on TB prevention and treatment in LMICs, but this was at least $2 billion less than the amount needed to fully implement the global TB strategy.[69] About 84% of this TB financing was from domestic sources, including out-of-pocket payments by people with TB and their families. Middle-income countries like Brazil and China fully fund their own TB programs, but the TB control programs in lower-income countries like India, Nigeria, and Ethiopia need additional support from international donors in order to make progress toward achieving global TB goals.[69]

▶ 8.9 Antimicrobial Resistance

Antibiotic medications that cure bacterial infections are a core part of many infectious disease control programs. There are also antimicrobial medications for other types of disease-causing agents, including antivirals, antiparasitics, and antifungal medications. A pathogen is sensitive to a medication if it is vulnerable to it. Bacteria are usually susceptible to certain types of antibiotics, and they will be killed when they are exposed to correct doses of the right classes of these medications. However, a growing number of these agents have developed resistance to at least some of the types of antibiotics that were once effective against them.[84] A pathogen is resistant to a medication if can withstand treatment with

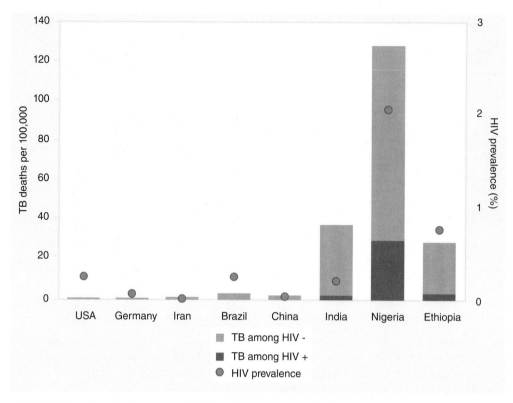

FIGURE 8–24 TB mortality: Deaths per 100,000 residents in 2015 (including cases among people with HIV infection).

Data from *Global tuberculosis report 2016*. Geneva: WHO; 2016.

it. Drug susceptibility testing (DST) can determine whether an infectious agent is sensitive or resistant to particular antimicrobials.

Antimicrobial resistance (AMR), or drug resistance, occurs when a pathogen that used to be susceptible to a particular type of therapeutic agent mutates in a way that makes the medication ineffective. The misuse and overuse of antibiotics are driving the development of AMR.[85] If someone has a mild bacterial infection, such as bronchitis or a mild ear infection, and takes antibiotics for only a few days rather than finishing the entire prescription, or if that person skips a few doses, that person will have killed off the susceptible, weaker bacteria, but the hardier bacteria will survive. This is a process that biologists call selection. The remaining bacteria may have developed resistance to the misused medication, which

means that it will be harder for that person to fight off the infection with common antibiotics. Worse yet, that person could spread this hardier strain to other people, for whom the common first-line antibiotics will not work at all. Antibiotics are also frequently overused in cattle, pigs, poultry, and other animal populations raised for food production.[86] Another misuse of antimicrobials is taking antibiotics for viral infections like the common cold. The individual taking the medications is not being helped by the antibiotic, and instead is killing off the body's helpful bacteria and allowing potentially harmful bacteria that are already in the body to proliferate. These stronger bacteria may develop drug resistance, necessitating that the infected person take yet another antibiotic.

Drug-resistant TB (DR-TB) is a growing global health problem. Among those who test positive for TB and begin treatment, the **default rate**, the proportion of people who are diagnosed but do not complete the full course of treatment, is high in some places. People who develop DR-TB as a result of defaulting on their treatment put their own lives at risk, and they also cause anyone they infect to have potentially life-threatening DR-TB. Multidrug-resistant TB (**MDR-TB**) is a TB strain that does not respond to two of the standard antibiotic therapies, rifampicin and isoniazid.[87] New concerns are arising about extensively drug-resistant TB (**XDR-TB**) that is resistant to rifampicin, isoniazid, fluoroquinolones, and at least one second-line injectable TB drug.[88] In 2015, about 3.9% of new cases of TB and 21% of previously treated cases were rifampicin-resistant TB (RR-TB) or MDR-TB, but in some countries and regions, the proportion is higher (**FIGURE 8–25**).[69] The MDR-TB rates are especially high in Eastern Europe and Central Asia. MDR-TB can be treated using a directly observed therapy approach (through a protocol sometimes called DOTS-Plus), but the medications are more expensive and the course of treatment is much longer, up to 2 years rather than 6 months.[89]

A **healthcare-associated infection (HAI)**, also called hospital-acquired infection or a **nosocomial infection**, is an infection that

is contracted while receiving care in a hospital, nursing or rehabilitation center, or another medical facility. HAIs include central line associated bloodstream infections, catheter associated urinary tract infections, surgical site infections, ventilator-associated pneumonia, *Clostridium difficile* infections, and others.[90] Some HAIs are drug resistant, such as MRSA. Methicillin-resistant *Staphylococcus aureus* (**MRSA**) is very difficult to treat, and it can cause severe "flesh-eating" infections (necrotizing fasciitis) and bloodstream infections. The first cases of MRSA were reported within months of methicillin being released for use as an antibiotic in 1960.[91] MRSA is now common in hospitals (where it is called hospital-acquired or HA-MRSA), but the infection can also be transmitted by unsterilized sports equipment and other everyday items that cause community-acquired MRSA (CA-MRSA).[92] Handwashing (by healthcare workers, patients, and visitors), the use of personal protective equipment, clean laundry, sterilized equipment, environmental sanitation, and waste management help prevent the spread of HAIs.[93] Patient risk is also reduced by avoiding unnecessary medical procedures and minimizing the use of invasive medical devices. Antimicrobial stewardship programs that ensure that patients are prescribed the right medications at the right doses for the right durations and through the right routes serve to limit the risk of adverse outcomes of HAIs, including drug-resistant infections.[94]

Inappropriate access to and use of medications in one nation can rapidly cause a global antimicrobial resistance problem.[95] Public health threats from drug resistance come from DR-TB, MRSA, drug-resistant types of Enterobacteriaceae (such as cephalosporin- and fluoroquinolone-resistant *E. coli* and cephalosporin- and carbapenem-resistant *Klebsiella pneumoniae*), penicillin-resistant *Streptococcus pneumoniae*, fluoroquinolone-resistant *Salmonella* and *Shigella*, and cephalosporin-resistant *N. gonorrhoeae*.[96] They also come from numerous other agents, including multidrug-resistant *Acinetobacter*, drug-resistant *Campylobacter*, vancomycin-resistant *Enterococcus* (VRE), multidrug-resistant *Pseudomonas*

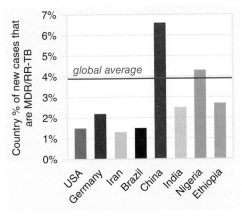

FIGURE 8–25 Percentage of new TB cases in 2015 that were multidrug-resistant (MDR-TB) and rifampicin-resistant (RR-TB).

Data from *Global tuberculosis report 2016*. Geneva: WHO; 2016.

aeruginosa, and others.[97] AMR prevention strategies include preventing infections so that antibiotics are not needed, expanding the use of diagnostic tests to ensure that appropriate antibiotics are prescribed, reducing the overuse of antibiotics to treat diseases in humans and livestock, and developing new types of antibiotics.[98] A new "superbug" that evolves anywhere in the world poses a threat to the whole world, so all countries must be committed to taking steps to prevent pathogens from developing resistance to new antibiotic medications and acting to address the challenges of containing the AMR strains already in circulation.[99]

▶ # References

1. Brandt AM. How AIDS invented global health. *N Engl J Med.* 2013;368:2149–52.
2. *Results report 2016.* Geneva: The Global Fund; 2016.
3. Horton R, Lo S. Investing in health: Why, what, and three reflections. *Lancet.* 2013;382:1859–61.
4. Maartens G, Celum C, Lewin SR. HIV infection: Epidemiology, pathogenesis, treatment, and prevention. *Lancet.* 2014;384:258–71.
5. *WHO case definitions of HIV for surveillance and revised clinical staging and immunological classification of HIV-related disease in adults and children.* Geneva: WHO; 2007.
6. The International AIDS Society Scientific Working Group on HIV Cure. Towards an HIV cure: A global scientific strategy. *Nat Rev Immunol.* 2012;12:607–14.
7. Chaiyachati KH, Ogbuoji O, Price M, Suthar AB, Negussie EK, Bärnighausen T. Interventions to improve adherence to antiretroviral therapy: A rapid systematic review. *AIDS.* 2014;28(Suppl 2): S187–204.
8. Safrit JT, Fast PE, Gieber L, Kuipers H, Dean HJ, Koff WC. Status of vaccine research and development of vaccines for HIV-1. *Vaccine.* 2016;34:2921–5.
9. Gray GE, Laher F, Doherty T, et al. Which new health technologies do we need to achieve an end to HIV/AIDS? *PLoS Biol.* 2016;14:e1002372.
10. Jaffar S, Grant AD, Whitworth J, Smith PG, Whittle H. The natural history of HIV-1 and HIV-2 infections in adults in Africa: A literature review. *Bull World Health Organ.* 2004;82:462–9.
11. Holmes C, Hallett T, Walensky R, Bärnighausen T, Pillay Y, Cohen M. Effectiveness and cost-effectiveness of treatment as prevention for HIV (Chapter 5). *Disease control priorities.* 3rd ed. *Major infectious diseases (Volume 6).* Washington DC: IBRD/World Bank; 2017.
12. *Consolidated guidelines on the use of antiretroviral drugs for treating and preventing HIV infection: Recommendations for a public health approach.* 2nd ed. Geneva: WHO; 2016.
13. Faria NR, Rambaut A, Suchard MA, et al. The early spread and epidemic ignition of HIV-1 in human populations. *Science.* 2014;346:56–61.
14. *Pneumocystis* pneumonia—Los Angeles, 1981. *MMWR Morb Mortal Wkly Rep.* 1981;30:250–2.
15. Jaffe HW, Bregman DJ, Selik RM. Acquired immune deficiency syndrome in the United States: The first 1000 cases. *J Infect Dis.* 1983;148:339–45.
16. Gallo RC, Montagnier L. The discovery of HIV as the cause of AIDS. *N Engl J Med.* 2003;349:2283–5.
17. Danforth K, Baxi S, Wideman D, Padian N. Global mortality and morbidity from HIV/AIDS (Chapter 2). *Disease control priorities.* 3rd ed. *Major infectious diseases (Volume 6).* Washington DC: IBRD/World Bank; 2017.
18. GBD 2015 HIV Collaborators. Estimates of global, regional, and national incidence, prevalence, and mortality of HIV, 1980–2015: The Global Burden of Disease Study 2015. *Lancet. HIV* 2016;3:e361–87.
19. *Global health sector response to HIV, 2000–2015: Focus on innovations in Africa.* Geneva: WHO; 2015.
20. Andrews G, Skinner D, Zuma K. Epidemiology of health and vulnerability among children orphaned and made vulnerable by HIV/AIDS in sub-Saharan Africa. *AIDS Care.* 2006;18:269–76.
21. *AIDS by the numbers 2016.* Geneva: UNAIDS; 2016.
22. *Fast-Track: Ending the AIDS epidemic by 2030.* Geneva: UNAIDS; 2014.
23. Quinn TC, Overbaugh J. HIV/AIDS in women: An expanding epidemic. *Science.* 2005;308:1582–3.
24. Higgins JA, Hoffman S, Dworkin SL. Rethinking gender, heterosexual men, and women's vulnerability to HIV/AIDS. *Am J Public Health.* 2010;100:435–45.
25. *Integrating gender into HIV/AIDS programmers in the health sector: Tools to improve responsiveness to women's needs.* Geneva: WHO; 2009.
26. *Consolidated guidelines on HIV prevention, diagnosis, treatment and care for key populations.* Geneva: WHO; 2016.
27. *Global health sector strategy on HIV, 2016–2021: Towards ending AIDS.* Geneva: WHO; 2016.
28. Denison JA, O'Reilly KR, Schmid GP, Kennedy CE, Sweat MD. HIV voluntary counseling and testing and behavioral risk reduction in developing countries: A meta-analysis, 1990–2005. *AIDS Behav.* 2008;12:363–73.
29. *Consolidated guidelines on HIV testing services—5 Cs: Consent, confidentiality, counselling, correct results and connection.* Geneva: WHO; 2015.
30. *"15 by 15": A global target achieved.* Geneva: UNAIDS; 2015.

31. *90–90–90: An ambitious treatment target to help end the AIDS epidemic.* Geneva: UNAIDS; 2014.

32. John-Stewart G, Peeling R, Levin C, Garcia P, Mabey D, Kinuthia J. Prevention of mother-to-child transmission of HIV and syphilis (Chapter 6). *Disease control priorities.* 3rd ed. *Major infectious diseases (Volume 6).* Washington DC: IBRD/World Bank; 2017.

33. De Cock KM, Fowler MG, Mercier E, et al. Prevention of mother-to-child HIV transmission in resource-poor countries: Translating research into policy and practice. *JAMA.* 2000;283:1175–82.

34. Siegfried NL, van der Merwe L, Brocklehurst P, Sint TT. Antiretrovirals for reducing the risk of mother-to-child transmission of HIV infection. *Cochrane Database Syst Rev.* 2007;(1):CD003510.

35. *Guideline: Updates on HIV and infant feeding: The duration of breastfeeding, and support from health services to improve feeding practices among mothers living with HIV.* Geneva: WHO/UNICEF; 2016.

36. *Guidelines on post-exposure prophylaxis for HIV and the use of co-trimoxazole prophylaxis for HIV-related infections among adults, adolescents and children: Recommendations for a public health approach.* Geneva: WHO; 2014.

37. *WHO technical update on pre-exposure prophylaxis (PrEP).* Geneva: WHO; 2015.

38. Murphy EM, Greene ME, Mihailovic A, Olupot-Olupot P. Was the "ABC" approach (abstinence, being faithful, using condoms) responsible for Uganda's decline in HIV? *PLoS Med.* 2006;3:e379.

39. Boily MC, Baggaley RF, Wang L, et al. Heterosexual risk of HIV-1 infection per sexual act: A systematic review and meta-analysis of observational studies. *Lancet Infect Dis.* 2009;9:118–29.

40. *Global strategy for the prevention and control of sexually transmitted infections 2006–2015: Breaking the chain of transmission.* Geneva: WHO; 2007.

41. *Joint strategic action framework to accelerate the scale-up of voluntary medical male circumcision for HIV prevention in eastern and southern Africa 2012–2016.* Geneva: WHO/UNAIDS; 2011.

42. Sawires SR, Dworkin SL, Fiamma A, Peacock D, Szekeres G, Coates TJ. Male circumcision and HIV/AIDS: Challenges and opportunities. *Lancet.* 2007; 369:708–13.

43. Wodak A, Cooney A. Do needle syringe programs reduce HIV infection among injecting drug users: A comprehensive review of the international evidence. *Subst Use Misuse.* 2006;41:777–813.

44. Kurth AE, Celum C, Baeten JM, Vermund SH, Wasserheit JN. Combination HIV prevention: Significance, challenges, and opportunities. *Curr HIV/AIDS Rep.* 2011;8:62–72.

45. Khan JG, Bollinger L, Stover J, Marseille E. Improving the efficiency of the HIV/AIDS policy response: A guide to resource allocation modeling (Chapter 9). *Disease control priorities.* 3rd ed. *Major infectious diseases (Volume 6).* Washington DC: IBRD/World Bank; 2017.

46. Kates J, Wexler A, Lief E. *Financing the response to HIV in low- and middle-income countries: International assistance from donor governments in 2015.* Menlo Park CA: The Henry J. Kaiser Family Foundation/UNAIDS; 2016.

47. *PEPFAR 2016 Annual Report to Congress.* Washington DC: U.S. Department of State; 2016.

48. Chesson HW, Mayaud P, Aral SO. Sexually transmitted infections: Impact and cost-effectiveness of prevention (Chapter 10). *Disease control priorities.* 3rd ed. *Major infectious diseases (Volume 6).* Washington DC: IBRD/World Bank; 2017.

49. *WHO guidelines for the treatment of Chlamydia trachomatis.* Geneva: WHO; 2016.

50. *WHO guidelines for the treatment of Neisseria gonorrhoeae.* Geneva: WHO; 2016.

51. *Global health sector strategy on sexually transmitted infections 2016–2021: Towards ending STIs.* Geneva: WHO; 2016.

52. Unemo M, Nicholas RA. Emergence of multidrug-resistant, extensively drug-resistant and untreatable gonorrhea. *Future Microbiol.* 2012;7:1401–22.

53. *WHO guidelines for the treatment of Treponema pallidum (syphilis).* Geneva: WHO; 2016.

54. Hook EW 3rd. Syphilis. *Lancet.* 2017;389:1550–7.

55. Newman L, Kamb M, Hawkes S, et al. Global estimates of syphilis in pregnancy and associated adverse outcomes: Analysis of multinational antenatal surveillance data. *PLoS Med.* 2013;10:e1001396.

56. *WHO guidelines for the treatment of genital herpes simplex virus.* Geneva: WHO; 2016.

57. Looker KJ, Magaret AS, Turner KME, Vickerman P, Gottlieb SL, Newman LM. Global estimates of prevalent and incident herpes simplex virus type 2 infections in 2012. *PLoS One.* 2015;10:e114989.

58. Looker KJ, Magaret AS, May MT, et al. Global and regional estimates of prevalent and incident herpes simplex virus type 1 infections in 2012. *PLoS One.* 2015;10:e0140765.

59. Plummer M, de Martel C, Vignat J, Ferlay J, Bray F, Franceschi S. Global burden of cancers attributable to infections in 2012: A synthetic analysis. *Lancet Glob Health.* 2016;4:e609–16.

60. Bruni L, Diaz M, Barrionuevo-Rosas L, et al. Global estimates of human papillomavirus vaccination coverage by region and income level: A pooled analysis. *Lancet Glob Health.* 2016;4:e453–63.

61. Poole DN, McClelland RS. Global epidemiology of *Trichomonas vaginalis. Sex Transm Infect.* 2013;89: 418–22.

62. Orion E, Matz H, Wolf R. Ectoparasitic sexually transmitted diseases: Scabies and pediculosis. *Clin Dermatol.* 2004;22:513–19.

63. Garnett G, Krishnaratne S, Harris K, et al. Cost-effectiveness of interventions to prevent HIV acquisition (Chapter 7). *Disease control priorities*. 3rd ed. *Major infectious diseases (Volume 6)*. Washington DC: IBRD/World Bank; 2017.

64. Gottlieb SL, Low N, Newman LM, Bolan G, Kamb M, Broutet N. Toward global prevention of sexually transmitted infections (STIs): The need for STI vaccines. *Vaccine*. 2014; 32:1527–35.

65. Ferreira A, Young T, Mathews C, Zunza M, Low N. Strategies for partner notification for sexually transmitted infections, including HIV. *Cochrane Database Syst Rev*. 2013; (10):CD002843.

66. Dheda K, Barry CE 3rd, Maartens G. Tuberculosis. *Lancet*. 2015;387:1211–26.

67. Lönnroth K, Jaramillo E, Williams BG, Dye C, Raviglione M. Drivers of tuberculosis epidemics: The role of risk factors and social determinants. *Soc Sci Med*. 2009;68:2240–6.

68. Sepkowitz KA. How contagious is tuberculosis. *Clin Infect Dis*. 1996;23:954–62.

69. *Global tuberculosis report 2016*. Geneva: WHO; 2016.

70. BCG vaccine: WHO position paper. *Wkly Epidemiol Rec*. 2004;79:27–38.

71. *Systematic screening for active tuberculosis: An operational guide*. Geneva: WHO; 2015.

72. *Implementing the End TB Strategy: The essentials*. Geneva: WHO; 2015.

73. *Treatment of tuberculosis: Guidelines (4th edition)*. Geneva: WHO; 2010.

74. *The Stop TB Strategy: Building on and enhancing DOTS to meet the TB-related Millennium Development Goals*. Geneva: WHO; 2006.

75. Evans TG, Schrager L, Thole J. Status of vaccine research and development of vaccines for tuberculosis. *Vaccine*. 2016;34:2911–4.

76. *Guidelines on the management of latent tuberculosis infection*. Geneva: WHO; 2015.

77. *Global tuberculosis report 2015*. Geneva: WHO; 2015.

78. *The End TB Strategy: Global strategy and targets for tuberculosis prevention, care and control after 2015*. Geneva: WHO; 2014.

79. Bloom BR, Atun R, Cohen T, et al. Tuberculosis (Chapter 11). *Disease control priorities* 3rd ed. *Major infectious diseases (Volume 6)*. Washington DC: IBRD/World Bank; 2017.

80. *A guide to monitoring and evaluation for collaborative TB/HIV activities (2015 revision)*. Geneva: WHO; 2015.

81. Harries AD, Zachariah R, Corbett EL, et al. The HIV-associated tuberculosis epidemic: When will we act? *Lancet*. 2010;375:1906–19.

82. *WHO policy on collaborative TB/HIV activities: Guidelines for national programmes and other stakeholders*. Geneva: WHO; 2012.

83. *The Global Plan to Stop TB 2011–2015: Transforming the fight: Toward elimination of tuberculosis*. Geneva: WHO; 2011.

84. Goldbert DE, Siliciano RF, Jacobs WR. Outwitting evolution: Fighting drug-resistant TB, malaria, and HIV. *Cell*. 2012;148:1271–83.

85. *Global action plan on antimicrobial resistance*. Geneva: WHO; 2015.

86. *The OIE strategy on antimicrobial resistance and the prudent use of antimicrobials*. Paris: World Organisation for Animal Health (OIE); 2014.

87. *Guidelines for the programmatic management of drug-resistant tuberculosis*. Geneva: WHO; 2016.

88. Matteelli A, Roggi A, Carvalho ACC. Extensively drug-resistant tuberculosis: Epidemiology and management. *Clin Epidemiol*. 2014;6:111–8.

89. *Companion handbook to the WHO guidelines for the programmatic management of drug-resistant tuberculosis*. Geneva: WHO; 2014.

90. *National and state healthcare associated infections: Progress report (2014)*. Atlanta GA: CDC; 2016.

91. Grundmann H, Aires-de-Sousa M, Boyce J, Tiemersma E. Emergence and resurgence of meticillin-resistant *Staphylococcus aureus* as a public-health threat. *Lancet*. 2006; 368:874–85.

92. Stefani S, Chung DR, Lindsay JA, et al. Meticillin-resistant *Staphylococcus aureus* (MRSA): Global epidemiology and harmonization of typing methods. *Int J Antimicrob Agents*. 2012;39:273–82.

93. *Guidelines on core components of infection prevention and control programmes at the national and acute health care facility level*. Geneva: WHO; 2016.

94. Dellit TH, Owens RC, McGowan JE Jr, et al. Infectious Diseases Society of America and the Society for Healthcare Epidemiology of America guidelines for developing an institutional program to enhance antimicrobial stewardship. *Clin Infect Dis*. 2007;44:159–77.

95. Miller-Petrie M, Pant S, Laxminarayan R. Drug resistant infections (Chapter 18). *Disease control priorities*. 3rd ed. *Major infectious diseases (Volume 6)*. Washington DC: IBRD/World Bank; 2017.

96. *Antimicrobial resistance: Global report on surveillance*. Geneva: WHO; 2014.

97. *Antibiotic resistance threats in the United States, 2013*. Atlanta, GA: CDC; 2013.

98. Laxminarayan R, Duse A, Wattal C, et al. Antibiotic resistance: The need for global solutions. *Lancet Infect Dis*. 2013;13:1057–98.

99. Laxminarayan R, Sridhar D, Blaser M, Wang M, Woolhouse M. Achieving global targets for antimicrobial resistance. *Science*. 2016;353:874–5.

CHAPTER 9

Diarrheal, Respiratory, and Other Common Infections

Infectious diseases remain common causes of death in low-income countries, and more than one-third of the victims are children. Most deaths from diarrheal diseases, pneumonia, and other common childhood infections can be prevented with vaccinations, antibiotics, and other low-cost preventive and therapeutic interventions. Global health initiatives are enabling significant reductions in the child mortality rate from infectious diseases. Global cooperation is also critical for containing new strains of influenza and other pathogens with the potential to spark dangerous pandemics.

▶ 9.1 Infectious Diseases and Global Health

Infectious diseases caused by bacteria, viruses, fungi, and parasites cause millions of deaths every year. In the early and middle decades of the 20th century, new laboratory techniques led to the identification of many disease-causing microbes and the development of vaccines and antibiotics like penicillin. These discoveries generated a great deal of optimism and confidence about the ability of humans to control and eradicate communicable diseases. But scientists now recognize that even though modern science has provided a good understanding of the infectious disease process and has allowed for the development of therapies and cures for many types of infectious diseases,

microbes continue to adapt and emerge. Even with improved preventive and therapeutic techniques, infectious diseases continue to be a health risk in all populations in every part of the world. Developing new methods for the prevention, diagnosis, and treatment of infectious diseases remains an important part of global health.

Most people who live in high-income countries would correctly consider heart disease, cancer, or diabetes to be their number one health concern. Few would mention infectious diseases as a top priority for their own health, except when a major infectious disease outbreak is getting a lot of media attention. This happens occasionally when there are new fears about the emergence of a particularly bad influenza strain or there is an outbreak linked to a food product or restaurant chain. These worries usually fade quickly. But in most low-income countries, infectious diseases remain responsible for a

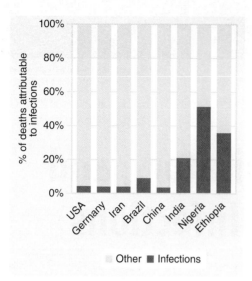

FIGURE 9-1 Infectious diseases cause a large proportion of deaths in lower-income countries.

Data from GBD Mortality and Causes of Death Collaborators. Global, regional, and national life expectancy, all-cause mortality, and cause-specific mortality for 249 causes of death, 1980–2015: A systematic analysis for the Global Burden of Disease Study 2015. *Lancet.* 2016; 388:1459–544.

large proportion of deaths (**FIGURE 9–1**).[1] These deaths disproportionately affect children, the poor, and other vulnerable population groups.

The burden from easily preventable infectious diseases falls especially hard on children,[2] who have a higher proportion of deaths from infectious diseases than adults (**FIGURE 9–2**).[3] An estimated 8.8 million people worldwide died from infections in 2015, including 3.1 million children under 14 years of age: 0.6 million neonates in their first month of life, 1.1 million post-neonatal infants, 1.0 million children between their first and fifth birthdays, and 0.4 million children between their fifth and fifteenth birthdays (**FIGURE 9–3**).[1] More than 99% of all infectious disease deaths in children occur in low- and middle-income countries, with low-income countries bearing a particularly disproportionate burden (**FIGURE 9–4**). The vast majority of these infections could have been prevented with inexpensive interventions like childhood vaccinations,

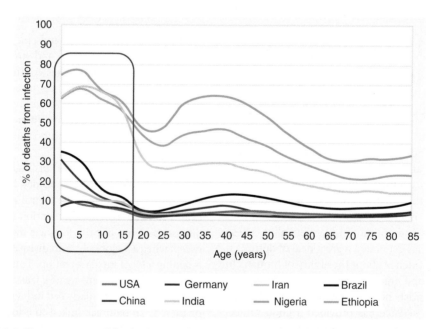

FIGURE 9-2 The percentage of deaths that are attributable to infectious diseases peaks in childhood.

Data from GBD Mortality and Causes of Death Collaborators. Global, regional, and national life expectancy, all-cause mortality, and cause-specific mortality for 249 causes of death, 1980–2015: A systematic analysis for the Global Burden of Disease Study 2015. *Lancet.* 2016;388:1459–544.

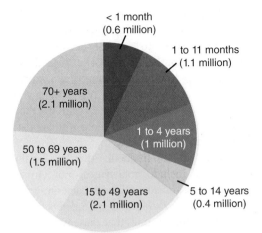

FIGURE 9–3 More than 3 million children died from infectious diseases in 2015.

Data from GBD Mortality and Causes of Death Collaborators. Global, regional, and national life expectancy, all-cause mortality, and cause-specific mortality for 249 causes of death, 1980–2015: A systematic analysis for the Global Burden of Disease Study 2015. *Lancet.* 2016;388:1459–544.

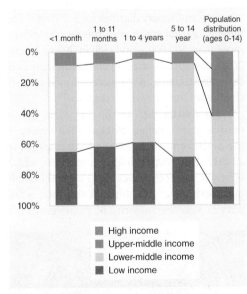

FIGURE 9–4 Nearly all infectious disease deaths among children (aged 0–14 years) occur in lower-income countries.

Data from GBD Mortality and Causes of Death Collaborators. Global, regional, and national life expectancy, all-cause mortality, and cause-specific mortality for 249 causes of death, 1980–2015: A systematic analysis for the Global Burden of Disease Study 2015. *Lancet.* 2016;388:1459–544.

reliable access to clean drinking water, and bednets to block mosquito bites. When prevention methods failed to stop the occurrence of an infection, the majority of deaths from these infectious diseases could still have been averted with antibiotic and other types of basic medical care.

The unnecessary burden of infectious diseases on children in low-income countries is more than sufficient reason for infectious disease prevention and control to remain a global health priority. One of the eight Millennium Development Goals was to reduce the mortality rate among children between birth and their fifth birthdays ("under-5" children) by two-thirds between 2000 and 2015 (MDG 4). The mortality rate dropped by more than half during that 15-year period, and infectious disease programs were critical contributors to the good progress made toward achieving this goal.[4] This trajectory will need to continue in order to achieve the Sustainable Development Goals target of ending preventable deaths of young children by 2030 (SDG 3.2).[5]

But infectious diseases are not just about children. They are equal-opportunity killers, and they can kill or disable people of all ages, all socioeconomic levels, and all geographies. Infectious diseases are spread through social networks, and the web of human contacts is becoming more complex as modern transportation allows people and products to travel almost anywhere in the world within a day. Infectious diseases can mutate, adapt, and disseminate themselves quickly, and that places everyone at risk.

Individuals, communities, health organizations, and governmental agencies all have a role to play in the control and prevention of infectious diseases. Individuals contribute to reducing the burden of infectious disease by engaging in healthy behaviors, such as washing their hands frequently and staying home from work or school when sick, so they do not continue the chain of transmission. Communities play key roles in environmental health, reducing infection transmission by increasing drinking water quality and the amount of water available to each person, ensuring access to sanitation facilities, promoting proper waste management, implementing policies that reduce air pollution, reducing mosquito populations through water drainage and insecticides, and controlling rodent and snail populations. Local and national governments implement food safety regulations, enforce zoning laws that restrict the number of individuals who can share a dwelling unit, require pet vaccination, and take other steps to minimize the infectious disease risks in the natural and built environments. At the national and international levels, scientists, policymakers, and others work together to create and disseminate technologies, such as new vaccines, and to track and address emerging infectious disease problems. One country alone cannot stop a pandemic. Infectious disease control requires international cooperation.

▶ 9.2 Diarrheal Diseases

Diarrhea is characterized by loose or liquid feces and an increased frequency of defecation, and it can quickly cause dehydration and death in young children. Severe **dehydration**, the excessive loss of water from the body, can cause low blood pressure (because fluid loss decreases blood volume), a fast and weak pulse, rapid breathing (but insufficient oxygen intake), sunken dry eyes, loss of skin elasticity, muscle contractions, convulsions, and delirium. Imbalances of sodium, potassium, bicarbonate, and other electrolytes can lead to kidney and heart failure, and eventually to death. In addition to diarrhea, people with gastroenteritis often have nausea, vomiting, cramps, and fever.

Infectious diarrhea affects all age groups, but it is especially dangerous in children.[6] About 1.7 billion cases of diarrhea occur in under-5 children each year, and diarrheal diseases remain a major cause of mortality in young children.[7] About 9% of the nearly

6 million children younger than 5 years old who died in 2015 succumbed to diarrhea, including nearly 16% of the deaths in children 1–59 months old.[3] Most of these deaths occurred in low-income countries. Diarrhea mortality rates are especially high among children who are undernourished, including those who are not breastfed and those who are deficient in vitamin A or zinc.[7]

The most frequent diarrhea-causing pathogens include rotaviruses, noroviruses, astroviruses, and adenoviruses; bacteria such as *Vibrio cholerae*, *Escherichia coli*, *Salmonella* species (including the ones that cause typhoid and paratyphoid), *Shigella*, *Campylobacter jejuni*, and *Aeromonas*; and protozoa, such as *Entamoeba histolytica*, *Giardia*, and *Cryptosporidium*.[8] These are all called **enteric** infections because they are infections of the intestinal tract.

Rotavirus is the most frequent cause of severe diarrhea in infants and young children.[9] Children with rotavirus infection typically have vomiting and watery diarrhea for 3–7 days.[10] The number of deaths from rotavirus decreased from more than 500,000 worldwide in 2000 to about 200,000 by 2015 as access to the vaccine increased, but rotavirus remains the most common cause of child death from infectious diarrhea.[11]

Norovirus, part of the calicivirus family (and formerly called Norwalk-like virus), is the most frequent cause of severe diarrhea in adults.[12] Norovirus is highly contagious, which is why it has been the cause of several notable outbreaks on cruise ships. Within just a few days at sea, the majority of passengers on a

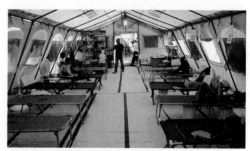

Cholera cots in a cholera treatment center.

ship can be ill.[13] Outbreaks have also occurred in daycare centers, restaurants, and other venues. Most people recover quickly from norovirus infection, but some may require hospital care for dehydration.

Cholera is an infection with *Vibrio cholerae* bacteria that causes large volumes of severe watery diarrhea to be produced from liquid secreted by the body into the small intestine.[14] A cholera cot is a simple bed with a hole cut in the center so that a bucket can be placed below the bed to capture the liquid being expelled from the intestines. Being able to quantify the amount of fluid lost allows an appropriate amount of water to be replaced through drinking or intravenous drips. Death can occur if the body's electrolyte balance cannot be maintained through fluid replacement. *Vibrio* can live in harsh environments, including ocean water and sewage, and the bacteria can survive for long periods of time.[15] A series of cholera pandemics in the 1800s was sparked by intensification of global trade.[16] The threat to human health and economic well-being posed by cholera was the impetus behind the creation of the International Sanitary Regulations that were the direct precursor to the International Health Regulations.[17] Today, many countries in sub-Saharan Africa (including Nigeria and Ethiopia) and a few countries in Asia (including India and a few provinces of China) are considered to be endemic for cholera, and nearly 3 million cholera cases

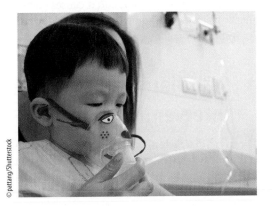

© pattang/Shutterstock

occur globally in a typical year.[18] Outbreaks periodically occur in other places, including in some countries in the Americas. An epidemic in Haiti after the devastating earthquake in 2010 was particularly notable because the origin of the outbreak was traced back to United Nations peacekeepers from Nepal who were participating in the international response to the disaster. This unfortunate event has led to changes in the protocols for UN deployments, including mandatory cholera vaccinations and higher standards for sanitation.[19]

Escherichia coli bacteria are very common, with *E. coli* present in most human intestines. Most types of *E. coli* are nonpathogenic, which means that they are not harmful and do not cause disease. However, some strains are pathogenic. These types of *E. coli* are described by the damage they cause, such as enterotoxigenic *E. coli* (ETEC), which is a common cause of diarrhea in children and travelers, and enteropathogenic *E. coli* (EPEC), which can be fatal in infants.[20] *E. coli* O157:H7, a Shiga toxin-producing *E. coli* (STEC), can cause hemolytic uremic syndrome, which is characterized by bloody diarrhea and kidney failure.[21] *E. coli* O157:H7 bacteria are spread via fecal contamination of food (such as produce or undercooked beef) and water (including swimming pools that are not properly maintained) and by person-to-person contact (typically in a daycare or other institutional setting).[22] **Food intoxication**, illness caused when ingested bacteria produce toxins in the body, is also caused by some other types of bacteria, including *Bacillus cereus*, *Clostridium perfringens*, and *Staphylococcus aureus*.[23]

Campylobacter, *Salmonella*, and *Shigella* are Gram-negative bacteria that are frequent causes of diarrhea. Campylobacteriosis, a disease of the small intestines caused by infection with *Campylobacter jejuni* and other species, is usually acquired through undercooked poultry and meat products.[24] *Salmonella* infections are divided into two main categories, typhoid fever and non-typhoidal *Salmonella*.[25] **Typhoid**

(*Salmonella* Typhi = *Salmonella enterica* serotype Typhi) causes severe diarrhea and a high fever. The symptoms of typhoid can persist for a month, and even with treatment, the disease can be fatal if it causes intestinal bleeding or perforation.[26] A typhoid vaccine is available, but it is not highly effective. An estimated 25 million cases of symptomatic typhoid fever occur globally every year,[27] and a small percentage of people infected with typhoid bacteria become chronic carriers of the pathogen. A **carrier** is a person with a persistent contagious infection who does not have symptoms of the disease but can pass the infectious agent on to others through stool. Carriers play an important role in sustaining typhoid transmission in communities, because typhoid does not have an animal or environmental reservoir.[28] There are more than 2600 serotypes of *Salmonella*, and they affect both the large and small intestines. The nearly 40 serotypes of *Shigella* typically affect only the colon.[29] **Dysentery** is bloody diarrhea, with the blood often mixed with mucus, and it can be caused by several different types of bacteria and parasites.[30] Bacillary dysentery is caused by *Shigella* bacteria. Amoebic dysentery is caused by *E. histolytica*, a protozoan.

Reliable access to and use of toilet facilities is important for reducing the community disease burden from *Entamoeba* species, cryptosporidiosis, giardiasis, and other protozoal causes of diarrhea.[31] **Cryptosporidiosis** is a waterborne protozoal disease (typically caused by *Cryptosporidium hominis* or *C. parvum*) that can be fatal in infants and immunocompromised adults.[32] The parasites are often found in livestock, and outbreaks in humans can occur when drinking water supplies become contaminated. A 1993 outbreak of cryptosporidiosis in Wisconsin, in the United States, was caused by a failure of the water treatment system. The outbreak caused more than 100 deaths in the city of Milwaukee and made more than 400,000 people sick.[33]

While most diarrheal infections resolve after a few days, some bacterial and parasitic infections can become chronic diseases. **Giardiasis** is an infection with *Giardia intestinalis* (also called

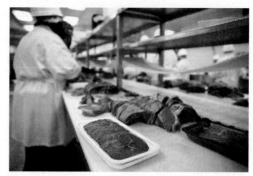

© El Nariz/Shutterstock

G. lamblia and *G. duodenalis*) that usually lasts for 3–6 weeks but can cause persistent diarrhea for several months or longer.[34] Other chronic foodborne infections include brucellosis and *Helicobacter pylori*. Brucellosis is caused by bacteria (*Brucella abortus* and *B. melitensis*) that are transmitted to humans through unpasteurized dairy products and contact with livestock. If untreated, the infection may cause chronic cyclic fevers.[35] Untreated *H. pylori* infection is associated with stomach ulcers.[36] *H. pylori* is also an example of a foodborne disease that does not cause diarrhea, as are listeriosis and botulism. *Listeria monocytogenes*, which can be acquired from processed meats and other foods, is of public health concern because pregnant women who contract the bacterium have an increased risk of miscarriages, stillbirths, and preterm delivery.[37] Botulism is a rare disease caused by ingesting toxins from *Clostridium botulinum* bacteria, usually in meals containing honey or improperly canned goods, and it causes cranial nerve palsies, descending paralysis, and the risk of respiratory failure and death.[38]

▶ 9.3 Diarrhea Interventions

Nearly all diarrheal infections are spread through **fecal-oral transmission**, which occurs when a person ingests products contaminated with fecal matter from animals or humans. Fecal-oral transmission is often described as being a function of the "5 Fs": fluids, fields, fingers, flies, and food.[39] When feces are not properly disposed of, they can contaminate drinking water (fluids) and soil (fields). The fecal matter can then get onto hands (fingers), especially the hands of young children who frequently touch the ground. Hands can transport the fecal matter to food when people do not wash their hands before preparing food or before eating. Insects (flies) can also spread feces to food and water, and flies thrive where fecal matter is in the open. The five Fs are sometimes expanded to a set of 6 Fs that includes fomites. A **fomite** is an inanimate object or surface that has been contaminated with infectious agents, such as a doorknob, stethoscope, clothing, or other item that has become coated in pathogenic microbes. Diarrhea prevention methods therefore include safe drinking water (fluids), access to toilets (fields), hand hygiene (fingers), insect control (flies), food safety (food), and surface disinfection (fomites).[40] (Diarrhea can also be caused by other conditions, such as inflammatory bowel disorders like Crohn's disease and ulcerative colitis, lactose intolerances and other food sensitivities that cause poor absorption of water, some antibiotics and other medications, and other conditions, but those are uncommon contributors to diarrhea mortality.[41])

Once a child has diarrhea, the most important method for preventing death is **oral rehydration therapy (ORT)**, drinking enough water to prevent or treat the dehydration caused by diarrhea. **Oral rehydration salts (ORS)**, also called oral rehydration solution, are a mixture of sugar, salt, and clean drinking water that replaces lost fluids and restores the balance of electrolytes in the blood. ORS packets are sometimes distributed at clinics, usually in a low osmolarity formula that contains sodium, chloride, glucose, potassium, and citrate.[42] Parents can also make their own ORS solution by mixing 8 teaspoons of sugar and one-half teaspoon of salt into one liter of boiled water.[43] Potassium can be added to the solution through fruit juice, coconut water, or mashed bananas. Children with diarrhea need to drink

ORT every time they pass watery stool for a total of at least one liter each day. If they also have vomiting, they need to drink more ORT to replace those lost fluids. **Continued feeding** is the process of encouraging children with diarrhea to eat the same foods that they normally consume (as long as they are not vomiting too much to keep food down) and continuing to breastfeed infants and young children as usual during their illness. ORT combined with continued feeding leads to the best health outcomes for children with diarrhea.[44]

A diverse package of cost-effective interventions is the best option for reducing the burden from diarrheal diseases in childhood. Interventions to reduce the incidence of diarrhea in children include improvements in access to a reliable source of safe drinking water, community-wide sanitation facilities for safely disposing of feces, and hygiene practices, including frequent handwashing with soap; breastfeeding and nutrition promotion; vitamin A and zinc supplementation; and vaccinations against rotavirus, measles, and (where available) cholera.[45] Interventions to reduce deaths in children who have diarrheal diseases include educating parents and communities about ORT and continued feeding as well as providing zinc treatment, probiotics, and antibiotics for diarrhea caused by dysenteric diseases for which antimicrobial therapy has been shown to be effective at reducing

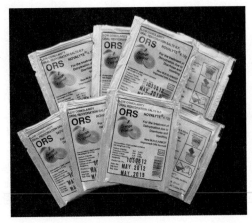

adverse outcomes.[45] After children recover from diarrhea, they should be encouraged to eat more food than normal to regain lost weight and lost nutrients. Undernutrition is a major underlying cause of child deaths from diarrhea and pneumonia, so this recovery period is critical for protecting children from the adverse outcomes of their next bout with an infectious disease.[46]

Although the numbers of cases and deaths from childhood diarrhea remain far above international targets, they are significantly better than the numbers from just 15 years ago.[47] The mortality rate from diarrhea among children younger than 5 years old decreased by more than 60% between 2000 and 2015, from 9.5 per 1000 live births to 3.8 per 1000 live births, and the number of deaths of children younger than 5 years old from diarrhea decreased from about 1.2 million in 2000 to 525,000 in 2015 (**FIGURE 9–5**).[3] *The Global Action Plan for Pneumonia and Diarrhea (GAPPD)*, initiated by the World Health Organization (WHO), UNICEF, and dozens of partner groups, aims to reduce the under-5 diarrhea mortality rate to less than 1 per 1000 live births by 2025.[44] Many of the low-income countries that have made significant progress in reducing deaths from diarrhea have current rates that are still considerably higher than this target level, but the trajectories show progress toward improvement (**FIGURE 9–6**).[48] Only about 41% of the world's under-5 children with diarrhea received ORT and continued feeding in 2015 (**FIGURE 9–7**),[49] roughly the same proportion as in 2000,[47] and increasing this rate is one of the key components of the GAPPD strategy.

Food safety is also critical for preventing dangerous cases of diarrhea in people of all ages. A diversity of bacterial and viral pathogens are frequent causes of foodborne outbreaks in countries across the globe, including brucellosis, campylobacteriosis, cholera, *E. coli*, listeriosis, *Mycobacterium bovis*, salmonellosis, shigellosis, typhoid, paratyphoid, hepatitis A virus, and norovirus.[50] Foodborne parasitic infections are less common in high-income countries than they are in low-income countries, but they do occur.[51] For example, the United States has

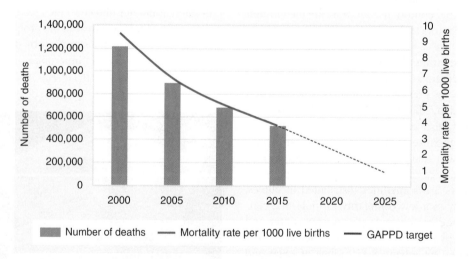

FIGURE 9–5 The diarrhea mortality rate in children aged 0–59 months has decreased significantly since 2000.

Data from Liu L, Oza S, Hogan D, Chu Y, Perin J, Zhu J, Lawn JE, Cousens S, Mathers C, Black RE. Global, regional, and national causes of under-5 mortality in 2000–15: An updated systematic analysis with implications for the Sustainable Development Goals. *Lancet* 2016; 388:3027–35.

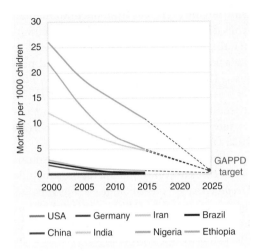

FIGURE 9–6 The diarrhea mortality rate per 1000 live births in children aged 0–59 months has decreased significantly in lower-income countries.

Data from Department of Evidence, Information and Research (WHO) and Maternal Child Epidemiology Estimation (MCEE) group. *WHO-MCEE estimates for child causes of death 2000–2015*. Geneva: WHO; 2016.

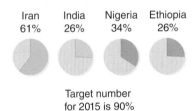

Target number
for 2015 is 90%

FIGURE 9–7 Percentage of children younger than 5 years old with diarrhea who receive oral rehydration salts (ORS).

Data from *State of the world's children 2016*. New York: UNICEF; 2016.

had foodborne outbreaks of giardiasis, cryptosporidiosis, cyclosporiasis (*Cyclospora cayetanensis*), and toxoplasmosis (*Toxoplasma gondii*).[52] For consumers, the key food safety practices include maintaining a clean kitchen area and practicing good hand hygiene, separating raw and cooked food, cooking food thoroughly, keeping food at safe hot or cold temperatures, and using safe water and food products.[53] Food producers, processors, distributors, and retailers also play critical roles in ensuring the safety of foods and beverages.[54]

▶ 9.4 Pneumonia

The main function of the body's respiratory system is the exchange of gases, which mostly means taking in oxygen and getting rid of carbon dioxide (**FIGURE 9–8**). When a person takes a breath, the air enters the lungs and fills tiny air sacs called alveoli. Each alveolus is wrapped in tiny blood vessels called capillaries and has a very thin surface so that gas exchange can take place. When a person inhales, oxygen is absorbed into the blood in those capillaries. This oxygenated blood is pumped into the heart and then to the rest of the body so that all of the cells can receive the oxygen they need to function properly. When the cells take in oxygen from nearby capillaries, they can also get rid of carbon dioxide and other waste products by dumping them into the blood. These products can then be released from the blood into the alveoli. When a person exhales, these wastes are expelled from the body. **Pneumonia** occurs when part of a lung fills with fluid. If the alveoli are filled with fluid, they cannot efficiently exchange oxygen and carbon dioxide. The symptoms of pneumonia usually include a

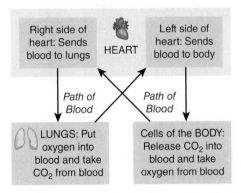

FIGURE 9–8 Path of blood through the heart, lungs, and body.

cough accompanied by difficult rapid breathing. People with pneumonia can feel like they are drowning as fluid fills their lungs and they develop **hypoxia**, an inadequate supply of oxygen in body tissues. A child with severe pneumonia may even turn bluish in color due to hypoxia.

The mortality rate from pneumonia among children younger than 5 years old decreased by more than 50% between 2000 and 2015, from 13.6 per 1000 live births to 6.6 per 1000 live births, and the number of deaths from pneumonia of children younger than 5 years old decreased from about 1.74 million in 2000 to 920,000 in 2015 (**FIGURE 9–9**).[3] However, pneumonia remains the most frequent cause of infectious disease death in under-5 children, with most deaths occurring in low-income countries.[47] In 2015, about 15.5% of the nearly 6 million children younger than 5 years old who died succumbed to pneumonia, and pneumonia was responsible for 6% of the deaths in newborns and 23% of the deaths in children 1–59 months old.[3] More

children die each year from pneumonia than from diarrhea, and more die from pneumonia than from other infectious causes like malaria, meningitis, HIV, measles, and pertussis (**FIGURE 9–10**).[3] *The Global Action Plan for Pneumonia and Diarrhea (GAPPD)* aims to reduce the under-5 pneumonia mortality rate to less than 3 per 1000 live births by 2025 (**FIGURE 9–11**).[44]

The agents that cause the highest number of cases of childhood pneumonia include *Streptococcus pneumoniae*, *Haemophilus influenzae* type b (Hib), respiratory syncytial virus (RSV), and influenza virus.[55] **Pneumococcus** is the disease caused by infection with *S. pneumoniae*,[56] and pneumococcus can cause severe pneumonia as well as ear infections and sinus infections.[57] Rarely, pneumococcus becomes an invasive disease when the bacteria cause blood infections (bacteremia) or infections of the brain and spinal cord (meningitis). "**Hib**" is a bacterial infection with *H. influenzae* type b.[58] The inclusion of *influenzae* in the name indicates that the bacterium causes an

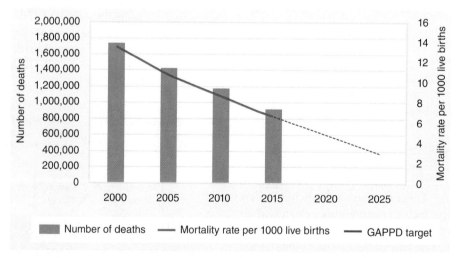

FIGURE 9–9 The pneumonia mortality rate in children aged 0–59 months has decreased significantly since 2000.

Data from Liu L, Oza S, Hogan D, Chu Y, Perin J, Zhu J, Lawn JE, Cousens S, Mathers C, Black RE. Global, regional, and national causes of under-5 mortality in 2000–15: An updated systematic analysis with implications for the Sustainable Development Goals. *Lancet.* 2016; 388:3027–35.

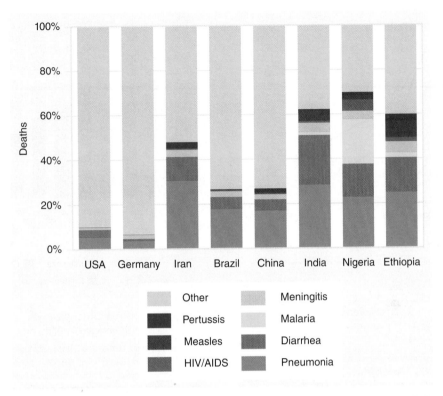

FIGURE 9-10 Percentage of deaths in children aged 1–59 months (post-neonatal under-5 mortality) caused by seven common infectious diseases in 2015.

Data from Liu L, Oza S, Hogan D, Chu Y, Perin J, Zhu J, Lawn JE, Cousens S, Mathers C, Black RE. Global, regional, and national causes of under-5 mortality in 2000–15: An updated systematic analysis with implications for the Sustainable Development Goals. *Lancet.* 2016; 388:3027–35.

influenza-like illness, but Hib is not influenza. Effective vaccines are available for both pneumococcus and Hib, which means that the deaths from these infections are completely preventable. **Respiratory syncytial virus (RSV)** is a common cause of severe pneumonia in preterm infants and other vulnerable babies,[59] and it accounts for a high proportion of cases of severe pneumonia in many higher-income countries (**FIGURE 9-12**).[55] Influenza is a viral respiratory infection that may lead to secondary bacterial pneumonia.[60] Other common causes of pneumonia include *Staphylococcus aureus* and *Klebsiella pneumoniae*.[61] Less-frequent pneumonia-causing pathogens include *Mycobacterium tuberculosis*, *Mycoplasma pneumoniae*, *Chlamydia pneumoniae*, *Legionella pneumophila*, Enterobacteriaceae, *Chlamydia psittaci*, *Coxiella burnetii* (which causes Q fever), *Pseudomonas aeruginosa*, and a diversity of respiratory viruses (such as adenoviruses and coronaviruses), among others.[62]

Bacterial pneumonia can often be cured by inexpensive oral antibiotics if treatment is sought soon after the onset of symptoms. However, only about 63% of the world's under-5 children with suspected pneumonia are taken to a healthcare provider (**FIGURE 9-13**),[49] and an even lower percentage are treated with antibiotics. More than

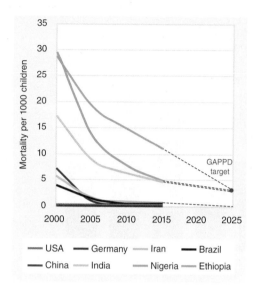

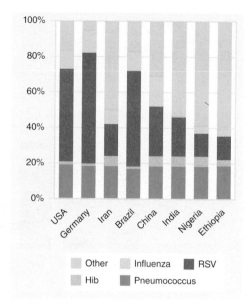

FIGURE 9–11 The pneumonia mortality rate per 1000 live births in children aged 0–59 months has decreased significantly in lower-income countries.

Data from Department of Evidence, Information and Research (WHO) and Maternal Child Epidemiology Estimation (MCEE) group. *WHO-MCEE estimates for child causes of death 2000–2015.* Geneva: WHO; 2016.

FIGURE 9–12 Common causes of severe pneumonia in children aged 0–59 months in 2010.

Data from Rudan I, O'Brien KL, Nair H, Liu L, Theodoratou E, Qazi S, Lukšić I, Fischer Walker CL, Black RE, Campbell H; Child Health Epidemiology Reference Group. Epidemiology and etiology of childhood pneumonia in 2010: Estimates of incidence, severe morbidity, mortality, underlying risk factors and causative pathogens for 192 countries. *J Glob Health* 2013; 3:010401.

10 million children are hospitalized each year because of severe pneumonia, but more than one-third of children with severe pneumonia are not treated in hospitals.[63] More than 80% of child pneumonia deaths occur outside of hospitals, and many of those children could have survived if they had received medical care.[63] Thus, an important component of improving child survival is educating caregivers about the importance of seeking medical care as soon as the symptoms of pneumonia appear, so that a course of antibiotics can be started. Antibiotics will not speed recovery from colds and other upper respiratory infections (like bronchitis) that are usually caused by viruses, but they are usually effective against early-stage bacterial pneumonia. Oxygen therapy may also help prevent cases of severe pneumonia from becoming fatal.[45]

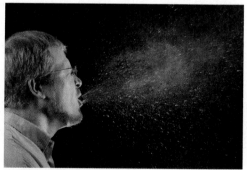

▶ 9.5 Other Respiratory Infections

Pneumonia is not the only respiratory infectious disease of public health concern.

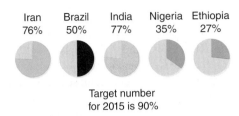

Iran	Brazil	India	Nigeria	Ethiopia
76%	50%	77%	35%	27%

Target number
for 2015 is 90%

FIGURE 9–13 Percentage of children younger than 5 years old with symptoms of pneumonia who receive care from a health facility or provider.

Data from *State of the world's children 2016*. New York: UNICEF; 2016.

An **acute respiratory infection (ARI)** is a short-term infection of the respiratory tract that typically has a rapid onset and resolves without becoming a chronic infection. ARIs are divided into two categories. Upper respiratory tract infections (URIs or URTIs) include acute infections of the nose, sinuses, pharynx, larynx (voice box), and trachea. Most URIs are considered mild, like the common cold and tonsillitis, but some can cause long-term damage. **Strep throat**, an illness caused by a type of Group A *Streptococcus*, is a common childhood infection that if left untreated can lead to complications such as scarlet fever or rheumatic fever, a condition that may cause permanent damage to the valves of the heart. **Lower respiratory infections (LRIs)** are acute respiratory infections of the bronchi and lungs, including infectious bronchitis and pneumonia. URIs are usually viral in origin, while LRIs are most often caused by bacteria.[64] Fungal pneumonias (such as aspergillosis, blastomycosis, and cryptococcosis) and parasitic pneumonias are uncommon compared to bacterial and viral respiratory infections, but they also occur.

Most respiratory infections are acquired through the air. **Airborne transmission** occurs when pathogens are aerosolized or suspended as droplets in the air and people inhale that contaminated air. Respiratory pathogens can also be transmitted through contact with hands or surfaces that have been contaminated by droplets expelled from the airways of infected persons when they sneeze or cough. For example, adenoviruses and the rhinoviruses that cause colds can live on some types of nonporous surfaces for days.[65] Some airborne pathogens are acquired from environmental sources rather than directly from infected humans.[66] For example, infection with *Legionellae* bacteria, called Legionnaires' disease when the symptoms are severe or Pontiac fever for milder disease, is acquired through the inhalation of moistened water from air conditioners, hot tubs, and humidifiers.[67] Some hantaviruses are acquired by inhaling aerosolized rat urine or feces when cleaning, and they can cause fatal hantavirus pulmonary syndrome.[68] Psittacosis, also called parrot fever, is acquired when bird owners inhale the dried droppings of pets infected with the bacterium *Chlamydophila psittaci*.[69] Coccidioidomycosis, also called valley fever, is caused by *Coccidioides immitis*, a fungus that lives in desert soil in places like the Southwest of the United States.[70] Histoplasmosis is caused by the fungus *Histoplasma capsulatum*, which is found in the Americas and elsewhere as a mold in soil containing bird or bat droppings.[71]

Prevention methods for respiratory infections include isolating infected persons and providing them with appropriate medical treatment; vaccinating members of vulnerable population groups against Hib, pneumococcus, and pertussis; reducing exposure to indoor air pollution and smoke, since polluted air damages the respiratory tract and increases susceptibility to respiratory diseases; reducing household overcrowding; using protective equipment at workplaces where occupational exposure to respiratory pathogens is likely; and encouraging frequent handwashing and the covering of the nose and mouth when coughing or sneezing.[45]

▶ 9.6 Influenza

Influenza is a highly contagious respiratory viral infection. Influenza viruses cause fevers and respiratory disease, and they can exacerbate existing medical conditions, especially lung and heart diseases, and lead to potentially fatal secondary infection with bacterial pneumonia.[60] ("Stomach flu" is not caused by influenza viruses.) Although the highest fatality rates from influenza are usually among the elderly and immunocompromised individuals, anyone who contracts influenza can die from it.

Seasonal influenza outbreaks occur every year, and the viruses that cause these epidemics are constantly mutating. When a novel strain of influenza emerges, it can cause pandemic influenza, sometimes shortened to just "pan flu."[72] The first influenza pandemic likely occurred in 1510, soon after the global shipping industry was launched, and other pandemics occurred in the 1730s, 1760s, 1780s, 1830s, 1840s, 1890s, and several times thereafter.[73] The term pandemic is a description of the geographic dispersion of a pathogen, and it is not necessarily an indicator of the severity of the infection,[74] but pandemic influenza strains can be dangerous. The most serious influenza pandemic in the 20th century occurred in 1918 and 1919 during World War I,[75] and that strain killed a disproportionate number of young adults as it spread through populations across the globe.[76] The emergence of a new strain of influenza can rapidly spark a global health crisis.

Two main types of influenza viruses cause epidemics in human populations, influenza A and influenza B. Influenza A viruses are further classified based on their surface antigens. An **antigen** is a foreign substance in the body that triggers an immune response, especially if the body's immune system has previously been exposed to the antigen and is therefore able to quickly recognize and neutralize it. The two key surface antigens for influenza A are

hemagglutinin (H) and neuraminidase (N). Influenza A strains are classified using abbreviations like H3N2 and H1N1 that are derived from the viruses' hemagglutinin and neuraminidase types. The dominant strain changes over time. H1N1 was the most common human influenza from 1918 until it was displaced by H2N2 in the late 1950s; H2N2 was displaced by H3N2 in the late 1960s.[77] A total of 17 types of influenza hemagglutinin types and 10 influenza neuraminidase types have been found in animals, but only a few have been found in humans.

Influenza viruses evade the immune systems of their hosts by changing their surface antigens so that the hosts' immune systems cannot recognize them. There are two processes by which surface antigens change, antigenic drift and antigenic shift.[78] **Antigenic drift** occurs when small genetic mutations bring about small changes in the antigens. Antigenic drift is the reason why infection with one version of H3N2 influenza might not confer immunity to another form of H3N2. Antigenic drift makes it necessary to develop a new influenza vaccine every year. **Antigenic shift** occurs when two very different types of influenza A viruses attack the same cell and the genetic material from both recombines to form a new type of influenza.[79] Antigenic shift led to the emergence in 1997 of an H5N1 strain of avian influenza ("bird flu") that spread rapidly through the bird populations in parts of Southeast Asia, affecting both domestic birds (such as ducks and chickens) and wild migrating fowl. The H5N1 strain of influenza was deemed to be a **highly pathogenic avian influenza (HPAI)** because it caused serious disease and high case fatality rates in affected birds.[80]

All infectious agents, whether newly emerging or long established in a population, are continually adapting and changing in ways that can make them more or less transmissible, infective, pathogenic, and virulent.[81] **Transmissibility** is the ease with which an

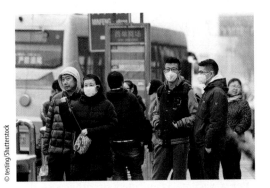

© testing/Shutterstock

infectious agent is passed from an infected host to another individual. **Infectivity** is the capacity of an infectious agent to cause infection in a susceptible host (one without immunity to the infection acquired from prior infection or vaccination) who is exposed to the agent. Infectivity is sometimes measured by calculating the **secondary attack rate**, the proportion of susceptible people exposed to a contagious person who contract the infection. **Pathogenicity** is the capacity of an infectious agent to cause disease in an infected host. **Virulence** is the ability of an infectious agent to cause severe disease or death in a host, and it is measured by the proportion of severe or fatal cases among all people who become ill. A virulent infection will have a high **case fatality rate**, because a high percentage of people who become ill from the infection will die from that infection. A mutation that causes greater transmissibility, infectivity, pathogenicity, or virulence in an influenza strain can pose a major threat to human populations globally.

Influenza viruses affect humans and also many types of animals, including chickens, ducks, pigs, horses, and even dogs, whales, and bats.[82] An infectious disease that usually occurs only in humans is called an **anthroponosis**. An infectious disease that usually occurs in animals and only occasionally infects humans is called a **zoonosis**. Some strains of influenza circulate in human populations, and some strains are zoonoses. Most strains of influenza

that affect humans originate in bird or mammal populations. When a virus mutates in a way that allows it to pass easily between humans and make humans severely ill, and it subsequently becomes established in human populations, that new strain is no longer a zoonosis.[83] For example, when a type of H1N1 "swine flu" began circulating widely in human populations in 2009, it ceased being an influenza of pigs and became a disease of humans.[84] Within months, human cases had been reported in 200 countries.[85] In 2013, an H7N9 influenza that primarily affects poultry caused several humans to become severely ill.[86] When H7N9, another strain of "bird flu," or another type of influenza not currently circulating in human populations further mutates in a way that allows it to be easily transmitted between humans, a pandemic may result.

Rapid laboratory tests are available to confirm the presence of influenza A or B viral antigens in the body fluids of people suspected to have influenza infections. People with suspected influenza who have not tested positive for the virus are said to have an **influenza-like illness (ILI)**. People who test positive for influenza can be prescribed antiviral medications that reduce the severity of symptoms from some strains of influenza. However, these medications do not cure the infection and they do not work against strains that have developed resistance to antivirals.[87]

Several public health strategies have been used to contain outbreaks of influenza and other dangerous infectious diseases, including isolation of sick people and quarantine of their contacts.[88] **Isolation** is the separation of people who have tested positive for a contagious infection from healthy people who are susceptible to the infection. Caregivers of people in isolation take precautions to protect themselves from infection with careful hygiene and **personal protective equipment (PPE),** such as gowns, gloves, facemasks, eye protection, and other barriers that prevent infection. The air supplies in isolation rooms may be filtered and vented away from places where people might gather. **Quarantine** is the restriction of freedom of movement for contacts of infected people because they may become contagious, even though they have no signs of infection at the time they are quarantined. Isolation is for sick people; quarantine is for healthy contacts of sick people. **Contact tracing** is the process of identifying the primary contacts of infected individuals (and, sometimes, the contacts of those primary contacts, who are called secondary contacts), so that they can be tested and monitored. Vaccination is also an important tool for reducing the burden from influenza, when there is an available vaccine that is effective at protecting people from the circulating strain.[89]

Influenza is a prime example of how global travel contributes to the rapid spread of newly mutated infectious agents. An infected person can fly to any part of the world in a day or two and spark an outbreak in a new location.[90] Globalization can also be beneficial for public health responses. Global communication systems may facilitate the containment of a pandemic by enabling public health officials to be alerted immediately to possible outbreaks of novel influenza strains. During the 2009 H1N1 pandemic, revised International Health Regulations guided the coordinated global response to the outbreak. Countries reported cases of H1N1 to the WHO, and WHO used its Pandemic Alert System to keep member nations and the public informed about the spread of the epidemic.[91] Coordinated capacity-building efforts initiated before the pandemic enabled pharmaceutical companies around the globe to expedite the development, testing, and manufacturing of H1N1 vaccines.[85] Local, national, and global preparedness plans implemented years before the emergence of H1N1 guided the response to the pandemic, and the lessons learned from H1N1 have been integrated into refined plans that are ready for implementation when the next major influenza pandemic emerges.

▶ 9.7 Immunization

Vaccination is the intentional delivery of a substance into the body in order to stimulate development of immunity against a particular disease. **Immunization** is the process of a person's immune system developing immunity against a particular infection. Vaccination is the action of delivering a vaccine to an individual; immunization is what happens in the body after a vaccine is injected or otherwise dispensed. A vaccine prompts the body's immune system to create antibodies specific to the antigens contained in the vaccine. An **antibody** is a protein produced by the human body (by B lymphocytes) in response to the presence of antigens. Antibodies can bind to antigens and destroy them. If a vaccinated person is later exposed to that same antigen when it is part of an infectious agent, the body's immune system will be able to quickly recognize the agent and destroy it before it has a chance to multiply.

Active immunity is present when the body's immune system produces antibodies against a specific infectious agent. This long-lasting protection against an infectious disease can be conferred by both infection and vaccination. By contrast, **passive immunity** is temporary protection from antibodies produced by another human or an animal, and it lasts only a few months.[92] Newborns and infants have some protection from maternal antibodies acquired transplacentally. For older children and adults, some protection can be conferred for a few weeks or months through blood products or immunoglobulin shots containing high concentrations of antibodies.

There are several different types of vaccines.[93] A **live attenuated vaccine** contains a pathogen that has been weakened using various laboratory techniques. A single dose of a live attenuated vaccine may be sufficient to confer lifelong immunity. However, live attenuated vaccines are not safe for some people with compromised immune systems, and they must be maintained at precise temperatures to maintain their effectiveness. If the cold chain is interrupted, as often occurs in places with unreliable electrical systems, the vaccine will be useless to the recipient. An **inactivated vaccine** contains a killed bacterium or an inactive virus that has been rendered harmless by heat, chemicals, or radiation. Inactivated vaccines are safer and more stable than live attenuated vaccines, but they are not as effective at stimulating an immune response. Multiple doses of inactivated vaccines may be required to confer and maintain immunity. An **adjuvant** is an ingredient added to some types of vaccines to boost the body's immune response to the vaccine. Some inactivated vaccines are whole-virus vaccines, and some are fractional vaccines that contain parts of a pathogen rather than the entire microbe. A toxoid vaccine is a fractional vaccine that protects from the toxins released by some bacteria, like the bacteria that cause diphtheria and tetanus. Subunit vaccines against bacteria and viruses have strong safety profiles, but they are a challenge to create. A conjugate vaccine is a fractional vaccine against a bacterial infection that is based on polysaccharides rather than proteins and has additional ingredients added to it to help infants' immune systems develop immunity. Other types of vaccines created through more complex laboratory methods are also available or in development.[94]

Vaccination programs are a key component of many infectious disease prevention and control strategies. New vaccines are often developed by partnerships of scientists, clinicians, pharmaceutical companies, nonprofit health organizations, and governments. These teams work together to select target diseases, create and test new vaccines, identify and educate the populations that would most benefit from the vaccine, and manufacture and deliver the vaccines to those populations. New vaccines undergo multiple rounds of testing

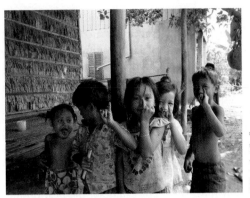

CDC/Jessica Curtis/Sue Chu

Ink marks the fingers of children vaccinated during an immunization campaign event.

before they are approved for widespread use. Pre-licensure studies demonstrate that the vaccine is safe and that it is efficacious in conferring immunity against the targeted disease.[95] There are three stages of clinical trials in humans.[96] Phase 1 trials enroll 20–100 healthy volunteers to test safety and dosage. Phase 2 trials enroll several hundred volunteers to further examine safety, dosage, and the timing of initial and follow-up shots. Phase 3 trials expand the number of participants to several thousand people. After a vaccine is approved, post-licensure studies continue to monitor safety and effectiveness.[97]

Licensed vaccines have undergone extensive testing to prove that they safe for most people.[93] An **adverse reaction** is a side effect of vaccination. The most typical adverse reactions are redness at the injection site, some local pain or swelling, and occasionally fevers or general achiness. Severe adverse reactions are extremely rare.[98] (The term **adverse event** is used to encompass both adverse reactions and other medical events that occur after vaccination but appear to be coincidental rather than being a result of the vaccine.[99]) However, there are some people who cannot receive particular vaccines. A **contraindication** is a condition that makes it unsafe for an individual to receive a particular vaccine. For example, a serious allergy to a component of a vaccine is a contraindication against that particular vaccine. Some vaccines may also be inappropriate for women who are pregnant or for people weakened by age, malnutrition, cancer treatments, immunosuppressive medications, or existing infections with other pathogens. A **precaution** is a condition that might make a vaccine ineffective at producing immunity or might increase the likelihood of an adverse reaction in a particular individual. For example, the best option for people with acute illnesses may be to wait until they have recovered before they receive a new vaccine.

When individuals receive a vaccination, they are not just protecting themselves from disease. They are also protecting the people around them who are unable to be vaccinated because of contraindications and those who are among the small percentage of vaccine recipients who do not develop immunity after vaccination. The theory of **herd immunity** says that reducing the proportion of a population that is susceptible to an infection protects the entire population, including those who are unable to receive vaccines.[100] Suppose that during an outbreak, each infected person exposes about ten other people to the infection. In a completely susceptible population, all ten of the exposed people might become infected, and each of those ten people could spread the infection to many others. But if 80% of the members of the population have been vaccinated, only two of the initial ten contacts are likely to result in infection, and those two newly infected people will not be able to spread the infection to many others. Herd immunity helps prevent epidemics.

▶ 9.8 Vaccine-Preventable Infections

The **Expanded Program on Immunization (EPI)** was established by the WHO in 1974 to ensure universal child access to vaccines

for six vaccine-preventable diseases: measles, polio, tuberculosis (BCG), diphtheria, tetanus, and pertussis.[101] (The tuberculosis vaccine Bacillus Calmette-Guérin protects against serious tuberculosis disease but is of limited value in preventing colonization with the bacteria that cause tuberculosis.[102] BCG is usually not used in high-income countries where the risk of tuberculosis infection is very low.) EPI continues to support child vaccination programs today. The number of recommended pediatric vaccinations has expanded significantly over the past 25 years.[103] About a dozen vaccines are now routinely recommended for children, including mumps, rubella, hepatitis B, influenza, Hib, pneumococcus, and rotavirus (**FIGURE 9–14**).

Measles is a very contagious viral infection.[104] The initial symptoms are a fever, cough, runny nose, and watery eyes. A few days later, small white spots (Koplik spots) appear on the inside of the mouth, then red spots show up on the face and progress down the trunk and extremities. Some children experience serious complications, such as pneumonia, encephalitis, deafness, brain damage, and death, especially if they are vitamin A deficient.[105] Before a measles vaccine was available, measles killed millions of children each year.[106] The number of measles deaths worldwide per year decreased from an estimated 650,000 in 2000 to 135,000 in 2015—a remarkable 80% reduction—as the percentage of infants receiving at least one dose of a measles-containing vaccine increased from 72% to 85% (**FIGURE 9–15**).[107] However, the vaccination rate remains lower than the target in many of the low-income countries where undernutrition is common and the risk of measles mortality is greatest (**FIGURE 9–16**).[49]

The measles vaccine is often distributed as part of a combination MMR (measles, mumps, rubella) vaccine. The most visible sign of **mumps** is swollen parotid salivary glands that cause the cheeks to swell, but

Vaccine	Type of Agent	Agent
Diphtheria	Bacterium	*Corynebacterium diphtheriae*
Hepatitis B	Virus	Hepatitis B virus (HBV, hepadnavirus family)
Hib	Bacterium	*Haemophilus influenzae* type B
Influenza	Virus	Influenza virus (orthomyxovirus family)
Measles	Virus	Measles virus (paramyxovirus family)
Mumps	Virus	Mumps virus (paramyxovirus family)
Pertussis (whooping cough)	Bacterium	*Bordetella pertussis*
Pneumococcal disease (pneumococcus)	Bacterium	*Streptococcus pneumoniae*
Polio	Virus	Poliovirus (picornavirus)
Rotavirus	Virus	Rotavirus (reovirus family)
Rubella (German measles)	Virus	Rubella virus (togavirus family)
Tetanus	Bacterium	*Clostridium tetani*

FIGURE 9–14 Routinely recommended childhood vaccinations.

mumps can also cause serious complications, including encephalitis, meningitis, deafness, and, in adolescent and adult males, testicular inflammation (orchitis) that may cause infertility.[108] **Rubella**, also called German measles, often causes just a mild rash, but when pregnant women contract it, the virus can cause miscarriages and serious birth defects associated with congenital rubella syndrome.[109]

A combination vaccine is usually used to confer protection against diphtheria, tetanus, and pertussis (**FIGURE 9–17**).[49] **Diphtheria** causes inflammation of the airway and the production of thick mucus that can become a fatal airway obstruction. The infection can also damage the body's nerves and the heart muscle.[110] Tetanus, also called lockjaw, causes painful muscle spasms throughout the body, starting in the muscles of the lower face.[111]

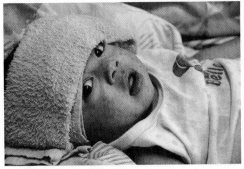

CDC/Molly Kurnit, M.P.H.

Measles.

Pertussis, also known as whooping cough, causes violent fits of coughing (paroxysms) punctuated by a "whoop" sound when inhaling.[112] Periodic coughing fits may persist for 10 weeks or longer, and they may be so vigorous that they cause rib fractures. Infants

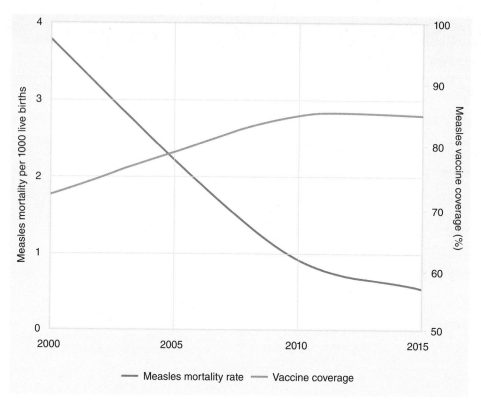

FIGURE 9–15 The measles mortality rate per 1000 live births in children aged 0–59 months decreased as the infant vaccine coverage increased.

Data from Department of Evidence, Information and Research (WHO) and Maternal Child Epidemiology Estimation (MCEE) group. *WHO-MCEE estimates for child causes of death 2000–2015*. Geneva: WHO; 2016.

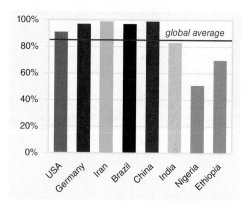

FIGURE 9–16 Percentage of infants receiving at least one dose of a measles-containing vaccine in 2015.

Data from *State of the world's children 2016*. New York: UNICEF; 2016.

who contract pertussis often do not cough, but instead suffer from bouts of **apnea** (long pauses in breathing) that may result in brain damage or death.[113]

Influenza,[114] Hib,[115] and pneumococcus[116] vaccines protect against respiratory infections, and rotavirus vaccines protect infants and young children from a type of severe gastroenteritis.[117] Some countries have opted not to include these vaccines in their childhood vaccination schedules, usually because of the cost of these recently developed products. In 2015, only about one in two infants received three doses of Hib vaccine, one in three infants received three doses of pneumococcal conjugate vaccine, and one in five infants received

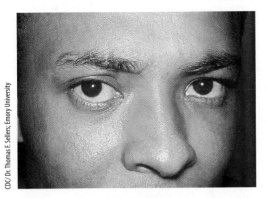

Jaundice caused by hepatitis A.

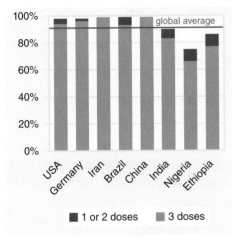

FIGURE 9–17 Percentage of infants receiving a diphtheria, tetanus, and pertussis (DTP) vaccine in 2015.

Data from *State of the world's children 2016*. New York: UNICEF; 2016.

the rotavirus vaccine (**FIGURE 9–18**).[49] Polio is a viral infection that causes paralysis in a small percentage of the people who contract it, and because it is the focus of a massive global eradication campaign, it is strongly recommended for all children.[118]

Other available vaccines that are recommended in some regions of the world, for some populations with high risk, and for some older age groups include anthrax, cholera,[119] hepatitis A,[120] human papillomavirus (HPV),[121] Japanese encephalitis,[122] meningococcus,[123] rabies,[124]

tick-borne encephalitis,[125] typhoid fever,[126] varicella-zoster (chickenpox and shingles),[127] and yellow fever[128] (**FIGURE 9–19**).[129] Additionally, several vaccines have been licensed in at least one country, such as ones for dengue[130] and hepatitis E,[131] and others are in advanced clinical trials, such as malaria,[132] and soon may be approved for public use. These vaccines may become more widely available after additional data demonstrate the safety and efficacy of the formulations.

Significant progress is being made in increasing access to vaccinations in low- and middle-income countries through partnerships like **Gavi**, the Vaccine Alliance (formerly GAVI, an acronym for Global Alliance for Vaccines and Immunization), which works with national governments across the income spectrum, WHO, UNICEF, The World Bank, charities like the Bill & Melinda Gates Foundation, and other entities to identify vaccine priorities and then procure and distribute the vaccines.[133] Further increases in vaccination coverage will require concurrent strengthening of health systems, disease surveillance coverage, laboratory testing capacity, health communications networks, and safety monitoring systems.[134]

▶ 9.9 Viral Hepatitis

Hepatitis is inflammation of the liver. Several types of viral hepatitis are of global public health concern, and each is caused by a very different type of virus that triggers liver inflammation (**FIGURE 9–20**).[135] About 1 million people each year die from acute or chronic viral hepatitis or the complications of chronic infection, including HBV- and HCV-associated liver cancers.[136]

Hepatitis A virus (HAV) is primarily spread through direct person-to-person contact and by ingestion of contaminated food and water.[137] HAV is an enteric pathogen that infects and replicates in the intestines. Young children who contract HAV typically have no

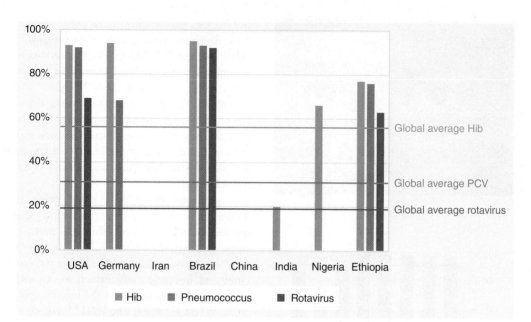

FIGURE 9–18 Percentage of infants receiving three doses of Hib (*Haemophilus influenzae* type B) vaccine, rotavirus vaccine, and three doses of pneumococcal conjugate vaccine in 2015.

Data from *State of the world's children 2016*. New York: UNICEF; 2016.

Vaccine	Type of Agent	Agent
Cholera	Bacterium	*Vibrio cholerae*
Hepatitis A	Virus	Hepatitis A virus (HAV, picornavirus family)
Hepatitis E	Virus	Hepatitis E virus (HEV, hepevirus family)
HPV	Virus	Human papillomavirus (HPV, papillomavirus family)
Japanese encephalitis	Virus	Japanese encephalitis virus (JEV, flavivirus family)
Meningococcal disease (meningococcus)	Bacterium	*Neisseria meningitidis*
Rabies	Virus	Rabies virus (rhabdovirus family)
Tick-borne encephalitis (TBE)	Virus	Tick-borne encephalitis virus (flavivirus family)
Typhoid fever	Bacterium	*Salmonella enterica* Typhi
Varicella zoster(chickenpox / shingles)	Virus	Varicella zoster virus (VZV, herpesvirus family)
Yellow fever	Virus	Yellow fever virus (flavivirus family)

FIGURE 9–19 Examples of other available vaccinations.

Disease	Viral Family	Primary Mode of Transmission	Risk of Chronic Disease?	Vaccine Preventable?
Hepatitis A	Picornavirus	Fecal-oral	No	Yes
Hepatitis B	Hepadnavirus	Parenteral	Yes	Yes
Hepatitis C	Flavivirus	Parenteral	Yes	No
Hepatitis E	Hepevirus	Fecal-oral	No	No

FIGURE 9–20 Major types of viral hepatitis.

symptoms, but older children and adults usually develop **jaundice**, a yellowing of the skin and sclera (the whites of the eyes) due to the build-up of bilirubin levels in the blood, and they typically suffer from fevers, gastrointestinal symptoms, and fatigue for about 8 weeks. A small proportion of people with hepatitis A develop life-threatening fulminant hepatitis, also called acute liver failure. Chronic HAV infection does not occur, and lifelong protection from the virus is conferred by infection and by vaccination. Most children in low-income countries contract HAV in very early childhood and develop immunity to the virus, but a large proportion of adults in high-income countries remain vulnerable to the infection.[138]

Hepatitis B virus (HBV) is transmitted through parenteral contact with blood or other body fluids as a result of a needle stick, an open wound (such as a cut or abrasion), or another tear in the skin or mucous membranes. The term **parenteral** describes the intake of a substance into the body through a route other than the digestive tract. HBV is also transmitted through sexual activity and through perinatal transmission in which the virus is passed from the mother to the neonate during delivery.[139] Hepatitis B can cause chronic liver disease.[140] Fewer than 5% of adults who contract HBV develop chronic infection, but about 95% of neonates do, and chronic HBV infection increases the risk of cirrhosis (scarring of the liver) and hepatocellular carcinoma, a type

of liver cancer.[141] Vaccination against HBV is contributing to a decrease in the prevalence of chronic hepatitis B disease (**FIGURE 9–21**), but the rates remain high in some parts of Africa, Asia, and South America.[142] Antiviral therapy can suppress the HBV virus but does not cure the infection, and HBV medications are not widely available in lower-income countries.[139]

Hepatitis C virus (HCV) is now transmitted primarily through injecting drug use.[143] HCV can also be transmitted sexually and from mother to child. Most people who contract HCV develop a chronic infection that substantially increases their risk of liver complications like cirrhosis and hepatocellular carcinoma. Several antiviral medications are available to suppress chronic HCV

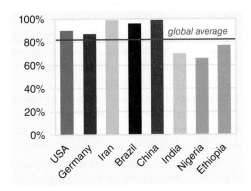

FIGURE 9–21 Percentage of infants receiving three doses of hepatitis B vaccine in 2015.

Data from *State of the world's children 2016*. New York: UNICEF; 2016.

infection, and some new medications completely eliminate the virus from most people who complete a course of treatment. However, these medications are too expensive to be widely available in lower-income countries or universally available in higher-income countries.[144] There is no vaccine against HCV, and the prevalence of chronic hepatitis C is increasing.[145]

Hepatitis E virus (HEV) is usually spread through contaminated water, and it is a common infection globally.[146] Most people who contract HEV have only mild disease, but pregnant women, especially those in the third trimester, have a significantly elevated risk of acute liver failure and a case fatality rate that might be as high as 20%.[147] Immunocompromised individuals may develop a chronic form of hepatitis E that causes rapid worsening of cirrhosis.[148] A vaccination against HEV has been licensed in China but is not yet available for wider use.[131]

▶ 9.10 Meningitis

Meningitis is an inflammation of the meninges, the membranes that cover the brain and spinal cord. Meningitis causes a severe headache and stiff neck along with other symptoms, such as confusion, nausea, sensitivity to light, and possibly sepsis (commonly called blood poisoning). **Encephalitis** is an acute inflammation of the brain. The symptoms of encephalitis are similar to those of meningitis, and include headaches, confusion, drowsiness, hallucinations, and seizures. When both meningitis and encephalitis occur in the same person, it is called meningoencephalitis.

Meningitis can be caused by a diversity of infectious agents, including fungi and parasites. Viral infections are the most common cause of meningitis, but bacterial meningitis is of greater concern because it has a higher case fatality rate.[149] The agents that cause bacterial meningitis include *Streptococcus pneumoniae* (pneumococcus), group B *Streptococcus*,

Neisseria meningitidis (meningococcus), *Haemophilus influenzae*, and *Listeria monocytogenes*, among others.[150] Three of those frequent causes are vaccine-preventable: pneumococcus, meningococcus, and Hib.

Meningococcus is the disease caused by infection with the bacterium *Neisseria meningitidis*, and it is one of the major causes of meningitis.[151] Meningococcus occurs worldwide, but rates of the disease have been particularly high in the "meningitis belt," an area that extends across the northern countries of sub-Saharan Africa from Senegal in the west to Ethiopia in the east.[152] Large outbreaks of meningococcus have historically occurred in these areas every few years during the dry season.[153] That pattern might be changing now that there is an effective vaccine against the primary cause of bacterial meningitis. The incidence of meningitis in the "meningitis belt" decreased rapidly after the introduction of meningococcus vaccine to the region in 2010.[154] However, cases are still occurring in countries across the region, and there is a need for continued surveillance to detect outbreaks early so that vaccination campaigns and other medical and public health measures can be implemented.[155]

▶ References

1. GBD 2015 Mortality and Causes of Death Collaborators. Global, regional, and national life expectancy, all-cause mortality, and cause-specific mortality for 249 causes of death, 1980–2015: A systematic analysis for the Global Burden of Disease Study 2015. *Lancet*. 2016;388:1459–544.
2. Babigumira J, Gelband H, Garrison LP Jr. Cost-effectiveness of strategies for the diagnosis and treatment of febrile illness in children (Chapter 15). *Disease control priorities*. 3rd ed. *Major infectious diseases (Volume 6)*. Washington DC: IBRD / World Bank; 2017.
3. Liu L, Oza S, Hogan D, et al. Global, regional, and national causes of under-5 mortality in 2000–15: An updated systematic analysis with implications for the Sustainable Development Goals. *Lancet*. 2016;388:3027–35.
4. *The Millennium Development Goals report 2015*. New York: UN; 2015.

5. United Nations. *Transforming our world: The 2030 Agenda for Sustainable Development.* New York: UN; 2015.

6. Keusch GT, Fischer-Walker C, Das JK, Horton S, Habte D. Diarrheal diseases (Chapter 9). *Disease control* priorities. 3rd ed. *Reproductive, maternal, newborn, and child health (Volume 2).* Washington DC: IBRD / World Bank; 2016.

7. Fischer-Walker CL, Rudan I, Liu L, et al. Global burden of childhood pneumonia and diarrhoea. *Lancet.* 2013;381:1405–16.

8. Platts-Mills JA, Babji S, Bodhidatta L, et al. Pathogen-specific burdens of community diarrhoea in developing countries: A multistate birth cohort study (MAL-ED). *Lancet Glob Health.* 2015;3:e564–75.

9. Lanata CF, Fischer-Walker CL, Olascoaga AC, Torres CX, Aryee MJ, Black RE. Global causes of diarrheal disease mortality in children <5 years of age: A systematic review. *PLoS One.* 2013;8:e72788.

10. Glass RI, Parashar UD, Bresee JS, et al. Rotavirus vaccines: Current prospects and future challenges. *Lancet.* 2006;368:323–32.

11. Tate JE, Burton AH, Boschi-Pinto C, Parashar UD. Global, regional, and national estimates of rotavirus mortality in children <5 years of age, 2000–2013. *Clin Infect Dis.* 2016;62(Suppl 2):S96–105.

12. Glass RI, Parashar UD, Estes MK. Norovirus gastroenteritis. *N Engl J Med.* 2009;361:1776–85.

13. Bert F, Scaioli G, Gualano MR, et al. Norovirus outbreaks on commercial cruise ships: A systematic review and new targets for the public health agenda. *Food Environ Virol.* 2014;6:67–74.

14. Sack DA, Sack RB, Nair GB, Siddique AK. Cholera. *Lancet.* 2004;363:223–33.

15. Almagro-Moreno S, Taylor RK. Cholera: Environmental reservoirs and impact on disease transmission. *Microbiol Spectr.* 2013;1:OH-0003-2012.

16. Lee K. The global dimensions of cholera. *Global Change Human Health.* 2001;2:6–17.

17. Lee K, Dodgson R. Globalization and cholera: Implications for global governance. *Glob Gov.* 2000;6:213–36.

18. Ali M, Nelson AR, Lopez AL, Sack DA. Updated global burden of cholera in endemic countries. *PLoS Negl Trop Dis.* 2015;9:e0003832.

19. Piarroux R, Frerichs RR. Cholera and blame in Haiti. *Lancet Infect Dis.* 2015;15:1380–1.

20. *Bad bug book: Foodborne pathogenic microorganisms and natural toxins handbook.* 2nd ed. Silver Spring MD: FDA Center for Food Safety and Applied Nutrition (CFSAN); 2014.

21. Tarr PI, Gordon CA, Chandler WL. Shiga-toxin-producing *Escherichia coli* and haemolytic uraemic syndrome. *Lancet.* 2005;365:1073–86.

22. Rangel JM, Sparling PH, Crowe C, Griffin PM, Swerdlow DL. Epidemiology of *Escherichia coli* O157:H7 outbreaks, United States, 1982–2002. *Emerg Infect Dis.* 2005;11:603–9.

23. Bennett SD, Walsh KA, Gould LH. Foodborne disease outbreaks caused by *Bacillus cereus, Clostridium perfringens,* and *Staphylococcus aureus*: United States, 1998–2008. *Clin Infect Dis.* 2013;57:425–33.

24. Kaakoush NO, Castaño-Rodríguez N, Mitchell HM, Man SM. Global epidemiology of *Campylobacter* infection. *Clin Microbiol Rev.* 2015;28:687–720.

25. Gal-Mor O, Boyle EC, Grassl GA. Same species, different diseases: How and why typhoidal and non-typhoidal *Salmonella enterica* serovars differ. *Front Microbiol.* 2014;5:391.

26. Wain J, Hendriksen RS, Mikoleit ML, Keddy KH, Ochiai RL. Typhoid fever. *Lancet.* 2015;385:1136–45.

27. Buckle GC, Fischer-Walker CL, Black RE. Typhoid fever and paratyphoid fever: Systematic review to estimate global morbidity and mortality for 2010. *J Glob Health.* 2012;2:010401.

28. Parry CM, Hien TT, Dougan G, White NJ, Farrar JJ. Typhoid fever. *N Engl J Med.* 2002;347:1770–82.

29. WHO Scientific Working Group. Enteric infections due to *Campylobacter, Yersinia, Salmonella,* and *Shigella. Bull World Health Organ.* 1980;58:519–37.

30. Pfeiffer ML, DuPont HL, Ochoa TJ. The patient presenting with acute dysentery: A systematic review. *J Infect.* 2012;64:374–86.

31. Speich B, Croll D, Fürst T, Utzinger J, Keiser J. Effect of sanitation and water treatment on intestinal protozoa infection: A systematic review and meta-analysis. *Lancet Infect Dis.* 2016;16:87–99.

32. Shirley DAT, Moonah SN, Kotloff KL. Burden of disease from cryptosporidiosis. *Curr Opin Infect Dis.* 2012;25:555–63.

33. Mac Kenzie WR, Hoxie NJ, Proctor ME, et al. A massive outbreak in Milwaukee of *Cryptosporidium* infection transmitted through the public water supply. *N Engl J Med.* 1994;331:161–7.

34. Escobedo AA, Hanevik K, Almirall P, Cimerman S, Alfonso M. Management of chronic *Giardia* infection. *Expert Rev Anti Infect Ther.* 2014;12:1143–57.

35. Dean AS, Crump L, Greter H, Hattendorf J, Schelling E, Zinsstag J. Clinical manifestations of human brucellosis: A systematic review and meta-analysis. *PLoS Negl Trop Dis.* 2012;6:e1929.

36. Kuipers EJ, Thijs JC, Festen HP. The prevalence of *Helicobacter pylori* in peptic ulcer disease. *Aliment Pharmacol Ther.* 1995;9(Suppl 2):59–69.

37. Ramaswamy V, Cresence VM, Rejitha JS, et al. Listeria: review of epidemiology and pathogenesis. *J Microbiol Immunol Infect.* 2007;40:4–13.

38. Sobel J. Botulism. *Clin Infect Dis.* 2005;41:1167–73.

39. Conant J, Fadem P. *Community guide to environmental health.* Berkeley CA: Hesperian Foundation; 2008.

40. Julian TR. Environmental transmission of diarrheal pathogens in low and middle income countries. *Environ Sci Process Impacts.* 2016;18:944–55.

41. Juckett G, Trivedi R. Evaluation of chronic diarrhea. *Am Fam Physician.* 2011;84:1119–26.

42. *Oral rehydration salts: Production of the new ORS.* Geneva: WHO/UNICEF; 2006.

43. *Where there is no doctor.* Berkeley CA: Hesperian Health Guides; 2017.

44. *Ending preventable child deaths from pneumonia and diarrhoea by 2025: The integrated Global Action Plan for Pneumonia and Diarrhoea (GAPPD).* New York: UNICEF/WHO; 2013.

45. Bhutta ZA, Das JK, Walker N, et al. The Lancet Diarrhoea and Pneumonia Interventions Study Group. Interventions to address deaths from childhood pneumonia and diarrhea equitably: What works and at what cost? *Lancet.* 2013;381:1417–29.

46. Chopra M, Mason E, Borrazzo J, et al. Ending of preventable deaths from pneumonia and diarrhoea: An achievable goal. *Lancet.* 2013;381:1499–506.

47. *One is too many: Ending child deaths from pneumonia and diarrhoea.* New York: UNICEF; 2016.

48. Department of Evidence, Information and Research (WHO) and Maternal Child Epidemiology Estimation (MCEE) group. *WHO-MCEE estimates for child causes of death 2000–2015.* Geneva: WHO; 2016.

49. *State of the world's children 2016.* New York: UNICEF; 2016.

50. Kirk MD, Pires SM, Black RE, et al. Global and regional disease burden of 22 foodborne bacterial, protozoal, and viral diseases, 2010: A data synthesis. *PLoS Negl Trop Dis.* 2015;12:e1001921.

51. Torgerson PR, Devleesschauwer B, Praet N, et al. World Health Organization estimates of the global and regional disease burden of 11 foodborne parasitic diseases, 2010: A data synthesis. *PLoS Negl Trop Dis.* 2015;12:e1001920.

52. Scallan E, Hoekstra RM, Angulo FJ, et al. Foodborne illness acquired in the United States: Major pathogens. *Emerg Infect Dis.* 2011;17:7–15.

53. *Five keys to safer food manual.* Geneva: WHO; 2006.

54. Codex Alimentarius Commission. *Food hygiene: Basic texts.* 4th ed. Rome: WHO/FAO; 2009.

55. Rudan I, O'Brien KL, Nair H, et al. Epidemiology and etiology of childhood pneumonia in 2010: Estimates of incidence, severe morbidity, mortality, underlying risk factors and causative pathogens for 192 countries. *J Glob Health.* 2013;3:010401.

56. O'Brien KL, Wolfson LJ, Watt JP, et al. Burden of disease caused by *Streptococcus pneumoniae* in children younger than 5 years: Global estimates. *Lancet.* 2009;374:893–902.

57. van der Poll T, Opal SM. Pathogenesis, treatment, and prevention of pneumococcal pneumonia. *Lancet.* 2009;374:1543–56.

58. Watt JP, Wolfson LJ, O'Brien KL, et al. Burden of disease caused by *Haemophilus influenzae* type b in children younger than 5 years: Global estimates. *Lancet.* 2009;374:903–11.

59. Nair H, Nokes DJ, Gessner BD, et al. Global burden of acute lower respiratory infections due to respiratory syncytial virus in young children: A systematic review and meta-analysis. *Lancet.* 2010;375:1545–55.

60. Gupta RK, George R, Nguyen-Van-Tam JS. Bacterial pneumonia and pandemic influenza planning. *Emerg Infect Dis.* 2008;14:1187–92.

61. Rudan I, Boschi-Pinto C, Biloglav Z, Mulholland K, Campbell H. Epidemiology and etiology of childhood pneumonia. *Bull World Health Organ.* 2008;86:408–16.

62. Prina E, Ranzani OT, Torres A. Community-acquired pneumonia. *Lancet.* 2015;386:1097–108.

63. Nair H, Simões EAF, Rudan I, et al. Global and regional burden of hospital admissions for severe acute lower respiratory infections in young children in 2010: A systematic analysis. *Lancet.* 2013;381:1380–90.

64. Ruuskanen O, Lahti E, Jennings LC, Murdoch Dr. Viral pneumonia. *Lancet.* 2011;377:1264–75.

65. Hall CB. The spread of influenza and other respiratory viruses: Complexities and conjectures. *Clin Infect Dis.* 2007;45:353–9.

66. Tang JW. The effect of environmental parameters on the survival of airborne infectious agents. *J R Soc Interface.* 2009;6(Suppl 6);S737–46.

67. Cunha BA, Burillo A, Bouza E. Legionnaires' disease. *Lancet.* 2015;387:376–85.

68. Jonsson BC, Moraes Figueiredo LT, Vapalahti O. A global perspective on hantavirus ecology, epidemiology, and disease. *Clin Microbiol Rev.* 2010;23:412–41.

69. Vanrompay D, Harkinezhad T, van de Walle M, et al. *Chlamydophila psittaci* transmission from pet birds to humans. *Emerg Infect Dis.* 2007;13:1108–10.

70. Kirkland TN, Fierer J. Coccidioidomycosis: A reemerging infectious disease. *Emerg Infect Dis.* 1996;2:192–9.

71. Kauffman CA. Histoplasmosis: A clinical and laboratory update. *Clin Microbiol Rev.* 2007;20:115–32.

72. Doshi P. The elusive definition of pandemic influenza. *Bull World Health Organ*. 2011;89:532–8.

73. Morens DM, Fauci AS. The 1918 influenza pandemic: Insights for the 21st century. *J Infect Dis*. 2007;195:1018–28.

74. Card AJ. Pandemicity and severity are separate constructs. *Am J Public Health*. 2012;102:e12.

75. Brundage JF, Shanks G. Deaths from bacterial pneumonia during the 1918–19 influenza pandemic. *Emerg Infect Dis*. 2008;14:1193–9.

76. Murray CJL, Lopez AD, Chin B, Feehan D, Hill KH. Estimation of potential global pandemic influenza mortality on the basis of vital registry data from the 1918–20 pandemic: A quantitative analysis. *Lancet*. 2006;368:2211–18.

77. Glezen WP. Emerging infections: Pandemic influenza. *Epidemiol Rev*. 1996;18:64–76.

78. Bouvier NM, Palese P. The biology of influenza viruses. *Vaccine*. 2008;26(Suppl 4):D49–53.

79. Webster RG, Govorkova EA. Continuing challenges in influenza. *Ann N Y Acad Sci*. 2014;1323:115–39.

80. Kalthoff D, Globig A, Beer M. (Highly pathogenic) avian influenza as a zoonotic agent. *Vet Microbiol*. 2010;140:237–45.

81. Barreto ML, Teixeira MG, Carmo EH. Infectious disease epidemiology. *J Epidemiol Community Health*. 2006;60:192–5.

82. Yoon SW, Webby RJ, Webster RG. Evolution and ecology of influenza A viruses. *Curr Top Microbiol Immunol*. 2014;385:359–75.

83. Reperant LA, Kuiken T, Osterhaus AD. Adaptive pathways of zoonotic influenza viruses: From exposure to establishment in humans. *Vaccine*. 2012;30:4419–34.

84. Novel Swine-Origin Influenza A (H1N1) Virus Investigation Team, Dawood FS, Jain S, Finelli L, et al. Emergence of a novel swine-origin influenza A (H1N1) virus in humans. *N Engl J Med*. 2009;360:2605–15.

85. Girard MP, Tam JS, Assossou OM, Kieny MP. The 2009 A (H1N1) influenza virus pandemic: A review. *Vaccine*. 2010;28:4895–902.

86. Gao R, Cao B, Hu Y, et al. Human infection with a novel avian-origin influenza A (H7N9) virus. *N Engl J Med*. 2013;368:1888–97.

87. Hayden FG, de Jong MD. Emerging influenza antiviral resistance threats. *J Infect Dis*. 2011;203:6–10.

88. Ferguson NM, Cummings DAT, Fraser C, Cajka JC, Cooley PC, Burke DS. Strategies for mitigating an influenza pandemic. *Nature*. 2006;442:448–52.

89. Osterholm MT, Kelley NS, Sommer A, Belongia EA. Efficacy and effectiveness of influenza vaccines: A systematic review and meta-analysis. *Lancet Infect Dis*. 2012;12:36–44.

90. Viboud C, Bjørnstad ON, Smith DL, Simonsen L, Miller MA, Grenfell BT. Synchrony, waves, and spatial hierarchies in the spread of influenza. *Science*. 2006;312:447–51.

91. Gostin LO. Influenza A (H1N1) and pandemic preparedness under the rule of international law. *JAMA*. 2009;301:2376–8.

92. Keller MA, Stiehm ER. Passive immunity in prevention and treatment of infectious diseases. *Clin Microbiol Rev*. 2000;13:602–14.

93. *Epidemiology and prevention of vaccine-preventable diseases*. 13th ed. Atlanta GA: CDC; 2015.

94. Plotkin SA. Vaccines: Past, present and future. *Nat Med*. 2005;11(Suppl 4):S5–11.

95. Chen RT, Orenstein WA. Epidemiologic methods in immunization programs. *Epidemiol Rev*. 1996;18:99–117.

96. Pickering LK, Orenstein WA. Development of pediatric vaccine recommendations and policies. *Semin Pediatr Infect Dis*. 2002;13:148–54.

97. Hanquet G, Valenciano M, Simondon F, Moren A. Vaccine effects and impact of vaccination programmes in post-licensure studies. *Vaccine*. 2013;31:5634–42.

98. Miller ER, Moro PL, Cano M, Schimabukuro T. Deaths following vaccination: What does the evidence show? *Vaccine*. 2015;33:3288–92.

99. Ellenberg SS, Chen RT. The complicated task of monitoring vaccine safety. *Public Health Rep*. 1997;112:10–21.

100. Fine PE. Herd immunity: History, theory, practice. *Epidemiol Rev*. 1993;15:265–302.

101. Casey RM, Dumolard L, Danovaro C, et al. Global routine vaccination coverage, 2015. *Wkly Epidemiol Rec*. 2016;91:537–43.

102. BCG vaccine: WHO position paper. *Wkly Epidemiol Rec*. 2004;79:27–38.

103. Feikin DR, Flannery B, Hamel MJ, Stack M, Hansen PM. Vaccines for children in low- and middle-income countries (Chapter 10). *Disease control priorities*. 3rd ed. *Reproductive, maternal, newborn, and child health (Volume 2)*. Washington DC: IBRD / World Bank; 2016.

104. Measles vaccines: WHO position paper. *Wkly Epidemiol Rec*. 2009;84:349–60.

105. Bester JC. Measles and measles vaccination: A review. *JAMA Pediatr*. 2016;170:1209–15.

106. Moss WJ. Measles. *Lancet*. 2012;379:153–64.

107. Patel MK, Gacic-Dobo M, Strebel PM, et al. Progress toward regional measles elimination—worldwide, 2000–2015. *Wkly Epidemiol Rec*. 2016;91:525–35.

108. Mumps virus vaccines: WHO position paper. *Wkly Epidemiol Rec.* 2007;82:51–60.

109. Rubella vaccines: WHO position paper. *Wkly Epidemiol Rec.* 2011;86:301–16.

110. Diphtheria vaccine: WHO position paper. *Wkly Epidemiol Rec.* 2006;81:24–32.

111. Tetanus vaccine: WHO position paper. *Wkly Epidemiol Rec.* 2006;81:198–208.

112. Pertussis vaccines: WHO position paper—August 2015. *Wkly Epidemiol Rec.* 2015;90:433–60.

113. Forsyth K, Plotkin S, Tan T, Wirsing von König CH. Strategies to decrease pertussis transmission to infants. *Pediatrics.* 2015;135:e1475–82.

114. Vaccines against influenza: WHO position paper—November 2012. *Wkly Epidemiol Rec.* 2012;87:461–76.

115. *Haemophilus influenzae* type b (Hib) vaccination position paper—July 2013. *Wkly Epidemiol Rec.* 2013;88:413–26.

116. Pneumococcal vaccines: WHO position paper. *Wkly Epidemiol Rec.* 2012;87:129–44.

117. Rotavirus vaccines: WHO position paper—January 2013. *Wkly Epidemiol Rec.* 2013;88:49–64.

118. Polio vaccines: WHO position paper—March 2016. *Wkly Epidemiol Rec.* 2016;91:145–68.

119. Cholera vaccines: WHO position paper. *Wkly Epidemiol Rec.* 2010;85:117–128.

120. WHO position paper on hepatitis A vaccines—June 2012. *Wkly Epidemiol Rec.* 2012;87:261–76.

121. Human papilloma vaccines: WHO position paper, October 2014. *Wkly Epidemiol Rec.* 2014;89:465–92.

122. Japanese encephalitis vaccines: WHO position paper—February 2015. *Wkly Epidemiol Rec.* 2015;90:69–88.

123. Meningococcal A conjugate vaccine: Updated guidance, February 2015. *Wkly Epidemiol Rec.* 2015;90:57–62.

124. Rabies vaccines: WHO position paper. *Wkly Epidemiol Rec.* 2010;85:309–20.

125. Vaccines against tick-borne encephalitis: WHO position paper. *Wkly Epidemiol Rec.* 2011;86:241–56.

126. Typhoid vaccines: WHO position paper. *Wkly Epidemiol Rec.* 2008;83:49–59.

127. Varicella and herpes zoster vaccines: WHO position paper, June 2014. *Wkly Epidemiol Rec.* 2014;89:265–88.

128. Vaccines and vaccination against yellow fever: WHO position paper—June 2013. *Wkly Epidemiol Rec.* 2013;88:269–84.

129. *Global vaccine action plan 2011–2020.* Geneva: WHO; 2013.

130. Dengue vaccine: WHO position paper—July 2016. *Wkly Epidemiol Rec.* 2016;91:349–64.

131. Hepatitis E vaccine: WHO position paper, May 2015. *Wkly Epidemiol Rec.* 2015;90:185–200.

132. Malaria vaccine: WHO position paper—January 2016. *Wkly Epidemiol Rec.* 2016;91:33–52.

133. *Keeping children healthy: The Vaccine Alliance progress report 2015.* Washington DC: Gavi; 2015.

134. *Global immunization vision and strategy 2006–2015.* Geneva: WHO/UNICEF; 2005.

135. *Global health sector strategy on viral hepatitis 2016–2021.* Geneva: WHO; 2016.

136. *Prevention & control of viral hepatitis infection: A strategy for global action.* Geneva: WHO; 2011.

137. Jacobsen KH, Koopman JS. Declining hepatitis A seroprevalence: A global review and analysis. *Epidemiol Infect.* 2004;133:1005–22.

138. Jacobsen KH, Wiersma ST. Hepatitis A virus seroprevalence by age and world region, 1990 and 2005. *Vaccine.* 2010;28:6653–7.

139. *Guidelines for the prevention, care and treatment of persons with chronic hepatitis B infection.* Geneva: WHO; 2015.

140. Hepatitis B vaccines: WHO position paper. *Wkly Epidemiol Rec.* 2009;84:405–19.

141. Trépo C, Chan HLY, Lok A. Hepatitis B virus infection. *Lancet.* 2014;384:2053–63.

142. Ott J, Stevens GA, Groeger J, Wiersma ST. Global epidemiology of hepatitis B virus infection: New estimates of age-specific HBsAg seroprevalence and endemicity. *Vaccine.* 2012;30:2212–9.

143. Webster DP, Klenerman P, Dusheiko GM. Hepatitis C. *Lancet.* 2015;385:1124–35.

144. *Guidelines for the screening, care and treatment of persons with hepatitis C infection.* Geneva: WHO; 2014.

145. Mohd Hanafiah K, Groeger J, Flaxman AD, Wiersma ST. Global epidemiology of hepatitis C virus infection: New estimates of age-specific antibody to HCV seroprevalence. *Hepatology.* 2013;57:1333–42.

146. Kamar N, Bendall R, Legrand-Abravanel F, et al. Hepatitis E. *Lancet.* 2012;379:2477–88.

147. Krain LJ, Nelson KE, Labrique AB. Host immune status and response to hepatitis E virus infection. *Clin Microbiol Rev.* 2014;27:139–65.

148. Hoofnagle JH, Nelson KE, Purcell RH. Hepatitis E. *N Engl J Med.* 2012;367:1237–44.

149. McGill F, Heyderman RS, Panagiotou S, Tunkel AR, Solomon T. Acute bacterial meningitis in adults. *Lancet.* 2016;388:3036–47.

150. Thigpen MC, Whitney CG, Messonier NE, et al. Bacterial meningitis in the United States, 1998–2007. *N Engl J Med.* 2011;364:2016–25.

151. Stephens DS, Greenwood B, Brandtzaeg P. Epidemic meningitis, meningococcaemia, and *Neisseria meningitidis.* *Lancet.* 2007;369:2196–210.

152. Molesworth AM, Thomson MC, Connor SJ, et al. Where is the meningitis belt? Defining an area at risk of epidemic meningitis in Africa. *Trans R Soc Trop Med Hyg.* 2002;96:242–9.

153. Agier L, Martiny N, Thiongane O, et al. Towards understanding the epidemiology of *Neisseria meningitidis* in the African meningitis belt: A multi-disciplinary overview. *Int J Infect Dis.* 2017;54:103–12.

154. Lingani C, Bergeron-Caron C, Stuart JM, et al. Meningococcal meningitis surveillance in the African meningitis belt, 2004–2013. *Clin Infect Dis.* 2015;61(Suppl 5):S410–5.

155. Meningococcal disease control in countries of the African meningitis belt, 2014. *Wkly Epidemiol Rec.* 2015;90:123–31.

CHAPTER 10

Malaria and Neglected Tropical Diseases

People who live in lower-income countries are frequently ill with malaria, intestinal worms, and a diversity of other infectious and parasitic diseases that are rare in high-income countries. These neglected tropical diseases (NTDs) maim, disable, and kill many of their victims, and they impede economic growth in affected communities and countries. Investments in controlling vectorborne diseases, treating common NTDs, supporting eradication campaigns, and containing emerging infectious diseases yield financial and security benefits for all partners.

▶ 10.1 Malaria, NTDs, and Global Health

Malaria has been the target of international public health efforts since the late 1800s, when scientists first discovered that the malaria parasite was transmitted to humans through the bites of infected mosquitoes. Initial research and development (R&D) investments by high-income countries focused on protecting military personnel and business interests in the tropics and on eliminating domestic threats posed by malaria.[1] The U.S. Centers for Disease Control and Prevention (CDC) is headquartered in Atlanta because the agency evolved from the national malaria control program.[2] Today, a diversity of governmental, charitable, and corporate partners are involved in developing and implementing control and elimination strategies for malaria and other debilitating infections.

Most countries where malaria still occurs are places where other dreadful tropical and parasitic diseases are also common. Many of these diseases are unimaginable to the typical person living in a high-income country, including parasites that cause body parts to swell to many times their normal size or leave their victims scarred and blind; disfiguring bacterial and protozoal infections that eat through skin, muscle, and even bones, causing permanent disability; and intestinal worms that can proliferate to completely block the digestive tract. A single photograph of any of these conditions would likely be enough to convince most people that these diseases deserve to be added to the list of priorities for global health funding. The need for prioritization becomes even clearer after seeing the epidemiological statistics showing that these conditions are far from rare. Nearly all of the 1 billion people from the world's lowest-income households—the so-called "bottom billion"[3]—have at least one of the bacterial, viral, or parasitic conditions that are classified by the World Health Organization (WHO) as neglected tropical diseases (**FIGURE 10–1**).[4]

Disease	Pathogen	Section
Dengue	Virus	10.5
Chagas disease	Protozoan	10.6
Human African trypanosomiasis (sleeping sickness)	Protozoan	10.6
Leishmaniases	Protozoan	10.7
Schistosomiasis	Helminth	10.8
Lymphatic filariasis	Helminth	10.9
Onchocerciasis (river blindness)	Helminth	10.10
Leprosy	Bacterium	10.11
Buruli ulcer	Bacterium	10.11
Trachoma	Bacterium	10.11
Rabies	Virus	10.12
Soil-transmitted helminthiases	Helminth	10.13
Taeniasis and neurocysticercosis	Helminth	10.14
Echinococcosis	Helminth	10.14
Yaws (and other endemic treponematoses)	Bacterium	10.14
Mycetoma	Bacterium/fungus	10.14
Foodborne trematodiases (clonorchiasis, opisthorchiasis, fascioliasis, and paragonimiasis)	Helminth	10.14
Dracunculiasis (guinea worm disease)	Helminth	10.15

FIGURE 10–1 Neglected tropical diseases recognized by the WHO.

Data from *Investing to overcome the global impact of neglected tropical diseases: 3rd WHO report on neglected tropical diseases*. Geneva: WHO; 2015.

Neglected tropical diseases (NTDs) are infectious diseases that primarily affect the poorest regions of the world and have not historically been a priority for funding agencies, pharmaceutical companies, or global policymakers.[5] The "big three" infectious diseases—HIV, tuberculosis, and malaria—have received the bulk of global health attention and financing in recent decades. The NTD designation is intended to call attention to infectious diseases that have been relatively invisible to the major players in global health even though they affect millions of people in the lowest-income countries and contribute to the cycle of poverty by causing long-term illnesses and disability.[6] "Neglected" does not mean infrequent, since NTDs affect more than one in six of the world's people. Neglected describes conditions that were overlooked, disregarded, and ignored as the field of global health emerged in the early 21st century.[7]

The Millennium Development Goal that called for the world to "combat HIV/AIDS, malaria, and other diseases" (MDG 6) has been expanded in the Sustainable Development Goals to call for commitments to "end the epidemics of AIDS, TB, malaria, and neglected tropical diseases" by 2030 and "combat hepatitis, water-borne diseases, and other communicable diseases" (SDG 3.3) (**FIGURE 10–2**).[8] Donors have answered this call by increasing their support for malaria and NTD control. In 2012, the London Declaration on Neglected Tropical Diseases, an ambitious plan to control 10 NTDs by 2020, was launched by WHO, the Bill & Melinda Gates Foundation, several multinational pharmaceutical companies, and other partners.[9] These groups have made commitments to help reduce infection transmission in endemic areas. In 2015 alone, pharmaceutical companies donated 1.5 billion doses of NTD treatments.[10] Many major drug companies are working with ministries of health and other organizations to create new NTD medications through product development partnerships like the Drugs for Neglected Diseases initiative.[11] These actions to recognize and address NTDs are a sign that NTDs are no longer being neglected. However, it will take

3.3.1	Number of new HIV infections per 1000 uninfected population
3.3.2	Tuberculosis incidence per 1000 persons per year
3.3.3	Malaria incident cases per 1000 persons per year
3.3.4	Number of new hepatitis B infections per 100,000 population per year
3.3.5	Number of people requiring interventions against neglected tropical diseases
3.8.1	Coverage of tracer interventions (universal health coverage of child immunization, antiretroviral therapy, tuberculosis treatment, and other health services)
3.b.1	Proportion of the population with access to affordable medicines and vaccines on a sustainable basis

FIGURE 10–2 Examples of Sustainable Development Goals targets focused on infectious diseases.

Data from United Nations Economic and Social Council. *Report of the Inter-Agency and Expert Group on Sustainable Development Goal Indicators* (E/CN.3/2016/2 /Rev.1). New York: UN; 2016.

continued commitments from global partnerships to alleviate the preventable burden that malaria and NTDs impose on the world's poorest children and families.

▶ 10.2 Parasites: Protozoa and Helminths

Many of the most burdensome tropical diseases, including malaria, are parasitic diseases. A **parasite** is a eukaryotic organism that survives by living in or on a host organism. A eukaryote consists of a complex cell or cells that have a membrane-bound nucleus. Bacteria and viruses are not eukaryotes, but fungi, plants, and animals are. Parasites can be acquired by walking barefoot in contaminated soil, wading in contaminated water, ingesting contaminated food or water, and being bit by parasite-infested insects. Some parasites only minimally affect their hosts, but others can cause serious illnesses and disability. Antiparasitic medications will kill many parasites, but the medicines may not be effective against all life stages of the parasites. For some parasitic infections, drug resistance means that medications that previously were effective treatments no longer work.

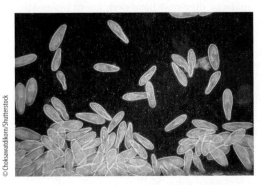

Paramecium are protozoa that are commonly found in environmental water sources.

There are two main types of eukaryotic parasites that affect human health: protozoa and helminths. A **protozoan** is a single-celled organism that has animal-like characteristics and often lives in water. Malaria is one of several diseases caused by protozoa. Protozoa are classified based on how they move and on the characteristics of their life cycles. For example, amoeba use pseudopods ("false feet") to move, flagellates have a "tail" that assists with motion, and ciliates have rows of hair-like projections that help the organisms move. A fourth category is for sporozoa, spore-forming protozoa. Some sporozoa (including the parasites that cause malaria) are apicomplexa that have complex life cycles involving both sexual and asexual reproduction.

A **helminth** is a multicellular endoparasitic worm that lives inside the body of its host. (Protozoa are also endoparasitic, living inside the body. In contrast, lice and the mites that cause scabies are ectoparasitic animals that live on the exterior surface of the body.[12]) Some worms are microscopic, but others grow to be several inches—or even several feet—long as they mature in the human body. Helminths are classified by shape as well as by their life cycles. There are three main types of helminths: nematodes, cestodes, and trematodes. A **nematode** is a cylindrically shaped roundworm. There are many types of nematodes that have humans as hosts, including filarial worms, guinea worms, hookworms, pinworms, roundworms, threadworms, and whipworms. Both cestodes and trematodes are flatworms in the platyhelminth phylum. A **cestode** is a tapeworm consisting of a mouthpiece (scolex) and numerous segments. Most tapeworms in humans (such as *Echinococcus* and *Taenia*) prefer to live in the human digestive tract, and some types of tapeworms can grow to be many feet long. A **trematode** is a fluke, and most trematodes have complex life cycles that involve two different animal hosts. In humans, trematodes infect a variety of body systems. For example, there are blood flukes (such as *Schistosoma*), liver flukes (such as *Clonorchis*), and lung flukes (such as *Paragonimus*). Some of these helminths have complex life cycles and undergo life stages in several different animal hosts and in the environment. An **intermediate host** is an animal host in which an immature parasite (a larva) develops but does not reach sexual maturity. A **definitive host** is the animal host in which a parasite reaches sexual maturity and reproduces.

▶ 10.3 Malaria

Malaria is a parasitic infection with protozoa from the **Plasmodium** species. There are five types of *Plasmodium* known to cause human infection: *Plasmodium falciparum, P. vivax, P. malariae, P. ovale,* and *P. knowlesi.* **Falciparum malaria** is the form most likely to cause life-threatening disease.[13] Nearly 90% of all malaria cases and deaths occur in sub-Saharan Africa, and nearly 99% of these cases are caused by *P. falciparum.* Outside of sub-Saharan Africa, about half of malaria cases are caused by *P. falciparum* and half by *P. vivax.*[14]

The parasites that cause malaria have a very complex life cycle that involves developmental stages in both humans and mosquitoes (**FIGURE 10–3**).[15] *Anopheles* mosquitoes need a bloodmeal in order to produce and lay eggs, and a female *Anopheles* mosquito acquires *Plasmodium* infection by biting an infected human. After the malaria parasites undergo several stages of development in the gut of the mosquito, they travel to the salivary gland of the mosquito and are injected into a human during a subsequent bloodmeal. After the parasites enter the bloodstream of the human, they move to the liver and reproduce rapidly. After several days of maturation, the parasites enter the bloodstream and invade the red blood cells that carry oxygen throughout the body. The parasites grow and divide inside the red blood cells. Every 2–3 days (depending on

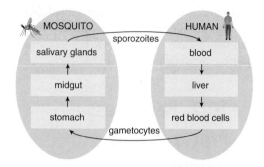

FIGURE 10–3 Life cycle of the *Plasmodium* parasites that cause malaria.

the species of *Plasmodium*), the red blood cells rupture, releasing parasites and toxins into the bloodstream and causing fever, chills, and anemia. The cycle can continue for 10–14 days, or longer if untreated.

Malaria usually causes cyclic fevers, headaches, joint pain, and other symptoms consistent with influenza-like illnesses, but it can cause organ failure and death. Although anyone can contract malaria, children and pregnant women have a higher risk of severe and fatal complications.[16] One common complication is severe **malarial anemia** due to the destruction of so many red blood cells that the body cannot adequately transport oxygen through the bloodstream.[17] Another complication in children is **cerebral malaria**, in which the infection causes seizures and coma (impaired consciousness).[18] If children survive cerebral malaria, they may have permanent brain damage and learning disabilities.[19] Adults who have grown up in endemic areas usually have some degree of resistance to severe malaria because of past infections.[20] However, susceptibility to malaria increases during pregnancy, and complications are common because pregnant women are often already anemic even before additional red blood cells are destroyed by *Plasmodium.*[21] As a result, babies born to mothers with malaria are at increased risk of low birthweight and other birth complications.[22]

People with malaria can usually be treated successfully with inexpensive antimalarial

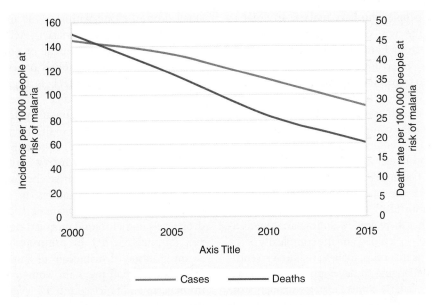

FIGURE 10-4 Global malaria cases and deaths decreased significantly between 2000 and 2015.
Data from *World malaria report 2015*. Geneva: WHO; 2015.

tablets, but malaria can cause weeks or even months of illness due to relapses and fatigue. Reinfection with malaria is common. In many tropical areas, the average child has several bouts of malaria each year. Each bout of malaria causes several days or weeks of absence from work or school and the inability to be productive at home. Infection is most common during the seasons when subsistence farmers grow and harvest their crops, and when malaria (or caring for people with malaria) keeps family members from being in the fields at this crucial time, it can result in long-term food insecurity for all members of the household.[23] The cost of lost productivity due to malaria extends to entire countries as well. Malaria-endemic countries have lower rates of economic growth than countries without malaria.[24]

More than 200 million cases of malaria occurred worldwide in 2015, and about 450,000 people died from the disease.[25] These numbers are large, but they represent a significant improvement from the year 2000.[26] The number of cases in 2015 was about one-third

lower than the number of cases in 2000, and the number of deaths decreased by nearly half during those 15 years (**FIGURE 10-4**).[14] The number of deaths in children younger than 5 years old decreased from about 725,000 to 300,000, and the percentage of malaria fatalities who were young children decreased from 85% to about 70%.[14] These improvements are attributed to expanded access to malaria prevention and treatment interventions.

▶ 10.4 Malaria Interventions

The only way that humans contract malaria is by being bit by an infected mosquito, and the only way that mosquitoes become infected is by biting an infected human. There are therefore two key sets of malaria control interventions. One set aims to reduce the likelihood of humans being bit by infected mosquitoes. The other set uses antiparasitic medications to treat people who have malaria in order to reduce the risk of mosquitoes contracting malaria from humans. Both types of interventions interrupt the mosquito–human–mosquito transmission cycle.

For decades, the drug of choice for treating malaria was chloroquine, but in most parts of the world, the common strains of malaria have become chloroquine-resistant and the medication is no longer effective. Strains of malaria are also becoming resistant to other pharmaceutical treatments, such as sulfadoxone/pyrimethamine (SP).[27] Widespread drug resistance means that there are few antimalarial medications that work today, and the complexity of the organisms that cause malaria makes it scientifically challenging to develop new therapeutic agents.[28] Malaria control experts strongly urge the use of **artemisinin-based combination therapy (ACT)** that combines at least two different antimalarial drugs (such as artemether plus lumefantrine or artesunate plus mefloquine), one of which is an artemisinin-based agent, because combination medications slow the emergence of drug resistance.[29]

Another component of successful malaria control programs is prescribing antimalarial medications only to people with laboratory-confirmed malaria (with just a few exceptions that have proven to be safe and cost-effective). A **rapid diagnostic test (RDT)** can detect the presence of a pathogen (or markers for a pathogen, such as the presence of specific antigens produced by malaria parasites) in a small drop of blood within 15–30 minutes.[30] If an RDT is positive for malaria, ACT can be prescribed. Prompt treatment of confirmed malaria reduces the likelihood of severe disease and death. If an RDT is negative for malaria, the febrile individual can be referred for additional clinical laboratory testing to determine the actual cause of the illness so that appropriate treatment can be prescribed.

Intermittent preventive treatment (IPT) is the use of "preventive chemotherapy" with antimalarial medications in vulnerable people so that they maintain therapeutic drug levels in their blood during times of high risk for malaria. **IPT in pregnancy (IPTp)** is the routine distribution of antimalarial medications to all pregnant women who live in malaria-endemic countries, even if the women do not have symptoms of malaria at the time of treatment.[31] IPTp medications are typically dispensed at two to four antenatal care visits during the second and third trimesters of pregnancy.[32] Presumptive treatment for malaria with IPTp is effective at increasing the average birthweight and survival rates of babies born to women in endemic areas who receive the recommended doses.[33] In very high-transmission areas, IPT of infants (IPTi) may also be a cost-effective intervention for reducing the burden from malaria.[34]

Although travelers from nonendemic areas to places where malaria is endemic generally take prophylactic (preventive) antimalarial drugs, these are not fully effective in preventing the disease. More importantly, it is not realistic or healthy to encourage prophylactic use among people who live in highly endemic areas. The financial cost would be high, long-term drug use could be detrimental to users' health, and the widespread use of antiparasitic agents would contribute to the development of more drug-resistant *Plasmodium* at a time when many species are no longer susceptible to existing antimalarial medications.

Because the mosquitoes that spread malaria bite primarily at dawn and dusk, one of

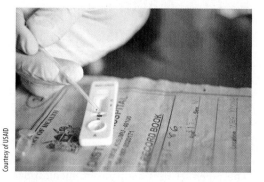

Rapid diagnostic test.

Courtesy of USAID

the most effective ways to prevent new malaria infections is the use of an **insecticide-treated net (ITN)**, a mesh sheet dipped in insecticides and then hung over a bed so that it provides a barrier between sleeping humans and mosquitoes while also killing any mosquitoes that land on it. Most ITNs need to be re-dipped in a pyrethroid insecticide every 6 months or so in order to maintain their effectiveness. A **long-lasting insecticidal net (LLIN)** is an ITN that has been impregnated with a pesticide that remains effective for 2 years or longer before requiring retreatment.[35] ITNs significantly reduce child mortality in malaria-endemic areas when they are used consistently.[36] It is also important for malaria patients to stay under a bednet so mosquitoes cannot bite them and become carriers of malaria. Since many adults who have grown up in malaria-endemic areas continue to have **parasitemia** (parasites in the blood) even when they are asymptomatic,[37] it is advisable for all children and adults who live in at-risk areas to consistently use ITNs. While many residents of households in regions where malaria is common still do not have ITNs or do not use them every night, the proportion of young children in sub-Saharan Africa who sleep under an ITN increased significantly after the year 2000 (**FIGURE 10-5**).[14] About two-thirds of the reduction in malaria cases between 2000 and 2015 is attributed to the scaled-up use of ITNs.[38]

Other barrier methods for insect bite protection include wearing clothes that cover the arms and legs during the times of the day when mosquitoes are most likely to bite and having screens or curtains cover the windows and doors of houses when it is possible to do this. Insect repellents like bug sprays, especially those that contain **DEET** (*N*,*N*-diethyl-*m*-toluamide), can also be helpful when they are affordable and are used appropriately.[39]

Malaria control efforts also aim to reduce the risk of mosquito bites by limiting the number of mosquitoes that live in proximity to human populations. Most cases of malaria occur in the tropics, where mosquitoes survive year-round. ***Anopheles* mosquitoes**,

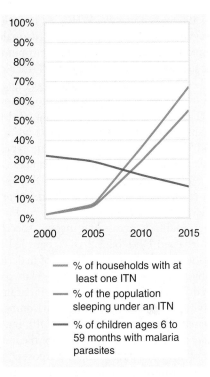

FIGURE 10-5 The percentage of under-5 children in sub-Saharan Africa who sleep under an ITN has increased rapidly.

Data from *World malaria report 2015*. Geneva: WHO; 2015.

the members of the genus of mosquitoes that spread malaria, deposit their eggs in relatively still but well-oxygenated water, so any places where water collects (like ponds, lakes, and puddles) can serve as mosquito habitats, especially during rainy seasons. Environmental changes related to road building, mining, logging, agriculture, and irrigation may also create breeding sites, further increasing the mosquito population.[40] These factors can make the environmental control of insect populations through land and water management or the widespread application of outdoor pesticides prohibitively expensive.

Until the middle of the 20th century, malaria was endemic across much of the globe, with cases reported as far north as Canada and Siberia. The Global Malaria Eradication Programme that was implemented between 1955 and 1969 was a massive WHO-led insecticide spraying program that eliminated malaria from dozens of countries.[41] One contributor to this success was the spraying of **DDT** (dichloro-diphenyl-trichloroethane) in large quantities over cities and crops to kill mosquitoes.[42] DDT does not easily degrade. It is a persistent organic pollutant (POP) that builds up in the food chain, eventually killing some types of birds and fish. The United States banned DDT in 1972 (in large part because of the uproar caused by Rachel Carson's book *Silent Spring*, which had been published in 1962), and many other countries across the income spectrum also enacted DDT bans.[43] DDT bans led to a drastic increase in the incidence of malaria in many countries.[44] In 2001, a global treaty sponsored by the UN Environment Programme (UNEP) and many private environmental organizations banned 11 other POPs, but the treaty made a special exemption for the indoor use of DDT for public health purposes.[45] Use of the chemical is now limited but not banned.

Since the reversal of the DDT ban, many communities in malaria-endemic areas have begun using DDT in homes. **Indoor residual spraying (IRS)** is the application of long-lasting insecticides to walls and other surfaces where mosquitoes might rest. When mosquitoes land on IRS-treated surfaces any time during the 6 months (or longer) after IRS has been applied, they absorb a lethal dose of the insecticidal chemical.[46] The environmental persistence that makes DDT a hazard when it is sprayed outdoors makes it appealing for in-home use as an insecticide. DDT sticks to the walls so that the pesticide only needs to be applied once or twice a year, and small amounts of DDT seem to be harmless to humans and household animals. DDT is also cheaper and more effective than most other pesticides.

DDT and other insecticides used for IRS only protect people from bites while they are indoors, and some mosquitoes are resistant to the effects of these chemicals. Still, the WHO now endorses the use of IRS for mosquito control in areas that have endemic or epidemic malaria transmission, and DDT could contribute, if used correctly, to preventing millions of malaria deaths.[47] Although still controversial, the policy changes that have enabled the reintroduction of DDT for home protection may end up being an example of how people with different views on the risks and benefits of an environmental intervention can find a middle ground that is acceptable to most parties involved.

While individuals and households bear much of the responsibility for implementing malaria control strategies, they are supported by national and global initiatives to develop, promote, and finance strategies for malaria prevention, diagnosis, treatment, and control.[48] For example, the **Roll Back Malaria** Partnership brings together the WHO, UNICEF, other multilateral organizations, national governments from malaria-endemic countries and donor countries, researchers, and representatives from foundations, nongovernmental organizations, academia, and the private sector in order to increase and sustain access to effective prevention and treatment technologies.[49] Other partnerships, such as the Medicines for Malaria Venture and the Malaria Vaccine Initiative, are focused on creating new preventive, diagnostic, and treatment tools.[50] Several vaccine candidates are in development.[51] Nonprofit organizations and advocacy groups like Malaria No More allow individual donors to contribute to malaria control efforts.[52] Continued financial, scientific, and social support for malaria elimination efforts will be necessary to reach the SDG goal of ending malaria by 2030.[53]

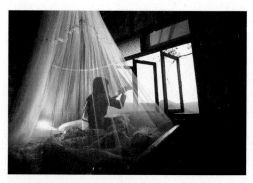
© Mr.Pornsatid/Shutterstock

▶ 10.5 Dengue and Other Arboviruses

Malaria is just one of many infections that are transmitted to humans by the bites of infected mosquitoes. A **vectorborne infection** is one that is transmitted to humans via an **arthropod**, such as an insect (like a mosquito, fly, or flea) or an arachnid (like a tick, louse, or mite). (An insect has six legs, an external covering made of chitin, a pair of antennae, and three body sections: a head, thorax, and abdomen. An arachnid has eight legs, an exoskeleton, compound eyes, and two body sections: a cephalothorax and an abdomen.) The **cycle of infection** describes how an infectious agent passes between different species. Some infections have a human–human–human cycle (like measles and sexually transmitted infections). Some have a vertebrate–vertebrate–vertebrate cycle and only occasionally affect humans (like rabies). A vectorborne infection has a human–arthropod–human cycle (or an animal–arthropod–animal cycle that occasionally affects a human). A wide variety of vectors can transmit infectious agents to humans (**FIGURE 10–6**).

Disease	Name of Pathogen	Type of Pathogen	Primary Vector (Genus)
African trypanosomiasis (sleeping sickness)	*Trypanosoma brucei*	Protozoan (flagellate)	Tsetse flies (*Glossina*)
Chagas disease	*Trypanosoma cruzi*	Protozoan (flagellate)	Reduviid bugs (*Triatominae*)
Leishmaniasis	*Leishmania*	Protozoan (flagellate)	Sandflies (*Lutzomyia* and *Phlebotomus*)
Loiasis (African eyeworm)	*Loa loa*	Helminth (filarial nematode)	Deer flies (*Chrysops*)
Lyme disease (borreliosis)	*Borrelia burgdorferi*	Bacterium	Ticks (*Ixodes*)
Lymphatic filariasis	*Wuchereria bancrofti, Brugia malayi, Brugia timori*	Helminth (filarial nematode)	Mosquitoes (*Culex*)
Malaria	*Plasmodium*	Protozoan (sporozoan)	Mosquitoes (*Anopheles*)
Onchocerciasis (river blindness)	*Onchocerca volvulus*	Helminth (filarial nematode)	Blackflies (*Simulium*)
Plague	*Yersinia pestis*	Bacterium	Fleas (*Xenopsylla*)
Rocky Mountain spotted fever	*Rickettsia rickettsii*	Bacterium (rickettsia)	Ticks (*Dermacentor*)
Tularemia	*Francisella tularensis*	Bacterium	Ticks
Typhus fever	*Rickettsia prowazekii*	Bacterium (rickettsia)	Body lice (*Pediculus*)

FIGURE 10–6 Examples of bacterial and parasitic vectorborne diseases.

A virus transmitted to humans by an arthropod is called an **arbovirus**, short for arthropod-borne virus. The pathogens that have recently caused large outbreaks of dengue fever, yellow fever, and Zika virus infections are arboviruses spread by mosquitoes. Some less common arboviruses, like the ones that cause Crimean-Congo hemorrhagic fever and tick-borne encephalitis, are spread by ticks (**FIGURE 10–7**). All arboviruses are viral infections. Bacterial and parasitic infections, like malaria, are not arboviruses because they are not viral.

Dengue fever is an arbovirus spread by the bites of infected **Aedes mosquitoes**, a genus of mosquito that thrives in urban areas. There are four distinct serotypes of dengue virus.[54] Infection with any one strain confers protection against future infections with that strain, but it does not protect against the other three dengue virus strains. Infection with a first strain is often asymptomatic, but it may cause a high fever, a severe headache, and pain in the eyes, joints, muscles, and bones. Infection with a second strain can lead to dengue hemorrhagic fever and dengue shock syndrome.[55] About 100 million people become ill from dengue virus infections each year, and many more have asymptomatic infections. The heaviest burdens are in South Asia, Southeast Asia, tropical South America, and some parts of tropical sub-Saharan Africa.[56] The geographic range of places where dengue is endemic has expanded significantly over the past several decades.[57] The countries already experiencing or at risk of dengue infection include Brazil, Nigeria, Ethiopia, and India as well as parts of the southern United States and southeastern China. Developing a tetravalent vaccine that is effective against all four serotypes has proven to be a major scientific challenge.[58] However, a dengue vaccine was licensed for the first time at the end of 2015, and there is hope that an effective tetravalent vaccine may soon be widely available for use as a preventive intervention.[59]

Yellow fever is a disease named for the jaundice that turns the skin and eyes of victims a bright yellow hue. About 1 in 20 people

Disease	Viral Family	Primary Vector (Genus)
Chikungunya	Togavirus	Mosquitoes (*Aedes*)
Crimean-Congo hemorrhagic fever (CCHF)	Bunyavirus	Ticks (*Hyalomma*)
Dengue fever	Flavivirus	Mosquitoes (*Aedes*)
Japanese encephalitis (JE)	Flavivirus	Mosquitoes (*Culex*)
Rift Valley fever (RVF)	Bunyavirus	Mosquitoes (*Aedes*)
Tick-borne encephalitis (TBE)	Flavivirus	Ticks (*Ixodes*)
West Nile (WN)	Flavivirus	Mosquitoes (*Culex*)
Yellow fever	Flavivirus	Mosquitoes (*Aedes*)
Zika	Flavivirus	Mosquitoes (*Aedes*)

FIGURE 10–7 Examples of arboviral diseases.

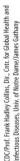

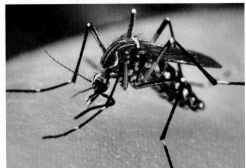

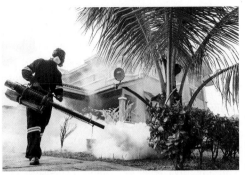

Aedes aegypti mosquito, the most common vector for dengue fever.

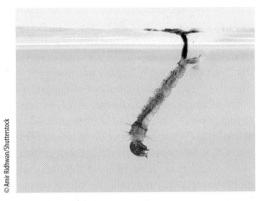

Aedes mosquito larva in water.

who contract the yellow fever virus die from it, usually as a result of hemorrhagic fever.[60] Epidemics of yellow fever occur primarily in tropical areas in South America and Africa, where the *Aedes* mosquitoes that transmit the yellow fever virus are common, but outbreaks have occurred in other regions.[61] Yellow fever is vaccine-preventable, and the global infectious disease control protocols spelled out in the International Health Regulations often mandate vaccination for travelers to and from places where outbreaks are occurring.[62]

Until recently, infection with Zika virus was considered to be such an inconsequential threat to human health that it was rarely tested for and only a few research papers had been published about it.[63] That perception changed dramatically in 2015, when

Zika virus spread to the Americas for the first time and an outbreak in Brazil was linked to a possible increase in the incidence of microcephaly in babies born to women who had been infected with Zika virus.[64] **Microcephaly** is an abnormally small head that is a sign of aberrant brain development. Concerns about Zika were exacerbated by the discovery that Zika virus could be transmitted not only through the bites of infected mosquitoes but also through sexual contact.[65]

West Nile virus is spread by *Culex* mosquitoes, and it typically cycles between mosquitoes and birds but occasionally affects humans.[66] Most people who become infected with West Nile virus have no symptoms or only mild symptoms, but a small percentage (<1%) develop severe neurologic complications.[67] West Nile virus was first identified in Africa, but outbreaks have occurred in many world regions. After the virus started circulating in the New York City metropolitan area in 1999,[68] the infection quickly spread across the continental United States.[69] Japanese encephalitis virus is closely related to West Nile virus. Like West Nile virus, most people who contract Japanese encephalitis virus are asymptomatic but a small proportion become seriously ill or die. Outbreaks of **Japanese encephalitis** occur regularly in Asia and Oceania even though the infection is vaccine-preventable.[70]

The dengue, yellow fever, Zika, West Nile, and Japanese encephalitis viruses are all in the flavivirus genus of the flavivirus family, but disease-causing viruses from other viral families are also spread by insects. For example, Rift Valley fever virus is in the phlebovirus genus of the bunyavirus family, and chikungunya virus is in the alphavirus genus of the togavirus family. **Rift Valley fever** is a zoonosis that can cause outbreaks of pregnancy loss in livestock herds. Most humans who contract Rift Valley fever virus have a mild infection, but a small percentage develop vision loss, meningoencephalitis, or hemorrhagic fever.[71] Chikungunya fever is notable because it can cause long-term disability. Most people with **chikungunya** virus infections suffer from weeks of severe pain in the joints of their arms and legs, but for some people the arthralgia and arthritis persist for months or even years.[72]

Vectorborne diseases can be at least partially contained through **vector control** interventions that reduce the size and density of arthropod populations. Vector control is typically achieved using insecticides and environmental modifications that limit the availability of insect breeding grounds. For example, community prevention efforts for dengue fever often focus on eliminating the standing water where the *Aedes* mosquitoes that transmit the virus breed.[73] Any small body of standing water, such as the water that collects in old cans and discarded tires, can become a breeding ground. One household that does not clean up its yard can put a whole neighborhood at risk, so all residents in a community must be involved in dengue prevention projects. Control of animal populations and waste management that keeps rodents and other mammals away from humans can help to control the spread of other types of vectorborne infections that are transmitted by arthropods that live on mammals.

▶ 10.6 Chagas Disease and Trypanosomiasis

Two of the NTDs recognized by the WHO and partner groups are caused by protozoa from the trypanosoma genus: Chagas disease and trypanosomiasis. **Chagas disease**, sometimes called American sleeping sickness, is an infection with *Trypanosoma cruzi* parasites that are spread by triatomines (also called reduviids, cone-nosed bugs, or "kissing bugs") that live in the cracks of walls and roofs of low-quality houses in Central and South America. The insects emerge at night to take bloodmeals from sleeping people. The feces of infected insects contain *T. cruzi* protozoa that can enter the human bloodstream through the wound left after the bloodmeal. Within a few days, a sore may develop at the site of the bite. This wound is often near the eye, where it may cause Romaña's sign, a swollen eyelid characteristic of acute Chagas disease.[74] About 20% to 30% of people who are infected with *T. cruzi* develop a chronic infection that over several decades causes severe damage to the heart (Chagas cardiomyopathy), digestive tract (gastrointestinal Chagas), or both.[75] Chagas-associated heart disease causes chronic heart failure and can induce fatal arrhythmias.[76] Vector control programs, screening of blood donors, and treatment with antiparasitic medications have reduced the incidence of new infections, but millions of people are already living with the damage caused by long-term infection.[74] Because many of those adults are people who have migrated to other countries and now live in North America, Europe, Japan, Australia, and other locations,[77] the need for improved Chagas disease care is a global one.

Human African **trypanosomiasis** (HAT), commonly called African sleeping sickness, is an infection with *Trypanosoma brucei*, which is transmitted to animals and humans by the bites of infected tsetse flies (biting flies from the *Glossina* genus).[78] Two subspecies of the protozoan can cause human disease. *T. b. rhodesiense* is found in eastern and southern Africa, and it is primarily a zoonotic infection that affects cattle and other mammals. (Animal African trypanosomiasis is sometimes called nagana.) Few human infections with *T. b. rhodesiense* have been diagnosed in recent years.[78] *T. b. gambiense* is found in western and central Africa, and it is primarily a human disease that

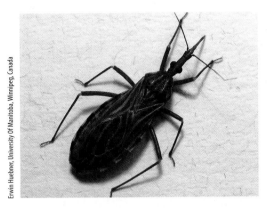

A triatomine (kissing bug), the vector for Chagas disease.

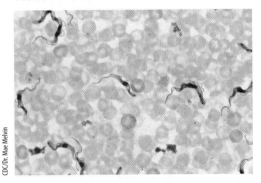

Trypanosoma brucei in blood.

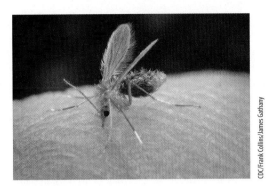

A phlebotomine sand fly, the vector for lieshmaniasis.

affects rural populations. Infected people experience chronic fevers and headaches in an initial hemolymphatic stage, and then the disease progresses to a meningoencephalitic stage that leads to coma and death if not treated. Without treatment, HAT is fatal within a few weeks or months for *T. b. rhodesiense* and about 3 years for *T. b. gambiense*.[79] The available treatments have limited efficacy, and they are often toxic, causing pain and dangerous side effects.[80] Although fewer than 20,000 cases of HAT are thought to occur each year, HAT is an important public health concern in affected regions because of the high case fatality rate.[78]

▶ 10.7 Leishmaniasis

Leishmaniasis is an infection with protozoa from various species of the *Leishmania* genus.

The parasites are transmitted to humans by female phlebotomine sandflies that need blood from a mammal in order to develop their eggs. Leishmaniasis occurs across parts of Asia (including India and China), North Africa and the Middle East (including Iran), Africa (including Ethiopia), and South America (including Brazil).[81] There are two common presentations of leishmaniasis disease. Cutaneous leishmaniasis causes lesions that can lead to permanent disfigurement, but they are not a life-threatening infection because they can be treated with wound care methods and antibiotics. Each year, about 700,000 to 1.2 million people develop cutaneous leishmaniasis.[82] Visceral leishmaniasis, also known as kala-azar, causes chronic fevers, weight loss, anemia, and swelling of the spleen and liver. People who are diagnosed as having visceral leishmaniasis are typically treated with combination antibiotic therapy.[83] Without treatment, visceral leishmaniasis is fatal within a few years. Each year, about 200,000–400,000 people develop visceral leishmaniasis, and about 20,000–40,000 people die from the disease.[82] Prevention and control strategies must be targeted to the particular types of *Leishmania* that are causing the disease in each affected country.[83]

▶ 10.8 Schistosomiasis

Schistosoma are trematodes that cycle between snails and humans.[84] Snails are the intermediate host for *Schistosoma*, which means that snails are hosts to immature parasites. Humans are the definitive host in which the parasites reach sexual maturity. Humans become infected by wading in water infested with parasite-infected snails while fishing, washing clothes, bathing, or doing other activities. Immature schistosomes are called cercariae, the name for the free-swimming larvae of trematodes. Schistosome cercariae penetrate through human skin, enter the blood supply, and then eventually travel to the veins of the intestines or bladder, where male–female pairs lay thousands of eggs. Some of those eggs become trapped in nearby tissues, where they trigger an inflammatory response that causes scarring. Some of the eggs pass through the abdominal tissues and enter the bladder or intestines. Infected humans who urinate or defecate in fresh water release those eggs into the environment, where the eggs hatch and release larvae called miracidiae. The larvae penetrate snails that live in the water, and within the snails, the miracidiae mature and produce cercariae. When cercariae leave the snails, they seek out a new human host and restart the cycle of infection.

Schistosomiasis, sometimes called bilharzia, is the disease caused by *Schistosoma* blood flukes. There are several different kinds of schistosomiasis.[85] *S. haematobium* occurs primarily in parts of Africa and the Middle East, and it causes urogenital schistosomiasis. Urogenital schistosomiasis instigates bloody urine (hematuria) and anemia in its early stages. If untreated, the resulting fibrous scarring of the bladder can lead to bladder cancer.[86] Chronic infection can also cause kidney damage. *S. mansoni*, which occurs in parts of South America and the Caribbean as well as in Africa and the Middle East, and *S. japonicum*, which occurs primarily in Asia, both cause intestinal schistosomiasis. Intestinal schistosomiasis induces abdominal pain, diarrhea, and bloody stool, and it can also cause enlargement of the liver and spleen (hepatosplenomegaly). In each species, the worms infect both snails and humans, and the parasites cycles between these two species.

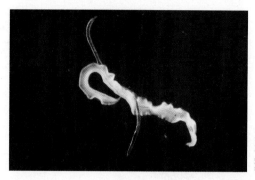

Coupled male and female *Schistosoma mansoni* parasites.

More than 230 million people worldwide are thought to have schistosomiasis.[85] An effective medication called praziquantel kills the parasites, but people who are treated for schistosomiasis are immediately susceptible to new infection when they come into contact with contaminated water. Each host in the cycle of infection must be considered for inclusion in an infection control plan. Molluscicides are sometimes used to kill the snails that live in infested waters, but snails will eventually move back into the waters, and new snail habitats are created when dams and irrigation systems are built. The prevalence of schistosomiasis increased significantly when the Aswan Dam was built on the Nile River in Egypt, when dams were built on the Senegal and Volta Rivers and in other locations in West Africa, and when small dams and irrigation projects have been introduced into villages in many parts of the world.[87] A comprehensive control plan includes snail control, treatment of existing cases with praziquantel, a community-wide sanitation program, and health education to encourage consistent use of toilets.[88]

▶ 10.9 Lymphatic Filariasis

Lymphatic filariasis (LF) is an infection with one of three types of filarial nematodes: *Wuchereria bancrofti*, *Brugia malayi*, and *B. timori*.[89] All three types of roundworms are transmitted by mosquitoes, and a diversity of mosquitoes can serve as vectors. Mosquitoes become infected by taking blood meals from humans who have immature nematode larvae, called microfilariae, circulating in their blood. After the larvae mature within the mosquito, they can be deposited in the skin of humans who are bitten during subsequent blood meals. The larvae mature into adults within the human lymph system. If the worms block the flow of lymph (tissue fluid), it can cause **lymphedema**, the swelling of body parts, usually the legs, due to retained lymph fluid in the tissues. Chronic lymphedema and poor hygiene can cause the skin of affected limbs to thicken and develop a coarse texture similar to that of an elephant's leg, a condition called **elephantiasis**. Males with lymphatic filariasis may also develop lymphedema of the scrotum, a condition called **hydrocele**. In 2015, more than 1 million people were living with LF-associated lymphedema and more than 500,000 men had hydrocele.[90]

Elephantiasis and hydrocele may cause permanent disfigurement and disability, and antihelminthic medications are ineffective in killing adult worms.[91] However, medications can kill microfilariae in the blood. Treatment of infected people is important for interrupting the cycle of infection by preventing new infections in mosquitoes. The WHO Global Programme to Eliminate Lymphatic Filariasis (GPELF) was launched in 2000, and it uses widespread distribution of antihelminthic medications in endemic places to reduce transmission rates.[92]

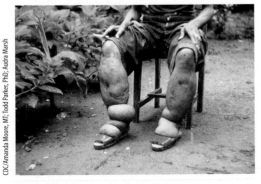

Elephantiasis caused by lymphatic filariasis.

Mass drug administration (MDA), also called **preventive chemotherapy**, is the distribution of safe medications to large population groups at regular time intervals as part of strategies for preventing and controlling infectious diseases. The main scientific limitation of MDA is that for most infections, the recipients are almost immediately susceptible to reinfection. To be effective, MDA must be repeated in endemic areas and must be accompanied by health education and environmental health programs.

GPELF and its partners were successful in limiting the number of people with circulating microfilariae in 2015 to about one-third the number in 2000.[92] That reduction represents significant progress toward elimination. However, there are still nearly 1 billion people living in endemic areas in South America (including Brazil), the Caribbean, Africa (including both Ethiopia and Nigeria), South and Southeast Asia (including India), and Oceania who remain at risk of contracting the worms that cause lymphatic filariasis.[90]

▶ 10.10 Onchocerciasis

Onchocerciasis, also known as river blindness, is caused by a filarial helminth called *Onchocerca volvulus* that is transmitted to humans by the bites of infected black flies (from the *Simulium* genus).[89] Adult worms form nodules in the subcutaneous tissue under the skin and release microfilariae into surrounding tissues. This causes a skin rash and intense itching, and it may also change the skin appearance, such as causing depigmentation of skin on the shins (a condition colloquially called leopard skin). If the microfilariae enter the eyes, they can scar the corneas and cause the host to become blind.

Preventive chemotherapy with an antiparasitic medication called ivermectin is used to kill microfilariae in people who live in onchocerciasis-endemic areas. Ivermectin is typically distributed to entire communities once or twice a year. MDA for onchocerciasis has been used since the 1970s by a variety of national,

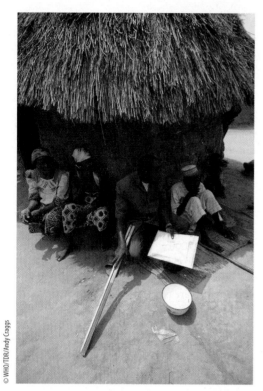

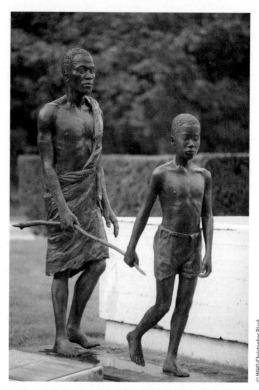

A community health center staff member shows village health workers how to use a stick to determine the right dosage for ivermectin, the drug used for onchocerciasis. The colors are related to size based on height. Each color signifies a different dosage.

Statue of an adult blinded by onchocerciasis (river blindness) and guided by a child.

regional, and global elimination initiatives.[93] In the Americas, onchocerciasis control efforts were so successful that by 2015 the disease was occurring in only a small rural area at the border between Brazil and Venezuela.[94] In sub-Saharan Africa, many countries were close to completely eliminating river blindness by 2015 and others were on track to achieve this goal within several years.[95] However, about 185 million people still required MDA for onchocerciasis in 2015 (including people living in Ethiopia and Nigeria).[94]

▶ 10.11 Leprosy, Buruli Ulcer, and Trachoma

Several bacterial diseases that have been recognized as problems for a long time but have

not been public health priorities are receiving new attention because of their designation as NTDs. Leprosy, also called Hansen's disease, was first described as a disease in ancient times, and it still exists.[96] **Leprosy** is the disease caused by *Mycobacterium leprae* infection. Chronic infection causes skin lesions, and about one in three people with leprosy suffer nerve damage.[97] When people have numb hands and feet, it is easy for them to accidentally burn or otherwise injure themselves. Those injuries may become infected, and those secondary bacterial infections may cause amputation of the digits. More than 200,000 cases of leprosy are diagnosed every year, including more than 125,000 cases in India, 30,000 cases in Brazil, 4,000 cases in Ethiopia, and 3,000 cases in Nigeria.[4] Historically, leprosy was a disfiguring disease that caused its victims to be ostracized from their communities. Today, the infection can

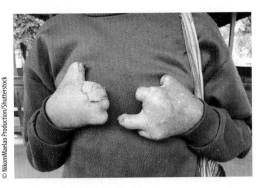

Amputations due to leprosy.

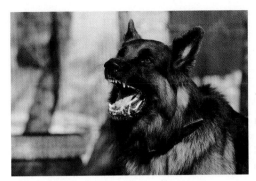

Dogs can spread rabies.

be treated with long-term courses of multiple types of antibiotics.[98]

Buruli ulcer, also called *Mycobacterium ulcerans* infection, causes necrotizing cutaneous lesions. The wound is often painless even if it is a large ulcer. Advanced cases may progress to osteomyelitis, contractures, and even amputation. The mode of transmission for the bacterium has not yet been confirmed, which makes the development of a prevention strategy impossible.[99] Early infection can be treated with wound care and antibiotics, but later stages of the disease require surgery to remove dead tissue, cover open wounds, and correct deformities.[100]

Trachoma is an eye infection with the bacterium *Chlamydia trachomatis* that can lead to blindness.[101] The bacteria are spread between people by person-to-person contact, shared clothes, and flies. Chronic infections scar the inside of the eyelid, and the inward turning of the eyelids (a condition called trichiasis) causes the eyelashes to scratch the eyeball and scar the cornea. Trachoma is a direct result of poor facial hygiene, and face washing is a core part of the WHO-recommended trachoma control plan called the **SAFE strategy**: Surgery to treat trichiasis, Antibiotics to kill the bacteria, Facial cleanliness encouraged by hygiene education, and Environmental improvements to ensure reliable access to water and sanitation.[102] In 2015, about 200 million people lived in places where trachoma is still endemic (including 75 million people in Ethiopia, 20 million people in Nigeria, tens of millions in India, and

2 million in Brazil), more than 3 million people had an urgent need for surgery to prevent blindness, and nearly 2 million people were blind or seriously visually impaired as a result of trachoma.[103] A global alliance estimated that it would cost about $1 billion to eliminate trachoma as a public health problem by 2020.[103]

▶ 10.12 Rabies

Rabies is an extremely virulent infection of the central nervous system caused by a virus in the lyssavirus genus of the rhabdovirus family. Humans contract the rabies virus when they are bitten by infected animals that are shedding the virus in their saliva. Rabies disease presents as either furious rabies, which is characterized by psychosis and cardiac arrest, or as paralytic rabies, which progresses through stages of ascending paralysis, coma, and death. No one who is bitten by a rabid animal survives without post-bite vaccination, a type of post-exposure prophylaxis (PEP). Each year, more than 10 million people receive rabies PEP within a few days after an animal attack, and this prevents hundreds of thousands of deaths.[104] Most of the 60,000 rabies deaths worldwide each year occur in low-income countries in Africa and Asia where access to PEP is limited.[105] These deaths are considered to be 100% preventable.

Rabies can occur in any mammal, including bats, and the rabies virus circulates in wild animal populations on every continent except

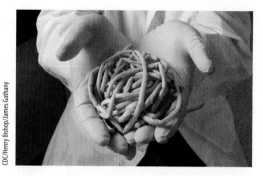

Ascariasis lumbricoides passed from the intestines of a young child.

Antarctica. Dogs are responsible for about 95% of human rabies cases, because dogs usually live in proximity to people.[106] Vaccinating pets is a key component of disease control strategies.[107] Pre-exposure prophylaxis of humans is recommended for veterinarians, animal handlers, and others who know they will have occupational exposure to animals that might have rabies.[108] Rabies cannot be eradicated because it circulates in wild animal populations. However, it is possible to prevent all human rabies deaths through expanded use of dog vaccinations, education promoting responsible pet ownership and bite prevention, and universal access to post-bite rabies treatment for humans.[109]

▶ **10.13 Soil-Transmitted Helminths**

A **soil-transmitted helminth** (STH), also called a geohelminth, is a nematode infection contracted through contact with soil mixed with feces that contain worm eggs.[110] A **reservoir** is the environmental home for an infectious agent. Some agents have an environmental reservoir and live in soil or water. STHs have a soil reservoir. Once the worms are inside a human host, most STHs are intestinal parasites. They increase the risk of malnutrition because nutrients from food go to the worms instead of the human host.

The parasites are also associated with stunted growth, low energy levels, reduced cognitive performance, school absences, and other adverse health and development outcomes.[111] The three most common STHs in humans are ascariasis, trichuriasis, and hookworm. Threadworm (*Strongyloides stercoralis*), pinworm (*Enterobius vermicularis*), and toxocariasis (*Toxocara* species) are also prevalent in humans.[112]

Ascariasis is the most common helminth infection in the world, and it occurs after a person swallows eggs from *Ascaris lumbricoides*. Ingested larvae hatch in the small intestine, penetrate the intestinal wall, and travel through the blood to the lungs, where they may be coughed up and swallowed and then develop into mature, egg-producing worms in the small intestine. Adult worms in the intestine grow, on average, to about a foot (30 centimeters) in length, and eggs passed in the stool may lead to infection in others if open defecation is practiced. Children with ascariasis can host hundreds of intestinal worms. That can cause distension of the abdomen, and it sometimes leads to obstruction of the intestines and subsequent peritonitis. More than 800 million people worldwide have ascariasis.[113]

Trichuriasis, also known as whipworm, occurs when *Trichuris trichiura* are residing in the large intestine. When the eggs that cause trichuriasis are swallowed, the eggs hatch in the small intestine. The released larvae mature in the colon into adults that are about 1.5 inches (4 centimeters) long. Trichuriasis can cause chronic digestive system symptoms associated with colitis, including bloody diarrhea (dysentery) and rectal prolapse. About 460 million people worldwide have whipworm.[113]

Hookworm, an infection caused by *Necator americanus* and *Ancylostoma duodenale*, is most often acquired by walking barefoot through contaminated soil. After the larvae penetrate human skin and pass through the bloodstream, heart, and lungs, they migrate to the gut, latch onto the wall of the small intestine, and mature into adults that are about 0.4 inches (1 centimeter) long. Because they are attached to the intestinal wall, hookworms cause the host to constantly lose small amounts of blood. This blood loss significantly increases the risk of anemia, especially in children and pregnant women. Globally, about 440 million children and adults have hookworm infection,[113] and about 90 million people have hookworm-associated anemia.[114]

Deworming medications are effective for treating all three of these STH infections, but re-infection can occur quickly when eggs from the worms remain in the local environment. Preventive chemotherapy, typically distributed to schoolchildren in endemic areas once or twice per year, is the primary current approach to STH prevention and control.[115] The concurrent distribution of four medications—praziquantel for schistosomiasis, ivermectin or diethylcarbamazine for lymphatic filariasis and onchocerciasis, azithromycin for trachoma, and albendazole or mebendazole for intestinal worms—can cost less than $1 per person per year in endemic areas when the drugs are distributed as part of an integrated control program.[116] However, even though the treatment is inexpensive on a per capita level, the total cost to include millions of people in MDA programs is greater than the health systems in many lower-income countries can afford. As of 2015, about 1.7 billion people lived in places where MDA programs for schistosomiasis, lymphatic filariasis, onchocerciasis (river blindness), and soil-transmitted helminths would be beneficial (**FIGURE 10–8**).[117] About 850 million people received preventive chemotherapy for one or more of those four NTDs in 2015, so about half of the global need for MDA was met (**FIGURE 10–9**).[117] In addition to MDA, community sanitation is helpful for reducing the disease burden from STHs because fewer helminth eggs will be in the soil if everyone consistently uses a toilet. However, sanitation facilities do not remove the eggs that are passed into the environment by infected livestock and other animals.

Country	Schistosomiasis	Lymphatic filariasis	Onchocerciasis	Soil-transmitted helminths
USA				
Germany				
Iran				
Brazil	🐌	🦟	🪰	🪱
China	🐌			🪱
India		🦟		🪱
Nigeria	🐌	🦟	🪰	🪱
Ethiopia	🐌	🦟	🪰	🪱

FIGURE 10–8 Use of mass drug administration for helminth diseases in featured countries.

Data from *Investing to overcome the global impact of neglected tropical diseases: 3rd WHO report on neglected tropical diseases*. Geneva: WHO; 2015.

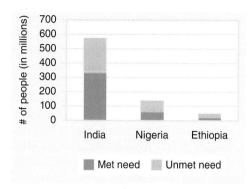

FIGURE 10–9 Many of the people in featured countries who would have benefited from participation in MDA programs did not receive preventive chemotherapy for an NTD in 2015.

Data from Preventive chemotherapy for helminth diseases: Progress report, 2014. *Wkly Epidemiol Rec.* 2016;91:93–103.

▶ 10.14 Other Neglected Tropical Diseases

Many of the recognized NTDs are helminthic diseases that thrive in tropical areas but can occur across a diversity of climates. *Taenia solium* is a tapeworm that undergoes early development in the muscle tissue of pigs and then matures in the intestines of humans who consume undercooked pork containing *T. solium* larvae. Pigs are the intermediate host, and humans are the definitive host for the worm. Pigs become infected by ingesting human feces containing tapeworm eggs. **Taeniasis** is the name for the disease caused by these tapeworms being present in human intestines. **Cysticercosis** is the name for the disease caused by the helminths forming cysts in muscle tissue or in other parts of the body. Taeniasis usually causes no symptoms in humans, but the tapeworms can cause serious problems if they invade the human nervous system.[118] **Neurocysticercosis** occurs when *T. solium* larvae, called cysticerci, trigger epileptic seizures and other problems associated with brain lesions.[119] About 1 in 25 people living in tropical countries of the Americas,

sub-Saharan Africa, and southern and eastern Asia have taeniasis, and about 15% have serological evidence of past infection, with considerable variation in levels by country.[120] About one in three people with epilepsy in endemic areas has seizures that are caused by neurocysticercosis.[121] The interventions for preventing and controlling cysticercosis include treatment of already infected pigs and humans with antihelminthic medications along with improved sanitation, vaccination of pigs, and meat inspection and other food safety practices.[122]

Echinocococcus granulosus is a tapeworm with a life cycle that requires an early developmental stage in sheep (or other livestock that serve as an intermediate host, such as cattle, goats, or pigs) followed by maturation in dogs (the definitive host). Humans are an accidental host who occasionally become infected from contact with dogs and develop **echinococcosis**. Most cases are asymptomatic. However, in some people the larvae cause cysts in the liver and lungs, a life-threatening condition called **hydatid cyst disease**.[123] Human cases of cystic echinococcosis can be treated with medication and surgery, and they can be prevented with responsible care of pets and stray dogs.[124] The cycling of the cestode between animals can be slowed with sheep vaccination, but echinococcosis remains an expensive zoonotic disease that occurs in nearly every world region.[125]

A treponematosis is an infection with bacteria from the *Treponema* genus. Three endemic treponematoses are on the NTD priority list: bejel (*Treponema pallidum* subspecies *endemicum*), which occurs in parts of Africa and the Middle East; pinta (*T. carateum*), which occurs in the Americas; and yaws (*T. pallidum* subspecies *pertenue*), which occurs in sub-Saharan Africa, southeast Asia (primarily Indonesia), and some Pacific Island nations.[126] Yaws is the most prevalent endemic treponematosis. **Yaws** causes skin lesions that may be disfiguring. If untreated, the infection can cause permanent disability by spreading to

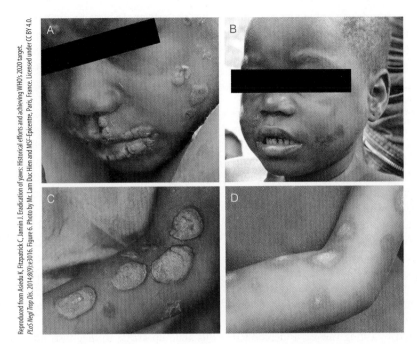

Yaws lesions before treatment (left) and 3 weeks after treatment (right) with a single dose of azithromycin.

bone and cartilage. A single dose of an antibiotic can cure yaws. The Global Yaws Control Programme that was implemented between 1952 and 1964 reduced the number of cases worldwide by 95% through mass treatment with penicillin injections.[127] There has been a resurgence of yaws in recent years, with thousands of cases reported.[128] In 2013, WHO approved a plan to attempt to eradicate yaws by 2020 by treating infected individuals with oral azithromycin.[129]

Mycetoma (also called Madura foot) is a chronic granulomatous inflammatory disease of the subcutaneous tissue of the foot (or other body part), and it is the newest addition to WHO's list of NTDs.[130] People with mycetoma have swollen, disfigured feet that ooze pus. Mycetoma is caused by a diversity of fungi (which cause eumycetoma) and by bacteria in the *Actinomycetes* order (which cause actinomycetoma).[131] Soil is thought to be the reservoir for the pathogens, and skin trauma is thought to provide a portal of entry.[130] The number of cases worldwide has not yet been determined, but most victims are young men.[131]

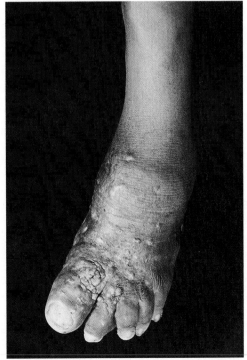

Mycetoma.

Treatment options include antibiotics and surgery. More research is required to understand the epidemiology of mycetoma and the options for prevention and control.

Four foodborne trematodiases are also included in the WHO list of NTDs: clonorchiasis, opisthorchiasis, fascioliasis, and paragonimiasis (FIGURE 10–10).[132] Most of these trematodes are parasites that have vertebrates or mollusks as hosts.[133] Clonorchiasis (*Clonorchis sinensis*), which occurs in many Asian countries, and opisthorchiasis (*Ophithorchis viverini* and *O. felineus*), which is found in countries in Asia and Europe, are caused by ingesting the larvae of liver flukes found in raw or undercooked fish. Fascioliasis (*Fasciola hepatica* and *F. gigantica*) is a liver fluke disease that is present in nearly every world region and is spread through vegetables. Paragonimiasis (various species of *Paragonimus*) is caused by a lung fluke acquired by eating raw or undercooked freshwater crabs and crayfish, and it occurs in parts of Africa, Asia, and the Americas.

A diversity of other helminth diseases—ones that have not been designated as NTDs, even though many are very common and cause health problems in humans—can be acquired by consuming contaminated food products, such as angiostryongyliasis (a roundworm of mollusks), diphyllobothriasis (a tapeworm of fish), fascioliasis and fasciolopsiasis (liver flukes from aquatic plants), and trichinosis or trichinellosis (a tapeworm of pork and other meats), or by ingesting food contaminated with feces, such as enterobiasis (pinworm), hymenolepiasis (a tapeworm), and toxocariasis (a roundworm). Some protozoa can also be transmitted through food. For example, toxoplasmosis (*Toxoplasma gondii*) is a sporozoan infection that can harm fetuses if the mother becomes infected while pregnant.[134] Most of these infections can be treated with antiparasitic drugs, but these medications are not always available to the populations that need them. When NTDs cannot be controlled with preventive chemotherapy, innovative and intensified disease management can be used to scale up access to diagnosis and treatment. Other contributors to NTD control include vector management (killing mosquitoes and other disease-transmitting insects), treating veterinary diseases that also affect humans, and increasing access to water and sanitation facilities.[135]

Country	Clonorchiasis	Opisthorchiasis	Fascioliasis	Paragonimiasis
USA			●	●
Germany		●	●	●
Iran			●	●
Brazil			●	●
China	●	●	●	●
India	●	●	●	●
Nigeria			●	●
Ethiopia			●	●

FIGURE 10–10 Presence of foodborne trematodiases.

Data from *Investing to overcome the global impact of neglected tropical diseases: 3rd WHO report on neglected tropical diseases*. Geneva: WHO; 2015.

▶ 10.15 Eradication

To **control** an infectious disease is to use public health interventions to reduce the incidence and prevalence of a condition to a substantially lower level within a community or a larger geopolitical area. Infection control measures like behavior change, environmental and vector control, vaccination, and mass drug administration can be used to limit the morbidity, disability, and mortality caused by an infectious disease in a local area. Control is achieved when the incidence or prevalence rates have dropped below a target threshold defined by the community, but a resurgence of the disease would likely occur if disease control measures ceased.[136] When control measures remove all risk of new infection in a defined geopolitical area, reducing the incidence to zero cases in that location, the **elimination** of the infection from that location has been achieved. For some infections, it is possible, at least in theory, to completely eradicate the infectious agent. **Eradication** is achieved when there is no risk of infection or disease anywhere in the world, even in the absence of immunization or other control measures. The term eradication should not be used to describe the elimination of a disease within a country or region when cases are still occurring in other places. Eradication is a term reserved for global elimination.

To be a candidate for eradication, the infectious agent must usually meet several criteria.[137] There must be an intervention that effectively interrupts the chain of transmission. If a vaccine is used as part of the eradication strategy, the vaccine should confer lifelong or long-term immunity to the infection. The disease should be highly pathogenic so that people who contract the disease have obvious symptoms and can easily be tracked. Additionally, eradication is more likely when the infection only occurs in humans. If both humans and animals serve as hosts for the infection, it may be impossible to monitor and contain all human and animal cases. Not all infections are appropriate

candidates for eradication. Eradication campaigns require large numbers of employees and structural support for intense months or years of interventions and for many years of follow-up surveillance. Because it takes considerable time, money, and organizational sophistication to achieve eradication, only diseases that are severe and for which there is a high likelihood of a successful campaign are targeted for eradication. A global eradication campaign cannot begin unless there is widespread political commitment to achieving success and a support system to ensure completion.

The only infectious disease of humans eradicated thus far is smallpox. (A livestock disease called rinderpest was declared eradicated in 2011.[138]) **Smallpox** was a viral disease that caused blisters to form over the body, starting on the face, then appearing on the extremities, and later showing up on the trunk.[139] There were

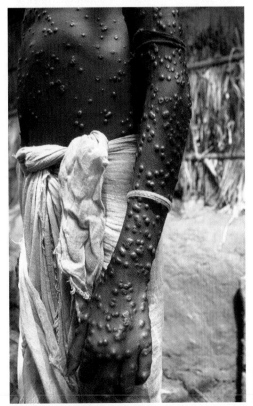

Smallpox.

two strains of the smallpox virus, which was in the poxvirus family of the orthopoxvirus genus. Variola major was the most common strain, and one in three people who contracted it died. Variola minor was the less common strain, but it had only a 1% case fatality rate. Nearly all smallpox survivors had severe scarring, and some were blind from corneal ulceration or had disabilities from skeletal complications.[140] An aggressive worldwide immunization campaign that included re-vaccination in areas where any new case of smallpox occurred led to the successful eradication of the disease in the late 1970s.[141] Because several laboratories stored samples of smallpox virus, the disease is not considered to be extinct. Eradication is achieved when an infectious agent is no longer circulating in humans. **Extinction** is complete when an agent no longer exists in nature or in the laboratory. There is some concern that viable smallpox virus could be obtained from a laboratory or corpse and used as a bioweapon.[142]

Two diseases are far along in the process toward eradication: dracunculiasis and polio. **Dracunculiasis**, also known as **guinea worm disease**, is a painful helminth infection.[143] People contract the guinea worm (*Dracunculus medinensis*) by drinking water that contains water fleas called copepods that are infected with worm larvae. Stomach acids kill ingested copepods and release guinea worm larvae, which migrate into the abdominal cavity of the human. A mature female guinea worm may grow inside the subcutaneous tissues of the human body to nearly 3 feet (1 meter) in length. Once the worm is mature, it forms a painful blister on the skin of its host. When the cyst ruptures, the worm begins to emerge from the human host's body. The blister is often near the foot, but the worm can also emerge from a wrist or another body part. It takes weeks for the worm to be extracted from the body, and a person with an emerging guinea worm is usually unable to work or go to school during this time because of the pain. The worm cannot simply be pulled out of the body, because if it breaks and part of the worm is left inside the body, serious infections like cellulitis and abscesses can result. Instead, the worm is often tied to a stick, and the guinea worm is coiled around the stick as the worm slowly makes its way out of the human's body, at a rate of an inch or so per day. Many people with an emerging worm only feel relief from the pain by putting their feet in cool water, but this causes the worm to release thousands of eggs. Those eggs can contaminate drinking water supplies and restart the cycle of infection.

There is no medication for dracunculiasis and no vaccine, and humans who have had guinea worm in the past do not develop immunity against the disease. Even so, the disease is nearing eradication thanks to a campaign led by The Carter Center that emphasizes health education over technology. Guinea worm education programs promote the filtering of drinking water to remove the copepods that host the worm larvae, and they also teach infected people to stay

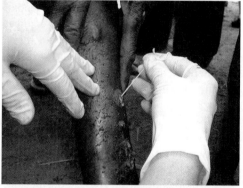

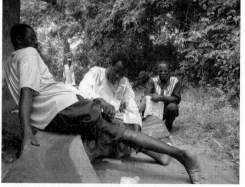

Guinea worm extraction.

out of water so they do not pass worm eggs to susceptible copepods. Every case of the disease is tracked as part of monitoring progress toward eradication. The number of cases of guinea worm disease diagnosed each year has dropped from an estimated 3.5 million cases in 1986, prior to the start of the eradication program, to less than 100,000 per year by 1997 to just 22 in 2015 (**FIGURE 10–11**).[144] The disease has been eliminated from many countries, including India in 2000 and Nigeria in 2013. However, as of 2015, cases were still occurring in Chad, Ethiopia, Mali, and South Sudan, countries that are located in both East Africa and West Africa, which meant that the disease had not yet been contained to a small geographic area.[144]

Polio, also called poliomyelitis or infantile paralysis, is a disease caused by infection with any of the three serotypes of poliovirus, a virus in the enterovirus genus. About 1 in 200 people who contract poliovirus develop a condition called acute flaccid paralysis,

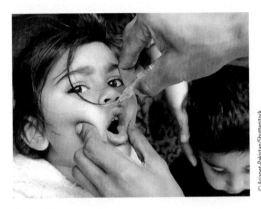

A child paralyzed by polio.

Oral polio vaccination.

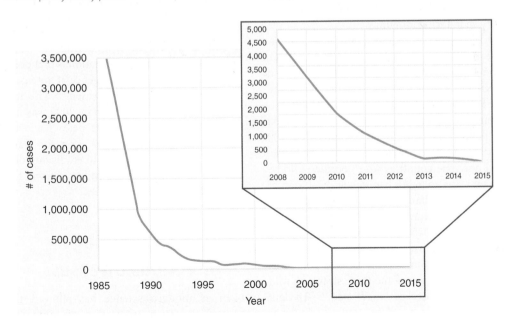

FIGURE 10–11 Number of cases of guinea worm globally each year.

Data from *Eradication of guinea worm disease: Case statement*. Atlanta GA: The Carter Center/WHO; 2016.

which is a sudden onset of weakness of the legs or a more widespread paralysis that might include weakness of the diaphragm, a muscle essential for breathing.[145] Some people who develop polio-related paralysis recover, but some die, some are left with permanent disabilities, and some who appear to recover develop post-polio syndrome years after their infection and have a recurrence of their muscle weakness.[146] The poliovirus is typically transmitted through fecal-oral transmission, and it can be spread through fecally contaminated food and water.

There is no cure for polio, but it is vaccine-preventable.[147] Oral polio vaccine (OPV) is a live attenuated virus administered by placing a drop of vaccine in the mouth. In very rare cases an OPV recipient can develop vaccine-associated paralytic poliomyelitis (VAPP) or the virus in the vaccine may mutate and become transmissible, causing small outbreaks of circulating vaccine-derived poliovirus (cVDPV).[148] Several doses of OPV are required for full protection to be conferred. A safe injectable inactivated polio virus (IPV) that carries no risk of VAPP is available, but IPV is not as effective as OPV in inducing immunity.

The Global Polio Eradication Initiative (GPEI) was launched in 1988 by WHO, The Rotary Foundation, the U.S. CDC, and UNICEF, along with other collaborators. Before the launch of the GPEI, more than 350,000 children in more than 125 countries were paralyzed by polio every year.[149] In 2015, fewer than 100 cases of paralytic polio occurred worldwide, and only two countries were considered to be endemic for polio, Afghanistan and Pakistan.[149] India was declared polio-free in 2014, and Nigeria was removed from the list of endemic countries in 2015. The term wild poliovirus (WPV) is used to distinguish naturally acquired cases of polio from vaccine-derived poliovirus cases. In 2015, one of the three strains of wild poliovirus was declared eradicated.[150] Trivalent (three-strain) vaccines were replaced by bivalent (two-strain) OPV formulations that contain only WPV1 and WPV3.[151]

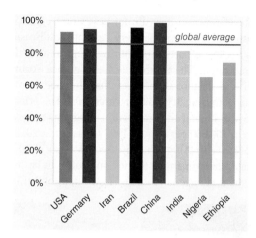

FIGURE 10–12 Percentage of infants receiving three doses of polio vaccine.

Data from *State of the world's children 2016*. New York: UNICEF; 2016.

Unfortunately, these successes do not necessarily mean that polio is on the verge of eradication. In 2016, Nigeria reported new cases of paralysis from wild poliovirus, and Nigeria was added back to the list of endemic countries.[152] Polio vaccination rates are alarmingly low in Nigeria; in India, the rates are below the global average even though India has an elevated risk for flare-ups because polio is still occurring in neighboring countries (**FIGURE 10–12**).[153] The expectation is that polio would make a quick resurgence if intensive global vaccination efforts ceased.[149] The initial goal of eradicating polio by 2000 was not achieved, and revised target dates have not been met either.[154] Sustained effort for many more years will be required to eradicate polio and permanently protect children from the risk of polio-induced disability.

▶ 10.16 Emerging Infectious Diseases

Even as modern science has allowed the control and even eradication of some diseases, other infectious diseases are becoming larger threats to human and animal health.

Outbreaks of **emerging infectious diseases (EIDs)** occur when a new pathogen begins to affect human populations or an existing pathogen changes the kind of disease it causes. The agent might evolve in a way that makes it easier to transmit to a susceptible person (increased transmissibility) and, therefore, more common (increased incidence). It might change so that it causes a new set of symptoms or more severe symptoms (increased virulence). In some cases, an infectious agent that usually affects only nonhuman hosts may adapt in a way that makes it infectious to humans. Sometimes, an infectious agent may change in a way that allows for a different portal of entry, perhaps developing the ability to spread through airborne transmission. Other infections, called reemerging infections, were controlled at some point in the past but are becoming problematic again.[155]

The U.S. Institute of Medicine has concluded that these new health threats derive from a complex interaction of genetic, biological, environmental, ecological, social, political, and economic factors (**FIGURE 10–13**).[156] As the world population increases (#6), humans and domestic animals move into previously uninhabited natural environments (#5) and are exposed to new plants, animals, and microbes. Alteration of the environment (#4), such as deforestation, dam building, and manipulation of wetlands, creates new environmental reservoirs for infectious agents and their hosts, and natural disasters (#3) like floods and droughts can alter the landscape and introduce new infectious agents to a region. Changes in dietary and other behaviors (#6) that become trendy and spread globally may also facilitate transmission. Urbanization facilitates emergence as people with different strains of infections interact with one another (#2) and create new habitats for vectors (#5). Technology is also speeding up the rate of emergence. Modern transportation (#8) has made it possible for an infectious person to travel nearly anywhere in the world within hours. Healthcare innovations (#7) have created

1	Microbial adaptation and change
2	Human susceptibility to infection
3	Climate and weather
4	Changing ecosystems
5	Economic development and land use
6	Human demographics and behavior
7	Technology and industry
8	International travel and commerce
9	Breakdown of public health measures
10	Poverty and social inequality
11	War and famine
12	Lack of political will
13	Intent to harm

FIGURE 10–13 Risk factors for EIDs as identified by the U.S. Institute of Medicine.

Data from Smolinski, MS, Hamburg MA, Lederberg J, editors. Committee on Emerging Microbial Threats to Health in the 21st Century. Institute of Medicine. *Microbial threats to health: Emergence, detection, and response.* Washington: The National Academies Press; 2003.

new risks and risk groups. Advanced medical therapies like the immunosuppressive drugs used by people who have had organ transplants and the technology for keeping premature infants alive have created new populations of highly susceptible people (#2). Healthcare-associated infections may be very hardy and difficult to treat, and antimicrobial resistance is increasing (#1). Other technological advances have created new places for infectious agents to grow and new methods of dispersion.

New infectious diseases can emerge anywhere in the world and spread quickly, so the distinction between local public health problems and global ones is increasingly limited. Nipah virus, which causes encephalitis, was first identified in 1999 when cases occurred in people in Malaysia and Singapore. In 2001, and in many years since then, Nipah virus caused outbreaks in Bangladesh and India.[157] Middle East respiratory syndrome (MERS) coronavirus was first identified in Saudi Arabia in 2012,[158] and the virus sparked an outbreak in South Korea in 2015.[159] The strain of H1N1 influenza that was first detected in Mexico in February 2009 had spread to dozens of countries by May of that year.[160] Some NTDs are also considered to be EIDs, such as dengue, which is occurring more often than it did in the past and has an increasing geographic range.[161] Systems for identifying and controlling emerging threats to human health no matter where they first occur are an important part of protecting the health of all of the world's people.

▶ # References

1. Keusch GT, Kilama WL, Moon S, Szlezák NA, Michaud CM. The global health system: Linking knowledge with action—Learning from malaria. *PLoS Med*. 2010;7:e100179.
2. Parascandola J. From MCWA to CDC: Origins of the Centers for Disease Control and Prevention. *Public Health Rep*. 1996;111:549–51.
3. Hotez PJ, Fenwick A, Savioli L, Molyneux DH. Rescuing the bottom billion through control of neglected tropical diseases. *Lancet*. 2009;373:1570–5.
4. *Investing to overcome the global impact of neglected tropical diseases: 3rd WHO report on neglected tropical diseases*. Geneva: WHO; 2015.
5. Feasey N, Wansbrough-Jones M, Mabey DCW, Solomon AW. Neglected tropical diseases. *Br Med Bull*. 2010;93:179–200.
6. Bhutta ZA, Sommerfeld J, Lassi ZS, Salam RA, Das JK. Global burden, distribution, and interventions for infectious diseases of poverty. *Infect Dis Poverty*. 2014;3:21.
7. Fitzpatrick C, Nwankwo U, Lenk E, de Vlas SJ, Bundy D. An investment case for ending neglected tropical diseases (Chapter 17). *Disease control priorities*. 3rd ed. *Major infectious diseases (Volume 6)*. Washington DC: IBRD/World Bank; 2017.
8. Fitzpatrick C, Engels D. Leaving no one behind: A neglected tropical disease indicator and tracers for

the Sustainable Development Goals. *Int Health*. 2016;8(Suppl 1):i15–18.
9. Molyneux DH. The 'neglected tropical diseases': Now a brand identity; responsibilities, context and promise. *Parasit Vectors*.2012;5:23.
10. *Reaching the unreached: 4th progress report of the London Declaration*. London: Uniting to Combat Neglected Tropical Diseases; 2016.
11. *An innovative approach to R&D for neglected patients: Ten years of experience & lessons learned by DNDi*. Geneva: DNDi; 2014.
12. Chosidow O. Scabies and pediculosis. *Lancet*. 2000;355:819–26.
13. Severe malaria. *Trop Med Int Health*. 2014;19(Suppl 1): 7–131.
14. *World malaria report 2015*. Geneva: WHO; 2015.
15. Aly ASI, Vaughan AM, Kappe SHI. Malaria parasite development in the mosquito and infection of the mammalian host. *Annu Rev Microbiol*. 2009;63: 195–221.
16. *Management of severe malaria: A practical handbook (3rd edition)*. Geneva: WHO; 2012.
17. Ghosh K, Ghosh K. Pathogenesis of anaemia in malaria: A concise review. *Parasitol Res*. 2007;101:1463–9.
18. Idro R, Marsh K, John CC, Newton CR. Cerebral malaria: Mechanisms of brain injury and strategies for improved neurocognitive outcomes. *Pediatr Res*. 2010;68:267–74.
19. Idro R, Jenkins NE, Newton CR. Pathogenesis, clinical features, and neurological outcomes of cerebral malaria. *Lancet Neuro*. 2005;4:827–40.
20. Doolan DL, Dobaño C, Baird JK. Acquired immunity to malaria. *Clin Microbiol Rev*. 2009;22:13–36.
21. Desai M, ter Kuile FO, Nosten F, et al. Epidemiology and burden of malaria in pregnancy. *Lancet Infect Dis*. 2007;7:93–104.
22. Steketee RW, Nahlen BL, Parise ME, Menendez C. The burden of malaria in pregnancy in malaria-endemic areas. *Am J Trop Med Hyg*. 2001;64(Suppl):28–35.
23. Chima RI, Goodman CA, Mills A. The economic impact of malaria in Africa: A critical review of the evidence. *Health Policy*. 2003;63:17–36.
24. Sachs J, Malaney P. The economic and social burden of malaria. *Nature*. 2002;415:680–5.
25. Shretta R, Liu J, Cotter C, et al. Malaria elimination and eradication (Chapter 12). *Disease control priorities*. 3rd ed. *Major infectious diseases (Volume 6)*. Washington DC: IBRD/World Bank; 2017.
26. *Achieving the malaria MDG target: Reversing the incidence of malaria 2000–2015*. Geneva: WHO /UNICEF; 2015.
27. Plowe CV. The evolution of drug-resistant malaria. *Trans R Soc Trop Med Hyg*. 2009;103(Suppl 10):S11–14.
28. Hemingway J, Shretta R, Wells TNC, et al. Tools and strategies for malaria control and elimination:

What do we need to achieve a grand convergence in malaria. *PLoS Biol.* 2016;14:e1002380.

29. *Guidelines for the treatment of malaria (3rd edition).* Geneva: WHO; 2015.

30. *Universal access to malaria diagnostic testing: An operational manual.* Geneva: WHO; 2011.

31. Menéndez C, D'Alessandro U, ter Kuile FO. Reducing the burden of malaria in pregnancy by preventive strategies. *Lancet Infect Dis.* 2007;7:126–35.

32. *WHO policy brief for the implementation of intermittent preventive treatment of malaria in pregnancy using sulfadoxine-pyrimethamine (IPTp-SP).* Geneva: WHO; 2013.

33. Eisele TP, Larsen DA, Anglewicz PA, et al. Malaria prevention in pregnancy, birthweight, and neonatal mortality: A meta-analysis of 32 national cross-sectional datasets in Africa. *Lancet Infect Dis.* 2012;12:942–9.

34. Conteh L, Sicuri E, Manzi F, et al. The cost-effectiveness of intermittent preventive treatment for malaria in infants in sub-Saharan Africa. *PLoS One.* 2010;5:e10313.

35. WHO Global Malaria Program. *Insecticide-treated mosquito nets: A WHO position statement.* Geneva: WHO; 2007.

36. Lengeler C. Insecticide-treated bed nets and curtains for preventing malaria. *Cochrane Database Syst Rev.* 2004; (2):CD000363.

37. Bousema T, Okell L, Felger I, Drakeley C. Asymptomatic malaria infections: Detectability, transmissibility and public health relevance. *Nat Rev Microbiol.* 2014;12:833–40.

38. Bhatt S, Weiss DJ, Cameron E, et al. The effect of malaria control on *Plasmodium falciparum* in Africa between 2000 and 2015. *Nature.* 2015;526:207–11.

39. Chen-Hussey V, Behrens R, Logan JG. Assessment of methods used to determine the safety of the topical insect repellent *N,N*-diethyl-*m*-toluamide (DEET). *Parasit Vectors.* 2014;7:173.

40. Yasuoka J, Levins R. Impact of deforestation and agricultural development on anopheline ecology and malaria epidemiology. *Am J Trop Med Hyg.* 2007;76:450–60.

41. Nájera JA, González-Silva M, Alonso PL. Some lessons for the future from the Global Malaria Eradication Programme (1955–1969). *PLoS Med.* 2011;8:e1000412.

42. Mendis K, Rietveld A, Warsame M, Bosman A, Greenwood B, Wernsdorfer WH. From malaria control to eradication: The WHO perspective. *Trop Med Int Health.* 2009;14:802–9.

43. Dunn R. In retrospect: Silent Spring. *Nature.* 2012;485:578–9.

44. Attaran A, Roberst DR, Curtis CF, Kilama WL. Balancing risks on the backs of the poor. *Nat Med.* 2000;6:729–31.

45. Sadasivaiah S, Tozan Y, Breman JG. Dichlorodiphenyltrichloroethane (DDT) for indoor residual spraying in Africa: How can it be used for malaria control? *Am J Trop Med Hyg.* 2007;77(Suppl 6): 249–63.

46. *Indoor residual spraying: An operational manual for indoor residual spraying (IRS) for malaria transmission control and elimination (2nd edition).* Geneva: WHO; 2015.

47. *The use of DDT in malaria vector control: WHO position statement.* Geneva: WHO; 2011.

48. Tediosi F, Lengeler C, Castro M, Shretta R, Wells T, Tanner M. Malaria control (Chapter 13). *Disease control priorities* 3rd ed. *Major infectious diseases (Volume 6).* Washington DC: IBRD/World Bank; 2017.

49. *The Global Malaria Action Plan for a malaria-free world.* Geneva: Roll Back Malaria Partnership; 2008.

50. Berdud M, Towse A, Kettler H. Fostering incentives for research, development, and delivery of interventions for neglected tropical diseases: Lessons from malaria. *Oxford Rev Econ Pol.* 2016;32:64–87.

51. Birkett AJ. Status of vaccine research and development of vaccines for malaria. *Vaccine.* 2016;34:2915–20.

52. Turner JW, Robinson JD. Malaria no more: Nothing but nets. *Health Commun.* 2014;29:1067–8.

53. *Global technical strategy for malaria 2016–2030.* Geneva: WHO; 2015.

54. Simmons CP, Farrar JJ, Nguyen V, Wills B. Dengue. *N Engl J Med.* 2012;366:1423–32.

55. Guzman MG, Halstead SB, Artsob H, et al. Dengue: A continuing global threat. *Nat Rev Microbiol.* 2010;8(Suppl 12):S7–16.

56. Bhatt S, Gething PW, Brady OJ, et al. The global distribution and burden of dengue. *Nature.* 2013;496:504–7.

57. Messina JP, Brady OJ, Scott TW, et al. Global spread of dengue virus types: Mapping the 70 year history. *Trends Microbiol.* 2014;22:138–46.

58. Schwartz LM, Halloran ME, Durbin AP, Longini IM Jr. The dengue vaccine pipeline: Implications for the future of dengue control. *Vaccine.* 2015;33:3293–8.

59. Vannice KS, Durbin A, Hombach J. Status of vaccine research and development of vaccines for dengue. *Vaccine.* 2016;34:2934–8.

60. Johansson MA, Vasconcelos PFC, Staples JE. The whole iceberg: Estimating the incidence of yellow fever virus infection from the number of severe cases. *Trans R Soc Trop Med Hyg.* 2014;108:482–7.

61. Monath TP, Vasconcelos PF. Yellow fever. *J Clin Virol.* 2015;64:160–73.

62. Simons H, Patel D. International Health Regulations in practice: Focus on yellow fever and poliomyelitis. *Hum Vaccin Immunother.* 2016;12:2690–3.

63. Hayes EB. Zika virus outside Africa. *Emerg Infect Dis.* 2009;15:1347–50.

64. Mlakar J, Korva M, Tul N, et al. Zika virus associated with microcephaly. *N Engl J Med.* 2016;374:951–8.

65. D'Ortenzio E, Matheron S, Yazdanpanah Y, et al. Evidence of sexual transmission of Zika virus. *N Engl J Med.* 2016;374:2195–8.

66. Murray KO, Mertens E, Desprès P. West Nile virus and its emergence in the United States of America. *Vet Res.* 2010;41:67.

67. Petersen LR, Brault AC, Nasci RS. West Nile virus: Review of the literature. *JAMA.* 2013;310:308–15.

68. Lindsey NP, Staples JE, Lehman JA, Fischer M. U.S. CDC. Surveillance for human West Nile Virus disease—United States, 1999–2008. *MMWR Surveill Summ.* 2010;59:1–17.

69. Kilpatrick AM. Globalization, land use and the invasion of West Nile virus. *Science.* 2011;334:323–7.

70. Campbell GL, Hills SL, Fischer M, et al. Estimated global incidence of Japanese encephalitis: A systematic review. *Bull World Health Organ.* 2011;89:766–74.

71. Ikegami T, Makino S. The pathogenesis of Rift Valley fever. *Viruses.* 2011;3:493–519.

72. Weaver SC, Lecuit M. Chikungunya virus and the global spread of a mosquito-borne disease. *N Engl J Med.* 2015;372:1231–9.

73. *Global strategy for dengue prevention and control 2012–2020.* Geneva: WHO; 2012.

74. Rassi A Jr, Rassi A, Marin-Neto JA. Chagas disease. *Lancet.* 2010;375:1388–402.

75. Bern C. Chagas' disease. *N Engl J Med.* 2015;373:456–66.

76. Pereira Nunes MC, Dones W, Morillo CA, Encina JJ, Ribeiro AL; Council on Chagas Disease of the Interamerican Society of Cardiology. Chagas disease: An overview of clinical and epidemiological aspects. *J Am Coll Cardiol.* 2013;62:767–76.

77. Schmunis GA, Yadon YE. Chagas disease: A Latin American health problem becoming a world health problem. *Acta Trop.* 2010;115:14–21.

78. Franco JR, Simarro PP, Diarra A, Jannin JG. Epidemiology of human African trypanosomiasis. *Clin Epidemiol.* 2014;6:257–75.

79. Brun B, Blum J, Chappuis F, Burri C. Human African trypanosomiasis. *Lancet.* 2010;375:148–59.

80. Lutje V, Seixas J, Kennedy A. Chemotherapy for second-stage human African trypanosomiasis. *Cochrane Database Syst Rev.* 2013; (6):CD006201.

81. Leishmaniasis is high-burden countries: An epidemiological update based on data reported in 2014. *Wkly Epidemiol Rec.* 2016;91:287–96.

82. Alvar J, Vélez ID, Bern C, et al. WHO Leishmaniasis Control Team. Leishmaniasis worldwide and global estimates of its incidence. *PLoS One.* 2012;7:e35671.

83. *Control of the leishmaniases: Report of a meeting of the WHO Expert Committee on the Control of Leishmaniases, Geneva, 22–26 March 2010.* Geneva: WHO Technical Report Series; 2010.

84. King CH. Toward the elimination of schistosomiasis. *N Engl J Med.* 2009;360:106–9.

85. Colley DG, Bustinduy AL, Secor WE, King CH. Human schistosomiasis. *Lancet.* 2014;383:2253–64.

86. Honeycutt J, Hammam O, Fu CL, Hsieh MH. Controversies and challenges in research on urogenital schistosomiasis-associated bladder cancer. *Trends Parasitol.* 2014;30:324–32.

87. Steinmann P, Keiser J, Bos R, Tanner M, Utzinger J. Schistosomiasis and water resources development: Systematic review, meta-analysis, and estimates of people at risk. *Lancet.* 2006;6:411–25.

88. Rollinson D, Knopp S, Levitz S, et al. Time to set the agenda for schistosomiasis elimination. *Acta Trop.* 2013;128:423–40.

89. Taylor MJ, Hoerauf A, Bockarie M. Lymphatic filariasis and onchocerciasis. *Lancet.* 2010;376:1175–85.

90. Global programme to eliminate lymphatic filariasis: Progress report, 2015. *Wkly Epidemiol Rec.* 2016;91:441–60.

91. *Lymphatic filariasis: Managing morbidity and preventing disability: An aide-mémoire for national programme managers.* Geneva: WHO; 2013.

92. Ramaiah KD, Ottesen EA. Progress and impact of 13 years of the Global Programme to Eliminate Lymphatic Filariasis on reducing the burden of filarial disease. *PLoS Negl Trop Dis.* 2014;8:e3319.

93. Boatin B. The Onchocerciasis Control Programme in West Africa (OCP). *Ann Trop Med Parasitol.* 2008;102(Suppl 1):13–7.

94. Progress report on the elimination of human onchocerciasis, 2015–2016. *Wkly Epidemiol Rec.* 2016;91:505–14.

95. Tekle AH, Zouré HG, Noma M, et al. Progress toward onchocerciasis elimination in the participating countries of the African Programme for Onchocerciasis Control: Epidemiological evaluation results. *Infect Dis Poverty.* 2016;5:66.

96. *WHO Expert Committee on Leprosy: 8th report.* Geneva: WHO; 2012.

97. Rodrigues LC, Lockwood DNJ. Leprosy now: Epidemiology, progress, challenges, and research gaps. *Lancet Infect Dis.* 2011;11:464–70.

98. Suzuki K, Akama T, Kawashima A, Yoshihara A, Yotsu RR, Ishii N. Current status of leprosy: Epidemiology, basic science and clinical perspectives. *J Dermatol.* 2012;39:121–9.

99. Merritt RW, Walker ED, Small PLC, et al. Ecology and transmission of Buruli ulcer disease: A systematic review. *PLoS Negl Trop Dis.* 2010;4:e911.

100. *Treatment of Mycobacterium ulcerans disease (Buruli ulcer): Guidance for health workers.* Geneva: WHO; 2012.

101. *Trachoma control: A guide for programme managers.* Geneva: WHO; 2006.

102. Emerson P, Frost L, Bailey R, Mabey D. *Implementing the SAFE strategy for trachoma control: A toolbox of interventions for promoting facial cleanliness and environmental improvement.* Atlanta GA: The Carter Center/International Trachoma Initiative; 2006.

103. *Eliminating trachoma: Accelerating towards 2020.* Geneva: WHO Alliance for the Global Elimination of Trachoma by 2020; 2016.

104. Knobel DL, Cleaveland S, Coleman PG, et al. Re-evaluating the burden of rabies in Africa and Asia. *Bull World Health Organ.* 2005;83:360–8.

105. Hampson K, Coudeville L, et al. Estimating the global burden of endemic canine rabies. *PLoS Negl Trop Dis.* 2015;9:e0003709.

106. Fahrion AS, Mikhailov A, Abela-Ridder B, Giacinti J, Harries J. Humans rabies transmitted by dogs: Current status of global data, 2015. *Wkly Epidemiol Rec.* 2016;91:13–20.

107. *WHO Expert Consultation on Rabies (2nd report).* Geneva: WHO Technical Report Series; 2013.

108. Rabies vaccines: WHO position paper. *Wkly Epidemiol Rec.* 2010;85:309–20.

109. *Global elimination of dog-mediated human rabies: Report of the Rabies Global Conference 10–11 December 2015.* Geneva: WHO/OIE (World Organization for Animal Health); 2016.

110. Bethony J, Brooker S, Albonico M, et al. Soil-transmitted helminth infections: Ascariasis, trichuriasis, and hookworm. *Lancet.* 2006;367:1521–32.

111. Bundy DA, Walson JL, Watkins KL. Worms, wisdom, and wealth: Why deworming can make economic sense. *Trends Parasitol.* 2013;29:142–8.

112. Knopp S, Steinmann P, Keiser J, Utzinger J. Nematode infections: Soil-transmitted helminths and trichinella. *Infect Dis Clin North Am.* 2012;26:341–58.

113. Pullan RL, Smith JL, Jasrasaria R, Brooker SJ. Global numbers of infection and disease burden of soil transmitted helminth infections in 2010. *Parsit Vectors.* 2014;7:37.

114. Bartsch SM, Hotez PJ, Asti L, et al. The global economic and health burden of human hookworm infection. *PLoS Negl Trop Dis.* 2016;10:e0004922.

115. *Helminth control in school age children: A guide for managers of control programmes.* 2nd ed. Geneva: WHO; 2011.

116. Hotez PJ, Molyneux DH, Fenwick A, et al. Control of neglected tropical diseases. *N Engl J Med.* 2007;357:1018–27.

117. Preventive chemotherapy for helminth diseases: Progress report, 2014. *Wkly Epidemiol Rec.* 2016;91:93–103.

118. *Preventable epilepsy: Taenia solium infection burdens economies, societies and individuals: A rationale for investment and action.* Geneva: WHO; 2016.

119. García HH, Gonzalez AE, Evans CAW, Gilman RH. Cysticercosis Working Group in Peru. *Taenia solium* cysticercosis. *Lancet.* 2003;362:547–56.

120. Coral-Almeida M, Gabriël S, Abatih EN, Praet N, Benitez W, Dorny P. *Taenia solium* human cysticercosis: A systematic review of sero-epidemiological data from endemic zones around the world. *PLoS Negl Trop Dis.* 2015;9:e0003919.

121. Ndimubanzi PC, Carabin H, Budke CM, et al. A systematic review of the frequency of neurocysticercosis with a focus on people with epilepsy. *PLoS Negl Trop Dis.* 2010;4:e870.

122. Thomas LF. *Landscape analysis: Control of Taenia solium.* Geneva: WHO; 2015.

123. Mandal S, Mandal MD. Human cystic echinococcosis: Epidemiologic, zoonotic, clinical, diagnostic, and therapeutic aspects. *Asian Pac J Trop Med.* 2012;5:253–60.

124. Macpherson CNL. Human behaviour and the epidemiology of parasitic zoonoses. *Int J Parasitol.* 2005;35:1319–31.

125. Budke CM, Deplazes P, Torgerson PR. Global socioeconomic impact of cystic echinococcosis. *Emerg Infect Dis.* 2006;12:296–303.

126. Marks M, Solomon AW, Mabey DC. Endemic Treponema diseases. *Trans R Soc Trop Med Hyg.* 2014;108:601–7.

127. Mitjà O, Asiedu K, Mabey D. Yaws. *Lancet.* 2013;381:763–73.

128. Mitjà O, Marks M, Donan DJ, et al. Global epidemiology of yaws: A systematic review. *Lancet Glob Health.* 2015;3:e324–31.

129. Asiedu K, Fitzpatrick C, Jannin J. Eradication of yaws: Historical efforts and achieving WHO's 2020 target. *PLoS Negl Trop Dis.* 2014;8:e3016.

130. van de Sande WWJ, Maghoub ES, Fahal AH, Goodfellow M, Welsh O, Zijlstra E. The mycetoma knowledge gap: Identification of research priorities. *PLoS Negl Trop Dis.* 2014;8:e2667.

131. van de Sande WW. Global burden of human mycetoma: A systematic review and meta-analysis. *PLoS Negl Trop Dis.* 2013;7:e2550.

132. Fürst T, Keiser J, Utzinger J. Global burden of human food-borne trematodiases: A systematic review and meta-analysis. *Lancet Infect Dis.* 2012;12:210–21.

133. Keiser J, Utzinger J. Emerging foodborne trematodiasis. *Emerg Infect Dis.* 2005;11:1507–14.

134. Torgerson PR, Mastroiacovo P. The global burden of congenital toxoplasmosis: A systematic review. *Bull World Health Organ.* 2013;91:501–8.

135. *Accelerating work to overcome the global impact of neglected tropical diseases: A roadmap for implementation.* Geneva: WHO; 2012.

136. Dowdle WR. The principles of disease elimination and eradication. *Bull World Health Organ.* 1998;76(Suppl 2): 22–5.

137. Hopkins DR. Disease eradication. *N Engl J Med.* 2013;368:54–63.

138. Morens DM, Holmes EC, Davis AS, Taubenberger JK. Global rinderpest eradication: Lessons learned and why humans should celebrate too. *J Infect Dis.* 2011;204:502–5.

139. Moore ZS, Seward JF, Lane JM. Smallpox. *Lancet.* 2006;367:425–35.

140. Breman JG, Henderson DA. Diagnosis and management of smallpox. *N Engl J Med.* 346:1300–8.

141. Henderson DA. Principles and lessons from the smallpox eradication programme. *Bull World Health Organ.* 1987;65:535–46.

142. Henderson DA, Inglesby TV, Bartlett JG, et al. Smallpox as a biological weapon: Medical and public health management: Working Group on Civilian Biodefense. *JAMA.* 1999;281:2127–37.

143. Cairncross S, Muller R, Zagaria N. Dracunculiasis (guinea worm disease) and the eradication initiative. *Clin Microbiol Rev.* 2002;15:223–46.

144. *Eradication of guinea worm disease: Case statement.* Atlanta GA: The Carter Center/WHO; 2016.

145. Hinman AR, Foege WH, de Quadros CA, Patriarca PA, Orenstein WA, Brink EW. The case for global eradication of poliomyelitis. *Bull World Health Organ.* 1987;65:835–40.

146. Howard RS. Poliomyelitis and the postpolio syndrome. *BMJ.* 2005;330:1314–18.

147. Polio vaccines: WHO position paper—March, 2016. *Wkly Epidemiol Rec.* 2016;91:145–68.

148. Minor P. Vaccine-derived poliovirus (VDPV): Impact on poliomyelitis eradication. *Vaccine.* 2009;27:2649–52.

149. *Polio Global Eradication Initiative: Annual report 2015.* Geneva: WHO; 2016.

150. Apparent global interruption of wild poliovirus type 2 transmission. *MMWR Morb Mortal Wkly Rep.* 2001;50:222–4.

151. Patel M, Orenstein W. A world free of polio: The final steps. *N Engl J Med.* 2016;374:501–3.

152. Roberts L. New polio cases in Nigeria spur massive response. *Science.* 2016;353:738.

153. *State of the world's children 2016.* New York: UNICEF; 2016.

154. *Polio eradication & endgame strategic plan 2013– 2018.* Geneva: WHO; 2013.

155. Morens DM, Folkers GK, Fauci AS. The challenge of emerging and re-emerging infectious diseases. *Nature.* 2004;430:242–9.

156. Smolinski, MS, Hamburg MA, Lederberg J, editors. Committee on Emerging Microbial Threats to Health in the 21st Century. Institute of Medicine. *Microbial threats to health: Emergence, detection, and response.* Washington DC: The National Academics Press; 2003.

157. Lo MK, Rota PA. The emergence of Nipah virus, a highly pathogenic paramyxovirus. *J Clin Virol.* 2008;43:396–400.

158. The WHO MERS-CoV Research Group. State of knowledge and data gaps of Middle East respiratory syndrome coronavirus (MERS-CoV) in humans. *PLoS Curr.* 2013;5:1.

159. Cowling BJ, Park M, Fang VJ, Wu P, Leung GM, Wu JT. Preliminary epidemiologic assessment of MERS-CoV outbreak in South Korea, May–June 2015. *Euro Surveill.* 2015;20:21163.

160. Neumann G, Noda T, Kawaoka Y. Emergence and pandemic potential of swine-origin H1N1 influenza virus. *Nature.* 2009;459:931–9.

161. Mackey TK, Liang BA, Cuomo R, Hafen R, Brouwer KC, Lee DE. Emerging and reemerging neglected tropical diseases: A review of key characteristics, risk factors, and the policy and innovation environment. *Clin Microbiol Rev.* 2014;27:949–79.

CHAPTER 11

Reproductive Health

Reproductive health services help babies get their healthiest start in life, keep women from dying during pregnancy and childbirth, and enable adults and adolescents to make informed decisions about family planning. They also support demographic goals, especially in lower-income countries where increased access to modern contraceptives has slowed the rate of population growth. However, limited access to skilled birth attendants in many lower-income countries means that many babies and mothers are still dying each year from preventable causes. Global goals for improving maternal and neonatal survival will not be met unless more resources are invested in reproductive health interventions.

▶ 11.1 Reproductive Health and Global Health

Reproductive health encompasses issues of fertility and infertility, contraception, pregnancy and childbirth, gynecologic and urologic health, and the prevention and treatment of sexually transmitted infections. Many reproductive health services are provided under the broader umbrella of **maternal and child health (MCH)** or maternal, newborn, and child health (MNCH) programs that promote health for pregnant women, newborns, infants, children, and adolescents. MCH programs often focus on helping babies and young children get their healthiest start in life. Women are included in MCH initiatives because the healthiest babies are born to women who were healthy before they conceived their offspring, who had access to

health services during pregnancy, and who had skilled birth attendants assist with delivery and the postnatal period. But reproductive health is not just about pregnancy, and it is relevant to both women and men of all ages. All adults and adolescents need to have access to reproductive health care and the tools to maintain their reproductive health.

Although there is nearly universal consensus on the merit of improving infant and child health, reproductive rights have long been a controversial global health topic because they require frank discussions about sexual behaviors and gender issues. Sustainable Development Goal (SDG) 3 focuses on health, and one of its targets is to "ensure universal access to sexual and reproductive health-care services, including for family planning, information, and education, and the integration of reproductive health into national strategies and programs" (SDG 3.7) (**FIGURE 11–1**).[1] SDG 5 focuses on gender equality, and one of its targets is to "ensure universal access to sexual and

3.1.1	Maternal deaths per 100,000 live births
3.1.2	Proportion of births attended by skilled health personnel
3.7.1	Percentage of women of reproductive family age (aged 15–49) who have their need for family planning satisfied with modern methods
3.7.2	Adolescent birth rate (aged 10–19) per 1000 women in that age group
5.2.1	Proportion of ever-partnered women and girls aged 15 years and older subjected to physical, sexual, or psychological violence by a current or former intimate partner in the past 12 months
5.2.2	Proportion of women and girls aged 15 years and older subjected to sexual violence by persons other than an intimate partner in the past 12 months
5.3.1	Percentage of women aged 20–24 years who were married or in a union before age 15 and before age 18
5.3.2	Percentage of girls and women aged 15–49 years who have undergone female genital mutilation/cutting
5.6.1	Proportion of women aged 15–49 years who make their own informed decisions regarding sexual relations, contraceptive use, and reproductive health care
5.6.2	Number of countries with laws and regulations that guarantee women aged 15–49 years access to sexual and reproductive health care, information, and education
11.7.2	Proportion of persons who were victims of physical or sexual harassment in the previous 12 months
16.2.2	Number of victims of human trafficking per 100,000 population
16.2.3	Percentage of young women and men aged 18–29 years who experienced sexual violence by age 18

FIGURE 11–1 Examples of Sustainable Development Goals targets related to reproductive and sexual health.
Data from United Nations Economic and Social Council. *Report of the Inter-Agency and Expert Group on Sustainable Development Goal Indicators* (E/CN.3/2016/2/Rev.1). New York: UN; 2016.

reproductive health and reproductive rights as agreed in accordance with the Programme of Action of the ICPD and the Beijing Platform for Action and the outcome documents of their review conferences" (SDG 5.6).[1] The International Conference on Population and Development (ICPD) was a United Nations (UN) meeting held in Cairo, Egypt, in 1994.[2] The Cairo Conference program of action emphasized **reproductive rights**, calling for women and their partners to have the freedom to decide how many children they want without interference from governments or other organizations.[3] This agenda raised concerns among a diversity of religious and social groups, with the Roman Catholic Church especially vocal about the promotion of contraception and possible increases in the number of abortions.[4]

The Beijing Platform for Action was the result of the 4th UN World Conference on Women, held in China in 1995.[5] The Beijing Conference vigorously advocated for gender equality and women's empowerment.[6] The political and religious implications of linking reproductive health with women's rights made both of these outcome documents controversial.[7] Reproductive health remains a hot topic in global health because there is not unanimous agreement on the value of reproductive rights, contraceptive use, and gender equity.

In the 20 years since those landmark UN conferences, significant progress has been made toward reducing the number of women who die in childbirth each year, increasing access to the tools for family planning, and protecting the rights of women. Billions of dollars have been invested in supporting reproductive, maternal, newborn, and child health (RMNCH) initiatives in low- and middle-income countries since 2000.[8] However, much more work will need to be done in order to meet the SDG targets for universal access to reproductive health care and reproductive rights by 2030. There is also increased attention being paid to **sexual health**, the enjoyment of safe, voluntary, and nonviolent sexual experiences, with the SDGs aiming to reduce the prevalence of sexual violence against women and girls (SDG 5.2). Integrated services for sexual, reproductive, maternal, and newborn health (SRMNH) provide more comprehensive health education and clinical care than programs focused solely on pregnant women and babies. The inclusion of both men and women in SRMNH services will help countries make faster progress toward achieving the SDGs.

▶ 11.2 The Fertility Transition

Demography is the study of the size and composition of human populations. The

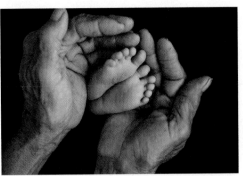

© DON016_STUDIO/Shutterstock

demographic transition describes the changes in population composition that accompany the shift toward lower birth and death rates that often occurs as populations move from being lower-income economies toward being middle-income and then higher-income economies (**FIGURE 11–2**).[9] Pre-transition populations have high birth rates and high death rates, and the population maintains a stable but relatively small number of people. During the early stages of the demographic transition, increased food security and improved health care reduce the death rate, but the birth rate stays high and the population size increases, sometimes drastically. In later stages, education, technology, economic growth, and other factors reduce the average number of offspring the typical female gives birth to—a process called the **fertility transition**—and the population begins to stabilize at its larger size. Eventually, prolonged low birth rates may lead to a slow decline in population size.

The total **fertility rate** is the average number of children a woman gives birth to during her childbearing years (**FIGURE 11–3**). The fertility rate has an impact on population health, not just the health of individual women, babies, and families. Countries with high fertility rates have a high percentage of children in their populations. Countries with low fertility rates have about as many older adults as children in their populations

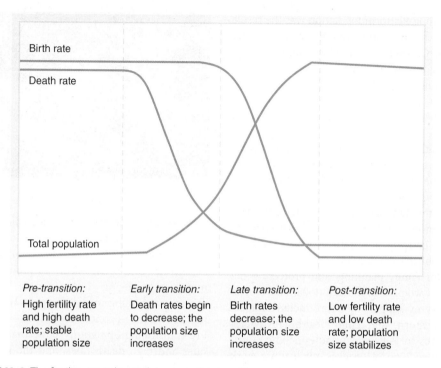

Pre-transition:	Early transition:	Late transition:	Post-transition:
High fertility rate and high death rate; stable population size	Death rates begin to decrease; the population size increases	Birth rates decrease; the population size increases	Low fertility rate and low death rate; population size stabilizes

FIGURE 11–2 The fertility, mortality, and demographic transitions.

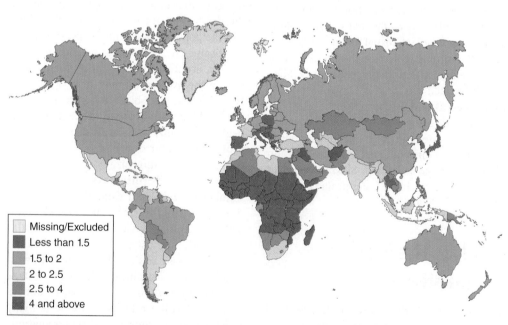

FIGURE 11–3 Total fertility rate (births per woman) (2015).

Data from *Human development report 2016*. New York: UNDP; 2015.

(**FIGURE 11–4**). If each woman has, on average, about two children, and those children live to adulthood, then each couple will produce only a **replacement population**. In other words, those two parents will produce two offspring, "replacing" themselves but not increasing the size of the population. In populations with fertility rates near 2, the population size will remain about the same from generation to generation. If the total fertility rate is greater than 2, then the size of the population will increase over time. If the fertility rate is less than 2, the number of people in the total population will begin to decrease and the average age of the population will increase. In the high-income and upper-middle-income countries where the fertility rate has fallen below the replacement rate, the population is expected to shrink over time if immigration does not boost the number of residents.

The fertility rate has decreased significantly in recent decades in most countries (**FIGURE 11–5**).[10] However, the fertility rates

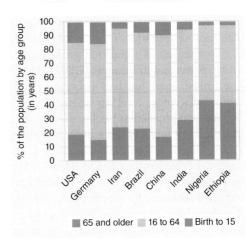

FIGURE 11–4 Higher-income countries have a high proportion of older adults and lower-income countries have a high proportion of children.

Data from *2016 world population data sheet*. Washington: Population Reference Bureau (PRB); 2016.

remain higher in low-income countries than in high-income countries. This means that the number of people living in low-income

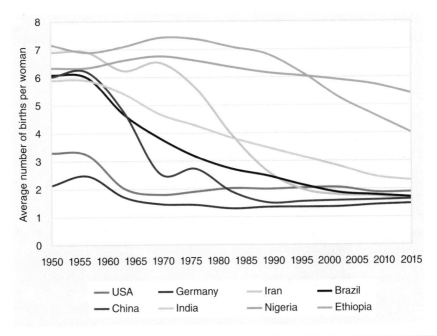

FIGURE 11–5 Fertility rates have decreased over time.

Data from United Nations Department of Economic and Social Affairs. *World population prospects: The 2017 revision*. New York: UN; 2017.

countries is growing at a faster rate than in high-income countries. This can be observed in a comparison of population growth in the United States and in Ethiopia (**FIGURE 11–6**).[10] The United States has had a fertility rate at about replacement level for about 50 years. The national population has increased during that time, but much of the growth is attributable to longer life spans and immigration. The number of children has stayed relatively stable over time, while the number of adults has increased substantially, especially the number of older adults. By contrast, Ethiopia's population has increased dramatically in recent decades, and most of this growth is attributable to a high birth rate. The number of children is increasing at about the same rate as the number of adults.

A **population pyramid** displays the number of males and females by age group in a population. Low-income countries like Ethiopia usually have a population pyramid with a wide base of many children that gradually narrows in older age groups (**FIGURE 11–7**). Countries with a triangle-shaped population pyramid are often concerned about population growth

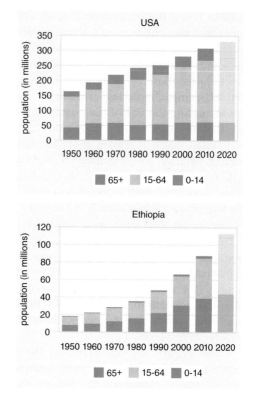

FIGURE 11–6 Population growth by age group.

Data from United Nations Department of Economic and Social Affairs. *World population prospects: The 2017 revision.* New York: UN; 2017.

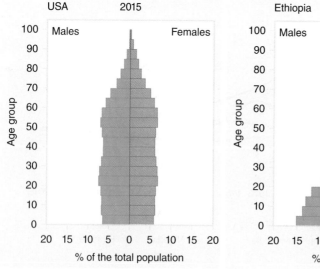
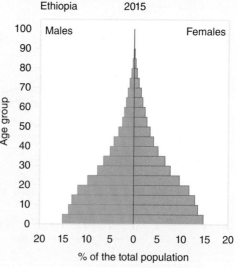

FIGURE 11–7 Examples of population pyramids (2015).

Data from United Nations Department of Economic and Social Affairs. *World population prospects: The 2017 revision.* New York: UN; 2017.

and are taking measures to encourage decreased fertility rates. High-income countries like the United States often have low fertility rates that make the population "pyramid" look more like a cube. Some of these countries with narrow bases of few children face a shrinking population size and are concerned about who will care for the aging population as the number of working adults for each older adult dwindles.

▶ # 11.3 Population Planning

The high fertility rates in some parts of the world have created concerns about global population growth and appropriate policies for promoting healthy fertility rates.[11] The goal of national population planning policies is to promote a population growth rate in line with desired demographic and socioeconomic profiles. Ideally, these policies help increase the health status of infants and children, reproductive-age adults, older adults, their families, and their communities.

In the high-income countries where fertility rates have remained below the replacement level for more than a generation and population aging is a major concern, the goal of population policies is to provide incentives for increased fertility (**FIGURE 11–8**).[12] In these low-fertility countries, policies promoting increased fertility, increased immigration, and older ages at retirement from the workforce are intended to reduce the economic burdens of caring for aging populations.[13] High-income countries often cover the full medical costs of pregnancy, support lengthy paid leaves from work for new parents, offer tax incentives that encourage childbearing, and provide subsidies to offset childcare costs.[14]

Upper-middle-income countries generally view their growth rates as satisfactory, but there is considerable diversity in how

Country	View on Population Growth and Fertility Level	Policy on Population Growth and Fertility Level	Government Support for Family Planning	Level of Concern about Population Aging
USA	Satisfactory	No intervention	Direct support	Major concern
Germany	Too low	Raise	No support	Major concern
Iran	Too low	Raise	No support	Major concern
Brazil	Satisfactory	No intervention	Direct support	Major concern
China	Satisfactory	Maintain	Direct support	Major concern
India	Too high	Lower	Direct support	Major concern
Nigeria	Too high	Lower	Direct support	Minor concern
Ethiopia	Too high	Lower	Direct support	Minor concern

FIGURE 11–8 Population policies in featured countries.

Data from United Nations Department of Economic and Social Affairs. *World population policies 2013*. New York: UN; 2013.

population policies are framed and implemented. These are obvious in a comparison of Iran, Brazil, and China. Iran's aging population has led to the government's recent adoption of a pro-natalist agenda that actively promotes higher fertility rates through support for marriage at younger ages, financial incentives to have more children, and access to treatment for infertility.[15] Brazil has experienced a significant decrease in fertility rates with minimal governmental intervention.[16] By contrast, China has had very active government involvement in limiting population growth. The "late, long, few" policy of the 1970s encouraged delayed childbearing, longer spacing between children, and fewer children, and it cut the total fertility rate in half.[17] China's one-child policy adopted in 1979 used economic and educational incentives to promote one-child families, especially in urban areas. Because there were exemptions to the policy for rural residents, for highly educated and wealthy parents, for parents who were both only children, and for some minority groups, the total fertility rate by the mid-1990s was closer to 1.8 children per couple rather than 1 child per couple, but this was sufficient to significantly slow population growth.[18] However, the program was controversial because of reports of forced abortions and sterilizations, infanticide (especially of females in rural areas), and other human rights abuses, even though these actions were contrary to the official policy.[19] Another concern was that the preference for sons over daughters may have made sex-selective abortions common enough to skew male/female birth ratios.[20] By 2015, China had achieved what it deemed to be satisfactory population growth and fertility rates, and the one-child policy was replaced with a much less restrictive policy.[21] Within China, some concern has been expressed about the many families with a "one-two-four" structure and only one grandchild to support two parents and four grandparents.[21] However, most young adults living in China today have a desire for small families, so the

fertility rate is expected to remain below the replacement rate.[22]

In most low- and lower-middle-income countries, population policies focus on encouraging reduced fertility rates because population growth levels are considered to be too high.[12] Countries with high fertility rates usually provide direct government support for the distribution of family planning information and contraceptives. They also promote female education, since women with more years of school generally have smaller families.[23] In addition to delays in marriage and first pregnancy, educated women are equipped to make better decisions about contraception and childbearing with their partners because they have the ability to read and act on information about good health practices, nutrition, disease prevention, and child-rearing strategies.[24] Reductions in fertility in places where the birth rate is well above the replacement level are usually associated with economic growth as reduced fertility rates increase the percentage of women who work outside the home.[25] However, even with policies promoting reduced fertility, the population of most low-income countries is expected to grow considerably over the next decades (**FIGURE 11–9**).[12]

▶ 11.4 Family Planning

All women and men of reproductive age need to have access to information about reproduction and contraception so they are better

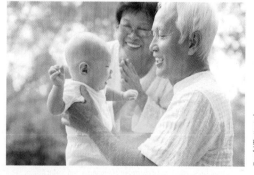

© szefei/Shutterstock

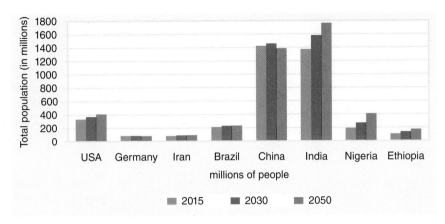

FIGURE 11-9 Projections of population growth in featured countries.
Data from *2016 world population data sheet*. Washington: Population Reference Bureau (PRB); 2016.

prepared to make decisions about sex and are able to prevent unwanted pregnancies, unsafe abortions, and sexually transmitted infections (STIs). **Family planning** is a process by which women and men make informed decisions about how many children they want to have, how many years apart they want those pregnancies to be, and the actions they will take to achieve these goals.[26]

Women and their babies are usually healthier when women have fewer pregnancies. Mothers, babies, and children also benefit from **birth spacing**, waiting until at least 2 years after the birth of one child before conceiving the next child.[27] When the time between the birth of one baby and the next one is short, the older baby is at risk for malnutrition because of being weaned from breastmilk at a young age and having fewer household resources per child, and the younger baby has an increased risk of low birthweight and preterm birth.[28] Family planning also has social and economic benefits because the adults in families with fewer children have more resources available to invest in each child and more years of productivity in the workforce.[8]

Complete sexual **abstinence**, refraining from sexual intercourse and other types of genital contact, is the only guaranteed way to prevent pregnancy. Some couples practice periodic abstinence and avoid intercourse during the days after ovulation, since the risk of conception is highest when an egg has just been released from an ovary. However, this is an imperfect method because it can be difficult for a woman to recognize when ovulation is imminent or has just occurred.

Contraception is the intentional prevention of pregnancy. Modern contraceptive methods include barriers, medications, and surgery (**FIGURE 11-10**). A **condom** is a physical barrier used to prevent sperm from coming into contact with an egg after sexual contact. Condoms also help protect against the spread of some types of STIs. Contraceptive sponges that are placed over the cervix prior to intercourse are another barrier method. Sponges are often used with spermicides to increase their effectiveness at preventing sperm from entering the uterus.

Oral contraceptives (birth control pills) prevent ovulation when taken as prescribed, so no eggs are released from the ovaries and a pregnancy cannot occur. In many parts of the world, oral contraceptives are called the "family planning pill" in recognition of their importance for birth spacing. Oral contraceptive pills must be taken at the same time every day, without skipping any doses, for this method to be effective. Some women prefer a longer-term

Type	Approach	Approximate Pregnancy Rate in 1st Year of Typical (Not Perfect) Use	Protection against STIs (Sexually Transmitted Infections)?	Notes
Complete abstinence	Abstinence	0%	Yes	No intercourse
Male sterilization (vasectomy)	Surgery	~0%	No	Permanent
Subdermal implant contraceptives	Hormones	~0%	No	Effective for about 3–5 years after implantation
Female sterilization (tubal ligation)	Surgery	<1%	No	Permanent
Intrauterine device (IUD)	IUD	<1%–2%	No	Effective for 5 or more years after insertion
Injection contraceptives	Hormones	<1%–3%	No	One injection every 1–3 months
Oral contraceptives	Hormones	8%	No	Pill must be taken daily to be effective
Transdermal (patch) contraceptives	Hormones	8%	No	The patch must be replaced weekly
Intravaginal (ring) contraceptives	Hormones	8%	No	The vaginal ring must be replaced monthly
Male condom	Barrier	15%	Yes	Must be used during every act of intercourse
Diaphragm or cervical cap with spermicide	Barrier 1 spermicide	20%	No	Must be used during every act of intercourse

Female condom	Barrier	21%	Some	Must be used during every act of intercourse
Spermicide alone	Spermicide	29%	No	Must be used during every act of intercourse
Periodic abstinence (fertility awareness-based methods)	Behavior	12%–25%	No	Requires daily monitoring of body functions and periods of abstinence
Withdrawal method	Behavior	27%	No	Must be used during every act of intercourse
No contraceptive method used	None	85%	No	

FIGURE 11–10 Contraceptive methods.

Data from Black KI, Gupta S, Rassi A, Kubba A. Why do women experience untimed pregnancies? A review of contraceptive failure rates. *Best Pract Res Clin Obstet Gynaecol* 2010; 24:443–55.

method of pregnancy prevention and choose hormonal contraceptives that are delivered through a weekly patch, monthly injections, or vials placed under the skin of the upper arm that release medication for up to 5 years.

An **intrauterine device (IUD)** prevents fertilization of eggs by creating a uterine environment that is unfavorable to sperm, which must pass through the uterus to reach unfertilized eggs.[29] IUDs may also inhibit the implantation of fertilized eggs in the endometrium that lines the uterus. Permanent **sterilization** is the use of surgical or medical procedures to intentionally make it difficult or impossible for a person to reproduce. Tubal ligation surgery for females and vasectomies for males are common sterilization procedures. Because only abstinence and condoms help to prevent the spread of STIs, all sexually active people of all ages are encouraged to consider the methods they will use to prevent contracting and

spreading STIs, even if they have taken steps to permanently prevent pregnancy.

Abortion is the termination or loss of a pregnancy. A **miscarriage** is the spontaneous loss of a pregnancy prior to the fetal age of viability. Miscarriages are also called **spontaneous abortions**. **Induced abortions** are chemically or surgically terminated pregnancies. Induced abortions are not a form of contraception. They terminate a pregnancy rather than prevent pregnancy. Increased access to contraception reduces the number of induced abortions by preventing unplanned pregnancies.

Even though there are many options for pregnancy prevention, many sexually active reproductive-age women and men worldwide do not use any contraceptive method (**FIGURE 11–11**).[12] The rates are especially low in the lowest-income countries. However, most countries and communities now recognize the importance of all adults and adolescents,

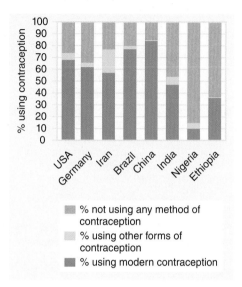

FIGURE 11–11 Percentage of married and partnered women aged 15–49 years who are using modern contraception (such as condoms, the pill, sterilization, or an IUD).

Data from *2016 world population data sheet*. Washington: Population Reference Bureau (PRB); 2016.

both males and females, understanding their options for contraception and family planning. The SDGs call for monitoring progress toward ensuring that all women of reproductive age have access to modern methods of family planning (SDG 3.7.1) and that the adolescent birth rate (births to females who are less than 20 years old) decreases (SDG 3.7.2).[1] Family planning programs target both women and men, because household reproductive decisions should involve both partners and because a woman whose partner does not want her to use contraception will often follow her partner's wishes. Although millions of people who would like to use modern forms of contraception still do not have access to family planning services, there are thousands of healthcare providers, governments, partners of the UN Population Fund, Planned Parenthood affiliates, and other organizations seeking to bring information and supplies to men and women worldwide who want to make informed reproductive decisions.

▶ **11.5 Infertility**

Infertility is the inability to become pregnant when sexually active and not using contraception or the inability to maintain a pregnancy through to a live birth. **Primary infertility** is infertility in a woman who has never had a live birth, and it is usually diagnosed when conception does not occur within a year of attempting to become pregnant. **Secondary infertility** is the inability to have additional offspring when attempting to conceive after giving birth. About 2% of women who are 20–44 years old have primary infertility after 5 years of attempting to conceive, and about 10.5% of women who have had a live birth have secondary infertility.[30] Infertility rates tend to be highest in the places with the highest fertility rates, because many cases of secondary infertility are attributable to complications from prior pregnancies.[31] More than 50 million couples worldwide with a female partner of childbearing age are unable to have a child after 5 years of attempting to become pregnant.[32]

Treatments for infertility include the use of medications to stimulate egg production, surgery to remove fibroids in the uterus and blockages in the fallopian tubes, medication and surgery to improve male reproductive function, and procedures like intrauterine insemination.[33] **Assisted reproductive technologies** (ART) are fertility treatments that handle eggs or embryos. The most common form of ART is **in vitro fertilization (IVF)** in which a woman's eggs are extracted from her ovaries, fertilized with sperm in a laboratory setting, and then the resulting embryos are transferred to the uterus. However, ART is costly even in high-income countries and it is not widely available to residents of lower-income countries. Treatment for infertility is a low priority for healthcare systems in countries with high birth rates. This may exacerbate the ostracism of women without children who live in cultures where having numerous children is the norm.[31]

▶ 11.6 Healthy Pregnancy

There are several ways to report a woman's reproductive history. **Gravidity** refers to the total number of times a woman has been pregnant, including miscarriages, abortions, stillbirths, and live births. **Fertility** is the total number of births, whether the result was a stillbirth or a live birth. **Parity** refers to the total number of live births. Because very few miscarriages and abortions are reported to healthcare professionals, most global health reports use fertility to measure pregnancies in a population. The goal of family planning is to minimize unplanned pregnancies (to reduce gravidity) and maximize the health of babies from pregnancies that do occur (so that parity is as close as possible to gravidity).[34]

Safe motherhood programs promote healthy pregnancies from the months prior to conception through the postpartum period.[35]

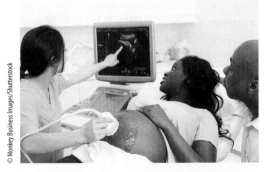

© Monkey Business Images/Shutterstock

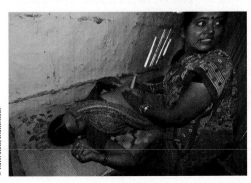

© Travel Stock/Shutterstock

Antenatal care check-ups, also called **prenatal care**, are routine preventive healthcare consultations during pregnancy that allow clinicians to identify and address potential health problems in a woman or fetus. These sessions are also times for clinicians to provide women and their partners with information about how to stay healthy, eat well, and recognize potential complications so they can be addressed as soon as possible. Women who have existing health problems, those who have a high-risk pregnancy or have experienced complications in previous pregnancies, and those who are having twins or higher numbers of children may require additional prenatal services.

Medical problems in the first trimester of pregnancy that require treatment include **hyperemesis gravidarum**, relentless nausea and vomiting that causes severe dehydration and significant weight loss; miscarriages that results in hemorrhage or infection; and **ectopic pregnancy**, in which a fertilized egg implants in the fallopian tubes or another location outside the uterus and the non-viable pregnancy puts the woman at risk of internal bleeding and death. As the pregnancy progresses, women may require treatment for anemia, hypertension, gestational diabetes, and other conditions. Most women are able to safely continue their normal routines throughout pregnancy, but premature labor and other complications may require reduced activity levels. For example, placental issues like **placenta previa**, in which the placenta covers part or all of the cervix and causes bleeding, or **placental abruption**, in which the placenta separates from the uterine wall prior to delivery, may necessitate extended periods of bedrest or emergency delivery.

Childbirth occurs in three stages. The first stage is labor, when contractions dilate the cervix to about 10 centimeters in diameter. The second stage is the delivery of the neonate. The third stage is the delivery of the **placenta**, also called the afterbirth, which is the organ that provides oxygen and nutrients to the fetus during fetal development. Complications can occur during any stage of labor.[36] During the first stage, problems may arise from unsatisfactorily slow progress of labor. For example, prolonged labor may occur when the fetus is poorly positioned, such as being in a transverse or breech position rather than head down. During the second stage, fetal distress (characterized by an abnormally slow or fast fetal heartrate) may occur, often as a result of the umbilical cord becoming compressed and cutting off the blood supply to the fetus. The mother is at risk of severe tearing during delivery. During the third stage, there is a risk of excessive bleeding that can lead to shock.

The presence of an obstetrician or gynecologist, another type of physician, a nurse midwife, a nurse, or another **skilled birth attendant (SBA)** who can recognize and treat potential complications during and after labor and delivery significantly reduces the risk of adverse outcomes for mothers and newborns. Nearly all deliveries in higher-income countries are attended by an SBA, but the rates are much lower in lower-income countries (**FIGURE 11–12**).[37] One in four births worldwide occurs without the assistance of an SBA, including half of all births in sub-Saharan Africa and South Asia.[38] A **traditional birth attendant (TBA)**, such as a lay midwife who has been trained through an apprenticeship rather than a formal educational program, may be able to handle uncomplicated births but does not have the advanced training to safely manage complications.[39]

When birth complications occur, it is important for women to have access to **emergency obstetric and newborn care (EmONC)**.[40] A basic EmONC (BEmONC)

facility can perform seven "signal functions": providing pregnant women with (1) intravenous or injected antibiotics, (2) anticonvulsants, and (3) uterotonic drugs to help the uterus contract after delivery; (4) using forceps or vacuum extraction to assist with delivery; (5) removing the placenta manually; (6) removing retained products of conception using tools; and (7) performing neonatal resuscitation using a bag and mask.[41] A comprehensive EmONC (CEmONC) facility can consistently implement all of the basic functions and also (8) provide blood transfusions and (9) perform caesarean sections. A **caesarean section** (often shorted to just "C-section") is the surgical delivery of a neonate through an incision in the mother's abdomen and uterus. A C-section rate of about 10%, and no more than 15%, is associated with the lowest maternal death rate.[42] The high C-section rates in many higher-income countries are evidence that many unnecessary surgeries are being performed as elective procedures. Lower rates in other countries raise concerns about the lack of access to advanced obstetric care leading to the unnecessary deaths of women and babies (**FIGURE 11–13**).[43] A safe C-section is performed by an obstetrician or surgeon with the assistance of an anesthesiologist, but there are few medical specialists in low-income countries who are able to provide these services (**FIGURE 11–14**).[44] This lack of access to advanced care contributes to pregnancy and childbirth remaining among the leading causes of death among women of reproductive age in low-income countries.[45]

The need for medical care does not end with delivery. Postnatal care ensures that

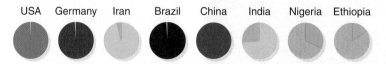

FIGURE 11–12 Proportion of births attended by skilled health personnel.

Data from *World health statistics 2016. Geneva*: WHO; 2016.

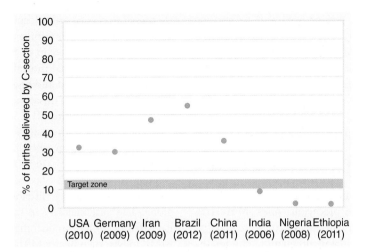

FIGURE 11-13 Percentage of babies delivered by caesarean section. The target range is about 10%–15%.

Data from Ye J, Zhang J, Mikolajczyk R, Torloni MR, Gülmezoglu AM, Betran AP. Association between rates of Caesarean section and maternal and neonatal mortality in the 21st century: a worldwide population-based ecological study with longitudinal data. *BJOG* 2016; 123:745–53.

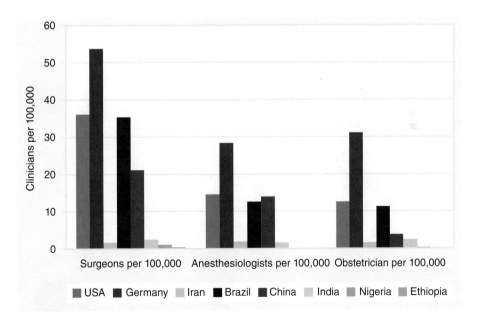

FIGURE 11-14 Medical specialists per 100,000 population.

Data from Holmer H, Lantz A, Kunjumen T, Finlayson S, Hoyler M, Siyam A, et al. Global distribution of surgeons, anaesthesiologists, and obstetricians. *Lancet Global Health* 2015;3(Suppl 2):S9–11.

mothers are recovering well and babies are healthy. Mothers and newborns should be carefully monitored in the hours after parturition and clinically examined several weeks later to check for problems.

▶ 11.7 Maternal Mortality and Disability

For many pregnant women, the hours of labor and delivery are precarious ones. **Maternal mortality** is death of women from pregnancy-related causes during pregnancy, childbirth, or the six weeks after delivery. About 300,000 women died from maternal causes in 2015.[46] That was a substantial reduction from the more than 500,000 women who died from pregnancy-related causes in 1990,[47] but the number remains far higher than it should be. Most maternal deaths could be prevented with increased access to obstetric care and increased access to contraception for women who want to plan their families but do not currently have the tools to do so.[48] Contraception helps prevent maternal mortality by reducing the rate of unintended and high-risk pregnancies that might lead to unsafe abortions or fatal pregnancy complications.[49]

The **maternal mortality rate (MMR)** is the number of women who die of pregnancy-related causes per 100,000 live births (**FIGURE 11-15**). The risks associated with pregnancy are not equally distributed across the globe. The vast majority of maternal mortality cases occur in low-income countries. The MMR in Nigeria is nearly 140 times higher than the MMR in Germany (**FIGURE 11-16**), and a Nigerian woman is more than 170 times more likely to die of maternal causes during her lifetime than a German woman (**FIGURE 11-17**).[47] There are also significant variations in the maternal mortality rate within most countries, with higher-income women experiencing a lower mortality rate than lower-income

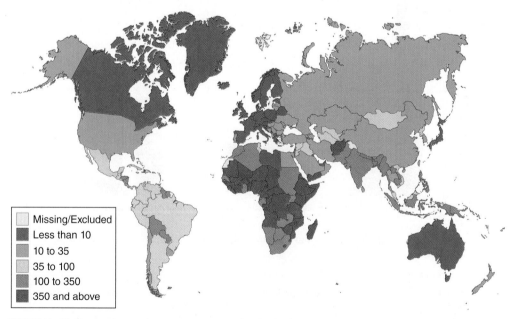

Missing/Excluded
Less than 10
10 to 35
35 to 100
100 to 350
350 and above

FIGURE 11-15 Maternal mortality ratio per 100,000 live births (2015).

Data from *Trends in maternal mortality, 1990 to 2015: Estimates by WHO, UNICEF, UNFPA, World Bank Group and the United Nations Population Division.* Geneva: WHO; 2015.

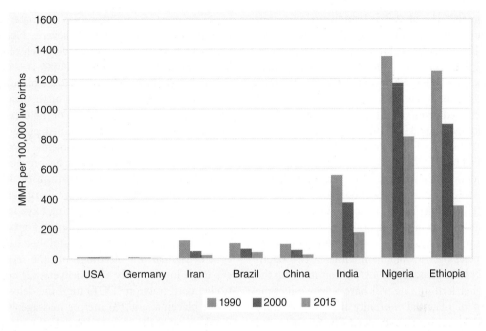

FIGURE 11–16 The MMR per 100,000 live births has decreased significantly, but disparities remain.

Data from *Trends in maternal mortality, 1990 to 2015: Estimates by WHO, UNICEF, UNFPA, World Bank Group and the United Nations Population Division.* Geneva: WHO; 2015.

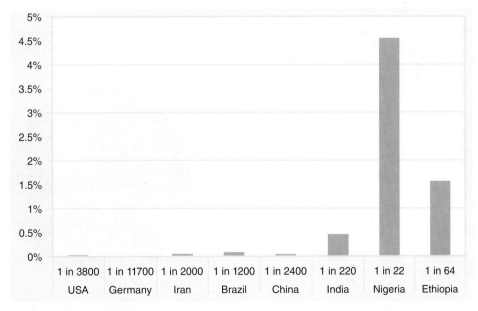

FIGURE 11–17 Lifetime risk of maternal mortality.

Data from *Trends in maternal mortality, 1990 to 2015: estimates by WHO, UNICEF, UNFPA, World Bank Group and the United Nations Population Division.* Geneva: WHO; 2015.

women.[50] The **obstetric transition** is the shift from a high MMR to a negligible rate that typically occurs with socioeconomic development.[51]

One of the Millennium Development Goals (MDGs) was to reduce the global MMR by 75% between 1990 and 2015.[52] The MMR decreased from about 385 per 100,000 live births worldwide in 1990 to 215 per 100,000 in 2015.[47] That 45% decrease fell short of the MDG target (**FIGURE 11–18**).[52] The lifetime risk of dying in childbirth also decreased during this 25-year period, from about 1 in 73 in 1990 to 1 in 180 in 2015.[47] (The calculation of lifetime risk accounts for both the risk of death per pregnancy and the average number of pregnancies over a woman's lifetime. If two countries have the same MMR, the country with the higher fertility rate will have a worse lifetime risk of maternal mortality than the country with the lower fertility rate.) The SDGs aim to reduce the MMR to fewer than 70 deaths per 100,000 live births (SDG 3.1).[1] Higher-income countries already have rates that are lower than the SDG target, but most lower-income countries have rates that are above the SDG target.

The most common causes of maternal mortality are hemorrhage (severe bleeding), hypertension (dangerously elevated blood pressure), and sepsis (**FIGURE 11–19**).[53] **Postpartum hemorrhage** is severe bleeding within several hours after giving birth, usually caused by uterine atony (failure of the uterine muscle to contract) or by retained placental tissue, trauma, or clotting problems.[54] Postpartum hemorrhage can often be prevented through the **active management of the third stage of labor**, which previously consisted of three actions: (1) injecting **oxytocin**, a hormone that strengthens uterine contractions during labor and delivery and then helps control postpartum bleeding, into the mother's thigh immediately after delivery, (2) controlled cord traction (CCT) until the delivery of the placenta, and (3) uterine massage after the delivery of the placenta to help the uterus contract. Newer protocols emphasize the importance of oxytocin but suggest that CCT be performed only by SBAs and that uterine massage be used only when the uterus is not contracting normally.[55]

Elevated blood pressure can occur at any time during pregnancy. **Preeclampsia** is characterized by worsening hypertension

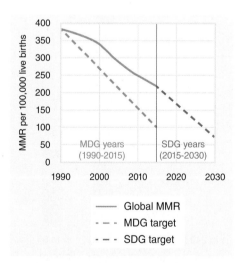

FIGURE 11–18 The MDG target for maternal survival was not met.

Data from *Trends in maternal mortality, 1990 to 2015: Estimates by WHO, UNICEF, UNFPA, World Bank Group and the United Nations Population Division*. Geneva: WHO; 2015.

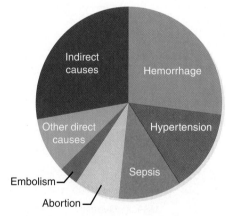

FIGURE 11–19 Causes of maternal mortality worldwide.

Data from Say L, Chou D, Gemmill A, Tunçalp Ö, Moller AB, Daniels J, Gülmezoglu AM, Temmerman M, Alkema L. Global causes of maternal death: A WHO systematic analysis. *Lancet* 2014; 2:e323–33.

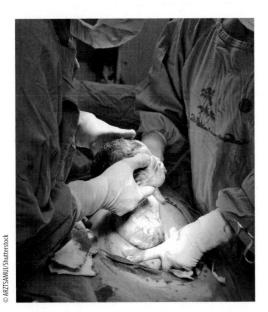

© ARZTSAMUI/Shutterstock

Caesarean section.

in the final months of pregnancy along with the presence of protein in the urine. Pregnant women with severe preeclampsia may sustain kidney and liver damage. When the condition progresses to eclampsia, seizures occur and there is a risk of organ failure and death. The only cure for preeclampsia is delivery of the fetus.[56] About 5% of pregnant women develop preeclampsia,[57] and many of those pregnancies require preterm deliveries that carry health risks for the babies but are necessary for the survival and health of the mother. **Sepsis**, sometimes called "blood poisoning," is widespread inflammation in the body that is triggered by the chemicals released by the body's immune system in response to an infection. Sepsis can lead to organ failure, shock, and death.

Women who survive pregnancy and delivery complications may be left with permanent disabilities.[58] For example, some women who are small, as is often the case with girls who become pregnant in their early teenage years, develop a condition called **obstructed labor**, which occurs when the unborn baby is wedged so tightly into the birth canal that blood flow to surrounding tissues is cut off and the tissues

start to die.[59] Women who are able to get to a hospital can have a caesarean section to deliver the baby before there is extensive damage. Women who do not have access to a surgeon may be in labor for several days. The outcome, if the woman survives, is often the formation of an **obstetric fistula**, a hole between the rectum or bladder and the vagina that constantly leaks urine or feces. Because of the odor, most women with an obstetric fistula are ostracized by their communities. Some women are left paralyzed because of nerve damage and many are left infertile. In nearly all of these cases, the baby is stillborn. More than 1 million women worldwide are estimated to be living with an obstetric fistula.[60] Fistulas can be surgically corrected, but the better option is preventing obstructed labor by delaying pregnancy until females are fully grown and ensuring access to medical professionals during delivery if help is needed.

▶ 11.8 Neonatal Health

About 140 million babies are born each year, and the vast majority of these babies are born healthy.[38] However, not all pregnancies result in a live birth or a healthy newborn. A **stillbirth** is the death of a fetus late in pregnancy but prior to delivery, typically defined as occurring after the 28th week of gestation and after the fetus already weighs at least 2.2 pounds (1000 grams).[61] There are about 18 stillbirths for every 1000 live births,[62] for a total of more than 2.5 million stillbirths worldwide each year (**FIGURE 11-20**).[63] Maternal infections or trauma, congenital abnormalities, umbilical cord and placental problems, uterine problems, and birth trauma cause some stillbirths, but there is often no identifiable reason for the stillbirth.[64] The term **perinatal mortality** encompasses stillbirths and deaths within the first 7 days (1 week) after a live birth. Some babies are extremely premature, suffer severe birth trauma, or have congenital abnormalities that are incompatible with survival, and these newborns may live for only a few minutes or hours after birth.[65]

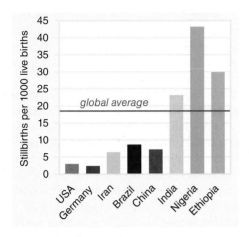

FIGURE 11–20 Stillbirth rate per 1000 live births.

Data from Blencowe H, Cousens S, Jassir FB, Say L, Chou D, Mathers C, et al. National, regional, and worldwide estimates of stillbirth rates in 2015, with trends from 2000: A systematic analysis. *Lancet Glob Health* 2016; 4:e98–108.

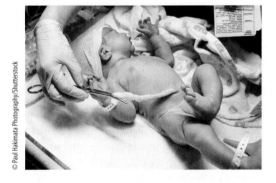

A **neonate** is a newborn within his or her first 28 days (4 weeks) after birth (**FIGURE 11–21**). An **infant** is a baby between birth and the first birthday. An **under-5 child** is a child between birth and the fifth birthday. The early neonatal period is the first week after birth, and early neonatal deaths alone account for more than one-third of all under-5 mortality (**FIGURE 11–22**). Neonatal deaths currently account for about 45% of all under-5 child mortality. The **neonatal mortality rate (NMR)** is the number of deaths of neonates per 1000 live births. The global NMR in 2015 was about 19 per 1000 live births, but the rate was lower in high-income countries and higher in low-income countries (**FIGURE 11–23**).[37] The SDGs aim to "end preventable deaths of newborns," setting a target of "all countries aiming to reduce neonatal mortality to at least as low as 12 per 1000 live births" (SDG 3.2).[1]

Of the two million neonates who died worldwide in 2015, about one-third of the deaths were attributed to preterm delivery, one-third to birth traumas, such as asphyxia, and one-third to infections and other causes (**FIGURE 11–24**).[66] A typical pregnancy is about 40 weeks long. **Preterm birth** is the delivery of a baby before the 37th week of pregnancy. About 10% of babies are born prematurely

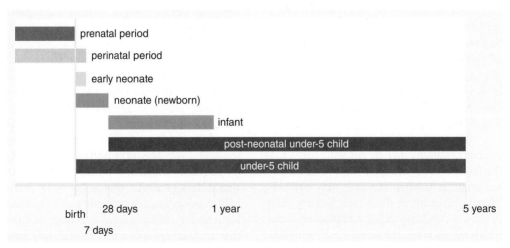

FIGURE 11–21 Age groups in early childhood.

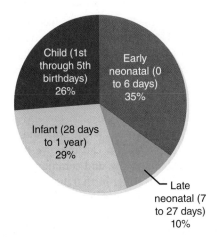

FIGURE 11-22 Neonates account for a large proportion of all under-5 child mortality.

Data from GBD 2015 Child Mortality Collaborators. Global, regional, national, and selected subnational levels of stillbirths, neonatal, infant, and under-5 mortality, 1980–2015: A systematic analysis for the Global Burden of Disease Study 2015. *Lancet* 2016; 388(10053):1725–74.

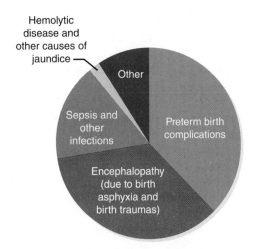

FIGURE 11-24 Causes of neonatal mortality.

Data from GBD 2015 Child Mortality Collaborators. Global, regional, national, and selected subnational levels of stillbirths, neonatal, infant, and under-5 mortality, 1980–2015: A systematic analysis for the Global Burden of Disease Study 2015. *Lancet* 2016; 388(10053):1725–74.

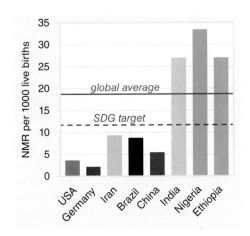

FIGURE 11-23 Neonatal mortality rates per 1000 live births.

Data from *World health statistics 2016*. Geneva: WHO; 2016.

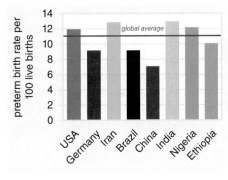

FIGURE 11-25 Preterm birth rate per 100 live births.

Data from Blencowe H, Cousens S, Oestergaard MZ, Chou D, Moller AB, Narwal R, Adler A, Vera Garcia C, Rohde S, Say L, Lawn JE. National, regional, and worldwide estimates of preterm birth rates in the year 2010 with time trends since 1990 for selected countries: A systematic analysis and implications. *Lancet* 2012; 379:2162–72.

(FIGURE 11-25), which results in about 15 million preterm babies being born each year.[67] Most cases of preterm birth are spontaneous, rather than being induced because of preeclampsia or other threats to the health of the mother or baby.[68] The causal factors for many of these spontaneous early deliveries remain poorly understood.[69] Each year, more than 1 million preterm babies die at a very young age.[70] Survivors, especially those with very low birthweights, may have long-term special needs related to learning disabilities, visual impairment, and other neurodevelopmental problems.[71] The best outcomes occur when the neonate has access to thermal care to keep the body temperature warm, prevention of infections through careful hygiene and appropriate use of antiseptics, assistance with consumption of breastmilk, and safe use of supplemental oxygen.[70] Babies in high-income countries usually have access to well-equipped neonatal intensive care units in hospitals. In resource-limited settings, the survival of preterm babies is enhanced by the use of kangaroo mother care: skin-to-skin contact between a mother and newborn, frequent breastfeeding, and early discharge from the hospital to reduce the risk of infection.[72]

Most babies who are born too early have **low birthweight (LBW)**, weighing less than 5.5 pounds (2500 grams) at birth. LBW can also occur in full-term babies, often as a result of their mothers being undernourished when they became pregnant and not taking in adequate nutrients during pregnancy.[73] The overall prevalence of LBW, including both preterm and full-term infants, is about 16% (**FIGURE 11–26**).[38] Many babies with LBW develop normally, but LBW babies, especially those with very low weights at birth, have an increased risk of neurodevelopmental difficulties, vulnerability to infections and other illnesses, and poor growth during infancy and childhood.[74]

About 1 in 400 newborns has **cerebral palsy** (CP), a neuromuscular disorder characterized by difficulties with movement, balance, and posture. The rate is highest in babies with very low birthweight.[75] While many of the symptoms of CP are permanent, they do not get worse over time. Physical therapy, occupational therapy, speech therapy, and other forms of rehabilitation can improve physical performance, mobility, and communication.[76] Some newborns suffer birth trauma like bruising, fractures, and nerve damage as a result of the physical pressures exerted on their bodies during delivery. For example, a brachial plexus injury to the nerves of the shoulder, arm, and hand can occur when shoulder dystocia occurs and a baby's shoulder is wedged behind the mother's pubic bone during delivery.[77] **Birth asphyxia** occurs when a full-term newborn fails to take a first breath immediately after delivery and is deprived of oxygen.[78] Neonatal resuscitation can save the lives of these newborns,[79] but they may have permanent brain damage because of the hypoxia.

A variety of infections can be fatal for newborns.[80] The most common infectious causes of death among newborns are neonatal sepsis, pneumonia, diarrhea, and neonatal tetanus.[59] Tetanus is an infection of special concern when babies are born in unclean environments, such as homes with dirt floors that allow the umbilical cord to come into contact with soil that might contain tetanus spores. The word **tetanus** means a sustained muscle contraction. Neonatal tetanus occurs when a neurotoxin from the bacterium *Clostridium tetani* causes painful muscle spasms in a neonate, starting as lockjaw that interferes with feeding and eventually affecting the full body and posing a significant risk of death.[81] Maternal immunization with tetanus toxoid prior to delivery protects both mothers and newborns.

Neonatal survival begins with universal access to prenatal care and intrapartum care provided by skilled birth attendants.[82] After birth, routine care for newborns includes keeping them warm, breastfeeding them at

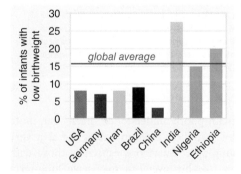

FIGURE 11–26 Percentage of infants with low birthweight (less than 2500 grams at birth).

Data from *State of the world's children 2016.* New York: UNICEF; 2016.

regular intervals starting soon after birth, and preventing infections through handwashing and hygienic cord care.[83] Babies with breathing difficulties, signs of infection, yellow skin suggesting jaundice, or other problems require clinical treatment.[84]

▶ 11.9 Gynecologic Health

Women's reproductive health is about much more than pregnancy care. For women of reproductive age, premenstrual syndrome (PMS), uterine fibroids, endometriosis, polycystic ovarian syndrome (PCOS), and genital prolapse are common gynecological disorders that can reduce the quality of life (**FIGURE 11–27**).[85] PMS is present when the physical discomfort, depressed mood, and other symptoms caused by hormonal changes during a menstrual cycle are severe enough to interfere with usual daily activities.[86] **Fibroids** are benign tumors in the uterus that can cause heavy bleeding and pelvic pain.[87] **Endometriosis** is present when some of the tissue that lines the uterus is located on the ovaries or in other parts of the abdominal cavity. That tissue bleeds with each menstrual cycle, often causing pain and resulting in the formation of scar tissue and adhesions.[88] PCOS is a hormonal disorder that is often characterized by irregular menstrual cycles, hirsutism (excess hair on the face), acne, and weight gain.[89] Genital prolapse occurs when the reproductive organs are displaced from their usual locations in the pelvis due to weak or damaged connective tissues, and it often causes urinary incontinence.[90] The symptoms of perimenopause, the years in which women transition into menopause and the end of menstrual cycles, may also create health challenges, including hot flashes, night sweats, and other signs of hormone changes.[91] Women of all ages are also at risk of a diversity of cancers of the reproductive system, including breast cancer, cervical cancer, uterine (endometrial) cancer, and ovarian cancer as well as benign breast diseases that cause pain or discomfort, sexual dysfunction, STIs, and gender-based violence.

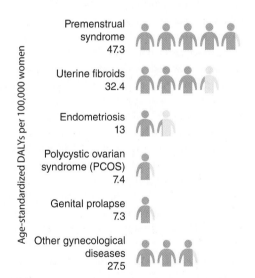

Age-standardized DALYs per 100,000 women

Premenstrual syndrome
47.3

Uterine fibroids
32.4

Endometriosis
13

Polycystic ovarian syndrome (PCOS)
7.4

Genital prolapse
7.3

Other gynecological diseases
27.5

FIGURE 11–27 Age-standardized disability-adjusted life years (DALYs) lost to gynecological diseases per 100,000 women (excluding cancers and pregnancy-related conditions).

Data from GBD 2015 DALYs and HALE Collaborators. Global, regional, and national disability-adjusted life-years (DALYs) for 315 diseases and injuries and healthy life expectancy (HALE), 1990–2015: A systematic analysis for the Global Burden of Disease Study 2015. *Lancet* 2016; 388:1603–58.

▶ 11.10 Men's Reproductive Health

Men may experience a variety of health issues related to reproduction and sexual function, including infertility, STIs, and cancers of the male reproductive system. Testicular cancer occurs very infrequently, but it has a higher incidence rate in younger men than in older men.[92] For older men, prostate health often becomes a significant health concern. **Benign prostatic hyperplasia (BPH)** is an enlargement of the prostate gland that may cause difficulty with urination and sexual performance, and it is very common among older men.[93] Many men with BPH go on to develop prostate cancer as they age, and treatments for prostate cancer may cause impotence.[94] Erectile dysfunction (ED) may also occur as a result of neurological conditions, diabetes, hypertension, cardiovascular disease, some types of medications, trauma, and a variety of other exposures and aging-related physiological conditions.[95] Medications and other tools may be helpful for treating ED.

▶ 11.11 Sexual Minority Health

Members of sexual and gender minority groups often have difficulty accessing high-quality health services. One of the steps toward improving access to health services is making sure that health and social service workers understand the various aspects of sexuality and gender and use appropriate terms when working with diverse clients.[96] **Sexual orientation** is a function of sexual attraction, identity, and behavior. Sexual attraction is about the type of person an individual desires sexually, romantically, emotionally, and in other ways. Heterosexual individuals are attracted to people of the opposite sex, homosexual individuals are attracted to people of the same sex, and bisexual individuals are attracted to both people of the opposite sex and the same sex. Sexual identity is about how people present their sexuality to others, with some people very private about their sexual identity and others very open. Sexual behavior is about the sexual actions in which a person engages. Some people choose to be celibate. Some people engage in sexual activities that do not align with their sexual attraction or identity. People with opposite-sex attractions may be involved in homosexual relationships, and people with same-sex

attractions may be involved in heterosexual relationships. For example, some **men who have sex with men (MSM)** do not identify as homosexual and are happily married to women. The term MSM emphasizes behavior rather than identity. All of these terms related to sexual orientation are in a different domain from terms related to **gender identity**, which is an individual's sense of maleness or femaleness. A **cisgender** person has a gender identity that aligns with the sex assigned to that person at birth. A **transgender** person has a gender identity that does not match the sex assigned at birth.

The term LGBT, which is an acronym for lesbian, gay, bisexual, and transgender, mixes terms about sexual orientation and gender identity. So does the longer acronym LGBTQIA, which adds terms for questioning, intersex, and asexual. But the grouping of these distinct categories highlights shared experiences of stigma and discrimination, including in healthcare settings.[97] Transgender people have a higher than typical risk of STIs, substance abuse, mental health disorders related to chronic stress, and injuries from violence.[98] Similarly elevated risks have been observed in sexual minority populations.[99] While some countries are enacting laws that protect the human rights of LGBT people and ensure equitable access to health services, other countries are moving in the opposite direction by codifying laws that discriminate against LGBT people and make it dangerous for LGBT people to seek medical care or be honest with their clinicians about their health needs.[100] Achieving the SDGs will require all adolescents and adults to have equitable access to health services (SDG 3.8), including reproductive health services (SDG 3.7), as well as having social, economic, and political inclusion (SDG 10.2) and freedom from violence (SDG 16.1). The SDGs cannot be achieved when sexual and gender majority and minority populations do not have equal access to health and safety.[1]

▶ References

1. United Nations. *Transforming our world: The 2030 Agenda for Sustainable Development.* New York: UN; 2015.

2. McIntosh CA, Finkle JL. The Cairo conference on population and development: A new paradigm? *Popul Dev Rev.* 1995;21:223–60.

3. United Nations. *International Conference on Population and Development Program of Action: 20th anniversary edition.* New York: UNFPA; 2014.

4. *Religion, women's health and rights: Points of contention and paths of opportunities.* New York: UNFPA; 2016.

5. Cook RJ, Fathalla MF. Advancing reproductive rights beyond Cairo and Beijing. *Int Family Plann Perspect.* 1996;22:115–21.

6. *The Beijing Declaration and Platform for Action turns 20.* New York: UN Women; 2015.

7. *Reproductive rights are human rights: A handbook for national human rights institutions.* New York: UNFPA; 2014.

8. Stenberg K, Sweeny K, Axelson H, Temmerman M, Sheehan P. Returns on investment in the continuum of care for reproductive, maternal, newborn, and child health (Chapter 16). *Disease control priorities.* 3rd ed. *Reproductive, maternal, newborn, and child health (Volume 2).* Washington DC: IBRD/World Bank; 2016.

9. Kirk D. Demographic transition theory. *Popul Studies.* 1996;50:361–87.

10. UN Department of Economic and Social Affairs. *World population prospects: The 2017 revision.* New York: UN; 2017.

11. Ezeh AC, Bongaarts J, Mberu B. Global population trends and policy options. *Lancet.* 2012;380:142–8.

12. *2016 world population data sheet.* Washington DC: Population Reference Bureau (PRB); 2016.

13. Harper S. Economic and social implications of aging societies. *Science* 2014;346:587–91.

14. Luci-Greulich A, Thévenon O. The impact of family policies on fertility trends in developed countries. *Eur J Popul.* 2013;29:387–416.

15. Ayatollah Ali Khamenei on Iran's population policy. *Popul Develop Rev.* 2014;40:573–5.

16. Amaral EFL, Almeida ME, Gonçalves GQ. *Characterization of fertility levels in Brazil, 1970-2010.* Santa Monica CA: RAND Labor and Population; 2015.

17. Hesketh T, Zhu WX. The one child family policy: The good, the bad, and the ugly. *BMJ.* 1997;314:1685–7.

18. Hesketh T, Lu L, Xing ZW. The effect of China's one-child family policy after 25 years. *N Engl J Med.* 2005;353:1171–7.

19. Hvistendahl M. Has China outgrown the one-child policy? *Science.* 2010;329:1458–61.

20. Zhu WX, Lu L, Hesketh T. China's excess males, sex selective abortion, and one child policy: Analysis of data from 2005 national intercensus survey. *BMJ.* 2009;338:b1211.

21. Abrahamson P. End of an era? China's one-child policy and its unintended consequences. *Asian Soc Work Pol Rev.* 2016;10:326–38.

22. Basten S, Jiang Q. Fertility in China: An uncertain future. *Popul Stud.* 2015;69:S97–105.

23. Upadhyay UD, Gipson JD, Withers M, et al. Women's empowerment and fertility: A review of the literature. *Soc Sci Med.* 2014;115:111–20.

24. Skirbekk V. Fertility trends by social status. *Demographic Res.* 2008;18:145–80.

25. Canning D, Schultz TP. The economic consequences of reproductive health and family planning. *Lancet.* 2012;380:165–71.

26. Stover J, Hardee K, Ganatra B, García Moreno C, Horton S. Interventions to improve reproductive health (Chapter 6). *Disease control priorities.* 3rd ed. *Reproductive, maternal, newborn, and child health (Volume 2).* Washington DC: IBRD/World Bank; 2016.

27. Moore Z, Pfitzer A, Gubin R, Charurat E, Elliott L, Croft T. Missed opportunities for family planning: An analysis of pregnancy risk and contraceptive method use among postpartum women in 21 low- and middle-income countries. *Contraception.* 2015;92:31–9.

28. Conde-Agudelo A, Rosas-Bermudez A, Castaño F, Norton MH. Effects of birth spacing on maternal, perinatal, infant, and child health: A systematic review of causal mechanisms. *Stud Fam Plann.* 2012;43:93–114.

29. Mishell DR Jr. Intrauterine devices: Mechanisms of action, safety, and efficacy. *Contraception.* 1998;58(3 Suppl):S45–53.

30. Mascarenhas MN, Flaxman SR, Boerma T, Vanderpoel S, Mathers CD, Stevens GA. Trends in primary and secondary infertility prevalence since 1990: A systematic analysis of demographic and reproductive health surveys. *Lancet.* 2013;381:S90.

31. Inhorn MC, Patrizio P. Infertility around the globe: New thinking on gender, reproductive technologies and global movements in the 21st century. *Hum Reprod Update.* 2015;21:411–26.

32. Mascarenhas MN, Flaxman SR. Boerma T, Vanderpoel S, Stevens GA. National, regional, and global trends in infertility prevalence since 1990: A systematic analysis of 277 health surveys. *PLoS Med.* 2012;9:e1001356.

33. Lindsay TJ, Vitrikas KR. Evaluation and treatment of infertility. *Am Fam Physician.* 2015;91:308–14.

34. Ezeh A, Bankole A, Cleland J, García-Moreno C, Temmerman M, Ziraba AK. Burden of reproductive

ill health (Chapter 2). *Disease control priorities. 3rd ed. Reproductive, maternal, newborn, and child health (Volume 2).* Washington DC: IBRD/World Bank; 2016.

35. Campbell OMR, Graham WJ; The Lancet Maternal Survival Series Steering Group. Strategies for reducing maternal mortality: Getting on with what works. *Lancet.* 2006;368:1284–99.

36. *Managing complications in pregnancy and childbirth: A guide for midwives and doctors.* Geneva: WHO; 2007.

37. *World health statistics 2016.* Geneva: WHO; 2016.

38. *State of the world's children 2016.* New York: UNICEF; 2016.

39. Lassi ZS, Kumar R, Bhutta ZA. Community-based care to improve maternal, newborn, and child health (Chapter 14). *Disease control priorities. 3rd ed. Reproductive, maternal, newborn, and child health (Volume 2).* Washington DC: IBRD/World Bank; 2016.

40. Black RE, Walker N, Laxminarayan R, Temmerman M. Reproductive, maternal, newborn, and child health: Key messages of this volume (Chapter 1). *Disease control priorities. 3rd ed. Reproductive, maternal, newborn, and child health (Volume 2).* Washington DC: IBRD/World Bank; 2016.

41. *Monitoring emergency obstetric care: A handbook.* Geneva: WHO/UNPF/UNICEF; 2009.

42. Betran AP, Torloni MR, Zhang JJ, Gülmezoglu AM. WHO working group on Caesarean section. WHO statement on Caesarean section rates. *BJOG.* 2016;123:667–70.

43. Ye J, Zhang J, Mikolajczyk R, Torloni MR, Gülmezoglu AM, Betran AP. Association between rates of Caesarean section and maternal and neonatal mortality in the 21st century: A worldwide population-based ecological study with longitudinal data. *BJOG.* 2016;123:745–53.

44. Holmer H, Lantz A, Kunjumen T, et al. Global distribution of surgeons, anaesthesiologists, and obstetricians. *Lancet Global Health.* 2015;3(Suppl 2): S9–11.

45. Bollinger LA, Kruk ME. Innovations to expand access and improve quality of health services (Chapter 15). *Disease control priorities. 3rd ed. Reproductive, maternal, newborn, and child health (Volume 2).* Washington DC: IBRD/World Bank; 2016.

46. GBD 2015 Maternal Mortality Collaborators. Global, regional, and national levels of maternal mortality, 1990–2015: A systematic analysis for the Global Burden of Disease Study 2015. *Lancet.* 2016;388(10053):1775–812.

47. *Trends in maternal mortality, 1990 to 2015: Estimates by WHO, UNICEF, UNFPA, World Bank Group and the United Nations Population Division.* Geneva: WHO; 2015.

48. Ahmed S, Li Q, Liu L, Tsui AO. Maternal deaths averted by contraceptive use: An analysis of 172 countries. *Lancet.* 2012;380:111–25.

49. Cleland J, Conde-Agudelo A, Peterson H, Ross J, Tsui A. Contraception and health. *Lancet.* 2012; 380:149–56.

50. Ronsmans C, Graham WJ; The Lancet Maternal Survival Series Steering Group. Maternal mortality: Who, when, where, and why. *Lancet.* 2008;368:1189–200.

51. Souza JP, Tunçalp Ö, Vogel JP, et al. Obstetric transition: The pathway towards ending preventable maternal deaths. *BJOG.* 2014;121(Suppl 1):1–4.

52. *The Millennium Development Goals report 2015.* New York: UN; 2015.

53. Say L, Chou D, Gemmill A, et al. Global causes of maternal death: A WHO systematic analysis. *Lancet.* 2014;2:e323–33.

54. Leduc D, Senikas V, Lalonde AB, et al. Active management of the third stage of labour: Prevention and treatment of postpartum hemorrhage. *J Obstet Gynaecol Can.* 2009;31:980–93.

55. Tunçalp Ö, Souza JP, Gülmezoglu M; World Health Organization. New WHO recommendations on prevention and treatment of postpartum hemorrhage. *Int J Gynaecol Obstet.* 2013;123:254–6.

56. Duley L. The global impact of pre-eclampsia and eclampsia. *Semin Perinatol.* 2009;33:130–7.

57. Abalos E, Cuesta C, Grosso AL, Chou D, Say L. Global and regional estimates of preeclampsia and eclampsia: A systematic review. *Eur J Obstet Gynecol Reprod Biol.* 2013;170:1–7.

58. Filippi V, Chou D, Ronsmans C, Graham W, Say L. Levels and causes of maternal mortality and morbidity (Chapter 3). *Disease control priorities. 3rd ed. Reproductive, maternal, newborn, and child health (Volume 2).* Washington DC: IBRD/World Bank; 2016.

59. Gülmezoglu AM, Lawrie TA, Hezelgrave N, et al. Interventions to reduce maternal and newborn morbidity and mortality (Chapter 7). *Disease control priorities. 3rd ed. Reproductive, maternal, newborn, and child health (Volume 2).* Washington DC: IBRD/ World Bank; 2016.

60. Adler AJ, Ronsmans C, Calvert C, Filippi V. Estimating the prevalence of obstetric fistula: A systematic review and meta-analysis. *BMC Pregnancy Childbirth.* 2013;13:246.

61. Lawn JE, Gravett MG, Nunes TM, Rubens CE, Stanton C; GAPPS Review Gropu. Global report on preterm birth and stillbirth: Definitions, description of the burden and opportunities to improve data. *BMC Pregnancy Childbirth.* 2010;10(Suppl 1):S1.

62. Blencowe H, Cousens S, Jassir FB, et al. National, regional, and worldwide estimates of stillbirth

rates in 2015, with trends from 2000: A systematic analysis. *Lancet Glob Health.* 2016;4:e98–108.

63. Liu L, Hill K, Oza S, et al. Levels and causes of mortality under age five years (Chapter 4). *Disease control priorities.* 3rd ed. *Reproductive, maternal, newborn, and child health (Volume 2).* Washington DC: IBRD/World Bank; 2016.

64. Aminu M, Unkels R, Mdegela M, Utz B, Adaji S, van den Broek N. Causes of and factors associated with stillbirth in low- and middle-income countries: A systematic literature review. *BJOG.* 2014;121 (Suppl 4):141–53.

65. Lawn J, Shibuya K, Stein C. No cry at birth: Global estimates of intrapartum stillbirths and intrapartum-related neonatal deaths. *Bull World Health Organ.* 2005;83:409–17.

66. GBD 2015 Child Mortality Collaborators. Global, regional, national, and selected subnational levels of stillbirths, neonatal, infant, and under-5 mortality, 1980–2015: A systematic analysis for the Global Burden of Disease Study 2015. *Lancet* 2016;388(10053):1725–74.

67. Blencowe H, Cousens S, Oestergaard MZ, et al. National, regional, and worldwide estimates of preterm birth rates in the year 2010 with time trends since 1990 for selected countries: A systematic analysis and implications. *Lancet.* 2012;379:2162–72.

68. Goldenberg RL, Culhand JF, Iams JD, Romero R. Epidemiology and causes of preterm birth. *Lancet.* 2008;371:75–84.

69. Voltolini C, Torricelli M, Conti N, Vellucci FL, Severi FM, Petraglia F. Understanding spontaneous preterm birth: From underlying mechanisms to predictive and preventive interventions. *Reprod Sci.* 2013;20:1274–92.

70. *Born too soon: The global action report on preterm birth.* Geneva: WHO; 2012.

71. Saigal S, Doyle LW. An overview of mortality and sequelae of preterm birth from infancy to adulthood. *Lancet.* 2008;371:261–9.

72. Conde-Agudelo A, Belizán JM, Diaz-Rossello J. Kangaroo mother care to reduce morbidity and mortality in low birthweight infants. *Cochrane Database Syst Rev.* 2011;(3):CD002771.

73. Kramer MS. Determinants of low birth weight: Methodological assessment and meta-analysis. *Bull World Health Organ.* 1987;65:663–737.

74. Hack M, Klein NK, Taylor HG. Long-term developmental outcomes of low birth weight infants. *Future Child.* 1995;5:176–96.

75. Oskoui M, Coutinho F, Dykeman J, Jetté N, Pringsheim T. An update on the prevalence of cerebral palsy: A systematic review and meta-analysis. *Dev Med Child Neurol.* 2013;55:509–19.

76. *World report on disability 2011.* Geneva: WHO; 2011.

77. Ouzounian JG, Korst LM, Miller DA, Lee RH. Brachial plexus palsy and shoulder dystocia: Obstetric risk factors remain elusive. *Am J Perinatol.* 2013;30:303–7.

78. Lawn JE, Manandhar A, Haws RA, Darmstadt GL. Reducing one million child deaths from birth asphyxia: A survey of health systems gaps and priorities. *Health Res Policy Syst.* 2007;5:4.

79. *Guidelines on basic newborn resuscitation.* Geneva: WHO; 2012.

80. Walker CL, Rudan I, Liu L, et al. Global burden of childhood pneumonia and diarrhea. *Lancet.* 2013;381:1405–16.

81. Roper MH, Vandelaer JH, Gasse FL. Maternal and neonatal tetanus. *Lancet.* 2007;370:1947–59.

82. Darmstadt GL, Bhutta ZA, Cousens S, Adam T, Walker N, Bernis L; Lancet Neonatal Survival Steering Team. Evidence-based, cost-effective interventions: How many newborn babies can we save? *Lancet.* 2005;365:977–85.

83. Gabrysch S, Civitelli G, Edmond KM, et al. New signal functions to measure the ability of health facilities to provide routine and emergency newborn care. *PLoS Med.* 2012;9:e1001340.

84. *Pregnancy, childbirth, postpartum and newborn care: A guide for essential practice.* 3rd ed. Geneva: WHO; 2015.

85. GBD 2015 DALYs and HALE Collaborators. Global, regional, and national disability-adjusted life-years (DALYs) for 315 diseases and injuries and healthy life expectancy (HALE), 1990–2015: A systematic analysis for the Global Burden of Disease Study 2015. *Lancet.* 2016;388:1603–58.

86. Yonkers KA, O'Brien S, Eriksson E. Premenstrual syndrome. *Lancet.* 2008;371:1200–10.

87. Khan AT, Shehmar M, Gupta JK. Uterine fibroids: Current perspectives. *Int J Womens Health.* 2014;6:95–114.

88. Vercellini P, Viganò P, Somigliana E, Fedele L. Endometriosis: Pathogenesis and treatment. *Nat Rev Endocrinol.* 2014;10:261–75.

89. Sirmans SM, Pate KA. Epidemiology, diagnosis, and management of polycystic ovary syndrome. *Clin Epidemiol.* 2014;6:1–13.

90. Abrams P, Andersson KE, Birder L, et al. Fourth International Consultation on Incontinence Recommendations of the International Scientific Committee: Evaluation and treatment of urinary incontinence, pelvic organ prolapse, and fecal incontinence. *Neurourol Urodyn.* 2010;29:213–40.

91. Burger H, Woods NF, Dennerstein L, Alexander JL, Kotz K, Richardson G. Nomenclature and endocrinology of menopause and perimenopause. *Expert Rev Neurother.* 2007;7(11 Suppl):S35–43.

92. Shanmugalingam T, Soultati A, Chowdhury S, Rudman S, Van Hemelrijck M. Global incidence and outcome of testicular cancer. *Clin Epidemiol.* 2013;5:417–27.

93. Gacci M, Eardley I, Giuliano F, et al. Critical analysis of the relationship between sexual dysfunctions and lower urinary tract symptoms due to benign prostatic hyperplasia. *Eur Urol.* 2011;60:809–25.

94. Park DL, Aron M, Rewcastle JC, Boyd SD, Gill IS. A model for managing erectile dysfunction following prostate cancer treatment. *Curr Opin Urol.* 2013;23:129–34.

95. Shamloul R, Ghanem H. Erectile dysfunction. *Lancet.* 2013;381:153–65.

96. Mayer KH, Bradford JB, Makadon HJ, Stall R, Goldhammer H, Landers S. Sexual and gender minority health: What we know and what needs to be done. *Am J Public Health.* 2008;98:989–95.

97. Daniel H, Butkus R; Health and Public Policy Committee of American College of Physicians. Lesbian, gay, bisexual, and transgender health disparities: Executive summary of a policy position paper from the American College of Physicians. *Ann Intern Med.* 2015;163:135–7.

98. Reisner SL, Poteat T, Keatley J, et al. Global health burden and needs of transgender populations: A review. *Lancet.* 2016;388:422–36.

99. Hatzenbuehler ML, McLaughlin KA, Keyes KM, Hasin DS. The impact of institutional discrimination on psychiatric disorders in lesbian, gay, and bisexual populations: A prospective study. *Am J Public Health.* 2010;100:452–9.

100. Beyrer C. Pushback: The current wave of anti-homosexuality laws and impacts on health. *PLoS Med.* 2014;11:e1001658.

CHAPTER 12

Nutrition

Some of the earliest international health campaigns focused on delivering food aid to starving children. Food insecurity and nutrient deficiencies continue to be public health priorities in many low-income countries. At the same time, most high- and middle-income countries are struggling with rising rates of obesity and dramatic increases in the prevalence of chronic diseases associated with being overweight. Global collaborations are seeking to end child undernutrition, prevent obesity in children and adults, and ensure food safety as international trade in food products intensifies.

▶ 12.1 Nutrition and Global Health

Nutrition is the consumption of food that allows the body to survive, grow, heal, and be healthy and the processing of those nutrients within the body. Nutrition is a key contributor to individual and population health status worldwide.[1] In the world's lowest-income communities, the primary nutritional concern is having too little food. Many children in these areas have stunted growth because they eat too few calories and too little protein, and many infants, children, adolescents, and adults have vitamin and mineral deficiencies because the starchy staple foods that form the bulk of their diets are low in nutritional quality. Food aid has been a key part of international health initiatives for many decades.[2] The continuing challenges of undernutrition are the target of Sustainable Development Goal (SDG) 2, which aims to "end hunger, achieve food security and improved nutrition, and promote sustainable agriculture."[3] One of the driving motivations for keeping nutrition as a global health priority is the ethical imperative to protect vulnerable children no matter where they happen to have been born.[4]

In middle-income and high-income communities, the biggest nutritional concern is usually obesity. People who live in wealthier areas have access to a great variety of nutritious foods, but they also eat more refined and processed foods along with more fats. Obesity-related health concerns like diabetes and hypertension are becoming more prevalent in industrialized and industrializing economies as more adults and children are physically inactive and overweight. The shift from having undernutrition and nutrient deficiencies as the most prevalent nutritional concerns in a population to having overweight and obesity as the dominant nutritional disorders is called the **nutrition transition**.[5] During the process of shifting from a pre-transition profile toward a post-transition profile, countries often experience a dual burden of nutritional problems, with undernutrition continuing to be prevalent among children, especially those living in rural areas and in low-income urban communities, while adult obesity becomes more common.[6] Thus, obesity is not just a problem of high-income countries, but one that affects countries across the income spectrum, including low-income countries. Collaborative efforts are needed to identify effective interventions for obesity prevention. Global cooperation is also required in order to ensure food safety as international trade in food products increases.

▶ 12.2 Macronutrients

Every person needs to eat on a regular basis to provide his or her body with energy and the materials needed to build and repair cells and tissues, fight infections, and stay warm. Healthy nutrition requires an appropriate amount of daily food that includes a diversity of types of nutrients. **Macronutrients** are nutrients such as carbohydrates, protein, and fats and oils that are required to be consumed in relatively large quantities because they provide energy.

Energy in food is typically measured in units of calories. One **calorie** of food (which is technically 1 kilocalorie, which is why food energy measurements are usually reported in "kcal" units) is equal to the amount of energy required to raise the temperature of 1 gram of water by 1 degree Celsius. The number of calories needed by a person each day varies based on age, sex, body size, activity level, climate, and pregnancy and lactation status.[7] A typical toddler requires about 1000 calories daily. Older children require approximately 1200–1800 calories per day. A typical adolescent girl might require about 1800 calories daily, while an adolescent boy might require 2200–3200 calories, depending on his level of activity. Young adult women require about 2000 calories per day when not pregnant or breastfeeding. Young adult men require 2400–3000 calories. The number of calories needed each day then decreases with aging. Older adult women need only about 1600 calories daily and older adult men require only about 2000 calories. In higher-income countries, the number of calories available per person each day far exceeds the required number of calories, but some low-income countries struggle to produce or import enough food to meet the daily requirements of their residents.[8]

Carbohydrates are chains of sugars. Carbohydrates are found in cereal grains like rice, maize, and wheat (the three most common staple foods in the world[9]), in starchy roots like potatoes and yams, and in fruits and vegetables. When the body requires a quick source of energy, the body's cells break down carbohydrates through a process called cellular respiration. The molecular units that form carbohydrates are called **saccharides**. Simple carbohydrates are made up of short chains of sugars that are easily absorbed into the bloodstream. The galactose found in milk and the glucose and fructose found in fruits and honey are monosaccharides ("one sugar"). Table sugar, or sucrose, is a disaccharide ("two sugar") composed of glucose and fructose. Lactose is a disaccharide composed of glucose and galactose. The complex carbohydrates (often classified as starches) found in whole grain products like whole wheat bread and oatmeal are made up of longer chains of sugars (polysaccharides) that take longer to digest.

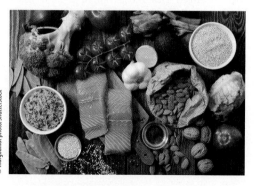

Eating complex carbohydrates keeps a person from feeling hungry longer than eating simple sugars. **Fiber**, a non-digestible complex carbohydrate found in unprocessed plant-based foods, is essential for healthy digestion because it provides bulk that moves food material through the intestines. Nutritionists recommend that carbohydrates account for 45%–65% of the daily calories consumed by the typical person.[7] In low-income countries, many people eat a starchy diet that exceeds this recommended proportion, even though they consume few nutrient-rich fruits and vegetables.[8]

Amino acids are organic compounds that contain carbon, hydrogen, oxygen, and nitrogen. **Proteins** are chains of amino acids. Amino acids from food are broken down and reassembled in the body's cells to form new proteins. The keratin that makes up hair and nails, the hemoglobin in blood that transports oxygen, the antibodies that help the body's immune system recognize and fight infection, the actin and myosin that contract and relax muscles, and the collagen in ligaments, tendons, and skin are all types of proteins. About 20 different kinds of amino acids are recognized as critical for human biochemistry. Humans are unable to produce several of these important amino acids, and those nine **essential amino acids** must be acquired from food. Proteins from animal-based foods are usually **complete proteins** that contain all of the essential amino acids. Plant proteins are usually incomplete proteins, but all of the amino acids can be consumed in one vegetarian meal by combining **complementary proteins**, like eating maize (corn) with beans or nuts with whole wheat bread. Nutritionists generally recommend that 10%–35% of daily calories for the typical person come from high-quality proteins.[7]

Fats and oils are both types of **lipids**, or fatty acids, which are hydrocarbon chains with other chemical groups at the ends of the chains. **Fats** are lipids of animal origin like butter and lard that are solid at room temperature. **Oils** are lipids of plant origin like corn oil and olive oil that are liquids at room temperature. Lipids contain more energy per gram than any other biological molecule and provide long-term energy storage, insulation, protective padding around internal organs, and assistance with nutrient absorption. They are needed for the processing of some vitamins (A, D, E, and K), and are used by the body to make other compounds, such as steroid hormones. Nutritionists recommend that about 20%–35% of calories consumed in a day should come from healthy fats and oils.[7] It is not uncommon for people who live in high-income countries to exceed the recommended proportion and for people who live in low-income countries to consume too few fats and oils (**FIGURE 12–1**).[8]

Not all fatty acids are equally healthy. The relative healthiness of lipids is often related to the amount of hydrogen they contain. **Unsaturated fatty acids** contain at least one double bond in the carbon chain. Both monounsaturated fats like those found in olive oil, avocados, and nuts

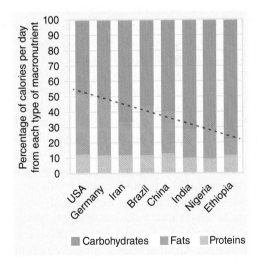

FIGURE 12–1 People living in higher-income countries eat more fats and fewer carbohydrates than people living in lower-income countries.

Data from *FAOSTAT food balance sheets 2013*. Rome: Food and Agriculture Organization of the United Nations; 2015.

and the polyunsaturated fats in cold water fish like salmon (which contain omega-3 fatty acids) seem to be protective against heart disease.[10] Saturated fatty acids are found in meat, butter, and other animal products, and they can contribute to blocked arteries. The term **saturated fatty acid** refers to the fact that the molecule is "saturated" with hydrogen, and no more hydrogen can be added to it because only single bonds exist between its carbon atoms. **Trans fats** are liquid oils that have been transformed into solid fats by adding hydrogen to them through the use of pressure. They are found in margarine and other processed foods and have been shown to raise "bad" (or "lousy") LDL (low-density lipoprotein) cholesterol while depleting "good" (or "healthy") HDL (high-density lipoprotein) cholesterol. When the LDL/HDL ratio is high, the excess fat in the blood is deposited on the walls of blood vessels as plaque.[11] When there is a lot of plaque lining the blood vessels, the resulting atherosclerosis increases the risk of having a heart attack or stroke.

Water is not a nutrient, but it is an essential part of the diet. Every cell in the body needs a way to take in oxygen and nutrients along with a way to get rid of carbon dioxide and waste. Blood is about 92% water, and it is the medium for transporting gases, nutrients, and wastes throughout the body. Blood volume is a function of the amount of water in the body. Without adequate blood volume, blood pressure drops and it is difficult for the body's cells to function. A person who loses a lot of blood due to an injury or a lot of water due to excessive vomiting or diarrhea can go into hypovolemic shock, shock caused by too little blood volume. Water also helps the body regulate its temperature by sweating and helps the body get rid of waste through urination and defecation. An adult loses about 2–3 quarts of water a day by urinating, sweating, and exhaling humidified air.[12] More may be lost in hot climates, during intense physical activity, or when a person has diarrhea. This lost water must be replaced to avoid dehydration. Severe dehydration can cause an acid-base imbalance in the blood and lead to organ failure (especially of the kidneys) and death.

▶ 12.3 Protein-Energy Malnutrition

Undernutrition is malnutrition resulting from deficiencies in the amount of food or types of nutrients eaten, or from poor absorption of the nutrients that have been consumed. For example, lack of protein in the diet means that the body does not have the amino acids it needs to repair itself, and too little fat in the diet means that fat-soluble vitamins cannot be processed. Even mild and moderate undernutrition can significantly increase a child's risk of illness and death due to infectious diseases.[13] Undernutrition contributes to more than one-third of under-5 child deaths from infectious diseases, including about three-quarters of diarrhea deaths, half of measles deaths, and more than two-fifths of pneumonia deaths.[14] At least one in five deaths of under-5 children can be attributed to undernutrition.[15] Improving access to nutrition is, therefore, a foundational requirement for achieving the other health goals spelled out in the SDGs. The SDGs aim to "end hunger and ensure access by all people, in particular the poor and people in vulnerable situations, including infants, to safe, nutritious, and sufficient food all year round" (SDG 2.1) and "end all forms of malnutrition" by achieving growth targets in children under 5 years of age and addressing "the nutritional needs of adolescent girls, pregnant and lactating women, and older persons" (SDG 2.2).[16]

Anthropometry is the measurement of the human body. Height, weight, waist circumference, body fat percentage, and other measurements can be useful indicators of a person's nutritional status. For children, height-for-age, weight-for-height, and weight-for-age are commonly used measures of healthy growth. A child with low height-for-age is classified as having **stunting**.[17] Stunting is an indicator of chronic malnutrition. A child with low weight-for-height (also called weight-for-length) is classified as having **wasting**. Wasting is a sign of acute malnutrition characterized by rapidly decreasing nutritional health status. There are a variety of definitions for what constitutes being underweight. For children, **underweight** is often defined as low weight-for-age.

Stunting and wasting are often used by global child nutrition initiatives as metrics for tracking progress toward achieving goals. The six global nutrition targets for 2025 approved by the World Health Assembly in 2012 aim to improve the nutritional status of the global population by (1) reducing the number of under-5 children who have stunting by 40%, so that fewer than 100 million young children in 2025 will have stunting, (2) reducing anemia in women of reproductive age by 50%, so that the prevalence is less than 15%, (3) reducing the percentage of newborns with low birthweight (less than 2500 grams) by 30%, (4) preventing a rise in the proportion of children who are overweight, (5) increasing the rate of exclusive breastfeeding in the first 6 months of life to at least 50%, and (6) reducing the prevalence of childhood wasting to less than 5%, which will require a reduction of nearly 40%.[18]

Global growth standards for children from birth through 60 months are provided by the World Health Organization (WHO).[19] The WHO growth charts can be used worldwide because scientific evidence shows that infants and children from geographically diverse regions experience very similar growth patterns when their health and nutritional needs are met.[20] The charts display the average measurements of healthy children of a particular age, and then use the distribution of measurements for healthy children to identify percentiles. For example, a child at the 85th height-for-age percentile is taller than 85% of healthy children globally and shorter than only 15% of healthy children. Since the distribution of anthropometric measurements follows a normal (bell-shaped) curve, these percentiles can be translated to z-scores. A

standard deviation is a statistical indicator for the width of a distribution, and a **z-score** is an indicator of how many standard deviations away from the mean an individual's measure is. A weight-for-height z-score of $z = 1$ indicates a child whose measurements falls one standard deviation above the mean. A z-score of 1 is equivalent to the child's weight-for-height being at the 84th percentile. A weight-for-height z-score of $z = -2$ indicates a child whose weight-for-height falls two standard deviations below the mean. A z-score of -2 is equivalent to being at the 2nd percentile of weight-for-height for healthy children. A child with a weight-for-height z-score below -3 is considered to have **severe acute malnutrition (SAM)** and require urgent medical care.[21] A child's **mid-upper arm circumference (MUAC)** or arm-circumference-for-age is another indicator of wasting. Children with a MUAC of less than 11.5 centimeters have severe acute malnutrition, and those with measurements between 11.5 and 12.5 centimeters have moderate acute malnutrition.[22]

FIGURE 12–2 shows a sample weight-for-age chart for girls.[23] The graph has age in months on the *x*-axis and weight on the *y*-axis. The graph allows a parent or healthcare worker to easily determine if a child of a particular age is underweight (below the 15th percentile) or severely underweight (under the 3rd percentile) for his or her age. The sample curve for "Child 1" shows a child of healthy weight. The sample curve for "Child 2" shows a seriously underweight child. Both children lost weight just after their first birthdays, probably due to diarrheal disease. For "Child 1," this was a minor event that barely influenced her growth. For "Child 2," this bout of diarrhea pushed her into severe malnutrition and could easily have caused her death. Children should be weighed often, especially when they are very young, so that growth trends can emerge. A child like "Child 2" who loses weight or fails to gain weight needs medical attention. (One limitation of many growth standards for children is that they require caregivers to know the birth date of the child, and many children

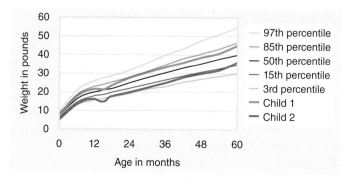

FIGURE 12–2 A sample child growth chart showing weight-for-age curves for girls from birth to the fifth birthday.

Percentile curve data from WHO Multicentre Growth Reference Study Group. *WHO child growth standards: Length/height-for-age, weight-for-age, weight-for-length, weight-for-height and body mass index-for-age: Methods and development.* Geneva World Health Organization; 2006.

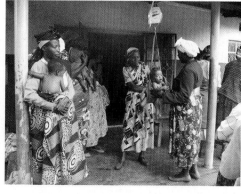

born at home or orphaned do not have a record of this date. When this information is not available, it can be difficult to determine if a child is growing well.)

Protein energy malnutrition (PEM) is a severe form of chronic undernutrition.[24] Severe PEM is also a sign of severe acute malnutrition. PEM can present as marasmus or as kwashiorkor. Children with **marasmus** are emaciated, weak, and lethargic because of long-term calorie deprivation. They look skeletal, have loose and wrinkled skin, and have too little energy to move or cry. Eventually, their body systems begin to fail. Children with **kwashiorkor** may have somewhat adequate calorie intake but lack the dietary protein necessary for healthy growth and development. Kwashiorkor is characterized by **edema**, fluid retention in extracellular spaces that causes swelling of the tissues in the arms, legs, and face.[25] Most children with kwashiorkor also have weak muscles and pale hair and skin, and they may have a distended abdomen because their nutrient-deficient bodies are retaining water and the abdominal walls are so weak that the internal organs sag out. Kwashiorkor is associated with early weaning, which often happens when an infant's mother becomes pregnant again soon after giving birth. Both marasmus and kwashiorkor increase susceptibility to infection and put children at risk of permanent disability and death.[26]

Infants with SAM require inpatient care so they can be fed specially formulated therapeutic milks and receive other medical treatments. Children with SAM who have no appetite and are suffering from medical complications also usually require inpatient hospital care so they can receive therapeutic nutrition, fluid and electrolyte management, and treatment for diarrhea, malaria, intestinal parasites, and other infections.[27] These undernourished children are typically fed **ready-to-use therapeutic food (RUTF)** that is high in energy and protein, often made from a peanut base.[28] Children with SAM who have an appetite and do not have other serious medical conditions can often be treated in

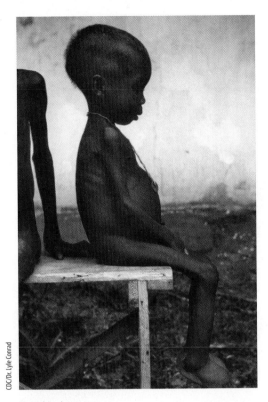

Kwashiorkor.

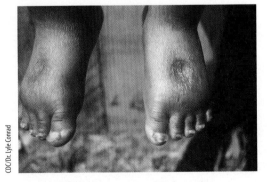

Pitting edema from kwashiorkor.

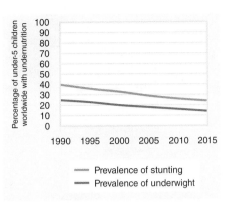

FIGURE 12-3 The nutritional status of children younger than 5 years old has improved significantly in recent years.

Data from *UNICEF-WHO-World Bank joint child malnutrition estimates.* New York: UNICEF/WHO/World Bank; 2012.

Significant progress toward reducing child hunger worldwide has been made over the past 25 years (**FIGURE 12-3**).[29] Even so, the statistics on childhood hunger remain alarming. Globally, about 150 million under-5 children have moderately or severely stunted growth, including more than one-third of children in sub-Saharan Africa and South Asia, about 20% in the Middle East and North Africa, and about 10% in East Asia and the Pacific, Latin America and the Caribbean, and Central and Eastern Europe (**FIGURE 12-4**).[29] About 30% of children in South Asia and 20% in sub-Saharan Africa are moderately or severely underweight, which tallies up to more than 90 million underweight under-5 children worldwide.[29]

Poverty is the underlying cause of nearly all cases of severe undernutrition in children. There are disparities in child nutritional status by country income level (**FIGURE 12-5**). There are also significant within-country differences in nutritional status. Children from lower-income households are much more likely than children from higher-income households in the same country to have serious nutritional problems (**FIGURE 12-6**).[29] Poverty creates a cycle of malnutrition and infectious disease that is hard to break. This reduction in child health and nutritional status can have long-term

community-based programs that offer RUTF and basic medical care.[22] Community-based management of acute malnutrition (CMAM) programs also provide care for children who have gained enough weight to be discharged from inpatient nutritional care but require continued monitoring.

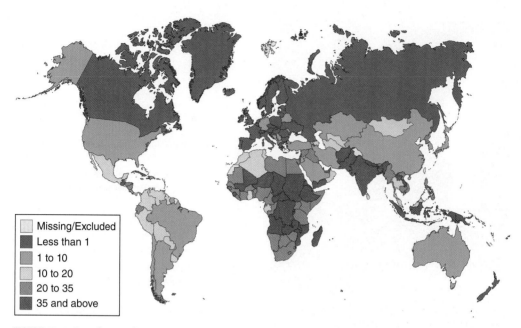

FIGURE 12–4 Prevalence of stunting in children younger than 5 years old (2005–2016).

Data from *World health statistics 2017*. Geneva: WHO; 2017.

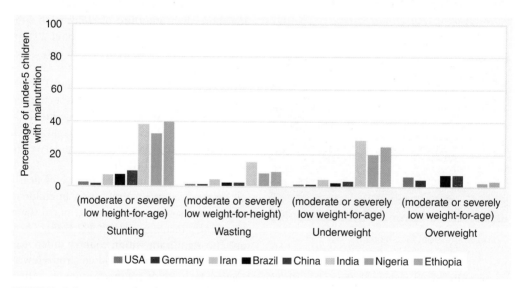

FIGURE 12–5 Percentage of under-5 children (aged 0–59 months) who are more than two standard deviations from the median of the WHO Child Growth Standards.

Data from *The state of the world's children 2016*. New York: UNICEF; 2016.

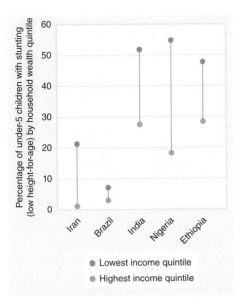

FIGURE 12-6 Children from poorer households have much higher rates of stunting than children in the same country who live in richer households.

Data from *The state of the world's children 2016.* New York: UNICEF; 2016.

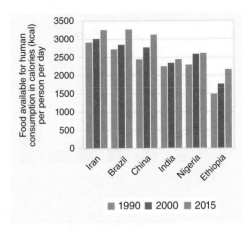

FIGURE 12-7 The number of daily food calories available for human consumption is increasing. (This figure presents the food available for human consumption after removing non-food use, such as exports, animal feed, and seed.)

Data from *FAO statistical pocketbook: World food and agriculture 2015.* Rome: FAO; 2015.

consequences. Adults who were undernourished as children tend to be shorter, less educated, less economically productive, and more likely to have low birthweight babies than adults who were not underfed in childhood.[30] Effective community-based strategies for improving child and family nutrition include promoting breastfeeding, educating about complementary feeding, providing of food supplements or conditional cash transfers to vulnerable households, and using WHO recommended case management strategies for clinically treating children with severe acute malnutrition.[31]

▶ 12.4 Food Security and Food Systems

Food security exists when the members of a household or community always have access to enough food to be healthy, active, and productive.[32] Food security is dependent on food being physically available, economically affordable,

and nutritionally valuable. The available food must also be safe to consume, culturally acceptable, and fairly allocated to individuals within households (such as ensuring that children receive adequate nutrition even when they eat from a shared dish more slowly than adults).[33] At the household level, access to food means being able to produce, purchase, or otherwise acquire an adequate quantity, quality, and variety of food during the entire year.[34] Food security is about the distribution and affordability of food as much as it is about food production.

In most countries, the number of food calories available has increased over the past few decades (**FIGURE 12-7**).[9] As access to calories increases, the prevalence of chronic undernourishment is decreasing (**FIGURE 12-8**).[9] The **Global Hunger Index (GHI)** is a metric that combines the percentage of the population that is undernourished, the percentage of children younger than 5 years old with wasting (low weight-for-height), the percentage of under-5 children with stunting (low height-for-age), and the mortality rate among under-5

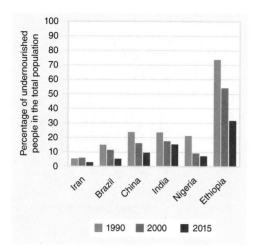

FIGURE 12–8 The percentage of the population with chronic food insecurity is decreasing.

Data from *The state of food insecurity in the world 2015.* Rome: FAO; 2015.

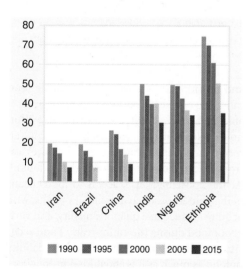

FIGURE 12–9 The Global Hunger Index has improved in most low- and middle-income countries.

Data from *2015 Global Hunger Index: Armed conflict and the challenge of hunger.* Bonn: International Food Policy Research Institute (IFPRI); 2015.

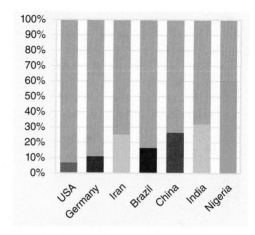

FIGURE 12–10 People in low-income countries spend a high share of their consumer expenditures on food.

Data from *Percent of consumer expenditures spent on food, alcoholic beverages, and tobacco that were consumed at home, by selected countries, 2015.* Washington: USDA Economic Research Service; 2016.

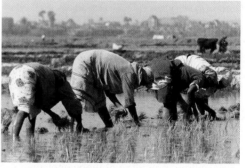

children. The GHI has improved in most low- and middle-income countries during the past 25 years (**FIGURE 12–9**).[35] However, there is still a significant burden from hunger in low-income countries, and pockets of food insecurity continue to exist in countries across the income spectrum. The risk of hunger is highest in places where food is expensive compared to incomes. The residents of lower-income countries spend a higher proportion of their incomes on food than people who live in higher-income countries (**FIGURE 12–10**).[36]

Some households and communities experience seasonal food insecurity as food stocks dwindle prior to a new harvest. Transitory food insecurity at the household level may also occur at unpredictable times due to unemployment or illness, or at the community or national level due to economic shocks or natural disasters. Members of food insecure households may report feeling hungry but not eating, worrying that their food will run out, running out of food and not having enough money to buy more, eating only a limited variety of low-cost foods, cutting the size of meals, skipping meals, and not eating for a whole day.[37] Sometimes, chronic food insecurity lasts for years, and widespread food insecurity may spiral into humanitarian catastrophes. No matter what the proximal cause is, most food insecurity is the result of chronic poverty. Poverty is both a cause of food insecurity and an outcome of it. Chronically undernourished people lack the strength and stamina to be productive, which further exacerbates the poverty that likely led to the initial food insecurity.[38]

During times of widespread hunger or **famine**, a large proportion of a population has very low food security for an extended period of time, often leading to mass migration and death.[39] Famines are partially attributable to demographics (such as population growth) and environmental factors (such as drought), but they are largely the result of economic and political dysfunction. Food shortages may occur because of reduced food production, but they also happen because of increased food prices and interruptions in the supply chain that transports food from producers to consumers. To quote Amartya Sen, a Nobel Prize winning economist from India, "starvation is a matter of some people not having enough food to eat, and not a matter of there being not enough food to eat."[40]

The **food system** encompasses the entire process of growing or producing food, processing and packaging food, distributing and selling food (which may require transportation and storage), and preparing and consuming food. SDG 2 emphasizes that the ability of people to have food security is dependent on healthy food systems. The overall goal is to "end hunger, achieve food security and improved nutrition, and promote sustainable agriculture," and the pathways toward ending hunger (SDG 2.1) and undernutrition (SDG 2.2) include increasing the agricultural productivity of small-scale food producers (SDG 2.3) and ensuring that food production systems

are sustainable and preserve ecosystem health (SDG 2.4).[3] A disruption in any of part of the food system may cause food insecurity.

As the world population increases and available croplands shrink, crop yields will have to increase to meet the growing demand for food. The best way to ensure that everyone is food secure is to increase food production while also increasing environmental protection.[41] This means developing new agricultural techniques or choosing to use time-tested techniques such as crop rotation that cause as little damage to the environment as possible and also increase yields.[42] Food supplies can be further maximized when as little food as possible is wasted, eaten by animals, or allowed to spoil during transportation and storage. Food distribution systems need to be strengthened so that those who are unable to produce enough food for their families have access to the surplus food produced by others. Additionally, trade policies that make it attractive for growers to produce crops for local consumption rather than export may help alleviate hunger.[43]

▶ 12.5 Micronutrients

Micronutrients are nutrients that the body requires in small amounts, and they include both vitamins and minerals. **Vitamins** are organic compounds that typically cannot be synthesized by the body. The B vitamins and vitamin C are water-soluble vitamins that are necessary for regulation of energy use and for critical cellular functions. These **water-soluble vitamins** are easily dissolved in the body but are not able to be stored in body tissues. They must be consumed daily for maximum health, and any excess amounts ingested in a day are excreted in the urine. Other vitamins are **fat-soluble vitamins** that are stored in body tissues. The fat-soluble vitamins (vitamins A, D, E, and K) contribute to bone health, vision, and other important body functions. People with too little fat in their diets or who have disorders that limit fat absorption from the intestines may have deficiencies of fat-soluble vitamins. People who consume too many fat-soluble vitamins, usually by overdosing on supplements, may accumulate elevated levels of these vitamins in their bodies.

Minerals are inorganic chemical elements. Macrominerals (also called major minerals) are needed in relatively large quantities. Trace minerals are required in very small amounts. As with any nutrient, either a deficiency or an excess of minerals can be harmful. Some people develop problems by overdosing on supplements. Others add too much salt to their foods, and excess sodium can increase the risk of high blood pressure in some adults.[44]

About 30 vitamins and minerals have been identified as essential components of the human diet (**FIGURE 12–11**). The best way to consume micronutrients is through food. When a person's diet does not provide enough nutrients or the body is not absorbing enough of the nutrients, nonfood sources may be helpful. One option is **supplementation** by taking a pill, tablet, or capsule that delivers one or several micronutrients. Another option is to add extra micronutrients to foods. **Enrichment** is the process of adding nutrients lost during handling, processing, or storage back to food products. **Fortification** is the process of adding micronutrients not

Vitamins		Minerals	
Water-Soluble Vitamins	**Fat-Soluble Vitamins**	**Macrominerals**	**Trace Minerals**
Thiamine (vitamin B_1)	Vitamin A (retinol, beta-carotene)	Calcium	Chromium
Riboflavin (vitamin B_2)	Vitamin D (cholecalciferol)	Chloride	Copper
Niacin (vitamin B_3)	Vitamin E (tocopherol)	Magnesium	Fluoride
Pantothenic acid (vitamin B_5)	Vitamin K	Phosphorus	Iodine
Pyridoxine (vitamin B_6)		Potassium	Iron
Biotin (vitamin B_7)		Sodium	Manganese
Folate (vitamin B_9, folic acid)		Sulfur	Molybdenum
Cobalamin (vitamin B_{12})			Selenium
Vitamin C (ascorbic acid)			Zinc

FIGURE 12–11 Essential vitamins and minerals.

naturally present in a food's ingredients to a food product. Common examples of enriched and fortified foods include vitamin A fortified sugar, vitamin D fortified milk, folic acid and iron-enriched flours, and iodized salt.[45] However, supplements and enriched and fortified foods may not provide vitamins and minerals in a form that has a high bioavailability. **Bioavailability** is the proportion of the nutrient consumed that is able to be absorbed and used by the body. Absorption can be increased by taking supplements with food.[46] For example, fat-soluble vitamins work best when taken with fat or oil, and iron absorption is boosted by vitamin C.

Vitamin and mineral deficiencies are a common form of undernutrition in both children and adults. Micronutrient deficiencies are sometimes called "hidden hunger" because they may not cause obvious symptoms but they do contribute to diminished health status.[47] A large proportion of the world's population is at risk of iodine, vitamin A, iron, zinc, and other deficiencies.[48] Most people with severe micronutrient deficiencies live in lower-income countries, but there are also pockets of micronutrient deficiencies in some high-income populations because of dietary habits. Providing pregnant women with supplemental iron, folate, iodine, and calcium significantly improves birth outcomes.[31] Ensuring that children receive adequate intake of iodine, iron, vitamin A, and zinc significantly improves child survival.[31]

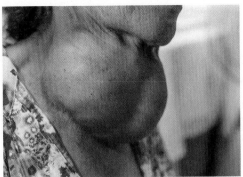

Goiter.

▶ 12.6 Iodine Deficiency Disorders

Iodine is an element that is critical for regulating **metabolism**, the rate at which a person's body uses energy. The thyroid gland, located in the neck, uses iodine to create thyroid hormones, which are the chemical messengers that control the body's metabolism. If there is too little iodine in the diet, there is not enough iodine in the blood for the thyroid gland to function properly. In response, the thyroid gland will enlarge as it tries to collect more iodine from the blood, and it will produce a **goiter**, a swollen neck resulting from an enlarged thyroid gland. A person with hypothyroidism who cannot produce enough thyroid hormones will have a low metabolism and will feel cold, tired, and apathetic. Babies born to mothers who have hypothyroidism may be stillborn or be born with **cretinism**, which is characterized by brain damage and stunted growth caused by a lack of maternal iodine during fetal development. Even relatively minor iodine deficiencies may cause impaired mental function in children and adults.[49] **Iodine deficiency disorders** (IDD) are among the most common causes of impaired cognitive function in the world.[50] About 30% of the world's population is estimated to have insufficient iodine intake.[51] Iodized salt is a cost-efficient way to reduce IDD, but only about two-thirds of the world's population uses it, and commercial salt may not reach the neediest households.[52]

▶ 12.7 Vitamin A Deficiency

Vitamin A is a fat-soluble vitamin that is critical for growth and vision. Vitamin A from animal sources is in the form of retinol, and plant-based vitamin A is in the form of beta-carotene. **Vitamin A deficiency** (VAD) is a major cause of preventable blindness in children. VAD initially causes **xerophthalmia**, a severe dryness of the eye. The first symptom of advanced VAD is night blindness. Untreated VAD can progress from the formation of Bitot's spots (dry patches on the conjunctiva, the whites of the eyes) to the ulceration and scarring of the cornea (keratomalacia). VAD also increases the risk of death from infectious diseases, especially measles and diarrhea.

The global prevalence of VAD has decreased significantly in recent years, but VAD remains one of the most common causes of preventable blindness in young children.[53] About 30% of the children aged 6–59 months who live in low- and middle-income countries are vitamin A deficient, with the highest burden in sub-Saharan Africa and South Asia.[54] These children are at risk of night blindness and other complications of xerophthalmia. Many pregnant women in very low-income countries are also severely vitamin A deficient, and a high proportion of pregnant women with VAD have night blindness.[55]

Yellow, orange, and dark green vegetables are the best dietary sources of vitamin A, in addition to some animal sources, such as liver. Because vitamin A is fat soluble and will only be absorbed by the body if it is eaten with fats or oils, dietary prevention of VAD requires a consistent source of both vegetables and oil. In some countries, milk, sugar, or other commercial products are fortified with vitamin A, but fortified foods are not available to all households that need them. Some genetically modified food products that are high in vitamin A are in development, but they are not yet widely available.[56] Oil-filled vitamin A capsule supplements are relatively inexpensive and have prevented hundreds of thousands of child deaths and many cases of blindness, but distribution can be a challenge and the benefits of the capsules only last for a few months, so frequent redistribution must occur.[57]

▶ 12.8 Iron Deficiency Anemia

Iron is a mineral that the body uses to make the red blood cells (RBCs) that carry oxygen from the lungs to the rest of the cells in the body. **Hemoglobin** is a molecule made from iron that holds the oxygen inside the RBCs. A person with too little iron is not able to make enough RBCs to efficiently transport oxygen. Symptoms of **anemia**, a deficiency of RBCs or hemoglobin, include pale skin, fatigue, weakness, shortness of breath, headaches, an increased heart rate, and a limited ability to concentrate at work or school. Anemia resulting from inadequate iron intake is called **iron deficiency anemia** (IDA).[58] Anemia may be caused by vitamin B$_{12}$ or folic acid deficiency, blood loss, inadequate production of RBCs, and infections that destroy RBCs, but IDA is by far the most common cause of anemia worldwide.[59] Children, pregnant women, and women who menstruate are at high risk for IDA.[60] Children need extra iron as their body grows and their blood volume increases. Pregnant women need extra iron as their blood volume expands and to reduce the risk of dying during childbirth. Menstruating women and women who have recently given birth may have depleted RBCs and iron from blood loss.

In total, more than 2 billion people worldwide have IDA, including more than 75 million people with severe anemia.[61] The prevalence of mild, moderate, and severe anemia has decreased in recent decades from an overall prevalence of about 40% in 1990 to 33% in 2010 (**FIGURE 12–12**).[61] However, even with those improvements, almost 50% of children, 40% of pregnant women, and 30% of nonpregnant women are anemic.[62] The public health burden from anemia in children (**FIGURE 12–13**) and women (**FIGURE 12–14**) tends to be mild in high-income countries, moderate in middle-income countries, and severe in low-income countries.[63]

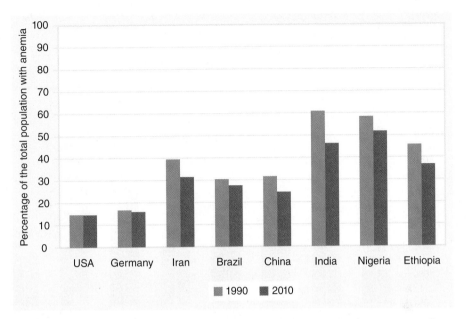

FIGURE 12–12 The percentage of the total population with anemia has decreased in many countries.

Data from Kassebaum NJ, Jasrasaria R, Naghavi M, Wulf SK, Johns N, Lozano R, Ragan M, Weatherall D, Chou DP, Eisele TP, Flaxman SR, Pullan RL, Brooker SJ, Murray CJL. A systematic analysis of global anemia burden from 1990 to 2010. *Blood* 2014; 123:615–24.

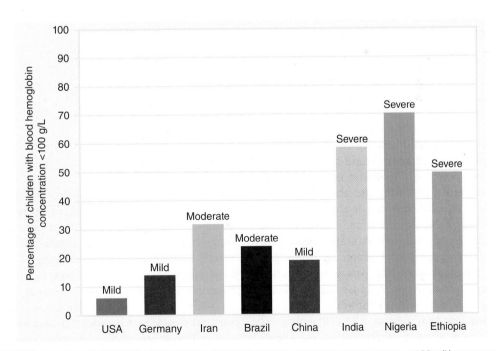

FIGURE 12–13 Anemia in children aged 6–59 months (blood hemoglobin concentration <100 g/L).

Data from *The global prevalence of anaemia in 2011*. Geneva: WHO; 2015.

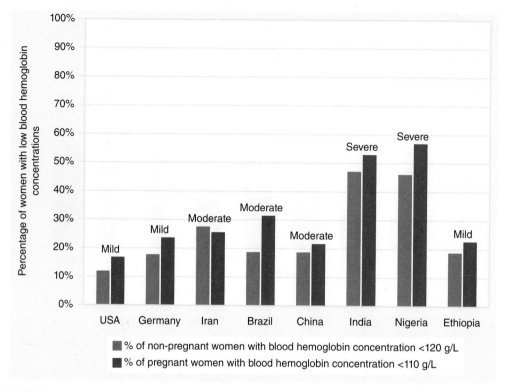

FIGURE 12-14 Anemia in women aged 15–49 years, by pregnancy status.
Data from *The global prevalence of anaemia in 2011*. Geneva: WHO; 2015.

The burden from IDA is highest in South Asia and sub-Saharan Africa.[62]

IDA can be prevented and treated by increasing iron intake. Iron is present in both plant and animal food sources. Heme iron is found in blood and meat from animals, birds, and fish, and about 15%–35% of consumed heme iron is absorbed by the body. Nonheme iron is found in plants, eggs, and milk, and less than 5% is absorbed.[64] Iron can also be taken as a supplement or added to fortified foods like pastas and flours.[65] Treating infections that cause internal bleeding (like hookworm, whipworm, and schistosomiasis) and destroy RBCs (like malaria) is also important for preventing and alleviating IDA.

▶ **12.9 Other Micronutrient Deficiencies**

A serious deficiency of any vitamin or mineral can cause significant impairment of a person's health status. For example, the B vitamins are critical for metabolism, and people with B vitamin deficiencies tend to lack energy. Each B vitamin plays a unique role in body function. **Thiamine** is a B vitamin that is necessary for nerve function. Thiamine deficiency is called **beriberi**. People with beriberi may have weakness and heart arrhythmias that can progress to heart failure.[66] **Riboflavin** is a B vitamin that contributes to skin and eye health. People with riboflavin deficiency often have sores at the corner of the mouth (called angular stomatitis), cracked lips, mouth and throat sores, and scaly skin.[67] **Niacin** is a B vitamin that is necessary for skin health and for digestive and nervous system function. Niacin deficiency is called **pellagra**. They key symptoms of pellagra include diarrhea, dementia, and a type of dermatitis in which the skin become scaly, darkens, and sloughs off the body.[68] Deficiencies of pantothenic acid, pyridoxine, biotin, and cobalamin can also cause serious health problems.

Folate is a B vitamin that is critical for growth, red blood cell production, and fetal development. The vitamin must be ingested daily because the chemical is not able to be stored by the body. Folate is naturally found in foods like liver and spinach. **Folic acid** is a synthetic form of folate that can be added to foods or supplements. Women of child-bearing age need to make sure that they have an adequate daily intake of folic acid because deficiency during the first weeks of pregnancy is associated with neural tube defects in developing fetuses.[69] The most common neural tube defects are anencephaly, a fatal condition in which the brain fails to develop, and spina bifida, in which the spinal cord does not develop properly. These defects occur very early in the pregnancy, usually before a woman knows she is pregnant, so it is recommended that all women who might become pregnant take a multivitamin.

Vitamin C is essential for collagen formation and iron absorption, and it is also involved in immune system function as well as being an antioxidant that reduces the free radicals in cells that may damage cell membranes. People with vitamin C deficiency develop **scurvy** that is characterized by bleeding gums, loose teeth, joint pain, and decreased immune system function.[70] Vitamin E is an antioxidant. Prematurely-born infants with vitamin E deficiency are at risk of hemolytic anemia.[71]

Vitamin K is critical for blood clotting. People who are vitamin K deficient may suffer from bleeding disorders.[72]

Calcium is a mineral used by the body for strengthening bones and teeth. It also plays critical roles in muscle and nerve function. Adolescents who consume too little calcium are at risk for developing osteoporosis as they age, and porous bones can lead to hip fractures and other life-threatening injuries later in life. **Vitamin D** is also necessary for bone health because it assists the body with calcium absorption. Vitamin D deficiency in children whose bones are still growing is called **rickets** or, more informally, "knock knees." Vitamin D deficiency in adults whose bones have stopped growing is called **osteomalacia** and can cause the bones to become soft and prone to breaking. Vitamin D, the "sun vitamin," can be made in the skin if the skin is exposed to sunlight for about 15 minutes daily, but adequate sun exposure is not always possible.[73] Vitamin D deficiency is a common problem among people who work indoors all day and avoid sun exposure, in places where women are expected to cover themselves in public, and seasonally among people who live far from the equator and experience several months of darkness and extreme cold each year.[74] Vitamin D deficiency is also common in older adults.[75]

Fluoride is a mineral that is essential for the development of strong teeth and bones. Increased availability of fluoride has dramatically improved dental health in high-income countries where fluoride is routinely added to toothpaste and many communities add small amounts of fluoride to drinking water as a public health measure to reduce the incidence of dental caries (cavities).[76] However, these tools for health are usually not available in lower-income countries.[77] Dental health is optimized by a level of fluoride exposure that is neither deficient nor excessive. Fluoride doses in toothpaste and water are intended to be the minimum concentration that improves health outcomes. High concentrations of fluoride are avoided because excess fluoride (fluorosis) can cause the teeth to stain and become pitted and weak when fluoride replaces some of the calcium in the teeth.

Zinc is a mineral that is important for immune function, growth, and child development. Any level of zinc deficiency can increase susceptibility to infection, slow wound healing, and increase the risk of death from diarrhea, malaria, and pneumonia. Zinc is found primarily in animal sources, so people who consume a mostly plant-based diet often benefit from taking zinc supplements or eating food fortified with zinc.[78] Zinc supplementation is especially effective as a public health intervention when it is provided to children suffering from diarrhea and other infections.[79] Many thousands of child deaths from these infections could be averted each year by reducing zinc deficiency in Africa and Asia.[80]

Deficiencies in other minerals can also impair growth, health, and healing.[81] Magnesium and phosphorus are required for maintaining skeletal health. Chloride, potassium, and sodium are all important for maintaining fluid balance within the body, and deficiencies can lead to fatigue, weakness, and serious complications related to electrolyte imbalances. Sulfur plays a role in stabilizing proteins. Chromium contributes to glucose tolerance. Copper is necessary for red blood cell production, so copper deficiency causes anemia. Manganese, molybdenum, and selenium all contribute to cell functioning.

▶ 12.10 Breastfeeding

Breastmilk contains all of the nutrients and water babies need, and it also includes digestive enzymes as well as antibodies and other immune factors that protect against harmful infections and promote health.[82] Many cases of undernutrition in infants and young children could be prevented by a simple set of nutritional interventions that include having infants consume only breastmilk during their first 6 months of life and then continuing to be nourished by breastmilk after solid foods are introduced into the infant's diet.[15]

New mothers should be encouraged to breastfeed their babies so that nutrients and disease-fighting antibodies will be delivered to them. **Colostrum**, the milk produced in the first days after giving birth, is especially beneficial because it contains large quantities of proteins and antibodies that stimulate the newborn's immune system development.[83] **Early breastfeeding**, breastfeeding within the first hours after giving birth, increases the neonatal survival rate.[84] In ideal circumstances, infants should be exclusively breastfed for the first 6 months of life. **Exclusive breastfeeding** means that breastmilk is the only substance the baby consumes, and that no supplemental water, juice, cow or goat milk, porridge, rice water, or any other foods are fed to the baby. After 6 months of exclusive breastfeeding, **complementary foods** should be introduced into the infant's diet while continuing breastfeeding until the baby's second birthday or later (**FIGURE 12–15**).[85] "Complementary" means that the foods accompany breastmilk and do not immediately replace it.[86] In 2015, less than half of newborns worldwide received breastmilk within 1 hour after birth (**FIGURE 12–16**), and less than 40% of infants younger than 6 months old were exclusively breastfed (**FIGURE 12–17**).[29] This low percentage contributes to illness and death from undernutrition and diarrhea.

Not all women are able to exclusively breastfeed. Some mothers do not produce

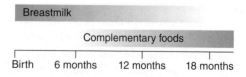

FIGURE 12–15 Global nutrition standards recommend exclusive breastfeeding for 6 months followed by the introduction of complementary foods with continued breastfeeding.

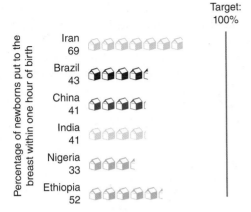

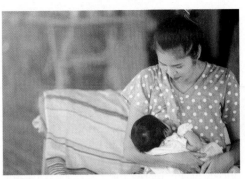

FIGURE 12–16 Early initiation of breastfeeding is low in low- and middle-income countries.

Data from *The state of the world's children 2016.* New York: UNICEF; 2016.

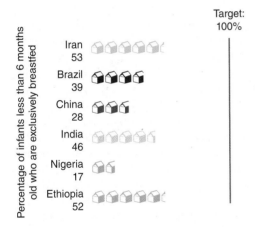

FIGURE 12–17 Few infants are exclusively breastfed in low- and middle-income countries.

Data from *The state of the world's children 2016.* New York: UNICEF; 2016.

adequate milk for their babies and have to supplement with formula at an early age. Some have HIV infection and do not want to risk passing the virus to their babies through breastmilk. Some have work schedules that do not allow them to feed their babies every few hours. Newborns whose mothers have died in childbirth are also not able to be breastfed by their biological mothers. Breastmilk substitutes for infants must provide hydration plus all of the essential nutrients. Commercial infant formula is usually the best substitute for breastmilk because cow's milk, tea, rice water, and other substitutes do not provide all the nutrients of breastmilk or infant formula. However, using infant formula can be a challenge for mothers and families who lack access to clean water, have difficulties reading and following the mixing instructions, or have limited incomes to pay for commercial products.

Additional concerns about the use of formula in lower-income countries stem from the marketing strategies used by Nestlé and other infant formula companies in the 1970s.[87] Hospital maternity wards in some developing countries were sponsored by formula companies, and new mothers would be sent home with formula samples and no breastfeeding education. New mothers who do not breastfeed will quickly lose the ability to produce milk and must then rely on breastmilk substitutes, so providing a limited amount of free formula may create a dependency on the product. Worse, some companies hired "milk nurses" to go into communities in nursing uniforms and advertise formula, implying that formula was better than breastmilk. In 1981, the World Health Assembly addressed these problematic marketing practices with their adoption of the **International Code of Marketing of Breast-milk Substitutes**. The Code stresses that breastmilk is the best option for feeding babies, and it requires new mothers who are given information about the use of infant formula to be informed about financial and health costs of formula adoption. The Code stipulates that marketing personnel should not directly contact pregnant women or new mothers, even if those salespeople are healthcare professionals; that health facilities should not promote formula use; and that samples of formula should not be distributed at hospitals or by retailers. Many of the major international formula producers have adopted the International Code of Marketing of Breast-milk Substitutes and no longer directly market to pregnant women or new mothers, but few countries have enacted laws that enforce the entire Code. For example, as of 2015, Brazil and India had fully implemented the Code, Iran and Nigeria had implemented many of the provisions, Germany and China had implemented only a few parts of the Code, and the United States and Ethiopia had enacted no legal measures based on the Code.[88]

Mothers need to be provided with the information to make an informed choice about whether to breastfeed and how long to breastfeed. Attitudes toward breastfeeding also need to be addressed because breastfeeding is discouraged in many cultures. Employers rarely have a private room available for mothers who would like to use a breast pump. Women are not always free to breastfeed in public areas, even the "public" areas of their own homes. New grandmothers who bottle fed their own babies may discourage their daughters from choosing breastfeeding. The advice that "breast is best" needs to be accompanied by conditions that support breastfeeding,[89] especially in places where breastfeeding is not the cultural norm.

▶ 12.11 Overweight and Obesity

Overnutrition is a form of malnutrition caused by excessive intake of calories and nutrients. A person who consistently takes in more calories than the body uses will gain weight, become overweight, and then develop obesity. Overweight and obesity are usually classified based on the **body mass index (BMI)**, a measure of body composition calculated by taking weight in kilograms and dividing it by the square of the person's height in meters.

$$BMI = \frac{Weight\ (kg)}{Height\ (m) \times Height\ (m)} = 703 \times \frac{Weight\ (lb)}{Height\ (in.) \times Height\ (in.)}$$

International classifications generally suggest that for adults a BMI of less than 18.5 indicates underweight, a BMI of 25–29.9 indicates **overweight**, and a BMI of 30 or greater indicates **obesity**.[90] For children and adolescents, BMI percentiles by age group are typically used to identify children who are overweight.[91] Additional anthropometric measures can complement the BMI by providing further information about health risks. For example, having a waist circumference greater than 35 inches for a woman or 40 inches for a man is associated with an increased risk of diabetes and heart disease.[92] The BMI and other anthropometric measurements have several limitations as a measure of health status.[93] The BMI does not adjust for the body fat percentage, so people who are trim but have a lot of muscle mass may be incorrectly classified as overweight. The BMI also does not measure physical fitness levels, and people with any BMI who have poor cardiovascular endurance are at risk of a diversity of adverse health outcomes. However, scientific studies consistently find that obesity is associated with an increased risk for many diseases, including type 2 diabetes, hypertension (high blood pressure), heart disease, strokes, gallstones and other digestive disorders, back pain, arthritis of the back and hip, and several types of cancer.[94]

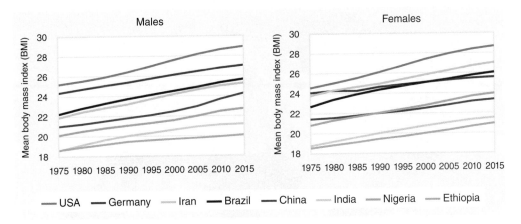

FIGURE 12-18 The average adult BMI is steadily increasing in most countries.

Data from NCD Risk Factor Collaboration (NCD-RisC). Trends in adult body-mass index in 200 countries from 1975 to 2014: A pooled analysis of 1698 population-based measurement studies with 19.2 million participants. *Lancet* 2016;387:1377–96.

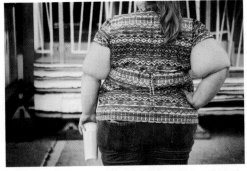

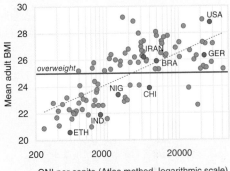

FIGURE 12-19 Higher gross national income per capita is associated with higher average adult body mass index (BMI). (The dots represent the 100 most populous countries. Note the use of the logarithmic scale on the x-axis.)

Data from *Global status report on noncommunicable diseases* 2014. Geneva: World Health Organization; 2014.

Over the past 25 years, most countries have had steady increases in adult BMIs (**FIGURE 12-18**).[95] The global prevalence of overweight and obesity among adults increased from about 29% in 1980 to about 39% in 2015.[96] By 2015, 10% of the world's people were obese.[97] Countries with higher average incomes tend to have higher average adult BMIs (**FIGURE 12-19**), but obesity is becoming a public health concern in nearly every region of the world (**FIGURE 12-20**). In many high-income countries and a growing number of middle-income countries, the average BMI among adults is greater than 25 (**FIGURE 12-21**), and the majority of adults are overweight or obese (**FIGURE 12-22**).[95] Overweight and obesity are also becoming common among children and adolescents (**FIGURE 12-23**).[96] In many countries, the rate of obesity doubled between 1990 and 2015 in both adult (**FIGURE 12-24**) and pediatric populations (**FIGURE 12-25**).[97]

Nutritional status is a function of biology and also of psychology and sociology.

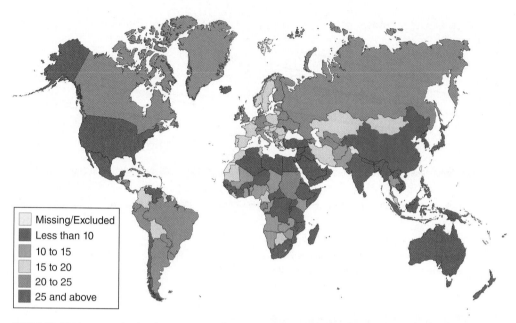

FIGURE 12–20 Age-standardized percentage of adults (aged 20+ years) who are obese (BMI ≥30) (2015).

Data from GBD 2015 Obesity Collaborators. Health effects of overweight and obesity in 195 countries over 25 years. *N Engl J Med* 2017; 377:13–27.

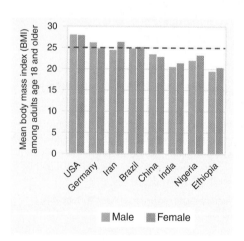

FIGURE 12–21 In some countries, the typical adult BMI as above the BMI>25 threshold for being classified as overweight or obese (2015).

Data from NCD Risk Factor Collaboration (NCD-RisC). Trends in adult body-mass index in 200 countries from 1975 to 2014: A pooled analysis of 1698 population-based measurement studies with 19.2 million participants. *Lancet* 2016; 387:1377–96.

Genetic changes do not explain why obesity has become so much more prevalent in recent decades. Genes influence metabolic rate, body shape (where a person carries excess weight), and the efficiency of the body at storing extra calories, but it takes generations for genetic adaptations to occur. By contrast, it takes only a short time to change dietary and exercise habits. The transition toward overnutrition as the dominant global nutrition concern is primarily a function of the dietary changes commonly associated with economic development.[98] These new practices often include increased portion sizes, more snacking, more meals eaten outside the home, replacing water with sweetened beverages, eating more animal protein, cooking with more oil, adding more sweeteners to the diet, and shifting from consuming whole grains to refined grains.[5]

The nutrition transition is also related to a variety of globalization processes, including

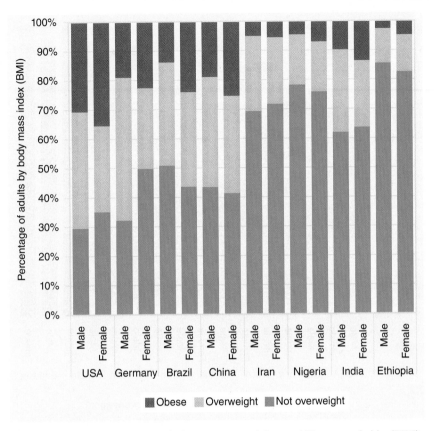

FIGURE 12-22 Prevalence of overweight and obesity among adults aged 20 years and older (2015).

Data from GBD 2015 Obesity Collaborators. Health effects of overweight and obesity in 195 countries over 25 years. *N Engl J Med* 2017; 377:13–27.

urbanization, new technologies, global media, and international transportation and trade. Besides having an impact on social and cultural eating behaviors, globalization influences cultural perceptions of physical beauty.[99] When the painters of the European Renaissance wanted to show beautiful, powerful women, they portrayed women with rolls of fat and rounded curves. In some cultures today, larger women are still seen as having ideal body shapes and greater weight is associated with perceived fertility. When resources are scarce, having greater weight is often a sign of wealth because it shows that the household has more than enough calories and does not have to expend so many of them

in physical labor. On the other hand, the women who model on the fashion runways in Paris and Milan and those who are Hollywood stars tend to be extremely skinny. In industrialized societies, being underweight is often an indication of wealth because richer households have the time and money to prepare healthy foods and exercise while working-class households rely on cheap fast foods and work long hours at jobs that are often sedentary.

Individuals and families seeking to reach and maintain target weights must adopt and sustain healthy behaviors. At the population level, policies that promote healthy diets and physical activity may help prevent and reduce

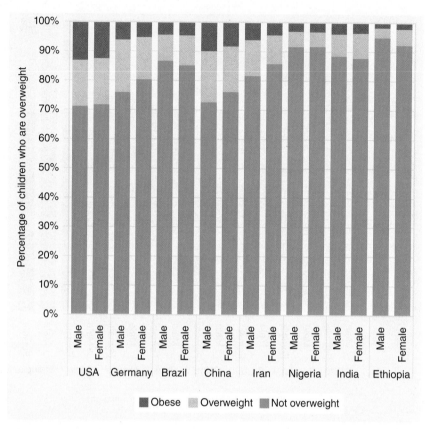

FIGURE 12–23 Prevalence of overweight and obesity in the pediatric population (aged 2–19 years) (2015).
Data from GBD 2015 Obesity Collaborators. Health effects of overweight and obesity in 195 countries over 25 years. *N Engl J Med* 2017; 377:13–27.

obesity. These may include health information campaigns, limits on the marketing of unhealthy food to children, taxes to increase the price of unhealthy foods, subsidies to lower the cost of healthy foods, and regulations that improve the nutrition information provided on food packages.[100]

▶ 12.12 Food Safety

The globalization of food systems is evident in changing eating habits, the increasing variety of foods on grocery store shelves, the growing number of international restaurant chains, and the global marketing of food products. International food markets have grown significantly in recent decades. For example, the proportion of food consumed in the United States that is imported increased from 12% in 1990 to nearly 20% 25 years later (**FIGURE 12–26**).[101] This increased cross-border trade in foods has created a new set of concerns about food safety.[102] Because these threats can only be addressed through international agreements, food safety has become a global health issue.

More than 2 billion cases of foodborne diseases and intoxications occur every year, and foodborne infectious diseases cause more than 1 million deaths each year.[103] A wide variety of foods have been implicated in outbreaks, including fruits and vegetables, meats and poultry, eggs, seafood, dairy products, bakery

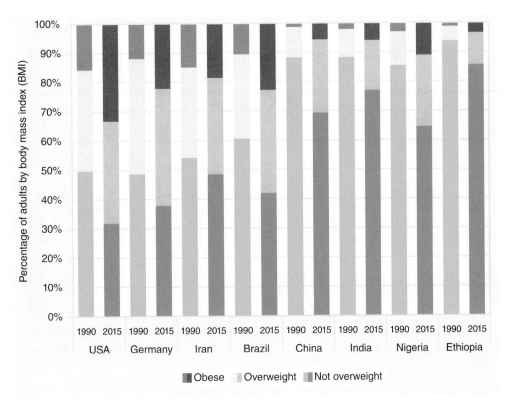

FIGURE 12–24 The prevalence of overweight and obesity among adults aged 20 years and older is increasing.
Data from GBD 2015 Obesity Collaborators. Health effects of overweight and obesity in 195 countries over 25 years. *N Engl J Med* 2017; 377:13–27.

items, and unpasteurized fruit juices.[104] The major causes of foodborne illness and death include norovirus, *E. coli*, *Salmonella*, *Campylobacter*, and hepatitis A virus.[105] In addition to microbial contamination, chemical contaminants are increasing threats to health.[106] Concerns have been raised about heavy metal poisoning from mercury in fish, pesticide residues, chemical additives and preservatives, and other substances.[107] Most outbreaks of foodborne diseases are caused by locally grown and processed foods, because most foods consumed around the world are still ones that were produced in the home countries of the people eating them, but an increasing number of large multinational foodborne outbreaks are being reported.[108]

Several simple food safety practices can help protect consumers at home and in restaurants, including careful cleaning, separation of uncooked and ready-to-eat foods, and keeping foods at appropriate temperatures.[109] However, food preparers have limited ability to combat some types of food contamination. Food producers, processors, distributors, and consumers all have a role to play in ensuring that foods remain safe along the supply chain. The **Codex Alimentarius** international food standards, which are compiled by scientific panels hosted by the United Nations, provide specific guidelines for keeping food products safe.[110] For example, **pasteurization**, a process of heating foods to kill the bacteria that might otherwise be present in milk, dairy and egg products, beer, fruit juices, and other products, is recommended for some food items. The hazard analysis and critical control point (HACCP) system is an approach to food

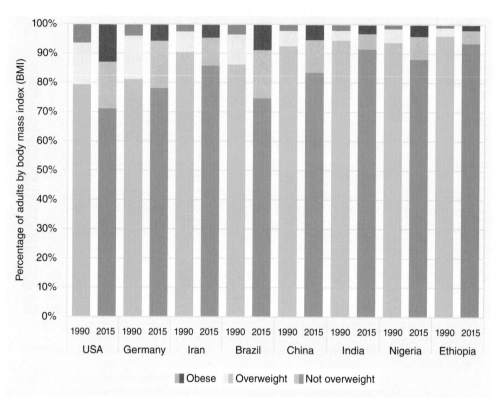

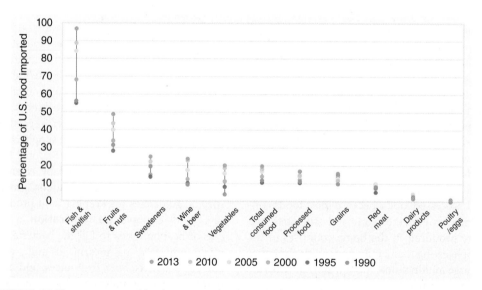

FIGURE 12–26 The percentage of foods consumed in the United States that are imported increased between 1990 and 2015.

Data from Jerardo A. Table 1: Import share of U.S. food consumption. *Import share of consumption.* Washington: USDA Economic Research Service; 2016.

safety that has been widely adopted by commercial food processors and distributors.[111] However, the Codex is not binding on countries or food producers, and the standards can be difficult to enforce.[112] Additionally, labeling requirements are not standardized across markets, and countries have different expectations about the use of additives and preservatives, fortification and enrichment with vitamins and minerals, and the use and labeling of genetically modified organisms (GMOs). As the food industry becomes increasingly global, it may become more difficult for governments and consumers to have confidence that their food supply is safe.

▶ **References**

1. *Global nutrition report 2016: From promise to impact: Ending malnutrition by 2030*. Washington DC: International Food Policy Research Institute (IFPRI); 2016.

2. Barrett BD, Maxwell DG. *Food aid after fifty years: Recasting its role*. New York: Routledge; 2005.

3. *The Sustainable Development Goals report 2016*. New York: United Nations; 2016.

4. Jonsson U. Nutrition and the convention on the rights of the child. *Food Policy*. 1996;21:41–55.

5. Popkin BM. Global nutrition dynamics: The world is shifting rapidly toward a diet linked with noncommunicable diseases. *Am J Clin Nutr*. 2006;84:289–98.

6. Popkin BM, Adair LS, Ng SW. The global nutrition transition: The pandemic of obesity in developing countries. *Nutr Rev*. 2012;70:3–21.

7. *2015–2020 dietary guidelines for Americans (8th edition)*. Table A7-1. Washington DC: U.S. Departments of Health and Human Services (HHS) and Agriculture (USDA); 2015.

8. *FAOSTAT food balance sheets 2013*. Rome: FAO; 2015.

9. *FAO statistical pocketbook: World food and agriculture 2015*. Rome: FAO; 2015.

10. Hu FB, Willett WC. Optimal diets for prevention of coronary heart disease. *JAMA*. 2002;288:2569–78.

11. Mensink RP, Zock PL, Kester AD, Katan MB. Effects of dietary fatty acids and carbohydrates on the ratio of serum total to HDL cholesterol and on serum lipids and apolipoproteins: A meta-analysis of 60 controlled trials. *Am J Clin Nutr*. 2003;77:1146–55.

12. Popkin BM, D'Anci KE, Rosenberg IH. Water, hydration and health. *Nutr Rev*. 2010;68:439–58.

13. Caulfield LE, de Onis M, Blössner M, Black RE. Undernutrition as an underlying cause of child deaths associated with diarrhea, pneumonia, malaria, and measles. *Am J Clin Nut*. 2004;80:193–8.

14. *Global health risks: Mortality and burden of disease attributable to selected major risks*. Geneva: WHO; 2009.

15. Black RE, Allen LH, Bhutta ZA, et al. Maternal and child undernutrition: Global and regional exposures and health consequences. *Lancet*. 2008; 371:243–60.

16. United Nations. *Transforming our world: The 2030 Agenda for Sustainable Development*. New York: UN; 2015.

17. Stevens GA, Finucane MM, Paciorek CJ. Levels and trends in low height-for-age (Chapter 5). *Disease control priorities*. 3rd ed. *Reproductive, maternal, newborn, and child health (Volume 2)*. Washington DC: IBRD/World Bank; 2016.

18. *Global nutrition targets 2025: Policy brief series*. Geneva: WHO; 2014.

19. WHO Child Growth Standards. *Length/height-for-age, weight-for-age, weight-for-length, weight-for-height and body mass index-for-age: Methods and development*. Geneva: WHO; 2006.

20. Onyango AW, de Onis M, Caroli M, et al. Field-testing the WHO Child Growth Standards in four countries. *J Nutr*. 2007;137:149–52.

21. Collins S, Dent N, Binns P, Bahwere P, Sadler K, Hallam A. Management of severe acute malnutrition in children. *Lancet*. 2006;368:1992–2000.

22. *WHO child growth standards and the identification of severe acute malnutrition in infants and children: A joint statement by the World Health Organization and the United Nations Children's Fund*. Geneva/New York: WHO/UNICEF; 2009.

23. WHO Multicentre Growth Reference Study Group. *WHO child growth standards: Length/height-for-age, weight-for-age, weight-for-length, weight-for-height and body mass index-for-age: Methods and development*. Geneva: WHO; 2006.

24. Grover Z, Ee LC. Protein energy malnutrition. *Pediatr Clin North Am*. 2009;56:1055–68.

25. Lenters L, Wazny K, Bhutta ZA. Management of severe and moderate acute malnutrition in children (Chapter 11). *Disease control priorities*. 3rd edition. *Reproductive, maternal, newborn, and child health (Volume 2)*. Washington DC: IBRD/World Bank; 2016.

26. Waterlow JC. Classification and definition of protein-calorie malnutrition. *Br Med J*. 1972;3:566–9.

27. *Guideline: Updates on the management of severe acute malnutrition in infants and children*. Geneva: WHO; 2013.

28. Brown KH, Nyirandutiye DH, Jungjohann S. Management of children with acute malnutrition in resource-poor settings. *Nat Rev Endocrinol*. 2009;5:597–603.

29. *The state of the world's children 2016.* New York: UNICEF; 2016.

30. Victora CG, Adair L, Fall C, et al. Maternal and child undernutrition: Consequences for adult health and human capital. *Lancet.* 2008;371:340–57.

31. Bhutta ZA, Ahmed T, Black RE, et al. What works? Interventions for maternal and child undernutrition and survival. *Lancet.* 2008;371:417–40.

32. *Trade reforms and food security: Conceptualizing the linkages.* Rome: FAO; 2003.

33. Jones AD, Ngure FM, Pelto G, Young SL. What are we assessing when we measure food security? A compendium and review of current metrics. *Adv Nutr.* 2013;4:481–505.

34. Barrett CB. Measuring food insecurity. *Science.* 2010;327:825–8.

35. *2015 Global hunger index: Armed conflict and the challenge of hunger.* Bonn: International Food Policy Research Institute (IFPRI); 2015.

36. *Percent of consumer expenditures spent on food, alcoholic beverages, and tobacco that were consumed at home, by selected countries, 2015.* Washington DC: USDA Economic Research Service; 2016.

37. Bickel G, Nord M, Price C, Hamilton W, Cook J. *Guide to measuring household food security.* Alexandria VA: USDA; 2000.

38. *An introduction to the basic concepts of food security.* Rome: FAO; 2008.

39. *Integrated food security phase classification: Technical manual version 1.1.* Rome: FAO; 2008.

40. Sen A. Ingredients of famine analysis: Availability and entitlements. *Q J Econ.* 1981;96:433–64.

41. Godfray HCJ, Beddington JR, Crute IR, et al. Food security: The challenge of feeding 9 billion people. *Science.* 2010;327:812–8.

42. Godfray HC, Crute IR, Haddad L, et al. The future of the global food system. *Philos Trans R Soc Lond B Biol Sci.* 2010;365:2769–77.

43. Maxwell S, Slater R. Food policy old and new. *Dev Policy Rev.* 2003;21:531–53.

44. Koliaki C, Katsilambros N. Dietary sodium, potassium, and alcohol: Key players in the pathophysiology, prevention, and treatment of human hypertension. *Nutr Rev.* 2013;71:402–11.

45. Nilson A, Piza J. Food fortification: A tool for fighting hidden hunger. *Food Nutr Bull.* 1998;19:49–60.

46. Yetley EA. Multivitamin and multimineral dietary supplements: Definitions, characterization, bioavailability, and drug interactions. *Am J Clin Nutr.* 2007;85:S269–76.

47. Ruel-Bergeron JC, Stevens GA, Sugimoto JD, et al. Global update and trends of hidden hunger, 1995–2011. *PLoS One.* 2015;10:e0143497.

48. Bailey RL, West KP Jr, Black RE. The epidemiology of global micronutrient deficiencies. *Ann Nutr Metab.* 2015;66(Suppl 2):22–33.

49. Li M, Eastman CJ. The changing epidemiology of iodine deficiency. *Nat Rev Endocrinol.* 2012;8:434–40.

50. Zimmermann MB, Jooste PL, Pandav CS. Iodine-deficiency disorders. *Lancet.* 2008;372:1251–62.

51. Andersson M, Karumbunathan V, Zimmermann MB. Global iodine status in 2012 and trends over the past decade. *J Nutr.* 2012;142:744–50.

52. Andersson M, de Benoist B, Rogers L. Epidemiology of iodine deficiency: Salt iodisation and iodine status. *Best Pract Res Clin Endocrinol Metab.* 2010;24:1–11.

53. Sherwin JC, Reacher MH, Dean WH, Ngondi J. Epidemiology of vitamin A deficiency and xerophthalmia in at-risk populations. *Trans R Soc Trop Med Hyg.* 2012;106:205–14.

54. Stevens GA, Bennett JE, Hennocq Q, et al. Trends and mortality effects of vitamin A deficiency in children in 138 low-income and middle-income countries between 1991 and 2013: A pooled analysis of population-based surveys. *Lancet Global Health.* 2015;3:e528–36.

55. *Global prevalence of vitamin A deficiency in populations at risk 1995–2005: WHO Global Database on Vitamin A Deficiency.* Geneva: WHO; 2009.

56. Moghissi AA, Pei S, Liu Y. Golden rice: Scientific, regulatory and public information processes of a genetically modified organism. *Crit Rev Biotechnol.* 2016;36:535–41.

57. Mayo-Wilson E, Imdad A, Herzer K, Yakoob MY, Bhutta ZA. Vitamin A supplements for preventing mortality, illness, and blindness in children aged under 5: Systematic review and meta-analysis. *BMJ.* 2011;343:d5094.

58. Lopez A, Cacoub P, Macdougall IC, Peyrin-Biroulet L. Iron deficiency anaemia. *Lancet.* 2016;387:907–16.

59. Tolentino K, Friedman JF. An update on anemia in less developed countries. *Am J Trop Med Hyg.* 2007;77:44–51.

60. *Essential nutrition actions: Improving maternal, newborn, infant and young child health and nutrition.* Geneva: WHO; 2013.

61. Kassebaum NJ, Jasrasaria R, Naghavi M, et al. A systematic analysis of global anemia burden from 1990 to 2010. *Blood.* 2014;123:615–24.

62. Stevens GA, Finucane MM, De-Regil LM, et al. Global, regional, and national trends in haemoglobin concentration and prevalence of total and severe anaemia in children and pregnant and non-pregnant women for 1995–2011: A systematic analysis of population-representative data. *Lancet Glob Health.* 2013;1:e16–25.

63. *The global prevalence of anaemia in 2011.* Geneva: WHO; 2015.

64. Zimmermann MB, Hurrell RF. Nutritional iron deficiency. *Lancet.* 2007;370:511–20.

65. Hurrell RF. How to ensure adequate iron absorption from iron-fortified food. *Nutr Rev.* 2002;60:S7–15.

66. Hiffler L, Rakotoambinina B, Lafferty N, Martinez Garcia D. Thiamine deficiency in tropical pediatrics: New insights into a neglected but vital metabolic change. *Front Nutr.* 2016;3:16.

67. Thakur K, Tomar SK, Singh AK, Mandal S, Arora S. Riboflavin and health: A review of recent human research. *Crit Rev Food Sci Nutr.* 2017;57:3650–60.

68. Frank GP, Voorend DM, Chamdula A, van Oosterhout JJ, Koop K. Pellagra: A non-communicable disease of poverty. *Trop Doct.* 2012;42:182–4.

69. Ami N, Bernstein M, Boucher F, Rieder M, Parker L. Folate and neural tube defects: The role of supplements and food fortification. *Pediatr Child Health.* 2016;21:145–54.

70. Grosso G, Bei R, Mistretta A, et al. Effects of vitamin C on health: A review of evidence. *Front Biosci.* 2013;18:1017–29.

71. Traber MG. Vitamin E inadequacy in humans: Causes and consequences. *Adv Nutr.* 2014;5:503–14.

72. DiNicolantonio JJ, Bhutani J, O'Keefe JH. The health benefits of vitamin K. *Open Heart.* 2015;2:e000300.

73. Wacker M, Holick MF. Sunlight and vitamin D: A global perspective for health. *Dermatoendocrinol.* 2013;5:51–108.

74. Holick MF. Vitamin D deficiency. *New Engl J Med.* 2007;357:266–81.

75. Autier P, Boniol M, Pizot C, Mullie P. Vitamin D status and ill health: A systematic review. *Lancet Diabetes Endocrinol.* 2014;2:76–89.

76. Harding MA, O'Mullane DM. Water fluoridation and oral health. *Acta Med Acad.* 2013;42:131–9.

77. Bagramian RA, Garcia-Godoy F, Volpe AR. The global increase in dental caries: A pending public health crisis. *Am J Dent.* 2009;22:3–8.

78. Fink G, Heitner J. Evaluating the cost-effectiveness of preventive zinc supplementation. *BMC Public Health.* 2014;14:852.

79. Penny ME. Zinc supplementation in public health. *Ann Nutr Metab.* 2013;62(Suppl 1):31–42.

80. Walker CLF, Ezzati M, Black RE. Global and regional child mortality and burden of disease attributable to zinc deficiency. *Eur J Clin Nutr.* 2009;63:591–7.

81. Freeland-Graves JH, Sanjeevi N, Lee JJ. Global perspectives on trace element requirements. *J Trace Elem Med Biol.* 2015;31:135–41.

82. Gura T. Nature's first functional food. *Science.* 2014;345:747–9.

83. Jones KDJ, Berkley JA, Warner JO. Perinatal nutrition and immunity to infection. *Pediatr Allergy Immunol.* 2010;21(4 Pt 1):564–76.

84. Debes AK, Kohli A, Walker N, Edmond K, Mullany LC. Time to initiation of breastfeeding and neonatal mortality and morbidity: A systematic review. *BMC Public Health.* 2013;13(Suppl 3):S19.

85. Das JK, Salem RA, Imdad A, Bhutta ZA. Infant and young child growth (Chapter 12). *Disease control priorities.* 3rd ed. *Reproductive, maternal, newborn, and child health (Volume 2).* Washington DC: IBRD/World Bank; 2016.

86. *From the first hour of life: Making the case for improved infant and young child feeding everywhere.* New York: UNICEF: 2016.

87. Brady JP. Marketing breast milk substitutes: Problems and perils throughout the world. *Arch Dis Child.* 2012;97:529–32.

88. *Marketing of breast-milk substitutes: National implementation of the International Code. Status report 2016.* Geneva: WHO; 2016.

89. Meedya S, Fahy K, Kable A. Factors that positively influence breastfeeding duration to 6 months: A literature review. *Women Birth.* 2010;23:135–45.

90. *Obesity: Preventing and managing the global epidemic.* Geneva: WHO; 2000.

91. Cole TJ, Lobstein T. Extended international (IOTF) body mass index cut-offs for thinness, overweight and obesity. *Pediatr Obes.* 2012;7:284–94.

92. Klein S, Allison DB, Heymsfield SB, et al. Waist circumference and cardiometabolic risk: A consensus statement from Shaping America's Health: Association for Weight Management and Obesity Prevention; NAASO, The Obesity Society; the American Society for Nutrition; and the American Diabetes Association. *Am J Clin Nutr.* 2007;85:1197–202.

93. Prentice AM, Jebb SA. Beyond body mass index. *Obes Rev.* 2001;2:141–7.

94. Field AE, Coakley EH, Must A, et al. Impact of overweight on the risk of developing common chronic diseases during a 10-year period. *Arch Intern Med.* 2001;161:1581–6.

95. NCD Risk Factor Collaboration (NCD-RisC). Trends in adult body-mass index in 200 countries from 1975 to 2014: A pooled analysis of 1698 population-based measurement studies with 19.2 million participants. *Lancet.* 2016;387:1377–96.

96. Ng M, Fleming T, Robinson M, et al. Global, regional and national prevalence of overweight and obesity in children and adults 1980–2013: A systematic analysis. *Lancet.* 2014;384:766–81.

97. GBD 2015 Obesity Collaborators. Health effects of overweight and obesity in 195 countries over 25 years. *N Engl J Med.* 2017;377:13–27.

98. Malik VS, Willett WC, Hu FB. Global obesity: Trends, risk factors and policy implication. *Nat Rev Endocrinol.* 2013;9:13–27.

99. Swami V, Frederick DA, Aavik T, et al. The attractive female body weight and female body dissatisfaction in 26 countries across 10 world regions: Results of the International Body Project I. *Pers Soc Psychol Bull.* 2010;36:309–25.

100. Cecchini M, Sassi F, Lauer JA, Lee YY, Guajardo-Barron V, Chisholm D. Tackling of unhealthy diets,

physical inactivity, and obesity: Health effects and cost-effectiveness. *Lancet.* 2010;376:1775–84.

101. Jerardo A. *Table 1: Import share of U.S. food consumption. Import share of consumption.* Washington DC: USDA Economic Research Service; 2016.

102. McEntire J. Foodborne disease: The global movement of food and people. *Infect Dis Clin North Am.* 2013;27:687–93.

103. Kirk MD, Pires SM, Black RE, et al. World Health Organization estimates of the global and regional disease burden of 22 foodborne bacterial, protozoal, and viral diseases, 2010: A data synthesis. *PLoS Med.* 2015;12:e1001921.

104. Dewaal CS, Hicks G, Barlow K, Alderton L, Vegosen L. Foods associated with foodborne illness outbreaks from 1990 through 2003. *Food Protection Trends.* 2006;26:466–73.

105. Havelaar AH, Kirk MD, Torgerson PR, et al. World Health Organization global estimates and regional comparisons of the burden of foodborne diseases in 2010. *PloS Med.* 2015;12:e1001923.

106. *Bad bug book: Foodborne pathogenic microorganisms and natural toxins handbook (2nd edition).* Silver Spring MD: FDA Center for Food Safety and Applied Nutrition (CFSAN); 2014.

107. Olson ED. Protecting food safety: More needs to be done to keep pace with scientific advances and the changing food supply. *Health Aff.* 2011;5:915–23.

108. Lynch MF, Tauxe RV, Hedberg CW. The growing burden of foodborne outbreaks due to contaminated fresh produce: Risks and opportunities. *Epidemiol Infect.* 2009;137:307–15.

109. *Five keys to safer food manual.* Geneva: WHO; 2006.

110. *Codex Alimentarius: Understanding Codex.* 4th ed. Rome: FAO/WHO; 2016.

111. Codex Alimentarius Commission. *Food hygiene: Basic texts.* 4th ed. Rome: WHO/FAO; 2009.

112. Livermore MA. Authority and legitimacy in global governance: Deliberation, institutional differentiation, and the Codex Alimentarius. *New York University Law Rev.* 2006;81:766–801.

CHAPTER 13

Cancer

Cancers are among the most common causes of adult death in every country. People who live in high-income countries have the highest likelihood of being diagnosed with cancer. Most cancer deaths worldwide occur in middle-income countries. The survival rates among people with cancer are lowest in low-income countries. Interventions like smoking cessation and treatment of chronic infections can prevent some cases of cancer, but for many types of cancer no preventive options are currently available. Reducing the global burden from cancer will require improving access to early diagnosis and creating more affordable and effective treatments.

▶ 13.1 Cancer and Global Health

Cancer is a major cause of disease, disability, and death in every country. Adults living in high-income countries are more likely to develop cancer than adults living in low-income countries. The higher incidence rate is partly due to the risk of cancer increasing with age. Average life expectancies are higher in high-income countries, so more people live long enough to develop cancer. The trend is also related to the lack of access to diagnostic tests in many lower-income countries. A person with cancer who lives in a high-income country is more likely to be tested for cancer and formally diagnosed than a person with the same type of cancer who lives in a low-income country. However, even after adjusting for differences in the age structures of populations and accounting for differential access to health services, people who live in high-income countries are more likely to be diagnosed with

cancer than people of the same age who live in low-income countries. That does not mean that cancer is not a significant problem in low-income countries. People in low-income countries who have cancer are more likely to die from the disease than people the same age who live in high-income countries. Cancers in low-income countries tend to be diagnosed at an advanced stage, and in many places there is limited access to cancer treatment.

Although there is significant diversity in which types of cancer cause the greatest burden by region and by country income level, all countries would benefit from discoveries that enable primary prevention of various types of cancer and from improvements in cancer diagnosis and treatment. Achieving these goals will require major investments in research. Global collaborations are the most efficient way to accelerate the process of making scientific breakthroughs, translating those findings into improved medical care, and increasing access to the new and existing tools for cancer prevention, screening, diagnosis, and treatment.

▶ 13.2 Cancer Biology

Cancer occurs when abnormal cells begin to reproduce uncontrollably, often invading nearby tissues and then spreading to other parts of the body. Cancers are also called **neoplasms**, a term derived from words meaning "new formation." Normal cells are genetically stable, and if mutations or other types of damage cannot be repaired, the cell will undergo a process of programmed cell death called **apoptosis**. Cancer cells, in contrast, are genetically unstable and undergo unlimited reproductive cycles.

Cells from a primary cancerous tumor that invade the walls of blood vessels or lymph vessels can travel to other parts of the body, proliferate (multiply) there, and form new tumors at that distant site. A secondary cancerous tumor at a new site is a **metastasis**. The cells in that secondary tumor will be the same as the cells at the primary cancer site. For example, a breast cancer metastasis in a lung will be composed of breast cells and not lung cells. Cancer cells can stimulate **angiogenesis**, the formation of new blood vessels, to nourish a new cancerous tumor. Not all tumors are **malignant** (cancerous). Some tumors are **benign** (noncancerous). Benign tumors usually remain encapsulated at their original site, and they do not metastasize.

There are several hundred different types of cancer. Each type has a unique set of causes, characteristics, and treatment approaches. Cancers are named for the part of the body where they originate and for the specific type of cell that has become cancerous. A **carcinoma** is a cancer that forms in epithelial tissues, which usually line the inside or outside of the body. A **sarcoma** is a cancer that arises from connective tissues like bones or muscles. Leukemias and myelomas are cancers that form from blood or in the bone marrow where blood is produced by the body.

Cancers are also classified based on whether the cancer cells remain noninvasive and local, if they have spread to regional lymph nodes, or if they have spread to distant parts of the body. There are several staging systems. One assigns a stage based on the TNM classification system, which categorizes the size of the original Tumor, the number of lymph Nodes near the primary tumor that have cancer cells in them, and whether Metastasis has occurred. Another classifies cancers using a four-stage scale. Precancerous lesions like carcinoma in situ are classified as Stage 0 cancers. Stage I cancers are localized. Stage II and III cancers have spread regionally. Stage IV cancers have spread to distant sites. The treatment approach recommended is based on the stage of the cancer at the time of diagnosis.

▶ 13.3 Cancer Epidemiology

About one in eight deaths worldwide each year is caused by cancer.[1] Each year, nearly 15 million people are diagnosed with cancer and more than 8 million people die of cancer.[2] About 30% of men and 20% of women who survive to their 80th birthdays will have developed some type of cancer, even after excluding the non-melanoma skin cancers that are typically not included in reports of cancer statistics because they are common but rarely fatal.[3]

The cancer diagnosis rate is higher in high-income countries than in low-income countries, even after adjusting for differences in the age structure of populations in those countries (**FIGURE 13-1**).[4] A person living in a high-income country is more than twice as likely to receive a cancer diagnosis as a person of the same age who lives in a low-income country. This is partly, but not entirely, due to richer people having more access to cancer screening and diagnosis. In contrast, cancer mortality rates are fairly similar across income groups (**FIGURE 13-2**).[4] That similarity in mortality rates, despite the differences in diagnosis rates, is a result of the survival rate in low-income countries being much lower than the survival rate in high-income countries. A person in a high-income country has a high likelihood of receiving a cancer diagnosis, but is likely to survive the disease. A person with cancer in a

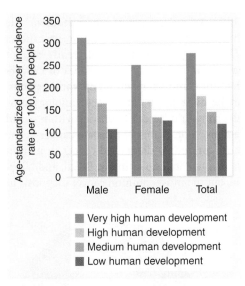

FIGURE 13–1 The age-standardized cancer incidence (diagnosis) rate is higher in high-income countries than in low-income countries.

Data from Ferlay J, Soerjomataram I, Ervik M, et al. *GLOBOCAN 2012: Estimated cancer incidence, mortality and prevalence worldwide in 2012 v1.0.* IARC CancerBase No. 11. Lyon: IARC; 2013.

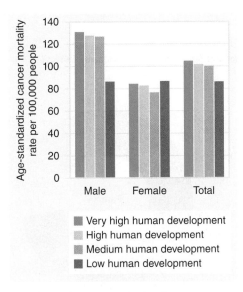

FIGURE 13–2 The age-standardized cancer mortality (death) rate is similar across most human development levels.

Data from Ferlay J, Soerjomataram I, Ervik M, et al. *GLOBOCAN 2012: Estimated cancer incidence, mortality and prevalence worldwide in 2012 v1.0.* IARC CancerBase No. 11. Lyon: IARC; 2013.

low-income country has a lower likelihood of that cancer being diagnosed, but a diagnosed individual in a low-income country is much less likely to survive that cancer than a person of the same age who lives in a high-income country.

Cancer mortality rates have been decreasing in high-income countries as diagnosis and treatment options improve, but cancer incidence rates and mortality rates are increasing in low- and middle-income countries as life expectancies in those areas increase.[5] While the percentage of cancers occurring in high-income areas remains disproportionately high compared to the percentage of people who live in high-income countries (**FIGURE 13–3**),

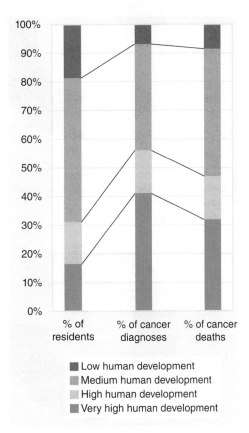

FIGURE 13–3 High-income countries have the highest burden from cancer.

Data from Ferlay J, Soerjomataram I, Ervik M, et al. *GLOBOCAN 2012: Estimated cancer incidence, mortality and prevalence worldwide in 2012 v1.0.* IARC CancerBase No. 11. Lyon: IARC; 2013.

the majority of cancer diagnoses and cancer deaths now occur in the middle-income countries where the majority of the world's people live.[4]

Globally, lung and prostate cancers are the most commonly occurring cancers in men and breast cancer is the most commonly occurring cancer in women.[3] Other common cancers include colorectal, stomach, liver, and cervical cancers (**FIGURE 13–4**).[2] Lung cancer is the most common cause of cancer death.[3]

Other common causes of cancer death include liver, stomach, colorectal, and breast cancers (**FIGURE 13–5**).[2] These global trends do not capture the diversity in the types of cancers that are common in different world regions, or the diversity of cancer epidemiology profiles among different countries within world regions.[6] For example, prostate cancer is the most commonly diagnosed cancer in men in the United States, Germany, Brazil, and Nigeria, but the most common cancer diagnosis in

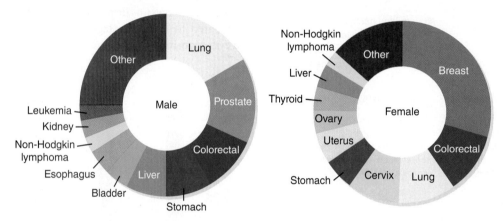

FIGURE 13–4 Distribution of worldwide cancer diagnoses by type and sex.

Data from Ferlay J, Soerjomataram I, Dikshit R, et al. Cancer incidence and mortality worldwide: sources, methods and major patterns in GLOBOCAN 2012. *Int J Cancer 2014;* 136:E359-86.

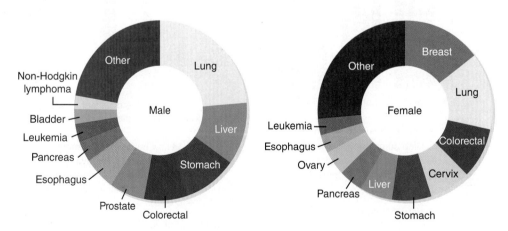

FIGURE 13–5 Distribution of worldwide cancer deaths by type and sex.

Data from Ferlay J, Soerjomataram I, Dikshit R et al. Cancer incidence and mortality worldwide: sources, methods and major patterns in GLOBOCAN 2012. *Int J Cancer 2014;* 136:E359-86.

men is stomach cancer in Iran, lung cancer in China, lip and oral cavity cancer in India, and colorectal cancer in Ethiopia (FIGURE 13–6).[4] There are similarly diverse variations in the most common causes of cancer mortality by country. While lung cancer is the most common cause of cancer death in men in the United States, Germany, China, and India, the most common cause of cancer death among men is stomach cancer in Iran, prostate cancer in Brazil and Nigeria, and leukemia in Ethiopia.[4]

Country	Rank	USA	Iran	Germany	Brazil	China	India	Nigeria	Ethiopia
Most Commonly Diagnosed Cancers in Men	#1	Prostate	Stomach	Prostate	Prostate	Lung	LOC	Prostate	CRC
	#2	Lung	Bladder	CRC	Lung	Liver	Lung	Liver	KS
	#3	CRC	Prostate	Lung	CRC	Stomach	Stomach	NHL	Leukemia
Most Common Causes of Cancer Death in Men	#1	Lung	Stomach	Lung	Prostate	Lung	Lung	Prostate	Leukemia
	#2	Prostate	Lung	CRC	Lung	Liver	Stomach	Liver	CRC
	#3	CRC	Esophagus	Prostate	Stomach	Stomach	Mouth	NHL	KS
Most Commonly Diagnosed Cancers in Women	#1	Breast	Breast	Breast	Breast	Lung	Breast	Breast	Breast
	#2	Lung	CRC	CRC	Cervix	Breast	Cervix	Cervix	Cervix
	#3	CRC	Stomach	Lung	CRC	Stomach	CRC	Liver	Ovary
Most Common Causes of Cancer Death in Women	#1	Lung	Breast	Breast	Breast	Lung	Breast	Breast	Breast
	#2	Breast	Stomach	Lung	Lung	Stomach	Cervix	Cervix	Cervix
	#3	CRC	Esophagus	CRC	CRC	Liver	CRC	Liver	Ovary

FIGURE 13–6 The most common cancer diagnoses and causes of cancer mortality in featured countries.

Data from Ferlay J, Soerjomataram I, Ervik M, et al. *GLOBOCAN 2012: Estimated cancer incidence, mortality and prevalence worldwide in 2012 v1.0.* IARC CancerBase No. 11. Lyon: IARC; 2013.

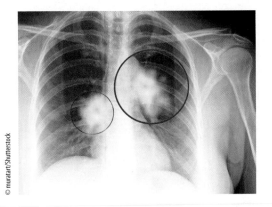

© muratart/Shutterstock

Lung cancer.

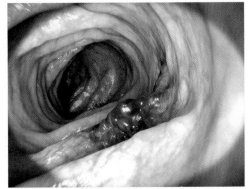

© Juan Gaertner/Shutterstock

Colorectal cancer.

▶ # 13.4 Cancer Risk Factors and Prevention

Cancer is a genetic disease, but it usually results from mutations rather than inheritance.[7] Those mutations can occur via numerous pathways.[8] Tobacco use increases the risk of cancers of the lungs, mouth, pharynx, larynx, esophagus, pancreas, urinary bladder, and kidneys.[9] Occupational exposures to carcinogens increase the risk of various types of cancers by damaging cells. For example, benzene increases the risk of leukemia; asbestos has been linked to a kind of lung cancer called mesothelioma; and arsenic, cadmium, chromium, and other chemicals increase the risk of cancers of the lungs, bronchi, and trachea.[10] Environmental hazards, such as air pollution, residential radon, and arsenic in drinking water, may also induce cellular damage.[11] An unhealthy diet, obesity, and physical inactivity may impair cellular function.[7] Additionally, chronic infections may cause more than 2 million cancers worldwide each year (**FIGURE 13−7**),[12] contributing to more than one in four cancers in lower-income areas and about one in 14 cancers in in higher-income areas.[13]

One of the key steps toward reducing the global burden from cancer will be identifying more ways to prevent cancer from developing. Primary prevention interventions are usually designed to reduce the prevalence of a **risk factor**, an exposure or characteristic that increases the likelihood of developing a

Infection	Associated Cancer(s)
Clonorchis sinensis	Cholangiosarcoma (bile duct cancer)
Epstein–Barr virus (EBV)	Hodgkin's lymphoma, Burkitt's lymphoma, nasopharyngeal carcinoma
Helicobacter pylori	Stomach cancer
Hepatitis B virus (HBV)	Liver cancer
Hepatitis C virus (HCV)	Liver cancer
Human herpes virus type 8 (HHV-8)	Kaposi sarcoma
Human papillomavirus (HPV)	Cervical cancer, oropharyngeal cancers, anogenital cancers
Human T-cell lymphotropic virus (HTLV)	Adult T-cell leukemia and lymphoma
Opisthorchis viverrini	Cholangiosarcoma (bile duct cancer)
Schistosoma haematobium	Bladder cancer

FIGURE 13−7 Examples of cancers associated with chronic infections.

Data from Plummer M, de Martel C, Vignat J, Ferlay J, Bray F, Franceschi S. Global burden of cancers attributable to infections in 2012: A synthetic analysis. *Lancet Glob Health* 2016;4:e609−16.

particular disease. Risk factors may be biological, behavioral, environmental, or other types of exposures or characteristics (**FIGURE 13–8**).[14] For most types of cancer, age is the strongest risk factor. Older adults have a higher rate of cancer diagnosis and death than younger people (**FIGURE 13–9**). Nearly 60% of cancer diagnoses and 70% of cancer deaths worldwide

Health-Related Behaviors	Nutritional Exposures	Environmental Exposures	Untreated Medical Conditions
■ Tobacco use ■ Physical inactivity ■ Unsafe sex ■ Alcohol abuse ■ Injecting drug use	■ Obesity and overweight ■ Child underweight ■ Low fruit and vegetable intake ■ Suboptimal breastfeeding ■ Vitamin A deficiency ■ Zinc deficiency ■ Iron deficiency	■ Indoor smoke from solid fuels ■ Unsafe water, sanitation, and hygiene ■ Urban outdoor air pollution ■ Occupational risks ■ Lead exposure	■ High blood pressure ■ High blood glucose ■ High cholesterol ■ Unmet contraceptive need

FIGURE 13–8 Common risk factors for adverse health outcomes.

Data from *Global health risks: Mortality and burden of disease attributable to selected major risks*. Geneva: WHO; 2009.

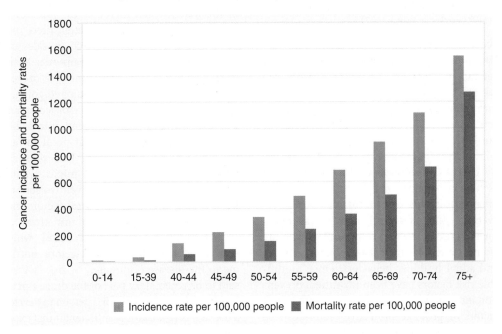

FIGURE 13–9 The cancer incidence and mortality rates worldwide increase with age. (Non-melanoma skin cancers are not included in these rates.)

Data from Ferlay J, Soerjomataram I, Ervik M, et al. *GLOBOCAN 2012: Estimated cancer incidence, mortality and prevalence worldwide in 2012 v1.0.* IARC CancerBase No. 11. Lyon: IARC; 2013.

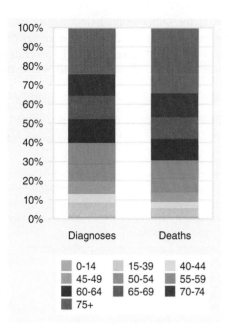

FIGURE 13–10 Most cancer deaths occur in older adults.

Data from Ferlay J, Soerjomataram I, Ervik M, et al. *GLOBOCAN 2012: Estimated cancer incidence, mortality and prevalence worldwide in 2012 v1.0.* IARC CancerBase No. 11. Lyon: IARC; 2013.

occur in people who are at least 60 years old (**FIGURE 13–10**). Age, ethnicity, and heritable genetic markers for particular diseases are examples of **nonmodifiable risk factors** that cannot be changed through health interventions. Because aging is not modifiable, the burden from cancers associated with aging will increase as life expectancies increase. By contrast, **behavioral risk factors**, such as tobacco smoking and exercise habits, and other **modifiable risk factors** can be altered, even if making lifestyle changes is challenging for the individuals and communities who are trying to reduce their hazardous exposures and adopt healthier behaviors. Once modifiable risk factors have been identified, prevention interventions that reduce exposure to risk factors or promote protective factors can be tailored to particular populations.[15]

A **causal factor** is an exposure that has been scientifically tested and shown to occur before the disease outcome and contribute

directly to its occurrence. Confirming causation requires more than just laboratory experiments and statistics. It also requires logical thinking. Some of the major criteria used to evaluate the likelihood that an exposure causes a disease are the strength of the association, the presence of a dose–response relationship between the exposure and outcome, and the consistency of the risk across numerous studies (**FIGURE 13–11**).[16] There is no expectation that all of these criteria have to be met for an exposure to be considered causal, but the evidence for causality is stronger when more criteria are met.

Cancer prevention campaigns can be effective even when an exposure has not been proven to directly cause cancer but appears to be part of a causal pathway. Consider the statistical association between hot weather and an increased rate of shark attacks. This association is statistically significant, but that does not prove that hot weather causes sharks to fall into a frenzy. A more likely explanation is that hot weather increases the number of humans in the water, which increases the number of humans attacked. For that matter, there may be an association between ice cream sales and shark attacks. Banning ice cream sales at the beach would probably not do much to prevent shark attacks, unless people stopped going to beaches because of the absence of ice cream. But identifying the link between hot temperatures and shark injuries might point toward the types of conditions that lead to shark attacks, and that knowledge might eventually translate into effective preventive actions. Both proximal and distal causal factors may be targets of cancer prevention initiatives.

Many diseases are **multicausal**, which means that many different risk factors contribute to the disease occurring.[17] A risk factor is said to be a necessary part of the disease pathway if it must be present for a person to develop a disease. A risk factor is sufficient if that exposure or characteristic by itself can cause disease. Some exposures are necessary but not sufficient on their own to cause disease. Some exposures are sufficient but not necessary.

Temporality	Did the exposure happen before the onset of disease?
Strength of association	Is the statistical association between the exposure and outcome strong?
Dose–response relationship/ biological gradient	Do people with a higher level of exposure have a higher risk of the outcome than people with a lower level of exposure?
Cessation	Does stopping the exposure reduce the risk of the outcome?
Specificity	Are the exposure and outcome both narrowly defined rather than general concepts?
Theoretical plausibility	Is there a reasonable biological explanation for why the exposure might cause the outcome?
Consistency	Has a potentially causal relationship between the exposure and outcome been observed in other studies and other populations?
Coherence	Is a causal relationship between the exposure and outcome congruent with other knowledge about the variables?
Consideration of alternate explanations	Are there reasons why what appears to be a causal relationship might not actually be causal?

FIGURE 13–11 Criteria for evaluating whether an exposure causes a disease or other health outcome.

Cancers are often the result of several risk factors being present together, not just one exposure. A diversity of sets of exposures may lead to the development of cancer. That multicausality means that there are many possible pathways for the primary prevention of cancer.

A global **risk transition** is occurring in which the risk factors accounting for the largest proportion of preventable morbidity and mortality are shifting.[18] In pre-transition populations, exposures like undernutrition, unsafe water, and indoor air pollution that increase the risk of childhood infectious diseases are the dominant risk factors. In post-transition populations, exposures like obesity, physical inactivity, and tobacco use that increase the risk of chronic diseases, including many types of cancer, are the dominant risk factors.

Today, about one-third of cancer deaths are attributed to nine modifiable lifestyle and environmental factors: overweight and obesity, low fruit and vegetable intake, physical inactivity, smoking, alcohol use, unsafe sex, urban air pollution, indoor smoke from household use of solid fuels, and contaminated injections in healthcare settings.[19] These risk factors associated with cancer are ones that can be modified at the individual, community, or broader population levels.

However, if one-third of cancers are linked to these common modifiable risk factors, that means that two-thirds are not. Even with advances in prevention science, only about half of cancers occurring globally today are ones that could be prevented with current scientific knowledge and technologies.[20] Many types of cancers have no currently known modifiable risk factors. For cancers that have known risk factors, alternative causal pathways can still lead to cancer. About 5% of the genetic mutations that lead to cancer are inherited, about 30% are due to environmental and other modifiable exposures, and about two-thirds are random mutations.[21] It is rarely possible to know with certainty which particular factors led to a particular case of cancer. For example, many people who develop lung cancer have never smoked,[22] and people who smoke for decades may develop lung cancer as a result of a mutation that is unrelated to tobacco exposure. Even people who follow all the scientific guidance about cancer prevention must remain vigilant about screening and seeking medical care for symptoms that might indicate the presence of cancer.

▶ 13.5 Cancer Screening and Diagnosis

When cancer cannot be prevented, the next best option is to detect cancer at an early stage through screening. **Screening** is a type of secondary prevention in which all members of a well-defined group of people are encouraged to be tested for a disease based on evidence that members of the population are at risk for the disease and early intervention improves health outcomes. The goal of cancer screening programs is to identify precancerous lesions or early-stage, localized cancers in people who have no symptoms of a particular cancer (**FIGURE 13–12**). When diagnostic tests are conducted in people who already have signs and symptoms of cancer in order to confirm the presence of cancerous cells, those tests are diagnostic tests and are not screening tests.

A good screening test will have a high **diagnostic accuracy**, with nearly 100% of test results being true positives or true negatives, and almost no results being false positives or false negatives. A good screening test will also have nearly 100% sensitivity and specificity. The **sensitivity** of a test is the proportion of people who truly have the disease who test positive for the disease. The **specificity** of a test is the proportion of people who are truly free of the disease who test negative for it. Additionally, a good screening test will have positive and negative predictive values near 100%. The **positive predictive value (PPV)** is the proportion of people who test positive for the disease who truly have the disease. The **negative predictive value (NPV)** is the proportion of people who test negative for the disease who truly do not have the disease. The PPV and NPV are based, in part, on the percentage of

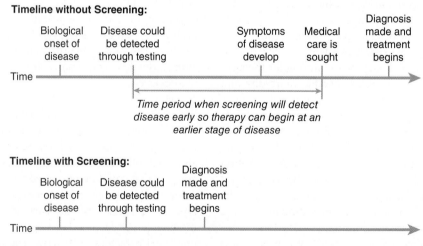

FIGURE 13–12 Timeline for the natural history of disease.

people in the population being tested who have the disease. A test will have a higher PPV in a population with a high prevalence of disease than in one with a low prevalence.

A variety of cancer screening tests are available (**FIGURE 13–13**). The recommended cancer screenings vary by country, by age group, by sex, and by other population characteristics. **Population-based screening** targets large groups of people, like all women aged 40–79 years. **High-risk screening** targets people who are known to have an elevated risk of cancer due to family history (genetics), occupational exposures, tobacco use, or other risk factors. Inherited mutations are responsible for relatively few cases of cancer, and most people diagnosed with cancer do not have a family history of that type of cancer. However, people with a family history may benefit from

being screened more often than is recommended for the general population and starting screening at a younger age than is typically recommended.

Diseases that are targeted by screening programs are usually severe, treatable, and relatively common (**FIGURE 13–14**). Decisions about when to implement a screening program and which population subgroups to target are made by health professionals, policymakers, and communities after considering the most important local health conditions. In lower-income countries, the most cost-effective cancer screening tests include clinical breast exams and cervical cancer visualization.[23] A more extensive set of screening tests are cost-effective in higher-income countries that have higher cancer incidence rates and spend more money on cancer treatment.[24]

Type of Cancer	Examples of Screening Tests
Breast cancer	■ Breast self-examination (BSE) ■ Clinical breast examination (CBE) ■ Mammography
Cervical cancer	■ Papanicolaou test (Pap smear, cervical cytology) ■ Visual inspection with acetic acid (VIA)
Colorectal cancer	■ Fecal occult blood test (FOBT) ■ Flexible sigmoidoscopy ■ Colonoscopy
Esophageal cancer	■ Endoscopy
Oral cancers	■ Physical examination of the mouth
Prostate cancer	■ Digital rectal examination (DRE) ■ Prostate-specific antigen (PSA) test
Skin cancers	■ Physical examination of the skin

FIGURE 13–13 Examples of cancer screening tests.

Data from Sankaranarayanan R. Screening for cancer in low- and middle-income countries. *Ann Global Health* 2014; 80:412–7; and *Recommendations for primary care practice*. Rockville, MD: U.S. Preventive Services Task Force (USPSTF); 2017.

The disease is life threatening.

There is an early asymptomatic stage of the disease in which early diagnosis is possible with an available test.

Early diagnosis significantly improves survival rates or other outcomes.

The screening test has high sensitivity and high specificity.

The screening test is acceptable to the target population.

The target population has access to additional testing and treatment if a screening test indicates the likely presence of disease.

The disease is relatively common in the target population.

Economic analyses have demonstrated that the screening program is likely to be cost-effective.

FIGURE 13-14 Characteristics of good screening programs.

▶ 13.6 Cancer Treatment

A comprehensive cancer care plan includes access to prevention, screening, diagnosis, various types of treatment, and psychosocial support for people with cancer and their caregivers.[25] Comprehensive cancer care also requires access to **palliative care**, which focuses on pain management and quality of life.[26] The three most common cancer treatments are surgery, chemotherapy, and radiation therapy.

Surgery is an operation to confirm whether a disease is present or to remove a tumor or other part of the body. Cancer surgery typically involves sedating a patient with anesthesia, making an incision through the skin with a scalpel in a sterile environment, excising cancerous tissues, and then closing the wound with sutures or staples. Some cancer surgeries are diagnostic. A **biopsy** of a small sample of cells or tissues may be collected through an incision or with a needle so that the specimen can be examined for the presence or absence of cancer. After a diagnosis is confirmed, a surgical procedure may be used to stage the cancer. The areas around the primary tumor, including nearby lymph nodes, may be examined. When cancers are localized, surgery can entirely remove a cancerous lesion or tumor. Some surgical procedures reduce the mass of a tumor prior to initiating other forms of therapy. Surgery can also be used to address the complications of advanced cancer, such as intestinal obstructions, and to reduce discomfort and pain. Additionally, reconstructive surgery can restore function and appearance after successful cancer treatment.

More than 100 different types of **chemotherapy** agents are available to kill cancerous cells, slow the growth of cancerous masses, and keep cancer from spreading to other parts of the body. Chemotherapeutic medications can be delivered orally, intravenously, by injection, or via other mechanisms. They typically must be administered according to strict protocols for dosage and timing, often using several cycles of treatment and rest periods. Chemotherapy can be used alone for some types of cancers. For others, it may be used as neoadjuvant therapy to shrink tumors before surgery or radiation or as adjuvant therapy to kill any cancer cells remaining after other types of treatments. Chemotherapy often causes fatigue and may cause other side effects, such as nausea, skin and mouth sores, and hair loss.

Radiation therapy uses high-energy ionizing radiation to damage the DNA of actively dividing cells, which causes the cells to stop dividing or die. Because cancer cells usually divide quickly, they are more likely than healthy cells to be affected by radiation. Even so, healthy cells near the tumor may also be damaged. External beam radiation therapy uses photon beams (or other types of radiation, such as proton therapy) from a machine outside the body to deliver targeted radiation to particular sites. Internal radiation therapy, also called brachytherapy, implants a radioactive isotope in or near the tumor. Systemic radiation therapy injects radioisotopes into the body so they

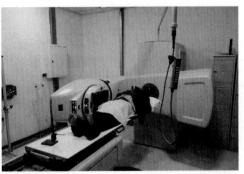
© International Atomic Energy Agency

can circulate throughout the body. Radiation may be used alone or in conjunction with other therapies. Fatigue and skin damage are common side effects, and there is a small risk of a secondary cancer being caused by the exposure to radiation.

There are significant disparities in access to cancer care by country income level (**FIGURE 13–15**). Rural residents often

Resource Environment	Basic	Limited	Enhanced	Maximal
Location	Low-income countries	Rural areas of middle-income countries	Urban areas of middle-income countries	High-income countries
Screening and treatment of precancerous conditions	Limited availability	Limited availability	Available	Available
Surgery	Limited availability	Limited availability	Widely available	Widely available
Chemotherapy	Not available	Limited availability	Available	Available
Radiation therapy	Not available	Limited availability	Widely available	Widely available

FIGURE 13–15 Typical resources for cancer care by country income level and location.

Data from Horton S, Gauvreau CL. Cancer in low- and middle-income countries: An economic overview (Chapter 16). *Disease control priorities. Cancer (Vol. 3).* 3rd ed. Washington: IBRD / World Bank; 2015.

have fewer options for cancer treatment than urban residents. Surgery is widely available in high-income countries, but may be inaccessible in rural areas of middle-income countries and almost completely unavailable in low-income countries.[27] Chemotherapy may be so expensive in low- and middle-income countries that it is not available to most cancer patients.[28] Radiation therapy is nonexistent in most low-income countries (**FIGURE 13–16**).[29] Advanced treatment options, such as immunotherapies (like the use of monoclonal antibodies) and stem cell transplants, are also not widely available.

Because accessible and affordable options for cancer care are limited in lower-income areas, survival rates for people diagnosed with cancer are significantly lower in low-income countries than in high-income countries (**FIGURE 13–17**).[30] These disparities in survival are present for cancers with relatively high 5-year survival rates in high-income countries (such as breast and prostate cancers) as well as for cancers with low 5-year survival rates in high-income countries (such as lung and liver cancers). Improved access to screening and diagnostic tests that allow cancer to be detected at an earlier, more treatable stage and increased access to advanced therapies would enable many more people to survive for many years after being diagnosed with cancer.

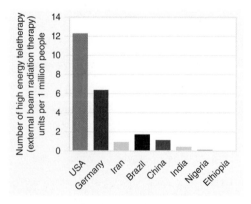

FIGURE 13–16 Access to radiation therapy is very limited in low- and middle-income countries.

Data from *Cancer country profiles 2014*. Geneva: WHO; 2015.

▶ 13.7 Lung Cancer

Lung cancer is the most common cause of cancer death globally.[3] More than 1 million men and about 500,000 women die from lung cancers each year.[31] There is wide variation in the lung cancer mortality rate for men and women by country and region. The highest rates are in Eastern Europe and Eastern Asia, and the lowest rates are in sub-Saharan Africa. This pattern closely mirrors the prevalence of tobacco smoking.[22] About 70% of lung cancer deaths are attributable to tobacco smoking.[32] Other risky exposures include indoor and outdoor air pollution and occupational hazards.[22]

The 5-year survival rate after a diagnosis of cancer of the lung, bronchus, or trachea remains below 20% even in the countries with the highest survival rates.[33] Because the treatment options for lung cancer are limited, the most effective lung cancer interventions focus on primary prevention. The most cost-effective interventions for reducing lung cancer incidence and mortality are tobacco control initiatives like warning labels and taxation.[34] Tobacco control initiatives also help reduce the incidence of lip, mouth, and other oral cancers.[35]

▶ 13.8 Breast Cancer and Cervical Cancer

Breast cancer is the most commonly diagnosed cancer in women, with about 1.7 million new cases detected worldwide each year.[36] Breast cancer is responsible for about 25% of cancer diagnoses and 15% of cancer deaths in women.[31] The diagnosis rate is higher in higher-income countries than it is in lower-income countries (**FIGURE 13–18**).[4] However, the mortality rate from breast cancer among all women (that is, the death rate calculated with the denominator including women with and without breast cancer) is higher in

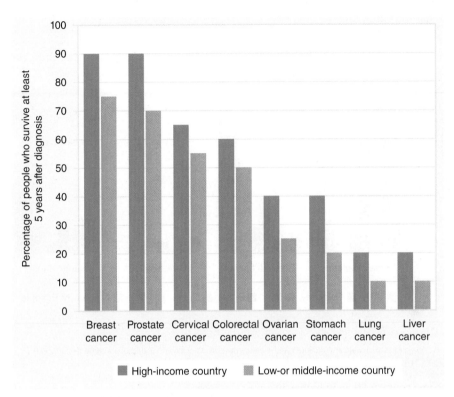

FIGURE 13–17 Cancer survival rates are higher in high-income than low-income countries, but the survival rate remains low for some cancers.

Data from Gelband H, Jha P, Sankaranarayanan R, Gauvreau CL, Horton S. Summary (Chapter 1). *Disease control priorities. Cancer (Vol. 3).* 3rd ed. Washington: IBRD / World Bank; 2015.

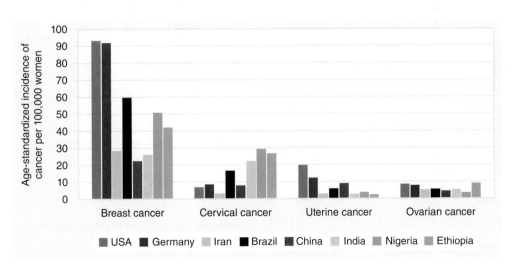

FIGURE 13–18 Incidence (diagnosis) rates of female reproductive cancers.

Data from Ferlay J, Soerjomataram I, Ervik M, et al. *GLOBOCAN 2012: Estimated cancer incidence, mortality and prevalence worldwide in 2012 v1.0.* IARC CancerBase No. 11. Lyon: IARC; 2013.

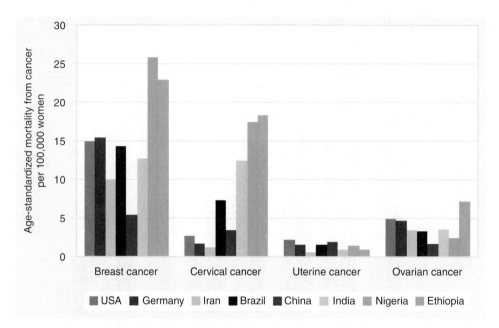

FIGURE 13–19 Mortality rates from female reproductive cancers.

Data from Ferlay J, Soerjomataram I, Ervik M, et al. *GLOBOCAN 2012: Estimated cancer incidence, mortality and prevalence worldwide in 2012 v1.0.* IARC CancerBase No. 11. Lyon: IARC; 2013.

lower-income countries than in higher-income countries (**FIGURE 13–19**).[4] Lower-income countries also have a higher breast cancer case fatality rate (that is, a higher proportion of women with breast cancer who die from the disease), and a lower survival rate among people diagnosed with breast cancer than is observed in higher-income countries. The lower survival rate is a result of both limited access to treatment and limited access to early diagnosis. Women diagnosed with breast cancer in higher-income areas usually have early stage breast cancers (Stage 0, I, or II), while women diagnosed with breast cancer in lower-income areas often have advanced stage breast cancers (Stage III or IV) (**FIGURE 13–20**).[36]

Early detection of breast cancer is associated with more favorable outcomes.[37] In low-income countries, the options for early detection are typically limited to clinical breast exams. In most middle-income and high-income areas, routine **mammography** (an X-ray of the breast that is generated using low-dose radiation) is available.[38]

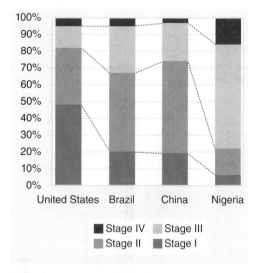

FIGURE 13–20 Stage of breast cancer at the time of diagnosis.

Data from *Global cancer facts & figures*. 3rd ed. Atlanta: American Cancer Society; 2015.

Treatment options also differ by country. For women with breast cancer who live in low-income countries, a mastectomy followed

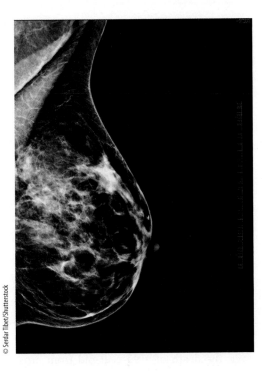

© Serdar Tibet/Shutterstock

by use of the drug tamoxifen is likely to be the best available option. In high-income countries, breast-conserving surgery followed by reconstruction is often offered, and a diversity of chemotherapy, radiation, endocrine therapies, and biological therapies provide additional pathways to long-term survival.[38]

Cancers of the female reproductive system are also significant contributors to the burden of disease in some populations. The uterine cervix is the lowest part of the uterus, and it is located at the top of the vagina. During pregnancy, the cervix helps protect the developing fetus. During delivery, the cervix relaxes to allow the baby to pass through the birth canal. The development of abnormal cervical cells, a condition called cervical dysplasia, is not uncommon among women of reproductive age. The majority of cervical dysplasia cases are associated with **human papillomavirus (HPV)**.[39] In most women, the viral infection will clear on its own. In some women, the infection becomes chronic and causes additional damage to the cervical

cells, eventually leading to **cervical cancer**.[40] As the malignant cells multiply, invasive cervical cancer may spread to nearby tissues and then metastasize to other organs. More than 500,000 women are diagnosed with cervical cancer each year.[4]

HPV vaccination is a primary prevention intervention that protects against cervical cancer, but it is not available in most lower-income countries.[41] Early detection of cervical dysplasia so that precancerous lesions can be treated is another way to prevent cervical cancer from developing. Pap smears in which cervical cells are collected and histologically examined in a cytology laboratory are the traditional form of cervical cancer screening, but this requires access to laboratory facilities. **VIA**, visual inspection with acetic acid, is a lower-cost option in which a diluted vinegar solution applied to the cervix with a cotton swab causes areas that are inflamed or have cellular damage to turn white.[42] Lesions that are observed during VIA screening can be treated with cryotherapy, a procedure that does not require surgery or general anesthesia.[43] Since women who have been vaccinated against the common strains of HPV are still at risk of cervical cancer from other causes, screening for cervical dysplasia is recommended for most women regardless of their HPV vaccination status.

In the high- and middle-income countries where screening for cervical cancer is routinely available, the incidence of cervical cancer has decreased significantly. In the low-income countries where cervical cancer screening is rarely available, cervical cancer continues to be a significant cause of death among reproductive-age women.[43] The cervical cancer diagnosis rate is considerably higher in lower-income countries than in higher-income countries. Most of the diagnosed cancers could have been prevented with early treatment of precancerous lesions found during screening examinations.[4]

Less common cancers of the female reproductive system include ovarian cancer and uterine cancer. **Ovarian cancer** is difficult to diagnose at an early stage, and survival rates for ovarian cancer remain low.[44] **Uterine cancer**, also called endometrial cancer, usually occurs in post-menopausal women. The outcomes are generally favorable in women who are able to receive surgery while the cancer is at an early stage.[45]

▶ 13.9 Prostate Cancer

Most older men develop benign prostatic hyperplasia (BPH), a noncancerous enlargement of the prostate gland that may make urination difficult.[46] A large proportion of men with BPH later develop **prostate cancer**, which may metastasize from the male reproductive gland to lymph nodes, bones, and other parts of the body. Increased age is the dominant risk factor for prostate cancer.[47] About one-third of 70-year-old men, half of 80-year-old men, and nearly 100% of 100-year-old men have cancerous cells in their prostates.[48]

Prostate cancer is the most frequently diagnosed cancer (other than non-melanoma skin cancers) among men in the Americas, Western Europe, Australia, and New Zealand, and the incidence rate is increasing in most world regions.[49] The rising diagnosis rates are partly explained by population aging. They are also the result of increased access to screening tests like digital rectal examination and prostate-specific antigen (PSA).[50] Although men in high-income countries have the highest likelihood of being diagnosed with prostate cancer, the mortality rate is highest in low-income countries.[49] Surgery and radiation therapy can be effective treatments for prostate cancer, but both are associated with adverse side effects related to urinary, bowel, and sexual function.[51]

Statistics about the 5-year survival rates for prostate cancer (as well as one-year, ten-year, and other survival rates) must be interpreted carefully because most prostate cancers occur in older men and most survival rates adjust for life expectancy. The typical 50-year-old man has a very high likelihood of surviving to his 55th birthday. If a 50-year-old is diagnosed with prostate cancer and dies from it a few years later, the prostate cancer would be considered to have caused a premature death. By contrast, a 90-year-old man is unlikely to survive to his 95th birthday even if he is very healthy on his 90th birthday. A death from prostate cancer after age 90 would not be classified as a premature death, since the decedent would have already far exceeded the average life expectancy for his birth cohort. A 90-year-old's death would be included in a count of prostate cancer deaths in his country, if the cause of death was determined to be prostate cancer rather than heart disease or another common cause of mortality in older men who might die with prostate cancer but not because of it. However, the death of a 90-year-old from prostate cancer would likely not be included in the calculation of age-standardized mortality and survival rates. This is why the United States reports a 99% survival rate for prostate cancer even though more than 25,000 American men die of prostate cancer each year (and more than 180,000 are diagnosed annually).[52] Prostate cancer mortality rates need to be considered alongside the counts of deaths in order to more fully understand the burden of disease on older men in the population.

▶ 13.10 Liver Cancer

Most cases of **liver cancer** currently occur in the places within East Asia, South Asia, and sub-Saharan Africa that have had historically high rates of hepatitis B virus (HBV) infection (**FIGURE 13–21**).[53] Chronic HBV infection, often acquired in infancy, can trigger a pathologic process that damages liver cells and leads to hepatocellular carcinoma (HCC), the most

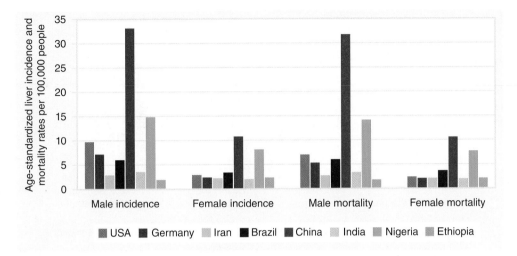

FIGURE 13–21 Liver cancer incidence (diagnosis) and mortality rates by sex.

Data from Ferlay J, Soerjomataram I, Ervik M, et al. *GLOBOCAN 2012: Estimated cancer incidence, mortality and prevalence worldwide in 2012 v1.0.* IARC CancerBase No. 11. Lyon: IARC; 2013.

common type of liver cancer.[54] Besides HBV, other major risk factors for liver cancer include hepatitis C virus (HCV), alcohol use, tobacco smoking, obesity, and exposure to aflatoxins, which are toxic molds found in some foods.[55] Some of these exposures are more common in men than women, and that accounts for the significant differences in liver cancer incidence by sex.

The best currently available option for preventing future cases of liver cancer is hepatitis B vaccine.[56] To prevent mother-to-child transmission of the virus, the first dose of the vaccine is typically given to neonates shortly after birth.[57] The vaccine prevents new HBV infections, but it does not stop cancer from developing in adults whose livers have already been scarred by chronic infection. The 5-year survival rate for liver cancer is less than 20% even in the countries with the most favorable outcomes,[33] so liver cancer will continue to be a common cause of cancer death among adults who already have liver damage. However, hepatitis B vaccination programs will reduce the incidence of HCC for future generations.

▶ 13.11 Esophageal, Stomach, and Colorectal Cancers

The incidence of cancers of the digestive tract—esophageal cancers, stomach cancers, and colon and rectal cancers—vary significantly by country (**FIGURE 13–22**). The highest incidence rates of **esophageal cancer** occur in Central and Eastern Asia and in eastern and southern Africa.[31] Most esophageal cancers are squamous cell carcinomas, and some are esophageal adenocarcinomas. The risk factors for squamous cell carcinomas are not well defined, but may include alcohol use, tobacco use, and nutritional exposures.[31] The major risk factors for esophageal adenocarcinomas are obesity and gastroesophageal reflux disease (GERD), which increases the risk of a precancerous condition called Barrett's esophagus that results from chronic acid reflux.[58] Early detection and treatment of Barrett's esophagus can help prevent the development of adenocarcinomas. The survival rates for esophageal cancer are low in all countries.[36]

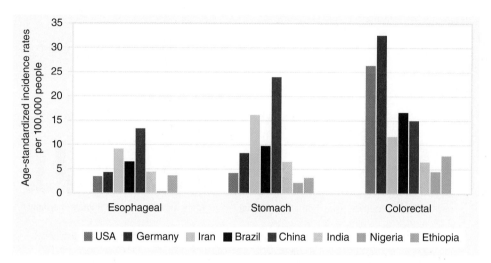

FIGURE 13–22 Esophageal, stomach, and colorectal cancer incidence (diagnosis) rates.

Data from Ferlay J, Soerjomataram I, Ervik M, et al. *GLOBOCAN 2012: Estimated cancer incidence, mortality and prevalence worldwide in 2012 v1.0.* IARC CancerBase No. 11. Lyon: IARC; 2013.

Stomach cancer rates are highest in Central and Eastern Asia, Eastern Europe, and South America.[36] For stomach cancers located near the esophagus (that is, for cardia gastric cancers), age, tobacco smoking, and obesity are associated with increased incidence.[59] For other stomach cancers (that is, for noncardia gastric cancers), age and *Helicobacter pylori* infection are risk factors, and dietary habits, such as low consumption of fruits, vegetables, and fiber and high intake of salty and smoked foods, may also influence the risk.[60] Because early-stage stomach cancer causes few symptoms, most stomach cancers are diagnosed at an advanced stage when survival rates are low.[36]

The incidence of **colorectal cancer** is highest in high-income countries.[61] Dietary factors like high intake of dietary fat, red meat, and processed meats may account for 30% to 50% of all colorectal cancers worldwide.[62] Colon and rectal cancers can be prevented through screening for polyps and removal of any observed precancerous lesions, but these procedures are expensive.[63] Colorectal cancer rates are decreasing in high-income countries where colonoscopies are widely available, but rates are increasing in some middle-income areas.[31]

▶ 13.12 Other Cancers

Cancer can occur in any part of the body, and a diversity of cancers contribute to the global burden of cancer. **Kidney cancer** diagnosis rates are rising in most countries, especially in Latin America.[64] The major known risk factors for kidney cancer are tobacco use, obesity, and hypertension.[65] **Pancreatic cancer** has a relatively low incidence rate, but it also has a very low survival rate. Tobacco use increases the risk of pancreatic cancer, but that exposure accounts for a low percentage of cases and few other risk factors have been identified.[66] Most cases of **bladder cancer** occur in men and are linked to tobacco use, since the toxins from smoke that are filtered out of the bloodstream by the kidneys are stored in the bladder prior to urination and may damage the cells lining the bladder.[67] Some urinary bladder cancers in Africa and Asia are linked to chronic infection with the parasitic worm that causes schistosomiasis.[68] Most skin cancers have a very low mortality rate, but **melanoma**, a cancer that originates in pigmented melanocytes in the skin, can be deadly. Most cases of malignant melanoma occur in people with pale skin who have a history of sunburns in childhood.[69] There is significant variability in the rates of **thyroid cancer** globally, but the general trend is that the rate of diagnosis is increasing but the mortality rate is decreasing.[70]

Non-Hodgkin **lymphoma** (NHL) is an immune system cancer that starts in the lymph nodes and is associated with some types of chronic infections.[71] The distribution of particular subtypes of NHL varies significantly between and within world regions.[72] **Leukemia** is a blood cancer that begins in the bone marrow where blood is produced by the body. There are many different types of leukemia, and different age groups experience different types of leukemia. Acute myelogenous leukemia (AML) and various types of chronic leukemias mostly affect older adults, while acute lymphoblastic leukemia (ALL) is the most common childhood cancer, responsible for about one-third of all cancers in children.[73] Although children younger than 15 years old probably account for less than 1% of all people with cancer worldwide, the proportion of child deaths that are attributable to cancer is increasing as deaths from infectious diseases decrease.[36] Reducing the burden of cancer on today's children as they age into adulthood and then older adulthood requires implementation of primary prevention interventions now to limit the uptake of tobacco use and excessive alcohol consumption in this population. Other interventions for preventing future cases of cancer include preventing and treating chronic infections, promoting healthy and active lifestyles, and minimizing the risks associated with occupational and environmental carcinogens.[74]

▶ References

1. Schottenfeld D, Beebe-Dimmer JL, Buffler PA, Omenn GS. Current perspective on the global and United States cancer burden attributable to lifestyle and environmental risk factors. *Annu Rev Public Health.* 2013;34:97–117.

2. Ferlay J, Soerjomataram I, Dikshit R, et al. Cancer incidence and mortality worldwide: Sources, methods and major patterns in GLOBOCAN 2012. *Int J Cancer.* 2014;136:E359–86.

3. Global Burden of Disease Cancer Collaborators. The global burden of cancer 2013. *JAMA Oncol.* 2015;1:505–27.

4. Ferlay J, Soerjomataram I, Ervik M, et al. *GLOBOCAN 2012 v1.0, Cancer incidence and mortality worldwide.* Lyon: IARC; 2013.

5. Torre LA, Siegel RL, Ward EM, Jemal A. Global cancer incidence and mortality rates and trends: An update. *Cancer Epidemiol Biomarkers Prev.* 2016;25:16–27.

6. Bray F, Ren JS, Masuyer E, Ferlay J. Global estimates of cancer prevalence for 27 sites in the adult population in 2008. *Int J Cancer.* 2012;132:1133–45.

7. *Food, nutrition, physical activity, and the prevention of cancer: A global perspective.* Washington DC: American Institute for Cancer Research/World Cancer Research Fund International; 2007.

8. Vineis P, Wild CP. Global cancer patterns: Causes and prevention. *Lancet.* 2014;383:549–57.

9. Sasco AJ, Secretan MB, Straif K. Tobacco smoking and cancer: A brief review of recent epidemiological evidence. *Lung Cancer.* 2004;45(Suppl 2):S3–9.

10. Driscoll T, Nelson DI, Steenland K, et al. The global burden of disease due to occupational carcinogens. *Am J Ind Med.* 2005;48:419–31.

11. Boffetta P, Nyberg F. Contribution of environmental factors to cancer risk. *Br Med Bull.* 2003;68:71–94.

12. Plummer M, de Martel C, Vignat J, Ferlay J, Bray F, Franceschi S. Global burden of cancers attributable to infections in 2012: A synthetic analysis. *Lancet Glob Health.* 2016;4:e609–16.

13. Oh JK, Weiderpass E. Infection and cancer: Global distribution and burden of diseases. *Ann Glob Health.* 2014;80:384–92.

14. Krieger N. Epidemiology and the web of causation: Has anyone seen the spider? *Soc Sci Med.* 1994;39:887–903.

15. Thun MJ, DeLancey JO, Center MM, Jemal A, Ward EM. The global burden of cancer: Priorities for prevention. *Carcinogenesis.* 2010;31:100–10.

16. Susser M. What is a cause and how do we know one? A grammar for pragmatic epidemiology. *Am J Epidemiol.* 1991;133:635–48.

17. Rothman KJ, Greenland S. Causation and causal inference in epidemiology. *Am J Public Health.* 2005;95(Suppl 1):S144–50.

18. *Global health risks: Mortality and burden of disease attributable to selected major risks.* Geneva: WHO; 2009.

19. Danaei G, Vander Hoorn S, Lopez AD, Murray CJ, Ezzati M; Comparative Risk Assessment collaborating group (cancers). Causes of cancer

in the world: Comparative risk assessment of nine behavioural and environmental risk factors. *Lancet.* 2005;366:1784–93.

20. *AACR cancer progress report 2016.* Philadelphia PA: American Association for Cancer Research (AACR); 2016.

21. Tomasetti C, Li L, Vogelstein B. Stem cell divisions, somatic mutations, cancer etiology, and cancer prevention. *Science.* 2017;355:1330–4.

22. Islami F, Torre LA, Jemal A. Global trends of lung cancer mortality and smoking prevalence. *Transl Lung Cancer Res.* 2015;4:327–38.

23. Sullivan T, Sullivan R, Ginsburg OM. Screening for cancer: Considerations for low- and middle-income countries (Chapter 12). *Disease control priorities.* 3rd ed. *Cancer (Volume 3).* Washington DC: IBRD/World Bank; 2015.

24. Smith RA, Manassaram-Baptiste D, Brooks D, et al. Cancer screening in the United States, 2014: A review of current American Cancer Society guidelines and current issues in cancer screening. *CA Cancer J Clin.* 2014;64:30–51.

25. Gospodarowicz M, Trypuc J, D'Cruz A, et al. Cancer services and the comprehensive cancer center (Chapter 11). *Disease control priorities.* 3rd ed. *Cancer (Volume 3).* Washington DC: IBRD/World Bank; 2015.

26. Krakauer E, Ali Z, Arreola H, et al. Palliative care in response to the global burden of remediable suffering (Chapter 12). *Disease control priorities.* 3rd ed. *Disease control priorities (Volume 9).* Washington DC: IBRD/World Bank; 2017.

27. Dare AJ, Anderson BO, Sullivan R, et al. Surgical services for cancer care (Chapter 13). *Disease control priorities.* 3rd ed. *Cancer (Volume 3).* Washington DC: IBRD/World Bank; 2015.

28. Horton S, Gauvreau CL. Cancer in low- and middle-income countries: An economic overview (Chapter 16). *Disease control priorities.* 3rd ed. *Cancer (Volume 3).* Washington DC: IBRD/World Bank; 2015.

29. Jaffray DA, Gospodarowicz MK. Radiation therapy for cancer (Chapter 14). *Disease control priorities.* 3rd ed. *Cancer (Volume 3).* Washington DC: IBRD/World Bank; 2015.

30. Gelband H, Jha P, Sankaranarayanan R, Gauvreau CL, Horton S. Summary (Chapter 1). *Disease control priorities.* 3rd ed. *Cancer (Volume 3).* Washington DC: IBRD/World Bank; 2015.

31. Torre LA, Bray F, Siegel RL, Ferlay J, Lortet-Tieulent J, Jemal A. Global cancer statistics, 2012. *CA Cancer J Clin.* 2015;65:87–108.

32. Bray F, Soerjomataram I. The changing global burden of cancer: Transitions in human development and implications for cancer prevention and control (Chapter 2). *Disease control priorities.* 3rd ed. *Cancer (Volume 3).* Washington DC: IBRD/World Bank; 2015.

33. Allemani C, Weir HK, Carreira H, et al. Global surveillance of cancer survival 1995–2009; analysis of individual data for 25,676,887 patients from 279 population-based registries in 67 countries (CONCORD-2). *Lancet.* 2015;385:977–1010.

34. Jha P, MacLennan M, Chaloupka FJ, et al. Global hazards of tobacco and the benefits of smoking cessation and tobacco taxes (Chapter 10). *Disease control priorities.* 3rd ed. *Cancer (Volume 3).* Washington DC: IBRD/World Bank; 2015.

35. Sankaranarayanan R, Ramadas K, Amarasinghe H, Subramanian S, Johnson N. Oral cancer: Prevention, early detection, and treatment (Chapter 5). *Disease control priorities.* 3rd ed. *Cancer (Volume 3).* Washington DC: IBRD/World Bank; 2015.

36. *Global cancer facts & figures.* 3rd ed. Atlanta GA: American Cancer Society; 2015.

37. Youlden DR, Cramb SM, Dunn NA, Muller JM, Pyke CM, Baade PD. The descriptive epidemiology of female breast cancer: An international comparison of screening, incidence, survival and mortality. *Cancer Epidemiol.* 2012;36:237–48.

38. Anderson BO, Lipscomb J, Murillo RH, Thomas DB. Breast cancer (Chapter 3). *Disease control priorities.* 3rd ed. *Cancer (Volume 3).* Washington DC: IBRD/World Bank; 2015.

39. Ho GY, Burk RD, Klein S, et al. Persistent genital human papillomavirus infection as a risk factor for persistent cervical dysplasia. *J Natl Cancer Inst.* 1995;87:1365–71.

40. Bulkmans NWJ, Berkhof J, Bulk S, et al. High-risk HPV type-specific clearance rates in cervical screening. *Br J Cancer.* 2007;96:1417–24.

41. Bruni L, Diaz M, Barrionuevo-Rosas L, et al. Global estimates of human papillomavirus vaccination coverage by region and income level: A pooled analysis. *Lancet Glob Health.* 2016;4:e453–63.

42. *Comprehensive cervical cancer control: A guide to essential practice.* 2nd ed. Geneva: World Health Organization; 2014.

43. Denny L, Herrero R, Levin C, Kim JJ. Cervical cancer (Chapter 4). *Disease control priorities.* 3rd ed. *Cancer (Volume 3).* Washington DC: IBRD/World Bank; 2015.

44. Lowe KA, Chia VM, Taylor A, et al. An international assessment of ovarian cancer incidence and mortality. *Gynecol Oncol.* 2013;130:107–14.

45. Amant F, Moerman P, Neven P, Timmerman D, Van Limbergen E, Vergote I. Endometrial cancer. *Lancet.* 2005;366:491–505.

46. Bostwick DB, Cooner WH, Denis L, Jones GW, Scardino PT, Murphy GP. The association of benign prostatic hyperplasia and cancer of the prostate. *Cancer.* 1992;70(1 Suppl):291–301.

47. Hsing AW, Chokkalingam AP. Prostate cancer epidemiology. *Front Biosci.* 2006;11:1388–413.

48. Haas GP, Delongchamps N, Brawley OW, Yang CY, de la Roza G. The worldwide epidemiology of prostate cancer: Perspectives from autopsy studies. *Can J Urol.* 2008;15:3866–71.

49. Center MM, Jemal A, Lortet-Tieulent J, et al. International variation in prostate cancer incidence and mortality rates. *Eur Urol.* 2012;61:1079–92.

50. Baade PD, Youlden DR, Krnjacki LJ. International epidemiology of prostate cancer: Geographical distribution and secular trends. *Mol Nutr Food Res.* 2009;53:171–84.

51. DeSantis CE, Lin CC, Mariotto AB, et al. Cancer treatment and survivorship statistics, 2014. *CA Cancer J Clin.* 2014;64:252–71.

52. *Cancer facts and figures 2016.* Atlanta GA: American Cancer Society; 2016.

53. Gelband H, Chen CJ, Chen W, et al. Liver cancer (Chapter 8). *Disease control priorities.* 3rd ed. *Cancer (Volume 3).* Washington DC: IBRD/World Bank; 2015.

54. El-Serag HB. Epidemiology of viral hepatitis and hepatocellular carcinoma. *Gastroenterology.* 2012;142:1264–73.

55. Bosetti C, Turati F, La Vecchia C. Hepatocellular carcinoma epidemiology. *Best Pract Res Clin Gastroenterol.* 2014;28:753–70.

56. Chang MH. Prevention of hepatitis A virus infection and liver cancer. *Recent Results Cancer Res.* 2014;193:75–95.

57. Franco E, Bagnato B, Marino MG, et al. Epidemiology and prevention in developing countries. *World J Hepatol.* 2012;4:74–80.

58. Rustgi AK, El-Serag HB. Esophageal carcinoma. *New Engl J Med.* 2014;371:2499–509.

59. de Martel C, Forman D, Plummer M. Gastric cancer: Epidemiology and risk factors. *Gastroenterol Clin N Am.* 2013;42:219–40.

60. Karimi P, Islami F, Anandasabapathy S, Freedman ND, Kamangar F. Gastric cancer: Descriptive epidemiology, risk factors, screening, and prevention. *Cancer Epidemiol Biomarkers Prev.* 2014;23:700–13.

61. Center MM, Jemal A, Smith RA, Ward E. Worldwide variations in colorectal cancer. *CA Cancer J Clin.* 2009;59:366–78.

62. Vargas AJ, Thompson PA. Diet and nutrient factors in colorectal cancer risk. *Nutr Clin Pract.* 2012;27:613–23.

63. Rabeneck L, Horton S, Zauber AG, Earle C. Colorectal cancer (Chapter 6). *Disease control priorities.* 3rd ed. *Cancer (Volume 3).* Washington DC: IBRD/World Bank; 2015.

64. Znaor A, Lortet-Tieulent J, Laversanne M, Jemal A, Bray F. International variations and trends in renal cell carcinoma incidence and mortality. *Eur Urol.* 2015;67:519–30.

65. Chow WH, Dong LM, Devesa SS. Epidemiology and risk factors for kidney cancer. *Nat Rev Urol.* 2010;7:245–57.

66. Raimondi S, Maisonneuve P, Lowenfels AB. Epidemiology of pancreatic cancer: An overview. *Nat Rev Gastroenterol Hepatol.* 2009;6:699–708.

67. Boffetta P. Tobacco smoking and risk of bladder cancer. *Scand J Urol Nephrol Suppl.* 2008;42(218):45–54.

68. Parkin DM. The global burden of urinary bladder cancer. *Scand J Urol Nephrol Suppl.* 2008;42(218):12–20.

69. Erdmann F, Lortet-Tieulent J, Schüz J, et al. International trends in the incidence of malignant melanoma 1953–2008: Are recent generations at higher or lower risk? *Int J Cancer.* 2013;132:385–400.

70. La Vecchia C, Malvezzi M, Bosetti C, et al. Thyroid cancer mortality and incidence: A global review. *Int J Cancer.* 2015;136:2187–95.

71. Shankland KR, Armitage JO, Hancock BW. Non-Hodgkin lymphoma. *Lancet.* 2012;380:848–57.

72. Müller AM, Ihorst G, Mertelsmann R, Engelhardt M. Epidemiology of non-Hodgkin's lymphoma (NHL): Trends, geographic distribution, and etiology. *Ann Hematol.* 2005;84:1–12.

73. Rodriguez-Abreu D, Bordoni A, Zucca E. Epidemiology of hematological malignancies. *Ann Oncol.* 2007;18(Suppl 1):i3–8.

74. Steward BW, Wild CP, editors. *World cancer report 2014.* Lyon: International Agency for Research on Cancer (IARC), WHO; 2014.

CHAPTER 14

Cardiovascular Diseases

Heart attacks, strokes, and other cardiovascular diseases are the leading cause of death in both men and women in every region of the world. They are also major contributors to disability and reduced quality of life. More than one-third of all deaths from cardiovascular diseases occur in people who are younger than 70 years old. Many of these cases of premature mortality could be prevented with increased access to medications that control hypertension and reduce cholesterol levels, smoking cessation tools, healthy nutrition, and other low-cost interventions.

▶ 14.1 Cardiovascular Disease and Global Health

A **cardiovascular disease (CVD)** is a disorder of the heart or blood vessels. The heart is the organ responsible for pumping blood throughout the body. Deoxygenated blood is returned through the vena cava to the right atrium of the heart, passes through the right ventricle, and is pumped to the lungs, where gas exchange occurs. After carbon dioxide and other wastes have been removed from the blood and oxygen has been added to the blood, the oxygenated blood is returned through the pulmonary veins to the left atrium of the heart, passes through the left ventricle, and is delivered to the rest of the body via the aorta. Arteries carry blood away from the heart, and veins carry blood back to the heart. Any problem with the structure or function of the heart or the major blood vessels can have detrimental effects on the whole body.

There are three key reasons why CVD is a concern shared by every country in the world: CVD is the most common cause of death for both men and women in nearly every country; the disability caused by common cardiovascular diseases like heart attacks and strokes is very expensive for families and nations; and much of the burden from CVD is preventable.

One in three deaths worldwide—about 18 million deaths each year—is attributable to cardiovascular diseases.[1] CVD is the #1 cause of mortality for women as well as for men, and there is a heavy burden from CVD in both high-income and low-income regions of the world (**FIGURE 14–1**). The prevalence of CVD increases with age. The overall (all-ages) CVD mortality rate per 100,000 residents is highest in high-income countries because those countries have the highest proportion of older adults in their populations. When mortality statistics are adjusted by applying the age-specific rates in each country to the global population and then calculating an age-standardized rate for each country, the adjusted mortality rates for CVD are higher in low- and middle-income

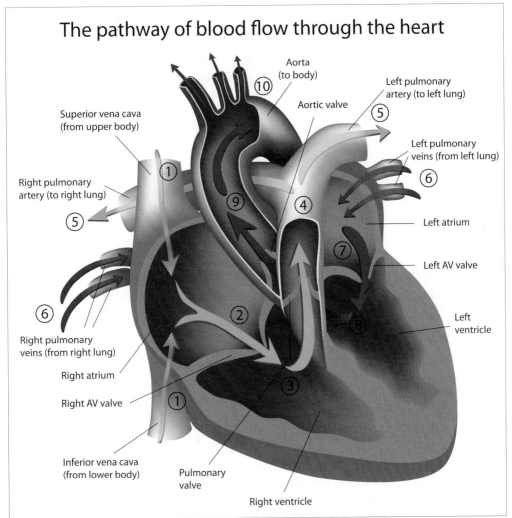

The pathway of blood flow through the heart

Aorta
(to body)

Left pulmonary
artery (to left lung)

Aortic valve

Superior vena cava
(from upper body)

Left pulmonary
veins (from left lung)

Right pulmonary
artery (to right lung)

Left atrium

Left AV valve

Right pulmonary
veins (from right lung)

Left
ventricle

Right atrium

Right AV valve

Inferior vena cava
(from lower body)

Pulmonary
valve

Right ventricle

© Alila Medical Media/Shutterstock

countries than in high-income countries (**FIGURE 14–2**).[1]

Globally, the age-standardized CVD mortality rate decreased slightly between 1990 and 2015. However, the number of deaths from CVD continued to increase because the total number of adults worldwide increased.[2] If most of the people dying from CVD were very old, the rise in the number of CVD deaths might not be considered problematic. Many adults report that their preference is to die in their sleep, without pain or suffering.[3] By this standard, dying quickly from a heart attack

or stroke would be considered preferable to a slow death from cancer, chronic respiratory diseases, or diabetes (or death after a long period of disability resulting from a CVD). If CVD fatalities always occurred among very old adults, then increasing the percentage of deaths that are attributable to CVD rather than to less preferred causes of death could be considered a public health improvement. That is not what is observed. More than one-third of CVD deaths occur in young and middle-aged adults (**FIGURE 14–3**). About 2% of people who die from CVD are in their 30s, about 5% are in

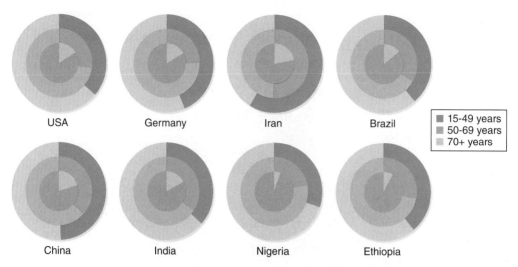

USA Germany Iran Brazil

■ 15-49 years
■ 50-69 years
■ 70+ years

China India Nigeria Ethiopia

FIGURE 14–1 CVD is the most common cause of adult mortality worldwide. This figure shows the percentage of deaths by age group that are due to CVD.

Data from GBD Mortality and Causes of Death Collaborators. Global, regional, and national life expectancy, all-cause mortality, and cause-specific mortality for 249 causes of death, 1980–2015: A systematic analysis for the Global Burden of Disease Study 2015. *Lancet* 2016; 388:1459-544.

their 40s, about 10% are in their 50s, and about 18% are in their 60s.[1] Only 63% of CVD deaths occur in people who are 70 years old or older. About 10.8% of 30-year-old men and 6.7% of 30-year-old women will die from CVD before their 70th birthdays.[2] Those individuals are dying prematurely, and preventing premature deaths is a global health priority. Specifically, the Sustainable Development Goals (SDGs) aim to "reduce by one-third premature mortality from noncommunicable diseases through prevention and treatment" by 2030 (SDG 3.4).[4]

Public health is not just about preventing premature mortality. It is also about promoting healthy lives and avoiding preventable disability. CVD contributes significantly to reduced health status in many adults. Most people with CVD do not live symptom-free and then, with no warning, drop dead from a heart attack or stroke. Nonfatal cardiovascular events may cause long-term impairment. People with **heart failure**, a chronic condition in which the heart is not able to pump enough blood to meet the body's need for oxygen,[5] may have symptoms like fatigue and shortness of breath that reduce their quality of life for many years.[6] People with **peripheral artery**

disease (PAD) have narrowed blood vessels that impair blood circulation and can cause severe leg pain and cramping when walking (a symptom called claudication).[7] Heart attack survivors may require months of rehabilitation and never regain the stamina they had before the infarction. Stroke victims may be permanently bedridden and unable to speak. CVD is expensive for affected individuals who incur healthcare expenses and cannot work, for family members who are physically and financially caring for relatives with CVD-related disability, and for communities and nations that provide social services and health care for people with long-term CVD.[8] Each year, CVD already costs the world more than $900 billion, including more than $400 billion in direct healthcare costs and about $500 billion in lost productivity. The annual costs of CVD will exceed $1 trillion by 2030.[9]

Much of the global burden from CVD could be prevented. About half of all CVD deaths—nearly 10 million deaths each year, including millions of deaths considered to be premature deaths based on the age of the deceased—are attributable to modifiable risk factors: uncontrolled hypertension (high blood

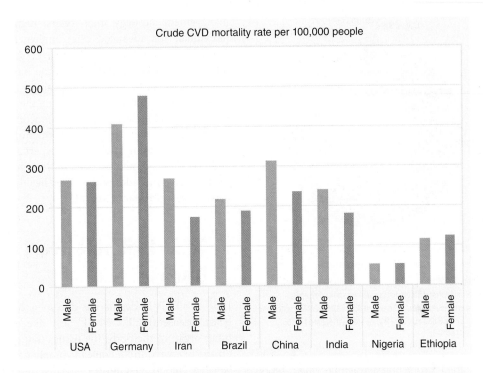

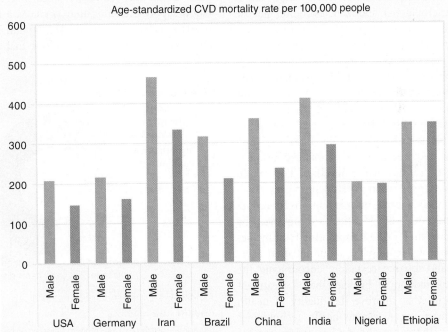

FIGURE 14–2 For people of the same age, the CVD mortality rate is usually higher in low- and middle-income countries than in high-income countries.

Data from GBD Mortality and Causes of Death Collaborators. Global, regional, and national life expectancy, all-cause mortality, and cause-specific mortality for 249 causes of death, 1980–2015: A systematic analysis for the Global Burden of Disease Study 2015. *Lancet* 2016; 388:1459-544.

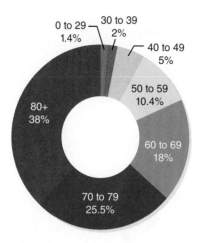

FIGURE 14–3 Percentage of global deaths from cardiovascular disease by age group.

Data from GBD Mortality and Causes of Death Collaborators. Global, regional, and national life expectancy, all-cause mortality, and cause-specific mortality for 249 causes of death, 1980–2015: A systematic analysis for the Global Burden of Disease Study 2015. *Lancet* 2016; 388:1459-544.

pressure), hypercholesterolemia (high blood cholesterol levels), and diabetes (blood glucose levels); tobacco use; a high body mass index (overweight and obesity); and the major behavioral contributors to these conditions, including physical inactivity and a diet high in salt, alcohol, processed meat, and trans fats and low in fruits, vegetables, fiber, and whole grains.[10] Mitigating these risk factors for CVD requires individuals to adopt healthier lifestyles,[11] and it also requires access to enhanced primary care for cardiovascular health.[12] The World Health Organization (WHO) promotes a six-component package of interventions for reducing the burden of CVD that is summarized by the acronym HEARTS: promoting Healthy lifestyles through counseling about nutrition, exercise, and tobacco cessation; encouraging the implementation of Evidence-based treatment protocols that improve the quality of health care; ensuring Access to health technologies (like stethoscopes and devices for measuring blood pressure) and essential medicines (like aspirin, cholesterol-lowering statins, and anti-hypertensive medications); using a Risk-based

management strategy that refers high-risk individuals for advanced care; implementing Team care and task-sharing in which community health workers support advanced medical professionals; and developing Systems for monitoring patient outcomes.[13] Achieving the SDG target of reducing the burden from noncommunicable diseases will require substantial investments in preventing and treating hypertension and CVD-related medical conditions, reducing tobacco use, and addressing other health and behavioral contributors to CVD.[14]

▶ 14.2 Ischemic Heart Disease

Half of all CVD deaths are due to ischemic heart disease (**FIGURE 14–4**).[1] Just like every other organ in the body, the tissues that make up the heart require a constant supply of oxygenated blood. **Ischemia** means reduced blood supply. Ischemia may occur as a result of **atherosclerosis**, the thickening and hardening of the walls of the arteries that carry

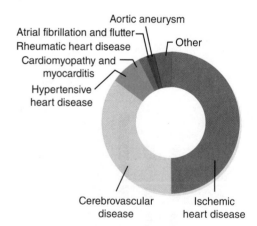

FIGURE 14–4 Distribution of causes of death from cardiovascular diseases.

Data from GBD Mortality and Causes of Death Collaborators. Global, regional, and national life expectancy, all-cause mortality, and cause-specific mortality for 249 causes of death, 1980–2015: A systematic analysis for the Global Burden of Disease Study 2015. *Lancet* 2016; 388:1459-544.

STAGES OF ATHEROSCLEROSIS

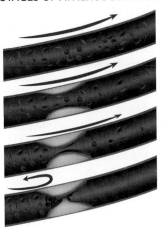

Healthy artery

Build-up begins

Plaque forms

Plaque ruptures; blood clot forms

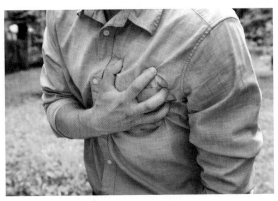

Anatomy of a heart attack

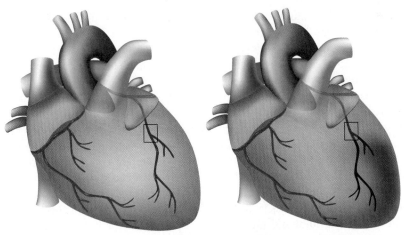

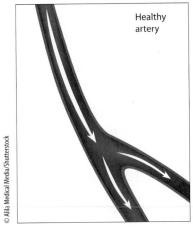

Healthy artery

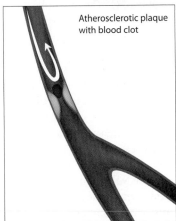

Atherosclerotic plaque with blood clot

oxygen-rich blood from the heart to the rest of the body, including to the heart muscle itself. As atherosclerotic plaque narrows the diameter of those blood vessels, the blood supply to the tissues fed by those arteries becomes limited. **Ischemic heart disease** (IHD), also called **coronary artery disease** (CAD) or coronary heart disease, occurs when atherosclerosis occurs in the arteries that provide blood to the heart, reducing blood flow to the heart muscle.[15]

The initial symptom of IHD might be **angina**, which is chest pain or tightness caused by the heart muscle not getting an adequate supply of oxygen. A **myocardial infarction**, or heart attack, happens when a blood vessel becomes mostly or fully occluded, either due to atherosclerosis or to blood clots forming on the plaque surface in an atherosclerotic vessel, and a portion of the heart muscle dies due to lack of oxygen.[16] In high-income countries, people with IHD may undergo **angioplasty** to physically open and unclog a blocked artery, or they may have **bypass surgery** that uses a healthy blood vessel from another part of the body to restore blood flow to the heart muscle by bypassing the damaged area. These surgical therapies are rarely available in low-income countries.

The best way to reduce the costs of IHD for individuals and for health systems is to invest in prevention. The major risk factors for IHD are the same behavioral and metabolic factors that apply to CVD as a whole: inactive lifestyles and unmanaged comorbidities like hypertension, elevated blood glucose levels, and hypercholesterolemia.[10] Medications can control high blood pressure, stabilize blood sugar levels in people with type 2 diabetes, and reduce blood levels of **cholesterol**, a waxy lipid (fat) that is a major component of the plaque that causes atherosclerosis. The medications deemed essential for cardiovascular health include antianginal agents that relax the muscles in the walls of arteries to increase blood flow, antiarrhythmic agents, antihypertensive agents, antithrombotic agents (blood thinners) like aspirin, and lipid-lowering

agents.[17] Many low- and middle-income countries do not yet have reliable stocks of all of these types of medications, but a variety of options are available for working with global partners to increase access to quality medications.[18] Health education provided to individuals and groups through community health organizations can help people become aware of their risk factors, adopt and sustain healthier behaviors, and access the medications they need to lower the risk of a heart attack.[19]

▶ **14.3 Cerebrovascular Disease (Strokes)**

Cerebrovascular disease is characterized by reduced blood flow to the brain. A **stroke** happens when cells in the brain die due to lack of oxygen.[20] The typical symptoms of a stroke include weakness on one or both sides of the face and body, confusion, trouble speaking (expressive aphasia) or understanding language (receptive aphasia), vision disturbances, a loss of balance, and a severe headache.

There are two common pathologic processes that cause strokes: ischemia and hemorrhage. An **ischemic stroke** occurs when a blocked blood vessel cuts off blood flow to a portion of the brain. This is a similar process to the pathology of heart attacks. Many ischemic strokes are due to blood clots in the blood vessels of the brain. Ischemic strokes are often preceded by **transient ischemic attacks (TIAs)**, sometimes called ministrokes or warning strokes, in which a temporary blockage of an artery causes stroke-like symptoms that quickly resolve. These episodes are signs that a person is at imminent risk of a severe stroke. The symptoms of an ischemic stroke are often permanent when the affected individual does not receive clot-busting intravenous thrombolytic medications within hours of the onset of an ischemic stroke.[13]

Brain Stroke

Ischemic Stroke

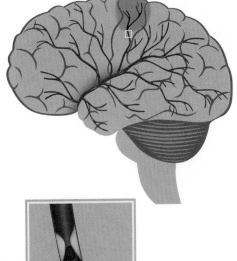

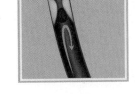

Blockage of blood vessels; lack of blood flow to affected area

Hemorrhagic Stroke

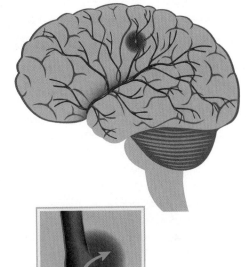

Rupture of blood vessels; leakage of blood

© Allia Medical Media/Shutterstock

A **hemorrhagic stroke** occurs when a blood vessel ruptures and causes bleeding in the brain. Globally, more people have ischemic strokes each year than hemorrhagic strokes, but the proportion of strokes that are due to hemorrhage rather than ischemia is not uniform across countries.[21] Because there is a higher case fatality rate for hemorrhagic strokes than for ischemic strokes,[22] the countries that have a higher proportion of strokes that are hemorrhagic tend to have higher death rates from stroke.

The relative burden from heart attacks and strokes also varies by country. In China, some other parts of Asia, and sub-Saharan Africa, the age-adjusted rates of death from strokes are often similar to or higher than the rates of death from IHD (**FIGURE 14–5**).[2] By contrast, in most high-income countries, strokes are a much less common cause of death than IHD.[1]

A large proportion of the global burden from stroke is attributed to modifiable risk factors, including health behaviors, metabolic conditions, and environmental exposures like air pollution.[23] One of the most well-established risk factors for stroke is uncontrolled high blood pressure.[24] Antihypertensive medications are a key component of primary prevention of stroke, along with the other common elements of CVD prevention plans.[25] For people who have already had strokes, access to emergency medical care and long-term rehabilitation is important for allowing the greatest chances for regaining function.[26] Rehabilitative care is scarce in most low- and middle-income countries,[27] and it is costly in most high-income countries.[28] More than half of stroke survivors have persistent physical and/or cognitive impairment.[26]

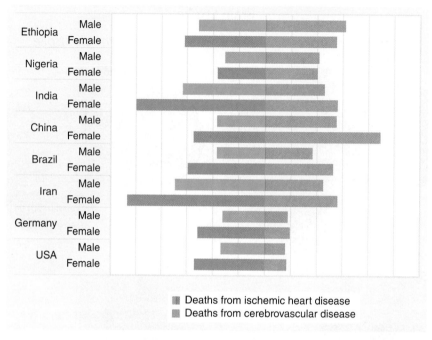

Deaths from ischemic heart disease
Deaths from cerebrovascular disease

FIGURE 14–5 Comparison of age-standardized mortality rates from ischemic heart disease (left) and cerebrovascular disease (right).

Data from GBD Mortality and Causes of Death Collaborators. Global, regional, and national life expectancy, all-cause mortality, and cause-specific mortality for 249 causes of death, 1980–2015: A systematic analysis for the Global Burden of Disease Study 2015. *Lancet* 2016; 388:1459-544.

▶ 14.4 Hypertension

Blood pressure is typically reported as a ratio of two numbers, like 110/70 or 130/85. The top number is the **systolic blood pressure** (SBP), the pressure in the blood vessels when the heart beats. The bottom number is the **diastolic blood pressure** (DBP), the pressure in the blood vessels when the heart is at rest between beats. The units are "millimeters of mercury" (mm Hg), a measurement of pressure. **Hypertension** is high blood pressure, and it is typically defined as having an SBP of 140 mm Hg or higher and/or a DBP of 90 or higher.[29]

Hypertension is common among both men and women worldwide (**FIGURE 14–6**).[30] About one in four men (24%) and one in five women (20%) has uncontrolled hypertension.[31] The rates of hypertension are even higher when adults taking medications to reduce their blood pressures are added to the calculations, with about 32% of men and 30% of women having hypertension.[32] Blood pressure typically increases with age (**FIGURE 14–7**).[33] Hypertension usually has no symptoms that are apparent to the individual with high blood pressure, but uncontrolled

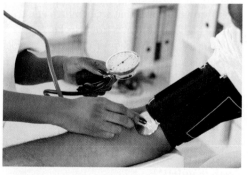

© Andrey_Popov/Shutterstock

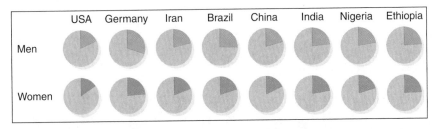

FIGURE 14–6 Hypertension is common among adults worldwide. This figure presents the age-standardized percentage of adults (aged 18+ years) with a systolic blood pressure of ≥140 mm Hg and/or a diastolic blood pressure of ≥90 mm Hg.

Data from Global status report on noncommunicable *diseases 2014*. Geneva: World Health Organization; 2014.

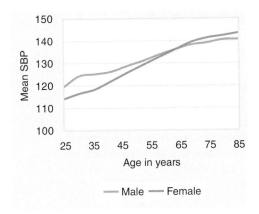

FIGURE 14–7 The mean systolic blood pressure increases with age.

Data from Forouzanfar MH, Liu P, Roth GA, et al. Global burden of hypertension and systolic blood pressure of at least 110 to 115 mm Hg, 1990–2015. *JAMA* 2017; 317:165-82.

hypertension significantly increases the risk of having a stroke. It also increases the likelihood of angina, heart attacks, heart failure, aneurysms, kidney failure, sexual dysfunction, and vision loss.[34]

Hypertension can be reduced to healthier levels with medications. More than 55% of people with high blood pressure who live in high-income countries take antihypertensive medication, but only about 30% of people with hypertension who live in low- and middle-income countries receive medications to reduce their blood pressure.[32] Ideally, this number would be 100% in all countries.

In high-income countries, the increased use of antihypertensive medications has led to a decrease in the mean SBP. In low- and middle-income countries, where these medications are not widely used, the mean SBP is increasing (**FIGURE 14–8**).[33]

Other strategies for reducing blood pressure include maintaining a healthy weight, exercising, avoiding tobacco and excess intake of alcohol, and reducing the amount of salt in the diet. The sodium in salt (sodium chloride) is associated with higher blood pressures, and reducing salt consumption helps control hypertension.[35] A lot of the salt that people consume comes from processed foods rather than from adding salt into their foods at mealtimes. Without being able to check food labels, people may not be aware of how much sodium they are ingesting. The SHAKE package of policies recommended by the WHO promotes salt intake of less than 5 grams per day via Surveillance of salt use; Harnessing industry to reduce salt in processed and prepared foods; Adopting standards for labeling and marketing; improving Knowledge about the value of low salt intakes; and developing a supportive Environment for healthy eating.[36]

Recent science suggests that it is healthiest to have an SBP below 115 mm Hg, which is significantly below the 140 mm Hg threshold for a hypertension diagnosis.[37] Blood pressure checks are one of the many health screening tests for which there is no obvious cutoff point

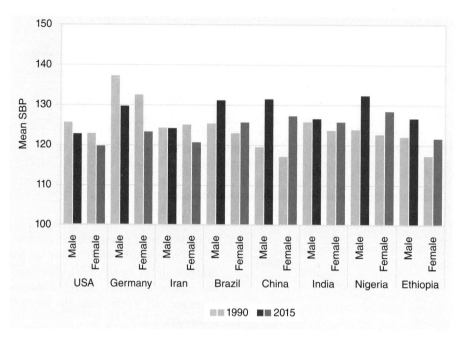

FIGURE 14-8 The age-standardized mean systolic blood pressure is decreasing in most high-income countries (because of antihypertensive medication use) and is increasing in most low- and middle-income countries.

Data from Forouzanfar MH, Liu P, Roth GA, et al. Global burden of hypertension and systolic blood pressure of at least 110 to 115 mm Hg, 1990–2015. *JAMA* 2017; 317:165-82.

to distinguish between a person with disease and a person without disease. Using an SBP cutoff of 130 mm Hg, or an even lower number, would result in a much higher prevalence of hypertension than using a cutoff of 140 mm Hg. For diseases with no treatment or with treatment that is expensive and potentially harmful, it is better to avoid false positive diagnoses by having a high threshold for declaring that a person has the condition. For diseases like hypertension that can often be easily managed and for which early intervention can prevent serious complications, it is better to have a low threshold for classifying an individual with a borderline test result as having the disease. In the past, the recommended cutoff for classifying a person as having hypertension was an SBP of 160 mm Hg or above. In the future, the threshold may be reduced to below 140 mm Hg.

▶ 14.5 Other Cardiovascular Diseases

Numerous other types of CVDs also contribute to disability and death worldwide.[38] An **aortic aneurysm** is a bulge in the aorta that can rupture and cause a rapid death from internal bleeding. **Cardiomyopathy** is a disease of the heart muscles that causes the heart to enlarge and become weaker. Cardiomyopathy is a common cause of heart failure. In dilated cardiomyopathy, the volume of the atria and ventricles inside the heart becomes larger as the heart muscle stretches out and thins. In hypertrophic cardiomyopathy, the cells in the heart muscle get bigger and the resulting thickening of the tissue may restrict blood flow through the heart. The cause of cardiomyopathy is often unknown, but some cases are inherited.[39]

Inflammation of the heart muscle is called carditis. **Rheumatic heart disease** is an inflammatory condition that causes irreversible damage to the heart and heart valves as a result of an untreated infection with group A *Streptococcus*, like strep throat or scarlet fever.[40] Most cases of rheumatic fever occur in children and adolescents.[41] Some types of carditis affect particular layers of the heart. The walls of the heart are composed of three layers of muscle: the endocardium on the inside, the myocardium in the middle, and the epicardium on the outside. Endocarditis is an inflammation of the inside of the heart that can cause damage to the heart valves. Myocarditis is inflammation of the myocardium that is typically caused by a viral infection.[42] Pericarditis is an inflammation of the fibrous sac that surrounds the heart.

An arrhythmia is an abnormal heartbeat that is too fast (tachycardia), too slow (bradycardia), or irregularly paced. The most common arrhythmia is **atrial fibrillation**, which occurs when the atria (the upper chambers of the heart) quiver fast and irregularly rather than contracting and relaxing at a regular pace.[43] People with atrial fibrillation may form blood clots in the heart because the blood stagnates in the atria instead of quickly being moved out of those chambers. If these clots enter the bloodstream and block a vessel in the brain, the blockage can cause a stroke. Use of blood thinning medications is recommended for people with atrial fibrillation to reduce the risk of stroke. While some of these arrhythmias occur because of the presence of other cardiovascular conditions, many cases present in people who are otherwise healthy. Ventricular tachycardia, in which the ventricles (the lower chambers of the heart) begin contracting extremely rapidly, can cause sudden death from cardiac arrest. The automated external defibrillators (AEDs) available in many public places in high-income countries are intended to save the lives of people who collapse due to a bout of ventricular tachycardia. Cardiac arrest is an "electrical" problem, in contrast to the "plumbing" problems that cause heart attacks. Both "electrical" and "plumbing" problems are major contributors to disease burden in countries across the income spectrum.

► References

1. GBD 2015 Mortality and Causes of Death Collaborators. Global, regional, and national life expectancy, all-cause mortality, and cause-specific mortality for 249 causes of death, 1980–2015: A systematic analysis for the Global Burden of Disease Study 2015. *Lancet.* 2016;388:1459–544.
2. Roth GA, Huffman MD, Moran AE, et al. Global and regional patterns in cardiovascular mortality from 1990 to 2013. *Circulation.* 2015;132:1667–78.
3. Meier EA, Gallegos JV, Thomas LP, Depp CA, Irwin SA, Jeste DV. Defining a good death (successful dying): Literature review and a call for research and public dialogue. *Am J Geriatr Psychiatry.* 2016;24:261–71.
4. United Nations. *Transforming our world: The 2030 Agenda for Sustainable Development.* New York: UN; 2015.
5. Huffman M, Roth G, Sliwa K, Yancy C, Prabhakaran D. Heart failure (Chapter 10). *Disease control priorities.* 3rd ed. *Cardiovascular, respiratory, and related diseases (Volume 5).* Washington DC: IBRD/World Bank; 2017.
6. Krum H, Abraham WT. Heart failure. *Lancet.* 2009;373:941–55.
7. Fowkes G, Naidoo N, Criqui M. Peripheral artery disease (Chapter 14). *Disease control priorities.* 3rd ed. *Cardiovascular, respiratory, and related diseases (Volume 5).* Washington DC: IBRD/World Bank; 2017.
8. Abejunde DO, Mathers CD, Adam T, Ortegon M, Strong K. The burden and costs of chronic diseases in low-income and middle-income countries. *Lancet.* 2007;370:1929–38.
9. Reddy S, Riahi F, Dorling G, Callahan R, Patel H. *Innovative approaches to prevention: Tackling the global burden of cardiovascular disease.* Doha: World Innovation Summit for Health; 2016.
10. Tzoulaki I, Elliott P, Kontis V, Ezzati M. Worldwide exposures to cardiovascular risk factors and associated health effects: Current knowledge and data gaps. *Circulation.* 2016;133:2314–33.
11. *Global atlas on cardiovascular disease prevention and control.* Geneva: WHO/World Heart Federation/World Stroke Organization; 2011.
12. Schwalm JD, McKee M, Huffman MD, Yusuf S. Resource effective strategies to prevent and treat cardiovascular disease. *Circulation.* 2016;133:742–55.

13. *Hearts: Technical package for cardiovascular disease management in primary health care.* Geneva: WHO; 2016.

14. Roth GA, Nguyen G, Forouzanfar MH, Mokdad AH, Naghavi M, Murray CJL. Estimates of the global and regional premature cardiovascular mortality in 2025. *Circulation.* 2015;132:1270–82.

15. Dugani C, Moran A, Bonow R, Gaziano T. Ischemic heart disease: Cost-effective acute management and secondary prevention (Chapter 8). *Disease control priorities.* 3rd ed. *Cardiovascular, respiratory, and related diseases (Volume 5).* Washington DC: IBRD/World Bank; 2017.

16. Reed GW, Rossi JE, Cannon CP. Acute myocardial infarction. *Lancet.* 2017;389:197–210.

17. *WHO model list of essential medicines (19th list).* Geneva: WHO; 2015.

18. Wirtz VJ, Kaplan WA, Kwan GF, Laing RO. Access to medications for cardiovascular diseases in low- and middle-income countries. *Circulation.* 2016;133:2076–85.

19. Yan L, Li C, Chen J, et al. Stroke (Chapter 9). *Disease control priorities.* 3rd ed. *Cardiovascular, respiratory, and related diseases (Volume 5).* Washington DC: IBRD/World Bank; 2017.

20. Prabhakaran S, Ruff I, Bernstein RA. Acute stroke intervention: A systematic review. *JAMA.* 2015;313:1451–62.

21. Roth GA, Johnson C, Abajobir A, et al. Global, regional, and national burden of cardiovascular diseases for 10 causes, 1990 to 2015. *J Am Coll Cardiol.* 2017;70:1–25.

22. Andersen KK, Skyhøj Olsen T, Dehlendorff C, Kammersgaard LP. Hemorrhagic and ischemic strokes compared: Stroke severity, mortality, and risk factors. *Stroke.* 2009;40:2068–72.

23. Feigin VL, Roth GA, Naghavi M, et al. Global burden of stroke and risk factors in 188 countries, during 1990–2013: A systematic analysis for the Global Burden of Disease Study 2013. *Lancet Neurol.* 2016;15:913–24.

24. Lawes CMM, Bennett Da, Feigin VL, Rodgers A. Blood pressure and stroke: An overview of published reviews. *Stroke.* 2004;35:776–85.

25. Strong K, Mathers C, Bonita R. Preventing stroke: Saving lives around the world. *Lancet Neurol.* 2007;6:182–7.

26. Teasell R, Hussein N, Foley N, Cotoi A. *Evidence-based review of stroke rehabilitation.* London, ON: Canadian Partnership for Stroke Recovery; 2015.

27. Brainin M, Teuschl Y, Kalra L. Acute treatment and long-term management of stroke in developing countries. *Lancet Neurol.* 2007;6:553–61.

28. Di Carlo A. Human and economic burden of stroke. *Age Ageing.* 2009;38:4–5.

29. Poulter NR, Prabhakaran D, Caulfield M. Hypertension. *Lancet.* 2015;386:801–12.

30. *Global status report on noncommunicable diseases 2014.* Geneva: World Health Organization; 2014.

31. NCD Risk Factor Collaboration (NCD-RisC). Worldwide trends in blood pressure from 1975 to 2015: A pooled analysis of 1479 population-based measurement studies with 19.1 million participants. *Lancet.* 2017;389:37–55.

32. Mills KT, Bundy JD, Kelly TN, et al. Global disparities of hypertension prevalence and control: A systematic analysis of population-based studies from 90 countries. *Circulation.* 2016; 134:441–50.

33. Forouzanfar MH, Liu P, Roth GA, et al. Global burden of hypertension and systolic blood pressure of at least 110 to 115 mm Hg, 1990–2015. *JAMA.* 2017;317:165–82.

34. *A global brief on hypertension: Silent killer, global public health crisis.* Geneva: WHO; 2013.

35. Sacks FM, Svetkey LP, Vollmer WM, et al. Effects on blood pressure of reduced dietary sodium and the Dietary Approaches to Stop Hypertension (DASH) diet. *N Engl J Med.* 2001;344:3–10.

36. *The SHAKE technical package for salt reduction.* Geneva: WHO; 2016.

37. Rapsomaniki E, Timmis A, George J, et al. Blood pressure and incidence of twelve cardiovascular diseases: Lifetime risks, healthy life-years lost, and age-specific associations in 1.25 million people. *Lancet.* 2014;383:1899–1911.

38. Watkins D, Hasan B, Mayosi B, et al. Structural heart disease (Chapter 11). *Disease control priorities.* 3rd ed. *Cardiovascular, respiratory, and related diseases (Volume 5).* Washington DC: IBRD/World Bank; 2017.

39. Seidman JG, Seidman C. The genetic basis for cardiomyopathy: From mutation identification to mechanistic paradigms. *Cell.* 2001;104:557–67.

40. Marijon E, Mirabel M, Celermajer DS, Jouven X. Rheumatic heart disease. *Lancet.* 2012;379:953–64.

41. Zühlke L, Karthikeyan G, Engel ME, et al. Clinical outcomes in 3343 children and adults with rheumatic heart disease from 14 low- and middle-income countries: Two-year follow-up of the Global Rheumatic Heart Disease Registry (the REMEDY Study). *Circulation.* 2016;134:1456–66.

42. Oakley CM. Myocarditis, pericarditis and other pericardial diseases. *Heart.* 2000;84:449–54.

43. Lip GYH, Tse HF, Lane DA. Atrial fibrillation. *Lancet.* 2012;379:648–61.

CHAPTER 15

Other Noncommunicable Diseases

When interventions targeted at children and young adults enable more people to live to older ages, the population-level burden from noncommunicable diseases (NCDs) increases. Chronic respiratory diseases, diabetes, chronic kidney disease, cirrhosis, and other NCDs are responsible for many early deaths in countries of all income levels. Nonfatal NCDs like migraines, lower back pain, arthritis, sensory disorders, and dental problems can cause significant reductions in quality of life. Behavior change, medications, tobacco control policies, and other interventions can facilitate healthy aging and reduce the disability associated with NCDs.

▶ 15.1 The Epidemiologic Transition and Global Health

The goal of public health is not to prevent death. Everyone will eventually die of something. The goal of public health is to prevent premature death—death before late adulthood—while promoting health across the lifespan. The **epidemiologic transition** (also called the epidemiological transition) is a shift from infectious diseases to chronic noncommunicable diseases being the primary cause of deaths and disability in a population. In pre-transition populations, the burden of disease falls heavily on children, with children accounting for a large percentage of deaths. In post-transition populations, most

deaths occur in older adults (**FIGURE 15–1**).[2] The epidemiologic transition often follows the demographic transition as the economic status of a population improves, the fertility rate decreases, the infant and child survival rates improve, and the population ages.[1] Moving the burden of illness, disability, and death from children and young adults to older adults is considered to be a good population-level health outcome.

Noncommunicable diseases (NCDs) are conditions that are not contagious, such as heart disease and other cardiovascular diseases (CVDs), cancers, chronic respiratory diseases, diabetes and other endocrine and metabolic disorders, kidney diseases, liver and digestive diseases, musculoskeletal and skin diseases, and some neurological and psychiatric disorders. Most noncommunicable conditions are chronic diseases that develop gradually and

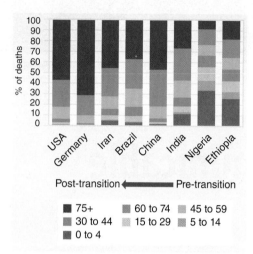

FIGURE 15–1 Percentage of deaths by age in featured countries (2015).

Data from United Nations Department of Economic and Social Affairs. *World population prospects: The 2017 revision.* New York: UN; 2017.

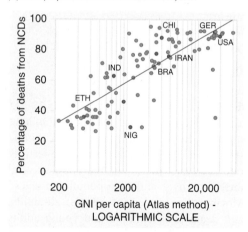

FIGURE 15–2 Higher gross national income per capita is associated with a higher percentage of deaths from NCDs. (The dots represent the 100 most populous countries. Note the use of the logarithmic scale on the x-axis.)

Data from *World development indicators 2016* (Table 2.20). Washington: World Bank; 2016.

last for a long time. The percentage of deaths from NCDs in a population generally increases with economic growth (**FIGURE 15–2**). Better economies facilitate longer life spans, and older adults in all countries usually die from NCDs (**FIGURE 15–3**).[3]

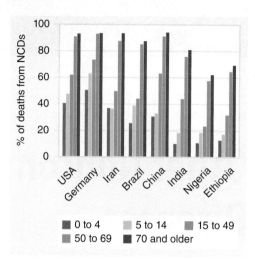

FIGURE 15–3 NCDs are the most common cause of death for older adults in every country (2015).

Data from GBD Mortality and Causes of Death Collaborators. Global, regional, and national life expectancy, all-cause mortality, and cause-specific mortality for 249 causes of death, 1980–2015: A systematic analysis for the Global Burden of Disease Study 2015. *Lancet* 2016; 388:1459–544.

Epidemiologic transition theory does not specify the economic threshold that triggers the increase of NCDs. It also does not provide details about the time line for the transition or the particular NCDs that become prominent at different times during the process. However, the epidemiologic transition does accurately describe the general trends observed in global health.[4] In high-income countries, the vast majority of deaths are attributable to NCDs (**FIGURE 15–4**).[3] In the lowest-income countries, infectious diseases of childhood remain a higher public health priority than NCDs in older adults. In most middle-income countries (and in some low-income countries), a transition toward a higher burden from NCDs has occurred over the past 25 years (**FIGURE 15–5**).[3] During these years of transition, many countries are experiencing a dual burden of disease (sometimes called a double burden), as children in some low-income communities within the country continue to have a significant burden from infectious diseases while many adults across the country experience a significant burden from NCDs.

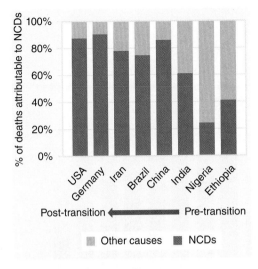

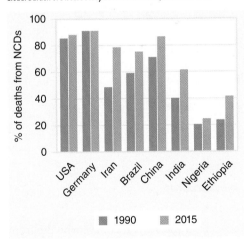

Health transitions theory helpfully highlights two important principles of global public health. One is the powerful influence that socioeconomic conditions have on the diseases experienced by individuals and populations. The epidemiologic transition describes the significant differences in health status that are observed when comparing populations with different income levels. These differences can be observed when comparing two countries with divergent economic profiles, and they are also sometimes evident when comparing states or provinces within the same country or comparing the health profiles of the richest and poorest residents within one country.[5]

The other key contribution of health transitions theory is that it emphasizes that every population at every income level has health concerns. Every country in the world experiences a mix of deaths from infections, NCDs, injuries, and other causes, even though the relative proportion of these causes of mortality differs according to the country's income level. Reducing deaths from infections, childbirth, and undernutrition is an excellent public health achievement because these conditions tend to kill children and young adults. But those averted deaths will be replaced with other causes of death because everyone dies. The majority of people who survive to their fifth birthdays will eventually die from an NCD.[3] As more children survive to adulthood and old age, the population health profile will shift toward a greater burden from CVDs, cancers, and other NCDs.[6] The epidemiologic transition does not reduce the costs of health care. It just shifts those costs to an older population with a different set of diseases and disabilities.

The need for strategies to reduce the burden from disability and premature death caused by NCDs in adult populations applies to countries across the income spectrum.[7] While the percentage of deaths from NCDs is highest in high-income countries, the age-standardized death rate from NCDs—a rate that adjusts for different population age structures in different countries—is higher

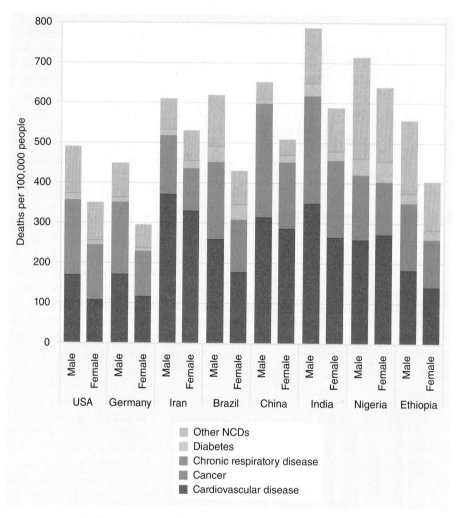

FIGURE 15-6 Age-standardized death rates from NCDs per 100,000 people.

Data from *Global status report on noncommunicable diseases 2014.* Geneva: World Health Organization; 2014.

in low- and middle-income countries than in high-income countries (**FIGURE 15-6**).[8] The Sustainable Development Goals (SDGs) aim to "reduce by one-third premature mortality from noncommunicable diseases through prevention and treatment" by 2030 (SDG 3.4).[9] The goal is not to reduce the number of deaths from NCDs. The goal is to increase the age at which people die from NCDs. A key metric for evaluating progress toward this goal is the percentage of people between 30 and 70 years of age who die from NCDs (**FIGURE 15-7**). The ultimate goal is to decrease this percentage to as close to 0% as possible, allowing adults to enjoy as many healthy years of life as possible before succumbing to an NCD in very old age. Achieving the socioeconomic and health goals spelled out in the SDGs will require both improved prevention of NCDs via risk factor reduction and improved case management for people with one or more NCDs.[10]

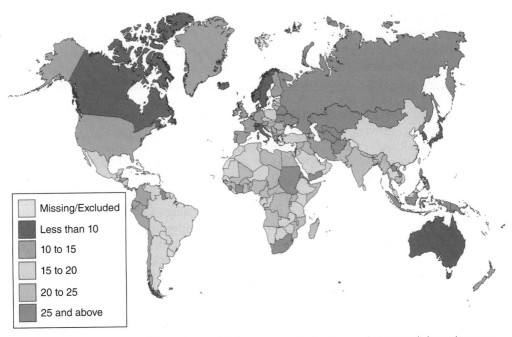

FIGURE 15–7 Probability (%) of dying from a CVD, cancer, chronic respiratory disease, or diabetes between ages 30 and 70 years (2015).

Data from *World health statistics 2017*. Geneva: WHO; 2017.

▶ 15.2 NCDs and Behavior Change

Modifiable risk factors are thought to be responsible for at least two-thirds of all deaths from NCDs.[11] NCDs that can be prevented through behavior change are sometimes called **lifestyle diseases** because they are associated with health-related behaviors, such as unhealthy diets, sedentariness, tobacco use, and heavy alcohol consumption.[12] These NCDs have also been called "diseases of affluence," a way of contrasting these conditions with the infectious diseases and undernutrition that are considered to be "diseases of poverty."[13] However, this is a false dichotomy. NCDs are the primary cause of disease burden in adult populations globally, regardless of the country's income level.

The *Global Action Plan for the Prevention and Control of Noncommunicable Diseases* endorsed by the World Health Assembly in 2013 spells out nine voluntary targets for NCD control in member countries.[14] The overall "25 × 25" target aims to achieve a 25% relative reduction in the rate of premature death from CVDs, cancers, diabetes, and chronic respiratory diseases (CRDs) by 2025 compared to 2010 rates.[15] Two targets focus on the tools required to achieve the 25 × 25 goal.[16] One calls for a higher proportion of adults to receive the medications and health counseling that can prevent heart attacks and strokes. The other aims to substantially increase the availability of affordable health technologies and essential medicines for NCDs. Two of the targets focus on modifiable biological risk factors for NCDs. One aims to halt the rise in obesity, which would contain the increase in diabetes prevalence. The other aims to reduce the prevalence of hypertension by 25%. Four of the targets focus on health behaviors linked to a diversity of NCDs: physical inactivity, harmful use of alcohol, salt intake, and tobacco use.[17] The goal is to achieve a 10% reduction in physical inactivity, a 10% reduction in harmful use of alcohol, a 30% reduction in mean salt (sodium) intake, and a 30% reduction in tobacco use.

In addition to those key activities—maintaining a healthy weight, controlling blood pressure, increasing exercise, drinking less alcohol, using less salt, and not smoking—there are hundreds of other relatively simple healthy behaviors that reduce the risk of an individual developing an NCD,[18] contracting an infectious disease, or becoming injured. There is an equally long list of actions that promote mental and social well-being. **Behavior change** is the process of adopting healthier habits and maintaining those new practices. There are many types of persistent behavior changes that are effective in reducing the risk of NCDs. Some are related to physical activity, such as deciding to start an exercise program, following through with increasing fitness levels through daily exercise, and maintaining that new routine for many years. Some are related to substance use, such as deciding to stop using tobacco products, following through with a smoking cessation plan, and remaining tobacco-free for many years after the initial decision. Some are focused on addressing existing health concerns, such as deciding to lose weight and then adopting a nutritious lower-calorie diet, shedding pounds, and maintaining the new, lower weight for many years. Behavior change is difficult because it requires a long-term commitment to a healthy lifestyle.

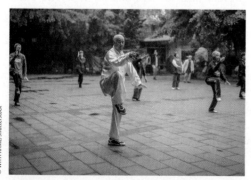

© WHYFRAME/Shutterstock

The ability of an individual or community to implement behavior change is not solely a function of knowledge or willpower. It is also dependent on access to the tools for health. Clinical care providers, community organizations, governments, and others involved in health education, health promotion, and health communication can all play a role in increasing knowledge about the risk of disease and the benefits of healthier behaviors, improving access to health resources, creating policies that facilitate healthier behaviors, and communicating with clients and constituents. Several theories about behavior change inform the work of health promoters.[19]

The **knowledge, attitudes, and practices (KAP)** model, also called the rational model, emphasizes the importance of health education for promoting behavior change.[20] In this model, attitudes include perceptions and beliefs, and practices include behaviors. Once individuals know why a behavior is healthy and believe that it is worth the effort to make a change, it is easier for them to choose to engage in healthier behaviors.

Self-efficacy is an individual's confidence in his or her ability to successfully complete a difficult task. The **health belief model** states that individual behavior change is a function of personal perceptions of the severity of the disease, beliefs about personal susceptibility to the disease, and beliefs about the likely benefits from adopting healthier behaviors as well as perceptions about the barriers to action and the self-efficacy to enact change.[21] In the health belief model, cues to action, such as news stories, reminder notices about health checkups, package warning labels, a friend's hospitalization, and referrals from clinicians, are important for triggering behavior change.

The **stages of change model**, also called the **transtheoretical model**, describes individual behavior change as a five-stage process from precontemplation to contemplation, preparation for action, action, and maintenance.[22] The **theory of reasoned action** says that follow-through on implementing plans for a healthier lifestyle is dependent on the individual's belief that the outcome of the change will be worth the effort and his or her confidence that others will support the change.[23] The **theory of planned behavior** builds on the theory of reasoned action by adding the importance of an individual's perceived self-efficacy and control over the change.[24]

Social cognitive theory acknowledges that behavior is a function of personal factors, behaviors, and environmental conditions, and recognizes that behavior change is about environmental realities as well as inner motivation.[25] The diffusion of innovations model describes a process of behavior change in communities that unfolds as new ideas and actions are adopted by community members.[26] Innovators demonstrate the benefits of the change, then early adopters generate enthusiasm for it. More and more residents decide to participate in the change. Finally, only a small number of residents remain who have not adopted it. The activated health education model describes a three-step process for engaging individuals in personal health assessments (the experiential stage), raising their knowledge of desirable health behaviors (the awareness phase), and then encouraging them to actively implement the change in their own lives (the responsibility phase).[27]

Physical activity provides a case study of the challenges associated with behavior change. The World Health Organization (WHO) recommends that children aged 5–17 years engage in at least 60 minutes of moderate or vigorous physical activity daily, that adults average at least 30 minutes of moderate or 15 minutes of vigorous physical activity daily along with strength-building exercises, and that older adults add balance training to their routines and maintain their physical activity levels for as long as they are able to do so.[28] **Physical inactivity** is the failure to regularly engage in exercise of moderate or vigorous intensity. About one in four adults worldwide completes less than 150 minutes of moderately intense (or more vigorous) physical activity each week. The rates of inactivity are especially high among

women (**FIGURE 15–8**).[8] Physical inactivity is associated with an increased risk of morbidity and mortality from numerous NCDs.[29]

A related but distinct concept is **sedentariness**, which is characterized by sitting for long durations each day. Sedentariness is often linked to screen time, the hours spent watching television or another electronic device, but sedentarism is also built into many work and school environments.[30] It is possible for a person to exercise enough to be classified as physically active and, at the same time, to sit enough to be considered to have a sedentary lifestyle.[31] For example, people who spend 8 hours a day at a desk job might be classified as sedentary even if they run 5 miles every day after work. Sedentariness is associated with an increased risk of NCDs, an increased likelihood of having other risk factors for NCDs, and a higher mortality rate.[32]

Although nearly everyone who is physically inactive or sedentary would benefit from adopting more active lifestyles, there are many barriers to behavior change. There may be perceived time

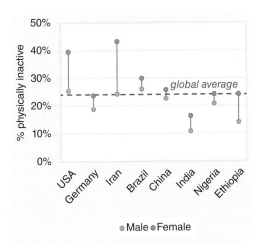

FIGURE 15–8 Many adults, especially women, are physically inactive. (The graph shows the age-standardized percentage of people aged 18 years and older with insufficient levels of physical activity rates. Standardized rates allow for direct comparison across populations with different age structures.)

Data from *Global status report on noncommunicable diseases 2014*. Geneva: World Health Organization; 2014.

barriers. Sleep, leisure, occupation, transportation, and home-based activities (a framework known as the SLOTH model) may be higher priorities than exercise.[33] There may be cultural barriers. For example, in places where women and older adults traditionally have not been physically active, they may feel uncomfortable being seen trying something outside the norms. There may be environmental barriers, especially in urban environments where homes are crowded, there are no sidewalks, and few parks, schoolyards, and sports facilities are available. Exercising more often is not just about learning that exercise is valuable, having the fortitude to establish a new exercise routine, and being physically able to do aerobic exercise. It is also dependent on having social support to make time for exercise and reduce periods of sedentariness, living in a community that considers exercise to be culturally acceptable, and having access to a safe and convenient environment in which to exercise.[34] Effective physical activity promotion campaigns combine community-, school-, and work-based health education and exercise programs with environmental and policy strategies that enable healthy practices to continue.[35]

pulmonary artery, which typically occurs secondary to other health issues), bronchiectasis, and interstitial lung diseases like sarcoidosis.[36] The CRD category typically does not include infectious diseases like tuberculosis, even when those infections last for many years, and it usually does not include lung cancers.

Asthma is a chronic, but reversible, inflammation of the airways that causes episodes of wheezing (especially when exhaling), coughing, chest tightness, and shortness of breath due to thickening of the airway wall and bronchospasms that narrow the diameter of the bronchi and bronchioles.[37] Cells in the airway may also secrete more mucus than normal, which can further restrict airflow. Symptoms can usually be managed with inhaled corticosteroids and bronchodilators, when those medications are locally available and affordable to the patient.[38] Avoiding potential environmental triggers of asthma attacks, such air pollution and cold air, may also reduce the severity of the disease. More than 300 million people worldwide have asthma, and it affects all age groups.[39] About 14% of children (**FIGURE 15–9**) and 9% of young adults have symptoms of asthma over the course

▶ 15.3 Chronic Respiratory Diseases

Chronic respiratory diseases (CRDs) are diseases of airway, bronchi, and lungs, such as asthma, chronic obstructive pulmonary disease, lung diseases associated with occupational exposures, sleep apnea, pulmonary hypertension (increased pressure in the

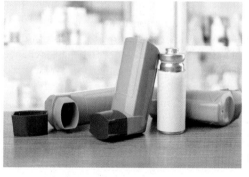

© Africa Studio/Shutterstock

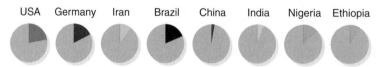

FIGURE 15–9 Percentage of 13- and 14-year-olds with current wheezing consistent with asthma.

Data from *The global asthma report 2014.* Auckland: Global Asthma Network; 2014.

of a year.[40] Asthma increases absenteeism from school and work, and it decreases learning, productivity, and quality of life.[41] Older adults often have symptoms of asthma in combination with other CRDs.[40] Severe asthma attacks can be fatal when medical care is not immediately available.

Chronic obstructive pulmonary disease (COPD) is a chronic, progressive disease that limits airflow and causes shortness of breath and productive coughing.[42] Two of the common presentations of COPD are chronic bronchitis and emphysema. **Bronchitis** is an inflammation of the bronchi that is characterized by a productive cough, narrowing of the airways, and excess mucus production. The chronic bronchitis

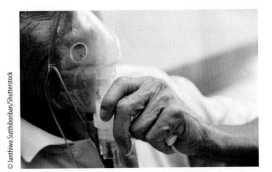

associated with COPD causes a persistent cough as airways progressively narrow and mucus clogs breathing passages. **Emphysema** occurs when the alveoli (the tiny air sacs in the lungs) lose elasticity and become distended or destroyed. This irreversible process reduces the surface area available for intake of oxygen and release of carbon dioxide.

Treatment can help manage some of the symptoms of COPD,[43] but the damage to the airways and lungs is not fully reversible with current therapies. Symptoms often worsen over time. More than 170 million adults worldwide have COPD, and the prevalence of COPD increases with age (**FIGURE 15–10**).[44] COPD is the primary cause of death for more than 3 million people annually, accounting for more than 5% of all deaths and more than 12% of deaths of adults aged 70 years and older.[44] The most prominent risk factor for COPD is tobacco smoking.[45] Although COPD is not curable, many cases could be prevented through avoidance of tobacco smoke, indoor and outdoor air pollution, and industrial chemicals.[46]

Pneumoconiosis is a restrictive lung disease caused by exposure to various types of

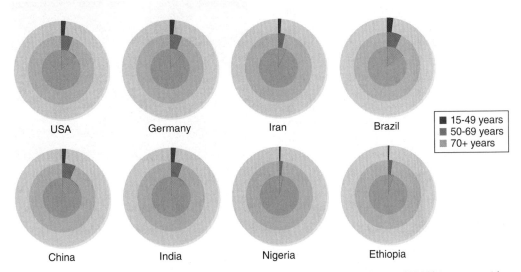

USA Germany Iran Brazil

■ 15-49 years
■ 50-69 years
■ 70+ years

China India Nigeria Ethiopia

FIGURE 15–10 The percentage of adults with chronic obstructive pulmonary disease (COPD) increases with age (2015).

Data from GBD Disease and Injury Incidence and Prevalence Collaborators. Global, regional, and national incidence, prevalence, and years lived with disability for 310 diseases and injuries, 1980–2015: A systematic analysis for the Global Burden of Disease Study 2015. *Lancet* 2016; 388:1545–602.

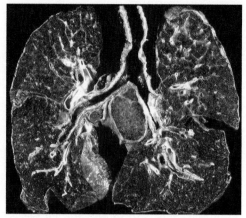

Coal worker's pneumoconiosis (anthracosilicosis).

occupational hazards. Obstructive lung diseases like asthma and COPD make it difficult for a person to exhale all the air in the lungs. By contrast, restrictive lung diseases like pneumoconiosis make it difficult for people to fully fill their lungs with air when they inhale. Both obstructive and restrictive lung diseases cause shortness of breath, especially with exertion. The most common form of pneumoconiosis is silicosis, which affects miners who inhale silica dust.[47] Other forms of pneumoconiosis include asbestosis, which is caused by prolonged periods of inhalation of asbestos fibers, and coal worker's pneumoconiosis (also called black lung disease). While pneumoconiosis is not a major cause of global mortality, it is important because most cases could be prevented with improved attention to worker safety, such as provision of face masks and hygiene facilities for washing dust off exposed skin.[48]

▶ 15.4 Tobacco Control

Tobacco smoke contains more than 5300 different compounds, including dozens of toxins and carcinogens.[49] The nicotine in tobacco is highly addictive. It is easy for new smokers to become dependent on tobacco and difficult for smokers who want to quit to do so successfully.[50] Smoking damages cells, stresses the cardiovascular system,[51] alters blood chemistry, destroys the cilia that help clear mucus out of the respiratory tract, and interferes with respiration.[52] Tobacco smokers and people frequently exposed to secondhand smoke sustain damage to nearly every body system.[53] Tobacco increases the risk of coronary artery disease, lung cancer, and stroke in adults, and it increases the risk of respiratory illnesses in children. Tobacco use is responsible for about one in eight deaths worldwide each year (**FIGURE 15–11**), including an estimated 69% of deaths from lung cancer, 47% of deaths from COPD, 36% of deaths from esophageal cancer, 27% of deaths from bladder cancer, 18% of deaths from ischemic heart disease, and 17% of deaths from strokes (**FIGURE 15–12**).[45]

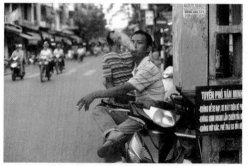

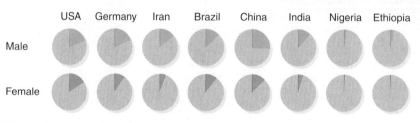

FIGURE 15–11 Percentage of deaths attributed to tobacco use (2015).

Data from GBD 2015 Risk Factors Collaborators. Global, regional, and national comparative risk assessment of 79 behavioural, environmental and occupational, and metabolic risks or clusters of risks, 1990–2015: A systematic analysis for the Global Burden of Disease Study 2015. *Lancet* 2016; 388:1649–724.

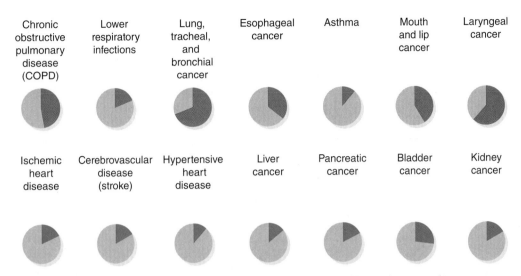

FIGURE 15-12 Proportion of deaths from various causes that are attributable to tobacco smoking.

Data from GBD 2015 Risk Factors Collaborators. Global, regional, and national comparative risk assessment of 79 behavioural, environmental and occupational, and metabolic risks or clusters of risks, 1990–2015: A systematic analysis for the Global Burden of Disease Study 2015. *Lancet* 2016; 388:1649–724.

Global efforts to reduce the morbidity and premature mortality from NCDs will not be successful without significant reductions in tobacco use.[54] Shared global concerns about the public health burden from tobacco use led to the adoption of the first global health treaty negotiated through the WHO,[55] the **Framework Convention on Tobacco Control (FCTC)**,[56] which aims to significantly reduce the global prevalence of tobacco use.[57] The call for a treaty was approved by the World Health Assembly (WHA) in 1995. After many rounds of negotiation, the FCTC was approved by the WHA in 2003 and put into force in 2005.[58] As of 2015, 180 UN members had become official parties to the FCTC and were actively working to implement the tobacco control measures stipulated in the agreement.[59] The FCTC has also been incorporated into the SDGs through a target that aims to "strengthen the implementation of the World Health Organization Framework Convention on Tobacco Control in all countries" (SDG 3.a).[9]

The key demand-side FCTC strategies that will reduce the desire of people to use tobacco products include increasing taxes on tobacco products (Article 6); banning smoking in government buildings, healthcare facilities, schools, public transportation, and other settings (Article 8); regulating the content of tobacco products (Articles 9 and 10); requiring bold health warning labels that cover a large portion of tobacco packaging (Article 11); providing education about tobacco control to health workers, educators, social workers, and other community leaders (Article 12); banning tobacco advertising (Article 13); and providing tobacco users with support for smoking cessation, such as offering nicotine replacement therapy and counseling (Article 14). The FCTC also includes

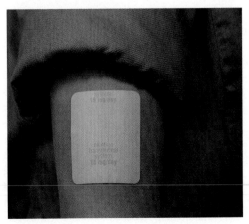

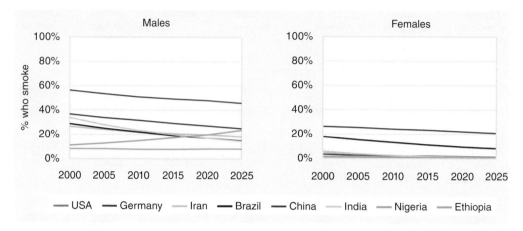

FIGURE 15-13 The percentage of adults (aged 15+ years) who are current tobacco smokers is decreasing in most, but not all, countries.

Data from *WHO global report on trends in prevalence of tobacco smoking*. Geneva: WHO; 2015.

supply-side measures that reduce the availability of tobacco products, such as eliminating illegal tobacco sales (Article 15); banning sales to minors (Article 16); and supporting alternative income-generating activities for people who currently depend on the tobacco industry for their livelihoods (Article 17). These strategies are operationalized with six actions summarized by the acronym MPOWER: Monitor tobacco use and prevention policies; Protect people from tobacco smoke; Offer help to quit tobacco use; Warn about the dangers of tobacco; Enforce bans on tobacco advertising, promotion, and sponsorship; and Raise taxes on tobacco.[60]

The percentage of people who smoke has decreased in most countries since the FCTC went into force in 2005, and the rate is expected to continue to gradually decline in most of these locations (**FIGURE 15-13**).[61] In 1980, about 41% of men and 11% of women worldwide were daily smokers. Thirty years later, these rates had dropped to about 31% and 6%, respectively.[62] However, this success is not uniform. The rate of tobacco use remains much higher among males than females (**FIGURE 15-14**), especially in middle-income countries, and the rates of tobacco use by males are increasing across West Africa (including in Nigeria) as well as in Egypt, Indonesia, and other countries.[61] There are now more than 900 million daily tobacco smokers worldwide,

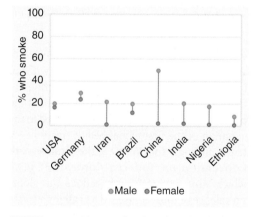

FIGURE 15-14 More males than females (aged 15+ years) are current tobacco smokers (2015).

Data from *WHO global report on trends in prevalence of tobacco smoking*. Geneva: WHO; 2015.

including nearly one in three adult males.[63] Population growth means that the number of daily smokers is increasing even as the percentage of adults who smoke decreases. About 5.8 trillion cigarettes are smoked each year (with more than 44% of those cigarettes smoked in China alone) (**FIGURE 15-15**).[63] While the number of cigarettes smoked per day by daily smokers has decreased in some countries, it is increasing in others (**FIGURE 15-16**).[62] There is a dose–response relationship between tobacco and health problems, with heavier consumption of tobacco associated with steadily worsening health outcomes.[49]

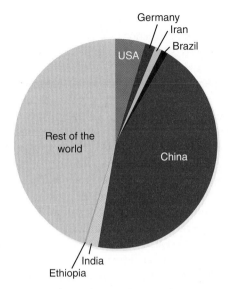

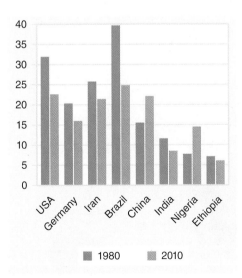

FIGURE 15–15 Distribution of where the cigarettes smoked worldwide are consumed.

Data from Eriksen M, Mackay J, Schluger N, Gomesthapeh FI, Drope J. *The tobacco atlas*, 5th ed. Atlanta: American Cancer Society / World Lung Foundation; 2015.

FIGURE 15–16 Number of cigarettes consumed each day by the average daily smoker in featured countries.

Data from Ng M, Freeman MK, Fleming TD, Robinson M, Dwyer-Lindgren L, Thomson B, Wollum A, Sanman E, Wulf S, Lopez AD, Murray CJL, Gakidou E. Smoking prevalence and cigarette consumption in 187 countries, 1980–2012. *JAMA* 2014; 311:183–92.

▶ 15.5 Diabetes

Insulin is a hormone produced by the pancreas that helps the body maintain a relatively constant level of glucose (sugar) in the bloodstream so cells have a relatively constant supply of energy. **Type 1 diabetes** (previously called juvenile-onset diabetes or insulin-dependent diabetes) occurs when the body does not produce enough insulin.[64] Type 1 diabetes typically has a sudden onset in childhood. **Type 2 diabetes** (formerly known as adult-onset diabetes or non-insulin-dependent diabetes) is characterized by the body developing insulin resistance and failing to respond appropriately to insulin even when the hormone is still being produced.[65] Type 2 diabetes typically has a gradual onset in adulthood. Both type 1 and type 2 diabetes are sometimes called diabetes mellitus. Type 2 diabetes is much more prevalent than type 1 diabetes.

Type 2 diabetes is considered to be a preventable disease because the major risk factors include obesity and related lifestyle characteristics, such as physical inactivity and an unhealthy diet. This connection is so strong that that some researchers refer type 2 diabetes as "diabesity."[66] People with type 1 diabetes are rarely overweight. People with type 2 diabetes are usually overweight or obese. **Gestational diabetes** is elevated blood sugar that is first diagnosed during pregnancy and typically resolves after delivery, but women who have had gestational diabetes have an increased likelihood of subsequently developing type 2 diabetes.[67]

Signs of the initial onset of diabetes may include excessive thirst, frequent urination,

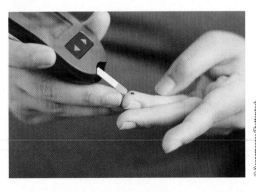

© Kwangmoozaa/Shutterstock

unexplained weight loss, and fatigue. Diagnosis is based on various types of blood sugar tests.[68] Fasting plasma glucose (FPG) levels of ≥126 mg/dL (7.0 mmol/L) at two points in time indicate diabetes. A random (non-fasting) plasma glucose level of ≥200 mg/dL (11.1 mmol/L) suggests diabetes but must be confirmed with other tests, such as a 2-hour oral glucose tolerance test (OGTT). Levels of glycated hemoglobin (HbA1c), a measure of the average plasma glucose over the 8–12 weeks prior to the test, are not diagnostic tests but provide insight about diabetes management.[69] People who have elevated blood glucose levels that are not above the threshold for a type 2 diabetes diagnosis may be classified as having a type of prediabetes, such as impaired glucose tolerance.[70]

The goal of diabetes management is to keep blood sugar levels from becoming too high (hyperglycemia) or too low (hypoglycemia).[71] When blood sugar levels are not carefully maintained, complications like blindness (from diabetic retinopathy), heart disease, kidney failure, nerve damage (diabetic neuropathy), and foot ulcers leading to amputation may develop over time.[72] People with type 1 diabetes require frequent insulin injections to maintain safe blood sugar levels. Waiting too long between injections allows a blood chemistry imbalance called diabetic ketoacidosis to develop as blood sugar levels increase and dehydration occurs. Untreated ketoacidosis can lead to seizures, coma, and death. For people with type 2 diabetes, the disease often can be controlled with weight loss, a careful diet, and sometimes also oral medications. Management of diabetes requires access to health and nutrition education, medication for diabetes and cardiovascular comorbidities, routine clinical examinations (including eye exams and foot checks), and referrals to advanced care when complications arise.

Diabetes and its complications have become major causes of disability and premature death in many high-income and middle-income countries (**FIGURE 15-17**). Between 1980 and 2015, the global diabetes prevalence rate nearly doubled from 4.7% to 8.5%, after standardizing the 1980 rates to the age distribution in 2015 (**FIGURE 15-18**).[73] By 2015, there were about 110 million people in China, 70 million people

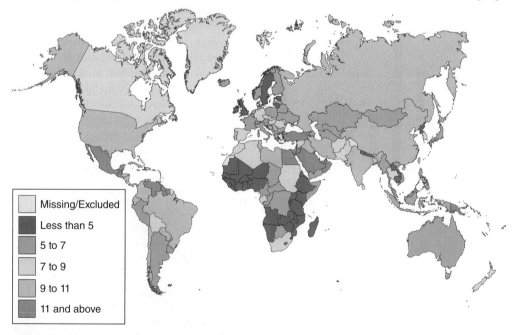

Missing/Excluded

Less than 5

5 to 7

7 to 9

9 to 11

11 and above

FIGURE 15-17 Prevalence of diabetes among adults aged 20–79 years (2015).

Data from *IDF diabetes atlas*, 7th ed. Brussels: IDF; 2015.

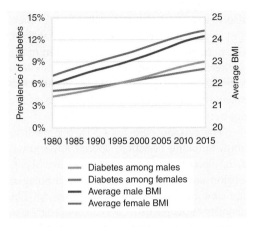

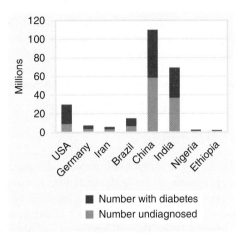

FIGURE 15–18 The global prevalence of obesity and diabetes are increasing.

Data from NCD Risk Factor Collaboration (NCD-RisC). Worldwide trends in diabetes since 1980: A pooled analysis of 751 population-based studies with 4.4 million participants. *Lancet* 2016; 387:1513–30

FIGURE 15–19 About half of adults who have diabetes have not been diagnosed (2015).

Data from *IDF diabetes atlas*, 7th ed. Brussels: IDF; 2015.

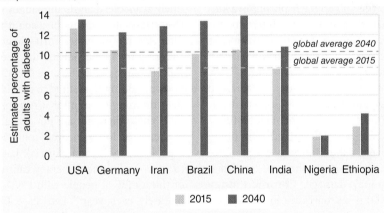

FIGURE 15–20 The prevalence of diabetes is expected to increase dramatically over the next 25 years.

Data from *IDF diabetes atlas*, 7th ed. Brussels: IDF; 2015.

in India, 29 million people in the United States, and 14 million people in Brazil living with diabetes.[74] These numbers are projected from population-based serosurveys that test the blood of randomly sampled people who are representative of the population as a whole. The percentage of participants in serological studies who have elevated blood sugar is usually higher than the percentage of survey participants who report that they have ever been diagnosed as having diabetes, because many people with diabetes are not aware of their condition. About half of adults with type 2 diabetes do not know that they have diabetes

(**FIGURE 15–19**).[74] People with diabetes who have not been clinically diagnosed are not receiving treatment for the condition, and they may develop complications that could have been prevented if their diabetes had been better managed.

The prevalence of diabetes is increasing in both higher- and lower-income countries as obesity and other risk factors become more prevalent.[75] The prevalence is expected to continue to climb in the coming decades, to 10.4% in 2040, as more people worldwide become obese (**FIGURE 15–20**).[74] The number of adults worldwide who are living with diabetes increased from 110 million in 1980 to 420 million in 2015.[71] If current trends continue, that number will rise to 640 million by 2040.[74]

▶ 15.6 Chronic Kidney Disease

The kidneys are responsible for several important functions in the body, including filtering toxins from the blood, maintaining fluid and electrolyte levels, helping control blood pressure, stimulating the production of red blood cells (by producing a hormone called erythropoietin), and supporting bone health. Wastes and excess fluid from the kidneys are excreted as urine. Each kidney is composed of about one million nephrons. When the nephrons in a kidney are damaged, their ability to filter blood is impaired. Kidney failure happens when kidneys are not functioning well enough for health.[76] Untreated kidney failure can cause death.[77]

Two tests are key indicators of decreased renal (kidney) function.[78] The glomerular filtration rate (GFR) is a measure of blood filtration efficiency that is determined from blood creatinine levels. Albuminuria is the presence of the protein albumin in the urine, and it is a sign of kidney damage. **Chronic kidney disease (CKD)** is a progressive loss of kidney function characterized by a reduced GFR and increased urinary albumin levels. The early stages of CKD are usually asymptomatic. As the kidney damage worsens, the individual may experience fatigue, itchiness, constipation, loss of appetite, pain, difficulty sleeping, anxiety, and other symptoms.[79]

At least 10% of the world's adults—more than 300 million people—are thought to have CKD.[44] The prevalence increases with age.[80] There are many different conditions that can cause CKD. Diabetes and hypertension are among the most common causes of CKD worldwide. In low-income regions, infections and environmental toxins (including harmful herbs used medicinally in some places) are also major contributors to CKD.[81] A glomerulus is a tiny filtering unit within a nephron. Glomerulonephritis is an inflammation of the glomeruli. Persistent inflammation can lead to CKD. Some types of CKD are genetic, like polycystic kidney disease, but most cases are not heritable.

There is no cure for CKD, but medications, smoking cessation, special low-sodium diets, management of comorbidities like hypertension and diabetes, and health technologies can slow the progression of the disease.[82] The majority of people with CKD do not progress to advanced disease, but they may still experience complications like adverse cardiovascular outcomes.[80] In high-income countries, two types of renal replacement therapy for people with end-stage renal disease are expensive but routinely available: dialysis and kidney transplants. **Dialysis** is the process of using a machine to filter the blood, either through hemodialysis (filtering the blood outside the body) or peritoneal dialysis (filtering the blood inside the body by adding clean fluid to the abdomen and then draining it out after it has absorbed toxins). These therapies are not available to most residents of lower-income countries (including China, India, and Nigeria). Lack of access to renal replacement therapy causes hundreds of thousands of people with CKD to die prematurely each year.[83] Late-stage CKD causes anemia and dramatically increases the risk of mortality from CVDs, so cardiologic care is a concurrent requirement for kidney patients.[84]

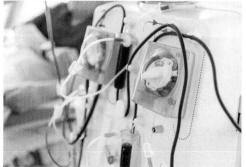

Hemodialysis.

© Aleksandr Ivasenko/Shutterstock

Not all kidney problems are chronic. Pyelonephritis is an inflammation of the kidneys caused by bacterial infections, and it usually resolves after antibiotic therapy.[85] An acute kidney injury, formerly called acute renal failure, is the sudden loss of kidney function caused by physical trauma, a poison (including overdoses of medications like nonsteroidal anti-inflammatory drugs), or another event.[86] Acute kidney injuries are most common among older adults with chronic diseases. In that population, an acute kidney injury is a life-threatening condition.[87]

▶ 15.7 Liver and Digestive Diseases

Liver and digestive diseases, excluding cancers, are responsible for about 4.5% of global deaths.[3] The liver has numerous important functions, including creating proteins that allow blood to clot, filtering toxins out of blood, and storing and releasing glucose and lipids into the bloodstream. The most common serious liver disorder is **cirrhosis**, irreversible scarring of the liver that impedes the flow of blood through the liver and prevents the liver from functioning normally.[88] Early stages of cirrhosis cause few symptoms, but the affected individual may feel fatigued and develop jaundice. As the liver becomes more scarred, fluid

may build up in the legs (edema) and then the abdomen may swell with excess fluid, a condition called ascites. Severe bleeding may occur when increased pressure in the portal vein (portal hypertension) causes the veins in the esophagus to expand (becoming esophageal varices) and possibly rupture. Cirrhosis may also damage to the kidneys, spleen, lungs, and other organs, and cirrhosis significantly increases the risk of liver cancer. A liver transplant is the only currently available cure for cirrhosis, but that option is not widely available.[89] About 2.8 million people worldwide are estimated to have cirrhosis and other chronic liver diseases.[44] About 1.3 million people die each year from them.[3] The most common causes of cirrhosis globally include alcohol abuse, hepatitis B virus, and hepatitis C virus.[90] More than twice as many men as women die from cirrhosis.[90] This disparity is largely attributable to higher rates of alcohol abuse by males.

Numerous digestive diseases contribute to the global burden of disease. Peptic ulcer disease is a painful wound in the lining of the stomach that may perforate and cause a fatal hemorrhage.[91] Gastritis and duodenitis are painful inflammations of the stomach and small intestine, respectively.[92] Pancreatitis is a severely painful inflammation of the pancreas that can cause multiple organ failure, shock, and death. Inflammatory bowel diseases, such as Crohn's disease and ulcerative colitis, cause chronic diarrhea and can significantly reduce quality of life.[93]

Several common digestive conditions—appendicitis, paralytic ileus and intestinal obstruction, intestinal hernias, and gallbladder and biliary diseases—often require surgical repairs. Appendicitis is an inflammation of the appendix that can perforate (rupture) and cause peritonitis, sepsis, and death. Intestinal obstructions prevent waste from passing through the intestines and out of the body, and they may cause bowel perforation, sepsis, and death. An abdominal hernia occurs when part of the intestine passes through the wall of the abdominal muscles, causing pain and possibly cutting off the blood supply to that

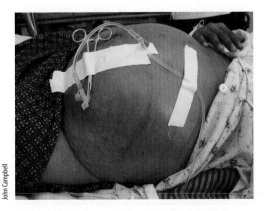

John Campbell

Draining ascites caused by cirrhosis of the liver.

part of the intestine. Exertion, such as lifting heavy objects, may increase the pain, so hernias may prevent affected individuals from doing manual labor. The gallbladder stores bile and releases it into the small intestine to facilitate the digestion of lipids (fats). Gallstones (cholelithiases) that block the bile ducts cause severe pain and jaundice. At least 150,000 people worldwide are thought to die each year because they lack access to emergency surgery for these digestive conditions.[94]

▶ # 15.8 Neurological Disorders

Neurological disorders are dysfunctions of the nervous system, such as epilepsy, migraines and other headache disorders, multiple sclerosis, Parkinson's disease, dementia, traumatic brain injuries, amyotrophic lateral sclerosis (ALS, also known as motor neuron disease), some types of infections that affect the nervous system, and other conditions. These conditions may cause physical impairments (such as paralysis, weakness, and mobility limitations), cognitive impairments, behavioral problems, and difficulties with communication and activities of daily living.[95] Together, neurological disorders are responsible for about 5% of the world's years lived with disability (YLDs).[96]

Epilepsy is a chronic seizure disorder characterized by episodes of excessive and abnormal electrical activity in the brain. Epileptic seizures may cause few observable symptoms, but some trigger muscle stiffness and jerking (tonic-clonic seizures) or loss of muscle tone (atonic seizures). About 65 million people worldwide have epilepsy, and the condition affects people of all ages.[97] Some cases of epilepsy are attributable to head trauma or other forms of brain damage. For most people with epilepsy, the etiology of the disorder is not known. Medications can prevent seizures in about 70% of people with epilepsy, and surgery can be curative in some people for whom

anti-epileptic medications are not effective.[98] However, the majority of people with epilepsy in lower-income countries are not receiving any treatment for the condition.[99] While treated epilepsy may cause almost no reduction in quality of life, some cases of epilepsy are severely disabling. Untreated epilepsy is associated with a significantly increased risk of premature death due to falls and other consequences of seizures.[100] Many people with epilepsy encounter stigma and discrimination because of their condition.[101]

Headache disorders are very common, with more than half of adults reporting that they have experienced a headache in the previous year.[102] Most headaches are relatively mild tension-type headaches or headaches related to acute infections or traumas, and these last only a short time.[103] However, some headache disorders cause moderate or severe pain and occur so frequently that they cause a significant reduction in productivity and quality of life.[104] A **migraine** is a recurrent severe headache that is often accompanied by nausea, vomiting, and sensitivity to light and sound. Common analgesics, such as aspirin or ibuprofen, are usually effective at reducing the pain from tension-type headaches. For migraines, specialized medications, such as ergotamine and sumatriptan, are necessary to control the pain. More than 10% of adults worldwide experience migraines, with women significantly more likely to have migraines than men.[102] Most people with headaches do not receive any clinical treatment for the disorder.[102]

Parkinson's disease and multiple sclerosis are both movement disorders. **Parkinson's disease** (PD) is a chronic, progressive, neurodegenerative disorder characterized by motor symptoms, such as slowed movement (bradykinesia), rigidity or stiffness in an arm or leg or other body part, and tremors when a limb is resting. In addition to problems with gait, balance, and other aspects of postural stability and movement, many people with PD eventually experience non-motor symptoms like depression and dementia.[105] PD is associated with the formation of Lewy bodies (clusters of alpha-synuclein proteins) in the brain and the loss of dopamine-producing neurons in a part of the midbrain called the substantia nigra.[106] A chemical precursor of the neurotransmitter dopamine (called L-DOPA or levodopa) helps manage the symptoms of PD, but long-term use can cause side effects, such as impairment of the ability to control voluntary movements (dyskinesia).[107] Up to 10 million people worldwide are thought to have PD.[108] Because the prevalence of PD increases with age, that number will increase substantially in the coming decades as the world's population ages.[109]

Most nerve cells are coated in myelin, an insulating material that helps speed up the transmission of signals between nerves. **Multiple sclerosis** (MS) is a chronic, progressive disease that causes inflammatory demyelination of the sheaths of nerve cells in the central nervous system. The symptoms may include vision disturbances, bladder or bowel control problems, pain, fatigue, walking difficulties, hand coordination problems, and memory issues and confusion. Most people with MS have a relapsing-remitting form of the disease characterized by periods of symptoms followed by periods of partially or fully recovered function.[110] A variety of medications can help reduce the frequency and severity of relapses.[111] Later on, many years after the initial episode, a progressive form of the disease typically develops. In this advanced stage, the symptoms usually persist and worsen over time.[112] The first symptoms of MS typically appear at about 30 years of age, which makes MS an important contributor to the global burden of neurological diseases in younger adults.[110] More than 2 million people worldwide have MS.[113] The disease is twice as common in women as in men.[114]

Scientists have not yet identified the primary causes of or risk factors for many neurological disorders, so they have not been able to develop effective prevention methods. Instead, the focus is on increasing access to treatment, supporting patients and their families, and helping to reduce the stigma associated with neurological disorders.

▶ 15.9 Genetic Blood Disorders

Genetics is the study of genes, genetic variation, and heredity, the passing of genes from parents to their biological offspring. Genes are sequences of nucleic acids that are part of the chromosomes found in the nucleus of every cell in the human body. This genetic material directs every function of the body, including cell replication, which is important for healing as well as for growth and development. Each cell contains identical DNA (deoxyribonucleic acid), although only some parts of the code are active in certain cells, which is why cells in a heart form different kinds of tissue than the cells that line the intestines. The differential expression of genetic code through activation or inactivation of genes is called **epigenetics**.[115]

Several types of genetic disorders can cause health problems. A chromosomal disorder is caused by the presence of an extra chromosome or by a missing part of a chromosome. Most people have 23 pairs of chromosomes, or 46 total. People with Down syndrome (trisomy 21) have an extra 21st chromosome and 47 total chromosomes.[116] People with Turner Syndrome are missing one of the two sex chromosomes, so they have only 45 chromosomes.[117] Multifactorial inheritance disorders (including many types of cancer and other NCDs) stem from a combination of inherited genes and genetic **mutations**, permanent changes in the sequence of bases that make up DNA that occur after birth in response to exposure to radiation, chemicals, pollutants, or other substances.

A **monogenic disorder** is the result of a child inheriting a single disease-causing gene from one or both parents. An **allele** is a version of a gene. Most genes have two alleles. A

genotype is the set of alleles a person inherits for a particular gene. An individual has a homozygous genotype if he or she inherited the same allele from both parents. An individual has a heterozygous genotype if he or she inherited two different alleles for a gene. A **phenotype** is the way a particular set of alleles is expressed in physical appearance, the way a person develops or functions physiologically, or disease status. Some alleles are **dominant**, which means that inheriting an allele from either parent will cause a person to display the phenotype associated with that allele. Huntington's disease, which causes a progressive degeneration of brain cells, is an example of an autosomal dominant genetic disorder.[118] An **autosomal gene** is one that is not located on the sex chromosome and is therefore not sex-linked. Some alleles are **recessive**, which means that a person must inherit a copy of the allele from both parents to display the phenotype associated with the allele. Cystic fibrosis, which causes excess production of mucus in the lungs and digestive tract, is an example of a recessive genetic disorder.[119]

Both thalassemia and sickle cell disease are autosomal recessive blood disorders that cause hemolytic anemia due to the breakdown of red blood cells. More than 5% of the global population may carry a gene for a hemoglobin disorder.[120] The rate of disease is lower than this percentage, because disease is only present when a person inherits the gene for a particular blood disorder from both parents. People who have just one copy of a gene for a hemoglobin disorder are said to have the trait for the disorder (such as thalassemia trait or sickle cell trait), and they are usually asymptomatic carriers. People who receive copies of the gene from both parents have blood disorders that cause anemia, jaundice, and an increased risk of heart failure and gallstones.

The various types of **thalassemia** are characterized by impaired production of hemoglobin, the molecules in red blood cells that carry oxygen.[121] Individuals who inherit thalassemia alleles from both parents and survive to birth often have a serious blood disease (such as alpha thalassemia intermedia or beta thalassemia major) that requires frequent transfusions of blood.[122] In some places, recipients of blood products may be exposed to bloodborne infectious diseases. Repeated transfusions also carry a risk of iron overload that can damage the body's organs and cause cardiac complications if chelation therapy is not used to remove excess iron from the body. Bone marrow transplants can cure thalassemia, but they are not routinely available in most countries. Thalassemias are prevalent across much of the Mediterranean region, Africa, and Asia.[120] More than 250 million people worldwide have thalassemia trait, and about 400,000 have a form of thalassemia.[44]

Sickle cell disease is a hemoglobinopathy, a genetic disorder that causes the hemoglobin in red blood cells to be malformed. People who inherit the sickle cell allele from one parent have sickle cell trait. People who inherit the allele from both parents have **sickle cell disease**, which causes some red blood cells to become misshapen. Rather than looking like donuts, the damaged erythrocytes look like crescents. These sickled cells can block small blood vessels. When the capillaries are blocked, the resulting ischemia can cause severe pain as well

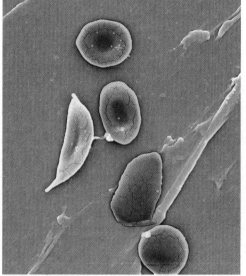

Sickle cell anemia.

as organ damage.[123] The sickle cell gene is most prevalent among people who live in Africa, people of African heritage, and people in who live in some parts of the Middle East and South Asia.[124] More than 400 million people worldwide have sickle cell trait, and about 4 million are estimated to have a sickle cell disorder.[44]

Other examples of genetic blood disorders include hemophilia and glucose-6-phosphate dehydrogenase (G6PD) deficiency. The various types of hemophilia are recessive genetic blood clotting disorders.[125] G6PD deficiency can cause impaired metabolism of red blood cells in some carriers.[126]

▶ 15.10 Musculoskeletal Disorders

Musculoskeletal disorders include problems of the muscles, bones, tendons, ligaments, and joints. These conditions account for a sizeable proportion of the world's YLDs, a metric that quantifies health-related losses in productivity after excluding the lost productivity attributed to premature mortality.[127] Low back and neck pain are the most common cause of YLDs worldwide. These disabling conditions affect more than 800 million people and account for about 12% of all YLDs.[44] As a comparison, all mental health and substance use disorders together are estimated to account for 19% of YLDs, infectious diseases about 14% of YLDs, iron-deficiency anemia about 6% of YLDs, and injuries about 5% of YLDs. People with severe back pain may be completely bedridden, and the pain may cause sleep disturbances, anxiety, and other aggravations.[128] For recent-onset back pain, the recommended course of treatment is anti-inflammatory medications coupled with remaining as active as possible. For chronic pain, analgesics and physical therapy are recommended.[129] Surgery is rarely the preferred option. Even "short-term" back pain usually persists for more than a month, and cases frequently become chronic.[130]

Arthritis is joint inflammation that often causes swelling and pain. Two common types of arthritis, osteoarthritis and rheumatoid arthritis, together account for about 2.5% of the world's YLDs.[44] **Osteoarthritis** (OA) is a degenerative disease that slowly causes loss of cartilage in the joints, causing pain, stiffness, and disability. The main joints affected include the knees, hips, and hands. The most prominent risk factors for OA are age, obesity, and a history of traumatic joint injuries.[131] Some cases can be managed with pain medication. In severe cases, hip or knee replacement may be the only option for restoring mobility. Because joint replacements are rarely available in lower-income countries, the proportion of OA cases that are severe is much higher in lower-income countries than it is in higher-income countries where people suffering from OA can access advanced therapies.[132]

Rheumatoid arthritis (RA) is a chronic inflammatory disease that damages the cartilage and bones in many joints. When treatment is accessed early after the onset of symptoms, many cases of RA can be managed with medications.[133] Without treatment, the disease is often disabling. RA is considered to be an autoimmune disorder. The immune system helps the body recognize and attack invaders like infectious agents and allergens. An **autoimmune disorder** like RA occurs when the body has difficulty distinguishing between "self" and "non-self" and begins to attack its

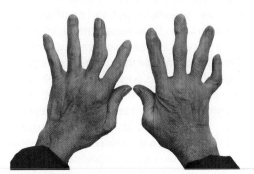

Rheumatoid arthritis.

© Gabdrakipova Dilyara/Shutterstock

own cells. Another example of an autoimmune disorder is systemic **lupus** erythematosus, which is often recognized by the "butterfly rash" it causes on the face. Lupus also causes swollen joints and affects numerous other body systems.[134] An autoimmune disorder is not an allergy. An **allergy** is an immune dysfunction in which the body is hypersensitive to foreign substances that are usually not harmful.

Other musculoskeletal disorders include osteoporosis, gout, and numerous less-common rheumatological conditions. **Osteoporosis** is a loss of bone density that significantly increases the risk of fractures of the hip, vertebrae, and other bones in older adults, especially women.[135] **Gout** is a painful swelling of a joint, usually the joint at the base of the big toe, due to elevated levels of uric acid in the blood. Gout especially affects older men.[136]

▶ **15.11 Sensory Disorders**

Nearly 300 million people worldwide are visually impaired, including about 40 million people who are blind and about 250 million people with low vision.[137] **Low vision** is defined as not being able to see better than 20/60 in the best eye even with glasses, which means that even with corrective lenses, the individual would need to be 20 feet away from an object to see it as clearly as the typical person could see the object from 60 feet away. **Blindness** is defined as having no light perception or having vision that even with glasses is no better than 20/400 in the best eye. These statistics for visual impairment do not include the hundreds of millions of people who have poor visual acuity because they do not have access to the corrective lenses that would remediate their vision to acceptable levels. About 40% of all visual impairment is due to severe refractive errors, such as extreme nearsightedness (myopia), farsightedness (presbyopia), or astigmatism (an anatomical defect that causes vision to be distorted or fuzzy).

Cost-effective interventions for uncorrected refractive errors, cataracts, and other common causes of vision impairment could eliminate the majority of the existing cases of reduced vision globally.[138] The age-standardized prevalence of vision impairment is decreasing as more people gain access to treatment.[139] However, the number of people with visual impairments has not declined. The number of older adults worldwide is increasing at a rate that offsets most of the gains in vision preservation and restoration.[139]

The majority of people with visual impairments are older adults. The vast majority of these adults live in lower- and middle-income countries.[140] Adults with untreatable or untreated visual impairments may experience reduced quality of life, mobility, and independence. Common causes of adult vision loss leading to blindness include cataracts, glaucoma, age-related macular degeneration, diabetic retinopathy, and infections like trachoma.[141] More than 1 in 3 cases of blindness worldwide is attributable to **cataracts**, which are present when the lenses of the eyes become cloudy.[142] Cataracts can be corrected with a simple surgical procedure that replaces the individual's cloudy lens with a clear artificial lens.[143] **Glaucoma** is elevated pressure within the eyeball that causes loss of peripheral vision. **Macular degeneration** occurs when a portion of the retina (a tissue at the back of the eyeball that receives visual images that are then sent to the brain via the optic nerve) deteriorates and causes loss of central vision. Glaucoma and macular degeneration are each responsible for about 1 in 15 cases of blindness.[142] Advanced medical care accessed before vision has been severely impaired can prevent many types of blindness. Some of this care can be provided at the primary health level, but there is a need to increase the number of vision care specialists, including ophthalmologists (physicians with advanced training in eye medicine and surgery), optometrists (vision testing specialists with advanced training), and opticians (technicians trained to fit corrective lenses). Many countries have severe shortages of vision health professionals.[144]

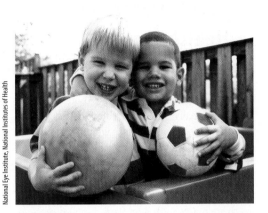

Normal vision.

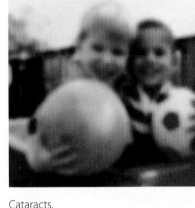

Cataracts.

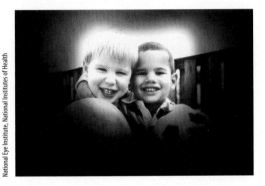

Glaucoma.

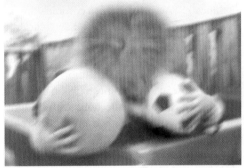

Macular degeneration.

More than 500 million people worldwide have a permanent reduction of hearing in the better ear of 35 decibels (dB) or more.[145] Hearing loss near this threshold for moderate hearing impairment makes it difficult to hear speech even at close distances. Age-related hearing loss (presbycusis) often makes it difficult for older adults to hear high frequencies. More severe hearing loss allows only very loud sounds to be heard. Even with the most powerful hearing aids, it may be difficult or impossible to follow a conversation. Profound hearing loss may allow only sound vibrations to be perceived.

The prevalence of hearing loss increases with age. About 1 in 70 children who are 5–14 years old has hearing loss, and this proportion increases to about 1 in 3 in adults aged 65 years and older.[145] Less than 10% of the people with severe hearing loss who would benefit from hearing aids are using them.[146]

About half of hearing loss cases could be prevented.[146] Hearing loss is often noise induced. High-intensity sounds damage the special surfaces (stereocilia) of cells in the ears that receive noise signals and transmit them to the brain.[147] Noise reduction, including the use of hearing protective gear, helps protect hearing. For children, preventing and treating infections is critical. Infectious diseases like measles, meningitis, and chronic ear infections can cause permanent hearing damage, and some of the antibiotics used to treat infections are lifesaving but may be ototoxic.[148]

▶ 15.12 Skin Diseases

The skin is the largest organ of the body. Skin protects the body from the environment and also provides insulation, regulates body temperature, takes in sensory information, and conducts other important functions. While skin and subcutaneous diseases are a rare cause of death, they cause more than 5% of health-related decreases in productivity each year as measured in YLDs.[44] Many people experience minor inconveniences from skin complaints like cuts, abrasions, blisters, other skin lesions, dandruff, and rashes. Some conditions are more disabling. Various types of dermatitis, including eczema, may cause urticaria (an itchy red rash or hives) and pruritis (itchiness).[149] Acne vulgaris is a chronic skin disease caused by blockages in the hair follicles.[150] Psoriasis is a chronic inflammatory condition characterized by patches of discolored skin plaques.[151] Scabies is an infestation with mites that can cause intense itchiness.[152] Skin problems can also be caused by infections with bacteria, viruses, and fungi. Cellulitis is a potentially dangerous condition that occurs when bacteria like *Staphylococcus* or *Streptococcus* spread from the skin into the bloodstream.[153] Malignant melanoma is a form of skin cancer that can be fatal. Other skin conditions, such as basal cell and squamous cell carcinomas, pyoderma (diseases that produce pus, such as impetigo), alopecia areata (hair loss due to autoimmune dysfunction), and decubitus ulcers (bedsores), may also cause reduced quality of life.

▶ 15.13 Dental and Oral Health

Oral health is an important part of overall health for both children and adults. Tooth decay is the most prevalent disease globally. About 2.5 billion people globally have untreated dental **caries**, colloquially called cavities, which are holes in teeth created by demineralization and decay.[154] The typical 12-year-old has at least one decayed tooth, and most decayed teeth remain untreated (**FIGURE 15–21**).[155] The number of damaged teeth increases with age. Periodontal disease, or **periodontitis**, occurs when poor oral hygiene

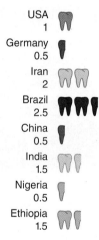

USA
1

Germany
0.5

Iran
2

Brazil
2.5

China
0.5

India
1.5

Nigeria
0.5

Ethiopia
1.5

FIGURE 15–21 Average number of decayed, missing, or filled permanent (adult) teeth among 12-year-olds in featured countries.

Data from *The challenge of oral disease: A call for global action. The oral health atlas*, 2nd ed. Geneva: FDI World Dental Federation; 2015.

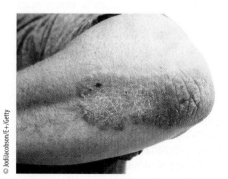

© Jodilacobson/E+/Getty

Psoriasis.

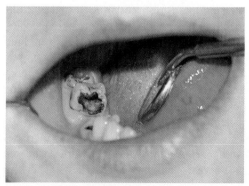

© TRIG/Shutterstock

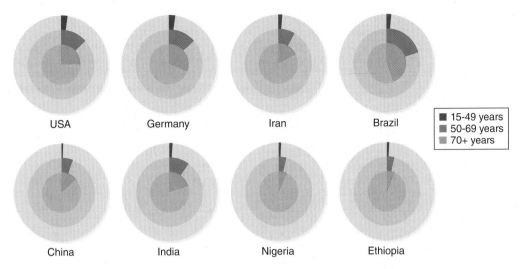

USA Germany Iran Brazil

- 15-49 years
- 50-69 years
- 70+ years

China India Nigeria Ethiopia

FIGURE 15–22 A large percentage of older adults have edentulism or severe tooth loss.

Data from GBD 2015 Disease and Injury Incidence and Prevalence Collaborators. Global, regional, and national incidence, prevalence, and years lived with disability for 310 diseases and injuries, 1990–2015: A systematic analysis for the Global Burden of Disease Study 2015. *Lancet* 2016; 388:1545–602.

and the presence of bacterial plaques cause chronic inflammation of the gums (a condition called gingivitis) that, if unresolved, can cause the teeth to become loose and fall out. More than 10% of adults worldwide have severe periodontitis.[156] At least 1 in 40 adults worldwide has **edentulism**, which means that they have lost most or all of their teeth.[157] The rate is especially high among the oldest adults, since they have had the longest time to develop periodontitis and suffer from its consequences (**FIGURE 15–22**). The major risk factors for poor oral health include poor oral hygiene; exposure to dietary sugars that feed the bacteria that cause caries; use of tobacco products that damage tissues in the mouth and throat; lack of exposure to fluoride, an element often added to toothpaste or drinking water because it strengthens teeth; and lack of access to dental care that can prevent minor dental problems from becoming severe.[155]

▶ References

1. Omran AR. The epidemiologic transition: A theory of the epidemiology of population change. *Milbank Mem Fund Q.* 1971;29:509–38.
2. United Nations Department of Economic and Social Affairs. *World population prospects: The 2017 revision.* New York: UN; 2017.
3. GBD 2015 Mortality and Causes of Death Collaborators. Global, regional, and national life expectancy, all-cause mortality, and cause-specific mortality for 249 causes of death, 1980–2015: A systematic analysis for the Global Burden of Disease Study 2015. *Lancet.* 2016;388:1459–544.
4. Caldwell JC. Population health in transition. *Bull World Health Organ.* 2001;79:159–70.
5. Braveman P, Tarimo E. Social inequalities in health within countries: Not only an issue for affluent nations. *Soc Sci Med.* 2002;54:1621–35.
6. Prabhakaran D, Anand S, Gaziano T, Wu Y, Mbanya JC, Nugent R. Cardiovascular, respiratory, and related conditions: Key messages on essential interventions to address its burden in low- and middle-income countries (Chapter 1). *Disease control priorities.* 3rd ed. *Cardiovascular, respiratory, and related diseases (Volume 5).* Washington DC: IBRD/World Bank; 2017.
7. Yach D, Hawkes C, Gould CL, Hofman KJ. The global burden of chronic diseases: Overcoming impediments to prevention and control. *JAMA.* 2014;291:2616–22.
8. *Global status report on noncommunicable diseases 2014.* Geneva: WHO; 2014.
9. United Nations. *Transforming our world: The 2030 Agenda for Sustainable Development.* New York: UN; 2015.
10. Beaglehole R, Bonita R, Horton R, et al. Priority actions for the non-communicable disease crisis. *Lancet.* 2011;377:1438–47.
11. *Global status report on noncommunicable diseases 2011.* Geneva: WHO; 2011.
12. *World health report 1997: Conquering suffering, enriching humanity.* Geneva: WHO; 1997.

13. Narayan KMV, Ali MK, Koplan JP. Global noncommunicable diseases: Where worlds meet. *N Engl J Med*. 2010;363:1196–8.

14. *Global Action Plan for the Prevention and Control of Noncommunicable diseases 2013–2020*. Geneva: WHO; 2013.

15. Kontis V, Mathers CD, Rehm J, et al. Contribution of six risk factors to achieving the 25×25 noncommunicable disease mortality reduction target: A modelling study. *Lancet*. 2014;384:427–37.

16. *Package of essential noncommunicable (PEN) disease interventions for primary health care in low-resource settings*. Geneva: WHO; 2010.

17. *Global health risks: Mortality and burden of disease attributable to selected major risks*. Geneva: WHO; 2009.

18. Mensah G, Prabhakaran D. Relationships among risk factors and the burden of cardiovascular diseases, diabetes, and chronic lung disease (Chapter 2). *Disease control priorities*. 3rd ed. *Cardiovascular, respiratory, and related diseases (Volume 5)*. Washington DC: IBRD/World Bank; 2017.

19. *Health education: Theoretical concepts, effective strategies and core competencies: A foundation document to guide capacity development of health educators*. Cairo: WHO Regional Office for the Eastern Mediterranean (EMRO); 2012.

20. Valente TW, Paredes P, Poppe PR. Matching the message to the process: The relative ordering of knowledge, attitudes, and practices in behavior change research. *Hum Commun Res*. 1998;24:366–85.

21. Rosenstock IM, Stretcher VJ, Becker MH. Social learning theory and the health belief model. *Health Educ Q*. 1988;15:175–83.

22. Prochaska JO, DiClemente CC. Transtheoretical therapy: Toward a more integrative model of change. *Psychother Theory Res Pract*. 1982;19:276–88.

23. Fishbein M. A theory of reasoned action: Some applications and implications. *Nebr Symp Motiv*. 1980;27:65–116.

24. Ajzen I. The theory of planned behavior. *Organ Behav Human Decision Processes*. 1991;50:179–211.

25. Bandura A. Health promotion from the perspective of social cognitive theory. *Psychol Health*. 1998;13:623–49.

26. Haider M, Kreps GL. Forty years of diffusion of innovations: Utility and value in public health. *J Health Commun*. 2004;9(Suppl 1):3–11.

27. Dennison D, Golaszewski T. The activated health education model: Refinement and implications for school health education. *J School Health*. 2002;72:23–6.

28. *Global recommendations on physical activity for health*. Geneva: WHO; 2010.

29. Lee IM, Shiroma EJ, Lobelo F, Puska P, Blair SN, Katzmarzyk PT. Effect of physical inactivity on major non-communicable diseases worldwide: An analysis of burden of disease and life expectancy. *Lancet*. 2012;380:219–29.

30. Bull F, Goenka S, Lambert V, Pratt M. Physical activity for the prevention of cardiometabolic disease (Chapter 5). *Disease control priorities*. 3rd ed. *Cardiovascular, respiratory, and related diseases (Volume 5)*. Washington DC: IBRD/World Bank; 2017.

31. Ekelund U, Steene-Johannessen J, Brown WJ, et al. Does physical activity attenuate, or even eliminate, the detrimental association of sitting time with mortality? A harmonized meta-analysis of data from more than 1 million men and women. *Lancet*. 2016;388:1302–10.

32. Katzmarzyk PT. Physical activity, sedentary behavior, and health: Paradigm paralysis or paradigm shift? *Diabetes*. 2010;59:2717–25.

33. Pratt M, Macera CA, Sallis JF, O'Donnell M, Frank LD. Economic interventions to promote physical activity: Application of the SLOTH model. *Am J Prev Med*. 2004;27(Suppl 3):136–45.

34. Bauman AE, Reis RS, Sallis JF, Wells JC, Loos RJF, Martin BW. Correlates of physical activity: Why are some people physically active and others not? *Lancet*. 2012;380:258–71.

35. Heath GW, Parra DC, Sarmiento OL, et al. Evidence-based intervention in physical activity: Lessons from around the world. *Lancet*. 2012;380:272–81.

36. *Global surveillance, prevention and control of chronic respiratory diseases: A comprehensive approach*. Geneva: WHO; 2007.

37. Martinez FD, Vercelli D. Asthma. *Lancet*. 2013;382:1360–72.

38. Burney P, Perez-Padilla R, Marks G, Wong G, Bateman E, Jarvis D. Chronic lower respiratory tract diseases (Chapter 15). *Disease control priorities*. 3rd ed. *Cardiovascular, respiratory, and related diseases (Volume 5)*. Washington DC: IBRD/World Bank; 2017.

39. Masoli M, Fabian D, Holt S, Beasley R. Global Initiative for Asthma (GINA) Program. The global burden of asthma: Executive summary of the GINA Dissemination Committee report. *Allergy*. 2004;59:469–78.

40. *The global asthma report 2014*. Auckland: Global Asthma Network; 2014.

41. Rabe KF, Adachi M, Lai CK, et al. Worldwide severity and control of asthma in children and adults: The global asthma insights and reality surveys. *J Allergy Clin Immunol*. 2004;114:40–7.

42. Decramer M, Janssens W, Miravitlles M. Chronic obstructive pulmonary disease. *Lancet*. 2012;179:1341–51.

43. *Prevention and control of noncommunicable diseases: Guidelines for primary health care in low-resource settings*. Geneva: WHO; 2012.

44. GBD 2015 Disease and Injury Incidence and Prevalence Collaborators. Global, regional, and national incidence, prevalence, and years lived with

disability for 310 diseases and injuries, 1980–2015: A systematic analysis for the Global Burden of Disease Study 2015. *Lancet*. 2016;388:1545–602.

45. GBD 2015 Risk Factors Collaborators. Global, regional, and national comparative risk assessment of 79 behavioural, environmental and occupational, and metabolic risks or clusters of risks, 1990–2015: A systematic analysis for the Global Burden of Disease Study 2015. *Lancet*. 2016;388:1649–724.

46. Mannino DM, Buist AS. Global burden of COPD: Risk factors, prevalence, and future trends. *Lancet*. 2007;370:765–73.

47. Leung CC, Yu ITS, Chen W. Silicosis. *Lancet*. 2012;379:2008–18.

48. Driscoll T, Nelson DI, Steenland K, et al. The global burden of non-malignant respiratory disease due to occupational airborne exposures. *Am J Ind Med*. 2005;48:432–45.

49. Tobacco smoking. *IARC monographs on the evaluation of carcinogenic risks to humans*. 2012;100E: 43–211.

50. Benowitz NL. Nicotine addiction. *N Engl J Med*. 2010;362:2295–303.

51. Roy A, Rawal I, Jabbour S, Prabhakaran D. Tobacco and cardiovascular disease: A summary of evidence (Chapter 4). *Disease control priorities*. 3rd ed. *Cardiovascular, respiratory, and related diseases (Volume 5)*. Washington DC: IBRD/World Bank; 2017.

52. *How tobacco smoke causes disease: The biology and behavioral basis for smoking-attributable disease: A report of the Surgeon General*. Atlanta GA: CDC; 2010.

53. *The health consequences of smoking: 50 years of progress: A report of the Surgeon General*. Atlanta GA: CDC; 2014.

54. Beaglehole R, Bonita R, Yach D, Mackay J, Reddy KS. A tobacco-free world: A call to action to phase out the sale of tobacco products by 2040. *Lancet*. 2015;385:1011–18.

55. Glynn T, Seffrin JR, Brawley OW, Grey N, Ross H. The globalization of tobacco use: 21 challenges for the 21st century. *CA Cancer J Clin*. 2010;60:50–61.

56. *WHO Framework Convention on Tobacco Control*. Geneva: WHO; 2005.

57. Shibuya K, Ciecierski C, Guindon E, Bettcher DW, Evans DB, Murray CJL. WHO Framework Convention on Tobacco Control: Development of an evidence based global public health treaty. *BMJ*. 2003;327:154–7.

58. Roemer R, Taylor A, Lariviere J. Origins of the WHO Framework Convention on Tobacco Control. *Am J Public Health*. 2005;95:936–8.

59. *2016 global progress report on implementation of the WHO Framework Convention on Tobacco Control*. Geneva: WHO; 2016.

60. Levy DT, Ellis JA, Mays D, Huang AT. Smoking-related deaths averted due to three years of policy progress. *Bull World Health Organ*. 2013;91:509–18.

61. *WHO Global Report on trends in prevalence of tobacco smoking*. Geneva: WHO; 2015.

62. Ng M, Freeman MK, Fleming TD, et al. Smoking prevalence and cigarette consumption in 187 countries, 1980–2012. *JAMA*. 2014;311:183–92.

63. Eriksen M, Mackay J, Schluger N, Gomesthapeh FI, Drope J. *The tobacco atlas*. 5th ed. Atlanta GA: American Cancer Society/World Lung Foundation; 2015.

64. Atkinson MA. Type 1 diabetes. *Lancet*. 2014;383:69–82.

65. Nolan CJ, Damm P, Prentki M. Type 2 diabetes across generations: From pathophysiology to prevention and management. *Lancet*. 2011;378:169–81.

66. Zimmet P, Alberti KGMM, Shaw J. Global and societal implications of the diabetes epidemic. *Nature*. 2001;414:782–7.

67. Imam K. Gestational diabetes mellitus. *Adv Exp Med Biol*. 2012;771:24–34.

68. *Definition and diagnosis of diabetes mellitus and intermediate hyperglycaemia*. Geneva: WHO/IDF; 2006.

69. *Use of glycated haemoglobin (HbA1c) in the diagnosis of diabetes mellitus: Abbreviated report of a WHO consultation*. Geneva: WHO; 2011.

70. Perreault L, Færch K. Approaching pre-diabetes. *J Diabetes Complications*. 2014;28:226–33.

71. *Global report on diabetes*. Geneva: WHO; 2016.

72. Ali M, Siegel K, Chandrasekar E, et al. Diabetes: an update on the pandemic and potential solutions (Chapter 12). *Disease control priorities*. 3rd ed. *Cardiovascular, respiratory, and related diseases (Volume 5)*. Washington DC: IBRD/World Bank; 2017.

73. NCD Risk Factor Collaboration (NCD-RisC). Worldwide trends in diabetes since 1980: A pooled analysis of 751 population-based studies with 4.4 million participants. *Lancet*. 2016;387:1513–30.

74. *IDF diabetes atlas*. 7th ed. Brussels: International Diabetes Federation (IDF); 2015.

75. Guariguata L, Whiting DR, Hambleton I, Beagley J, Linnenkamp U, Shaw JE. Global estimates of diabetes prevalence for 2013 and projections for 2035. *Diabetes Res Clin Pract*. 2014;103:137–49.

76. Dirks J, Anand S, Thomas B, et al. Kidney disease (Chapter 13). *Disease control priorities*. 3rd ed. *Cardiovascular, respiratory, and related diseases (Volume 5)*. Washington DC: IBRD/World Bank; 2017.

77. Levey AS, Coresh J. Chronic kidney disease. *Lancet*. 2012;379:165–80.

78. Webster AC, Nagler EV, Morton RL, Masson P. Chronic kidney disease. *Lancet*. 2017;389:1238–52.

79. Murtagh FE, Addington-Hall J, Higginson IJ. The prevalence of symptoms in end-stage renal disease: A systematic review. *Adv Chronic Kidney Dis*. 2007;14:82–99.

80. Zhang QL, Rothenbacher D. Prevalence of chronic kidney disease in population-based studies: Systematic review. *BMC Public Health*. 2008;8:117.

81. Jha V, Garcia-Garcia G, Iseki K, et al. Chronic kidney disease: Global dimension and perspectives. *Lancet*. 2013;382:260–72.

82. James MT, Hemmelgarn BR, Tonelli M. Early recognition and prevention of chronic kidney disease. *Lancet*. 2010;375:1296–309.

83. Liyanage T, Ninomiya T, Jha V, et al. Worldwide access to treatment for end-stage kidney disease: A systematic review. *Lancet*. 2015;385:1975–82.

84. Gansevoort RT, Correa-Rotter R, Hemmelgarn BR, et al. Chronic kidney disease and cardiovascular risk: Epidemiology, mechanisms, and prevention. *Lancet*. 2013;382:339–52.

85. Ramakrishnan K, Scheid DC. Diagnosis and management of acute pyelonephritis in adults. *Am Fam Physician*. 2005;71:933–42.

86. Lameire NH, Bagga A, Cruz D, et al. Acute kidney injury: An increasing global concern. *Lancet*. 2013;382:170–9.

87. Bellomo R, Kellum JA, Ronco C. Acute kidney injury. *Lancet*. 2012;380:756–66.

88. Lim YS, Kim WR. The global impact of hepatic fibrosis and end-stage liver disease. *Clin Liver Dis*. 2008;12:733–46.

89. Tsochatzis EA, Bosch J, Burroughs AK. Liver cirrhosis. *Lancet*. 2014;383:1749–61.

90. Mokdad AA, Lopez AD, Shahraz S, et al. Liver cirrhosis mortality in 187 countries between 1980 and 2010: A systematic analysis. *BMC Med*. 2014;12:145.

91. Lau JY, Sung J, Hill C, Henderson C, Howden CW, Metz DC. Systematic review of the epidemiology of complicated peptic ulcer disease: Incidence, recurrence, risk factors and mortality. *Digestion*. 2011;84:102–13.

92. Sugano K, Tak J, Kuipers EJ, et al. Kyoto global consensus report on *Helicobacter pylori* gastritis. *Gut*. 2015;64:1353–67.

93. Cosnes J, Gower-Rousseau C, Seksik P, Cortot A. Epidemiology and natural history of inflammatory bowel disease. *Gastroenterology*. 2011;140:1785–94.

94. Bickler SW, Weiser TG, Kassebaum N, et al. Global burden of surgical conditions (Chapter 2). *Disease control priorities*. 3rd ed. *Essential surgery (Volume 1)*. Washington DC: IBRD/World Bank; 2016.

95. *Neurological disorders: Public health challenges*. Geneva: WHO; 2006.

96. Thakur KT, Albanese E, Giannakopoulos P, et al. Neurological disorders (Chapter 5). *Disease Control Priorities*. 3rd ed. *Mental, neurological, and substance use disorders (Volume 4)*. Washington DC: IBRD/World Bank; 2015.

97. Ngugi AK, Bottomley C, Kleinschmidt I, Sander JW, Newton CR. Estimation of the burden of active and life-time epilepsy: A meta-analytic approach. *Epilepsia*. 2010;51:883–90.

98. Moshé SL, Perucca E, Ryvlin P, Tomson T. Epilepsy: New advances. *Lancet*. 2015;385:884–98.

99. *Atlas: Epilepsy care in the world*. Geneva: WHO; 2005.

100. Newton CR, Garcia HH. Epilepsy in poor regions of the world. *Lancet*. 2012;380:1193–201.

101. de Boer HM. Epilepsy stigma: Moving from a global problem to global solutions. *Seizure*. 2010;19:630–6.

102. *Atlas of headache disorders and resources in the world 2011*. Geneva: WHO; 2011.

103. Stovner LJ, Hagen K, Jensen R, et al. The global burden of headache: A documentation of headache prevalence and disability worldwide. *Cephalalgia*. 2007;27:193–210.

104. Headache Classification Committee of the International Headache Society (HIS). *The International Classification of Headache Disorders*. 3rd ed. (beta version). *Cephalalgia*. 2013;33:629–808.

105. Kalia LV, Lang AE. Parkinson's disease. *Lancet*. 2015;386:896–912.

106. Obeso JA, Rodriguez-Oroz MC, Goetz CG, et al. Missing pieces in the Parkinson's disease puzzle. *Nat Med*. 2010;16:653–61.

107. Calabresi P, Di Filippo M, Ghiglieri V, Tambasco N, Picconi B. Levodopa-induced dyskinesias in patients with Parkinson's disease: Filling the bench-to-bedside gap. *Lancet Neurol*. 2010;9:1106–17.

108. Dorsey ER, Constantinescu R, Thompson JP, et al. Projected number of people with Parkinson disease in the most populous nations, 2005 through 2030. *Neurology*. 2007;68:384–6.

109. Pringsheim T, Jette N, Frolkis A, Steeves TD. The prevalence of Parkinson's disease: A systematic review and meta-analysis. *Mov Disord*. 2014;29:1583–90.

110. Kister I, Bacon TE, Chamot E, et al. Natural history of multiple sclerosis symptoms. *Int J MS Care*. 2013;15:146–58.

111. Murray TJ. Diagnosis and treatment of multiple sclerosis. *BMJ*. 2006;332:525–7.

112. Tremlett H, Zhao Y, Rieckmann P, Hutchinson M. New perspectives in the natural history of multiple sclerosis. *Neurology*. 2010;74:2004–15.

113. Browne P, Chandraratna D, Angood C, et al. Atlas of multiple sclerosis 2013: A growing global problem with widespread inequity. *Neurology*. 2014;83:1022–4.

114. Alonso A, Hernán MA. Temporal trends in the incidence of multiple sclerosis: A systematic review. *Neurology*. 2008;70:129–35.

115. Goldberg AD, Allis CD, Bernstein E. Epigenetics: A landscape takes shape. *Cell*. 2007;128:635–8.

116. Mégarbané A, Ravel A, Mircher C, et al. The 50th anniversary of the discovery of trisomy 21: The past, present, and future of research and treatment of Down syndrome. *Genet Med.* 2009;11:611–16.

117. Bondy CA. Turner Syndrome Study Group. Care of girls and women with Turner syndrome: A guideline of the Turner Syndrome Study Group. *J Clin Endocrinol Metab.* 2007;92:10–25.

118. Roos RAC. Huntington's disease: A clinical review. *Orphanet J Rare Dis.* 2010;5:40.

119. 119 Strausbaugh SD, Davis PB. Cystic fibrosis: A review of epidemiology and pathobiology. *Clin Chest Med.* 2007;28:279–88.

120. Modell B, Darlison M. Global epidemiology of haemoglobin disorders and derived service indicators. *Bull World Health Organ.* 2008;86:480–7.

121. Rund D, Rachmilewitz E. Beta-thalassemia. *N Engl J Med.* 2005;353:1135–46.

122. Muncie HL, Campbell JS. Alpha and beta thalassemia. *Am Fam Physician.* 2009;80:339–44.

123. Rees DC, Williams TN, Gladwin MT. Sickle-cell disease. *Lancet.* 2010;376:2018–31.

124. Piel FB, Patil AP, Howes RE, et al. Global distribution of the sickle cell gene and geographical confirmation of the malaria hypothesis. *Nat Commun.* 2010;1:104.

125. Mannucci PM, Tuddenham EG. The hemophilias: From royal genes to gene therapy. *N Engl J Med.* 2001;344:1773–9.

126. Luzzatto L, Nannelli C, Notaro R. Glucose-6-phosphate dehydrogenase deficiency. *Hematol Oncol Clin North Am.* 2016;30:373–93.

127. Woolf AD, Pfleger B. Burden of major musculoskeletal conditions. *Bull World Health Organ.* 2003;81:646–56.

128. Hoy D, March L, Brooks P, et al. The global burden of low back pain: Estimates from the Global Burden of Disease 2010 study. *Ann Rheum Dis.* 2014;73:1309–15.

129. Chou R, Qaseem A, Snow V, et al. Diagnosis and treatment of low back pain: A joint clinical practice guideline from the American College of Physicians and the American Pain Society. *Ann Intern Med.* 2007;147:478–91.

130. Von Korff M, Saunders K. The course of back pain in primary care. *Spine.* 1996;21:2833–7.

131. Litwic A, Edwards M, Dennison E, Cooper C. Epidemiology and burden of osteoarthritis. *Br Med Bull.* 2013;105:185–99.

132. Cross M, Smith EU, Hoy D, et al. Severity of osteoarthritis in global populations. *Osteoarth Cartil.* 2014;22(Suppl 1):S208.

133. Smolen JS, Aletaha D, McInnes IB. Rheumatoid arthritis. *Lancet.* 2016;388:2023–38.

134. Yu C, Gershwin ME, Chang C. Diagnostic criteria for systemic lupus erythematosus: A critical review. *J Autoimmun.* 2014;48–49:10–3.

135. Leslie WD, Morin SN. Osteoporosis epidemiology 2013: Implications for diagnosis, risk assessment, and treatment. *Curr Opin Rheumatol.* 2014;26:440–6.

136. Smith E, Hoy D, Cross M, et al. The global burden of gout: Estimate from the Global Burden of Disease 2010 study. *Ann Rheum Dis.* 2014;73:1470–6.

137. Pascolini D, Mariotti SP. Global estimates of visual impairment: 2010. *Br J Ophthalmol.* 2012;96:614–8.

138. *Universal eye health: A global action plan 2014–2019.* Geneva: WHO; 2013.

139. Stevens GA, White RA, Flaxman SR, et al. Global prevalence of vision impairment and blindness: Magnitude and temporal trends, 1990–2010. *Ophthalmology.* 2013;120:2377–84.

140. *Global Initiative for the Elimination of Avoidable Blindness: Action plan 2006–2011.* Geneva: WHO; 2007.

141. *Global data on visual impairments 2010.* Geneva: WHO; 2012.

142. Bourne RR, Stevens GA, White RA, et al. Causes of vision loss worldwide, 1990–2010: A systematic analysis. *Lancet Glob Health.* 2013;1:e339–49.

143. Lee CM, Afshari NA. The global state of cataract blindness. *Curr Opin Ophthalmol.* 2017;28:98–103.

144. Chiang PP, O'Connor PM, Le Mesurier RT, Keeffe JE. A global survey of low vision service provision. *Ophthalmic Epidemiol.* 2011;18:109–21.

145. Stevens G, Flaxman S, Brunskill E, Mascarenhas M, Mathers CD, Finucane M. Global Burden of Disease Hearing Loss Expert Group. Global and regional hearing impairment prevalence: An analysis of 42 studies in 29 countries. *Eur J Public Health.* 2013;23:146–52.

146. *Millions of people in the world have hearing loss that can be treated or prevented.* Geneva: WHO; 2013.

147. Basner M, Babisch W, Davis A, et al. Auditory and non-auditory effects of noise on health. *Lancet.* 2014;383:1325–32.

148. Tucci D, Merson MH, Wilson BS. A summary of the literature of global hearing impairment: Current status and priorities for action. *Otol Neurotol.* 2010;31:31–41.

149. Nutten S. Atopic dermatitis: Global epidemiology and risk factors. *Ann Nutr Metab.* 2015;66(Suppl 1):8–16.

150. Williams HC, Dellavalle RP, Garner S. Acne vulgaris. *Lancet.* 2012;379:361–72.

151. Parisi R, Symmons DP, Griffiths CE, Ashcroft DM. Identification and Management of Psoriasis and Associated ComorbidiTy (IMPACT) project team. Global epidemiology of psoriasis: A systematic review of incidence and prevalence. *J Invest Dermatol.* 2013;133:377–85.

152. Chosidow O. Scabies. *N Engl J Med.* 2006;354:1718–27.

153. Carratalà J, Rosón B, Fernández-Sabé N, et al. Factors associated with complications and mortality in adult patients hospitalized for infectious cellulitis. *Eur J Clin Microbiol Infect Dis*. 2003;22:151–7.

154. Kassebaum NJ, Bernabé E, Dahiya M, Bhandari B, Murray CJL, Marcenes W. Global burden of untreated caries: A systematic review and metaregression. *J Dent Res*. 2015;94:650–8.

155. *The challenge of oral disease: A call for global action. The oral health atlas 2nd edition*. Geneva: FDI World Dental Federation; 2015.

156. Kassebaum NJ, Bernabé E, Dahiya M, Bhandari B, Murray CJL, Marcenes W. Global burden of severe periodontitis in 1990–2010: A systematic review and metaregression. *J Dent Res*. 2014;93:1045–53.

157. Kassebaum NJ, Bernabé E, Dahiya M, Bhandari B, Murray CJL, Marcenes W. Global burden of severe tooth loss: A systematic review and meta-analysis. *J Dent Res*. 2014;93(Suppl 7):S20–8.

CHAPTER 16

Mental Health

Each year about one in five people experiences a depressive disorder, an anxiety disorder, a substance use disorder, or another diagnosable mental health disorder. Mental illnesses are among the most common causes of disability in countries worldwide, and the people who have them often encounter stigma and discrimination. Although effective therapies for many mental health disorders exist, only a small proportion of people who would benefit from them are accessing mental healthcare services.

▶ 16.1 Mental Health and Global Health

Mental health disorders are a global health priority because they are very common worldwide and they cause significant reductions in quality of life. Approximately one in five people meets the criteria for a mental health disorder in any 1-year period.[1] Many of these individuals will have days of reduced productivity at work and home because of their mental health condition, and many will experience times when it takes extreme effort to perform routine daily activities.[2] Some people with severe mental illnesses will have extended periods of time when they have great difficulty with self-care, interpersonal relationships, and other life activities.[3] These challenges make mental health disorders the leading cause of disability worldwide,[4] accounting for about one-fifth of the years lived with disability (YLDs) generated each year by diminished function (**FIGURE 16–1**).[5]

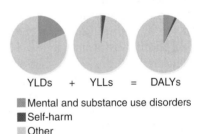

YLDs + YLLs = DALYs

■ Mental and substance use disorders
■ Self-harm
■ Other

FIGURE 16–1 Mental health disorders account for nearly one-quarter of years lived with disability (YLDs) worldwide.

Data from GBD 2015 Disease and Injury Incidence and Prevalence Collaborators. Global, regional, and national incidence, prevalence, and years lived with disability for 310 diseases and injuries, 1990–2015: A systematic analysis for the Global Burden of Disease Study 2015. *Lancet* 2016; 388:1545–602.

While there is some variation in regional prevalence rates, every part of the world bears a significant burden from mental health issues.[1] The most commonly diagnosed and disabling mental health conditions include schizophrenia, bipolar disorder, depressive disorders, anxiety disorders, and alcohol and drug use disorders (**FIGURE 16–2**).[5] However, even though these mental health disorders are known to be very common, most of these conditions remain poorly understood.[6] Mental illnesses likely arise from a complex set of genetic, biological, social, psychological, developmental, and environmental factors, but few risk factors have been conclusively identified.[7] The Grand Challenges in Global Mental Health initiative has identified critical gaps in our knowledge regarding the causes of mental health disorders, significant limitations in our ability to prevent mental health disorders through interventions across the lifespan, and major barriers to accessing mental health diagnoses and effective treatment.[8] Addressing these constraints would enable progress to be made toward achieving the Sustainable Development Goals (SDGs) targets that aim to "promote mental health and well-being" (SDG 3.4) and "strengthen the prevention and treatment of substance abuse, including narcotic drug abuse and harmful use of alcohol" (SDG 3.5).[9]

Mental health is also a global health priority because it is a human rights issue. Although medications and various types of therapy and support are effective at improving quality of life for people with neuropsychiatric conditions, most people who would benefit from these interventions are unable to access them.[10] In many communities, people with mental illness are maltreated. They may be imprisoned or involuntarily detained in hospitals for long periods of time without any legal recourse, they may be denied access to hospitalization when it is needed, and they may be subjected to various types of violence and abuse.[11] Poverty and discrimination exacerbate the challenges faced by many people with mental illnesses.[12] The global burden from mental health disorders will not be reduced without vigorous international commitments to work together to develop effective new treatments, increase access to specialty care, and reduce the stigma associated with mental illnesses.[13]

▶ 16.2 Schizophrenia

Schizophrenia is a mental health disorder characterized by distorted perceptions of reality.[14] People with schizophrenia and other psychotic disorders may experience delusions and hallucinations. **Delusions** are false beliefs that are irrational but seem very real to the person experiencing them. Some people with paranoid thinking firmly believe they are being robbed by family members or tracked by the police, even when in reality they are not being targeted. Some people with delusions believe they have superpowers. **Hallucinations** are sensory distortions that cause the affected person to hear, see, feel, smell, or taste something that in reality is not present. A person experiencing auditory hallucinations may hear the voices of people who are not actually nearby. People with schizophrenia may also express disorganized thinking and speech. These "positive" or psychotic symptoms are often accompanied by "negative" or deficit symptoms, such as a flat affect and low energy. Additionally, people with schizophrenia may exhibit cognitive issues, such as impaired decision-making and memory.

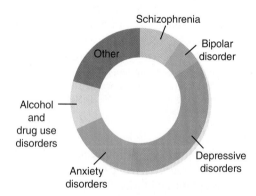

FIGURE 16–2 Global distribution of years lived with disability (YLDs) from various mental health disorders.

Data from GBD 2015 Disease and Injury Incidence and Prevalence Collaborators. Global, regional, and national incidence, prevalence, and years lived with disability for 310 diseases and injuries, 1990–2015: A systematic analysis for the Global Burden of Disease Study 2015. *Lancet* 2016; 388:1545–602.

Approximately 7 per 1000 people will be diagnosed with schizophrenia during their lifetimes.[15] Most initial diagnoses are made during early adulthood.[16] Antipsychotic medications are often effective in treating the most common psychotic symptoms. Psychosocial interventions, such as patient therapy, family support groups, and community-based rehabilitation, are also helpful in enabling people with schizophrenia to lead independent lives.[17] With medication and other therapies, many people with a schizophrenia diagnosis are able to achieve remission. However, relapses and chronic disability remain common.[18] One of the major barriers to favorable outcomes for people diagnosed with schizophrenia is limited access to psychiatric services. About two-thirds of people with schizophrenia and related disorders who live in low- and middle-income countries are not receiving specialized mental health care (**FIGURE 16–3**).[19]

Another challenge is the stigma associated with the disorder. **Stigma** is a term used to describe negative attitudes about members of a population group. Those negative perceptions often lead to discrimination, social exclusion, and other forms of marginalization. The majority of people with schizophrenia report having experienced rejection, avoidance, and other forms of interpersonal and social stigma.[20] The stigma of mental illnesses can be countered with education, social interactions between members of majority populations and stigmatized populations, and social activism that promotes more inclusive attitudes and behaviors.[21]

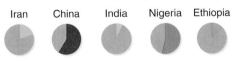

FIGURE 16–3 Proportion of people with schizophrenia who receive specialty mental health care.

Data from Lora A, Kohn R, Levav I, McBain R, Morris J, Saxena S. Service availability and utilization and treatment gap for schizophrenic disorders: A survey in 50 low- and middle-income countries. *Bull World Health Organ* 2012;90:47–54B.

▶ 16.3 Bipolar Disorder

Bipolar disorder, formerly called manic depression, is characterized by alternating periods of depression and mania or hypomania.[22] People with bipolar disorder experience dramatic shifts in mood, energy level, appetite and sleep habits, and self-image. These cycles may be relatively rapid, or they may occur slowly over a period of months. Antipsychotic medications can alleviate the symptoms of acute mania, which may include grandiose delusions, sleeplessness, euphoria, and irritability. Lithium and other pharmaceutical agents can help prevent relapses. These medications are most effective at managing the disorder when their use is combined with psychotherapy.[23]

It is likely that 1%–2% of adults have bipolar disorder, but it is difficult to ascertain the actual prevalence because diagnosis can be clinically challenging.[24] Many people who meet the clinical definition for bipolar disorder also meet the criteria for anxiety disorders and other comorbid (concurrent) mental illnesses. These complexities may make it difficult for people with bipolar disorder to receive an accurate diagnosis and access appropriate long-term management of their mental health conditions. Stigma associated with bipolar disorder in healthcare facilities, workplaces, and other settings may further reduce access to care and quality of life for people with the disorder and for their families.[25]

▶ 16.4 Depressive Disorders

Depressive disorder is characterized by sadness, hopelessness, loss of interest in usual activities, fatigue, poor concentration, and other negative thoughts, feelings, and physical symptoms that interfere with normal daily activities.[26] Major depressive disorder is sometimes called unipolar depressive disorder to

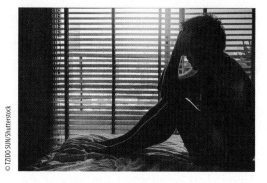

distinguish it from bipolar disorder. People with **unipolar depressive disorder** experience depression without the cycles of mania that affect people with bipolar disorder.

About 5% of adults worldwide meet the clinical definition of depression during the course of 1 year.[27] Most people with an episode of acute depression do not develop chronic depression. For about one in five people, especially those who were young when they first experienced depression and those with comorbid mental health disorders, the depression becomes a persistent depressive disorder.[28] Depression is a leading cause of disability globally because it affects so many people worldwide and it causes significant reductions in productivity at work, home, and school.[29] People with severe depression may not have the energy to get out of bed, eat, go to work, meet with friends, or conduct other routine daily activities.

The American Psychiatric Association guidelines published in the *Diagnostic and Statistical Manual of Mental Disorders (DSM-5)*, usually simply called "the DSM," spell out the defining features of dozens of mental health issues, including depression.[30] Children, adolescents, and adults can be clinically diagnosed as having mild, moderate, or severe depression based on criteria in the DSM.[31] However, the diagnosis of mental health disorders is, in part, dependent on cultural norms and perceptions.[32] Many disorders exist as part of a spectrum where

the distinction between what is classified as "normal" and what is classified as a "disorder" is blurry. This may help explain why there is variation in the country-specific prevalence rates of depression (**FIGURE 16–4**).[29] Countries with a higher prevalence of depression tend to include milder cases of depression in their statistics, while countries with a lower prevalence of depression tend to report only the moderate and severe cases of depression that cause significant impairment.[33]

Depression can be successfully treated with low-cost medications and psychotherapy, such as cognitive behavioral therapy.[34] **Cognitive behavioral therapy** (CBT) is a form of talk therapy in which a therapist helps an individual understand his or her thoughts, feelings, and behaviors and identify actions that can be taken to correct problems. Both amitriptyline (a tricyclic antidepressant) and fluoxetine (a selective serotonin reuptake inhibitor, or SSRI) are included in the World Health Organization's list of essential medicines,[35] and other types of antidepressants are also effective treatments. The barriers to accessing mental health care include perceptions that medication is not needed; structural barriers, such as the

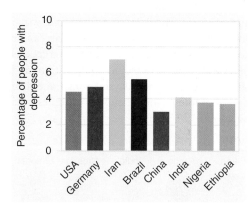

FIGURE 16–4 Percentage of the population with major depressive disorder each year.

Data from Ferrari AJ, Charlson FJ, Norman RE, Patten SB, Freedman G, Murray CJL, Vos T, Whiteford HA. Burden of depressive disorders by country, sex, age, and year: Findings from the Global Burden of Disease Study 2010. *PLoS Med* 2013; 10:e1001547.

financial costs and time constraints associated with seeking health services; and attitudinal barriers, such as the perception that treatment will be ineffective, the belief that the problem will resolve on its own with time, and concerns about stigma.[36] Because depression is linked with physical health—people with depression often report decreased overall health status, and people with chronic diseases have an elevated risk of depression—it can be beneficial for health systems to integrate depression screening, diagnosis, and treatment with care for other health conditions.[37]

▶ 16.5 Anxiety Disorders

Anxiety disorders are characterized by a disproportionate fear of imminent danger and worry about potential future threats.[30] There are several types of anxiety disorders. **Generalized anxiety disorder** is defined by persistent excessive worrying about numerous concerns, and it is often accompanied by sleep disturbances, muscle tension, and fatigue.[38] **Panic disorder** is defined by repeated panic attacks that last for several intense minutes and cause a racing heartbeat, dizziness or weakness, and other disturbing symptoms.[39] Other anxiety disorders include separation anxiety disorder, social anxiety disorder, agoraphobia, and other specific phobias.[30] Together, anxiety disorders are among the most common mental health issues globally,[40] and they are one of the leading causes of disability worldwide.[41] Antianxiety medications and CBT can be effective treatments for anxiety disorders.[7]

▶ 16.6 Alcohol and Drug Use Disorders

Addiction is a cognitive and neurological condition characterized by adverse behaviors related to physical or psychological dependence.[42] While the term addiction is primarily used to refer to dependence on substances, it is also used to describe some types of compulsive behaviors, such as excessive gambling.[43] The American Society of Addition Medicine has identified the ABCs of addiction as the inability to Abstain from harmful substances or behaviors, Behavior control impairment, Craving substances or experiences, Diminished recognition of the problems with individual functioning and interpersonal relationships, and dysfunctional Emotional responses.[44] Substance use disorders include misuse of alcohol, caffeine, cannabis, hallucinogens (including phencyclidine, more commonly called PCP), inhalants, opioids, sedatives, hypnotics, anxiolytics, stimulants, tobacco, and other substances.[30]

Excessive alcohol use causes cirrhosis and other forms of liver damage, significantly increases the risk of a diversity of cancers and other noncommunicable diseases, increases the risk of both unintentional injuries and intentional injuries, and increases the risk of premature mortality.[45] Men have a particularly high rate of adverse effects from alcohol use. Men on average drink more alcohol than women (**FIGURE 16–5**), and males are more likely than females to report binge drinking (**FIGURE 16–6**) and alcohol use disorders (**FIGURE 16–7**).[46] In many countries, more than 10% of the total disability among young and middle-aged adult men is attributable to alcohol use (**FIGURE 16–8**).[47]

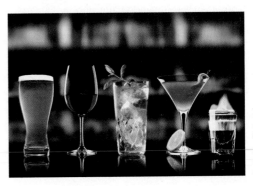

© petereleven/Shutterstock

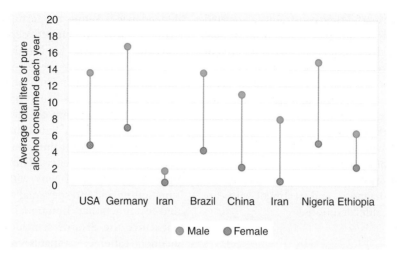

FIGURE 16–5 Males on average consume more liters of pure alcohol each year than females (aged 15+ years).

Data from *Global status report on noncommunicable diseases* 2014. Geneva: WHO; 2014.

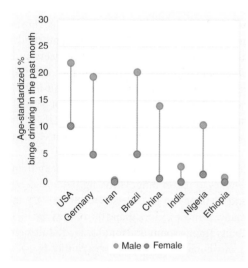

FIGURE 16–6 Males are more likely than females (aged 15+ years) to report binge drinking during the last month. (Heavy episodic drinking is defined as 60 grams of alcohol or more consumed during one occasion.)

Data from *Global status report on alcohol and health 2014*. Geneva: WHO; 2014.

The types of alcoholic beverages consumed vary by country (**FIGURE 16–9**), but it is the volume of pure alcohol ingested that predicts the health outcomes, not the particular type of alcoholic beverage consumed.[47]

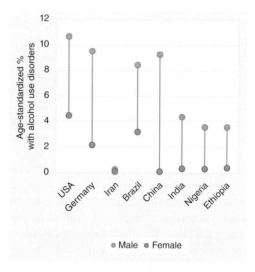

FIGURE 16–7 Age-standardized prevalence of alcohol use disorders among people aged 15 years and older. Alcohol use disorders include harmful use of alcohol and alcohol dependence.

Data from *Global status report on alcohol and health 2014*. Geneva: WHO; 2014.

Early detection and treatment of harmful drinking behaviors through community-based detoxification and self-help groups are cost-effective interventions for reducing the burden of alcohol use disorders.[48] Restrictions on alcohol sales, taxes on alcohol,

USA   Germany   Brazil   China   India   Nigeria

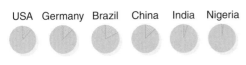

FIGURE 16-8 Percentage of disability-adjusted life years (DALYs) lost to alcohol among men aged 18–64 years.

Data from Rehm J, Mathers C, Popova S, Thavorncharoensap M, Teerawattananon Y, Patra J. Global burden of disease and injury and economic cost attributable to alcohol use and alcohol use disorders. *Lancet* 2009; 373:2223–33.

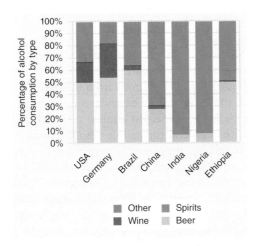

Other   **Spirits**
Wine   **Beer**

FIGURE 16-9 Types of alcoholic beverages consumed by liter of pure alcohol in featured countries.

Data from *Global status report on alcohol and health 2014.* Geneva: WHO; 2014.

and enforcement of laws banning driving while under the influence of alcohol have also been found to be effective at reducing alcohol abuse.[45]

Cannabis products, such as marijuana, are the most widely used illicit drugs worldwide, but the greatest disability is associated with injectable drugs, such as amphetamines, opioids (including heroin, morphine, and fentanyl), and cocaine.[49] A **person who injects drugs (PWID)**, also called an **injecting drug user (IDU)**, may face numerous negative health outcomes, including an increased risk of viral hepatitis, HIV infection, and premature mortality. These substances also harm relationships, decrease economic status, and increase the likelihood of participation in

criminal activity.[50] There is an additional and growing burden from the nonmedical use of prescription medications.[51] However, it can be difficult to measure the level of harm caused by problematic drug use because data about illegal activities are not easily gathered.[52] While many countries have attempted to reduce drug addiction problems through substance abuse awareness campaigns, enforcement of drug laws, and imprisonment of drug users, few policies and programs have proven to be effective at reducing the burden from harmful drug use.[50]

Substance abuse has a major adverse impact on public health in many countries. For example, of all people in the United States who were 12 years old or older in 2015, 25% reported binge drinking in the last month, 13.5% reported using marijuana in the last year, 4.7% reported misusing prescription pain relievers, 1.8% reported using cocaine or crack, 1.8% reported using hallucinogens, and 0.3% reported using heroin in the last year.[53] About 8.8% of the population met the criteria for a drug or alcohol use disorder, but only 10% of those individuals had received any treatment for the disorder in the last year. The number of people dying each year from opioid overdoses nearly quadrupled between 2000 and 2015.[53] In 2015 alone, nearly 50,000 people in the United States died from drug overdoses, with nearly 30,000 of those fatalities attributable to opioids (including prescription opioids and heroin). Opioid antagonist medications like naloxone and naltrexone are used by emergency medical personnel to reverse opioid overdoses, but many people die from overdoses before anyone is able to call for help.

▶ 16.7 Other Mental Health Disorders

Besides schizophrenia, bipolar disorder, major depressive disorder, and substance use disorders, numerous other mental health disorders have been identified. **Obsessive-compulsive disorder (OCD)** involves anxiety-inducing recurrent thoughts (obsessions) and repetitive behaviors intended to reduce distress or prevent bad events (compulsions). About 1%–1.5% of adults and 2.5%–3% of children and adolescents have OCD.[54] Medications and CBT can effectively treat OCD.[54]

Trauma and other stresses can increase the risk of a mental health disorder. The most common types of traumatic events include witnessing a death or a serious injury, losing a family member or friend to unexpected death, being mugged or threatened with a weapon, being involved in a serious motor vehicle collision, and having a life-threatening illness.[55] Other traumas include being exposed to war or other forms of collective violence, experiencing interpersonal or intimate partner violence, living through a natural disaster, and other types of personal and family traumas. **Posttraumatic stress disorder (PTSD)** occurs after a traumatic incident leads to nightmares or other types of distressing recollections of the event; avoidance of reminders of the traumatic event; and physiological signs of hyperarousal, such as hypervigilance and insomnia.[56]

Feeding and eating disorders present as disturbed eating behaviors. The word **anorexia** means a lack of appetite. **Anorexia nervosa** is a condition in which a person has a distorted body image and feels overweight even when emaciated. A person with anorexia nervosa follows a very restricted diet, exercises excessively, and may use laxatives and other methods of losing weight. Anorexia nervosa primarily affects adolescent females from high-income countries, and the disorder can lead to death if it is not treated successfully.[57] **Bulimia nervosa** occurs when a person engages in frequent binge–purge cycles, eating thousands of calories at one sitting, and then inducing vomiting and using laxatives to get rid of the ingested calories. **Binge-eating disorder** is characterized by repeated incidents of consuming large quantities of food without subsequent purging. In high- and upper-middle-income countries, about 1%

of people experience bulimia nervosa during their lifetimes and about 2% experience binge-eating disorder.[58]

A diversity of other mental health issues are described in DSM-5, including dissociative disorders, somatic disorders, sleep-wake disorders such as insomnia and narcolepsy, sexual dysfunctions, a variety of disruptive, impulse-control, and conduct (DIC) disorders, and personality disorders.[30]

▶ **16.8 Suicide**

Suicide is the intentional act of ending one's own life. Suicides are preventable, and numerous interventions from the individual to the societal level can help reduce the suicide rate.[59] Access to clinical mental health care is critical for people who are thinking or talking about ending their lives or are expressing hopelessness and ambivalence about living or dying. Community-based social support services, including crisis hotlines, can be lifesaving for people who have survived wars and disasters, have been displaced from their home communities or imprisoned, have encountered systemic discrimination, have been abused or bullied, have suffered chronic pain, or have experienced other forms of trauma and social disconnection. Policies that increase access to mental health services and decrease access to the common means of suicide, such as pesticides, other poisons, and firearms, can be effective at preventing self-harm.[59]

As awareness of suicide warning signs and effective prevention strategies has increased, the mortality rate from self-harm has decreased in most world regions.[60] However, suicide continues to be a significant cause of preventable mortality, with some countries bearing especially high burdens (**FIGURE 16–10**).[61] Globally, the proportion of deaths from suicide is highest among younger adults (**FIGURE 16–11**), but the rate of death from self-harm is highest among

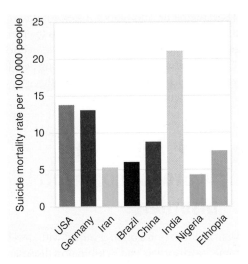

FIGURE 16–10 Suicide mortality rate per 100,000 people.

Data from *World health statistics 2016*. Geneva: WHO; 2016.

older adults (**FIGURE 16–12**).[60] The reason that young adults have a higher proportionate mortality rate from suicide is that the overall mortality rate in this age group is low. With few young adults dying from chronic diseases and other conditions each year, suicide stands out as a relatively common cause of mortality. By contrast, older adults have a high overall mortality rate, with many members of this age cohort dying each year from cardiovascular diseases, cancers, and other chronic conditions. Because the overall death rate is high, deaths from self-harm are a small percentage of all deaths of older adults, even in countries where the suicide rate is highest among the oldest people.[62]

Thinking about suicide is not uncommon. Each year about 2% of adults have thoughts about committing suicide (suicidal ideation), about 0.7% think about how they would commit suicide (suicidal planning), and about 0.4% make a suicide attempt (**FIGURE 16–13**).[63] The rates of suicidal ideating, planning, and attempting are similar in countries across the income spectrum. Most people who report having suicidal thoughts do not attempt suicide, and most suicide attempts do not result in death. Globally, there are about 20 suicide attempts and other potentially fatal acts of self-harm for every one reported suicide death.[64] However, it is important for all people who are thinking about suicide to address the thoughts, feelings, and behaviors that led to suicidal ideation. Trained mental health workers are best able to assist with this process.

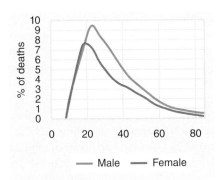

FIGURE 16–11 The percentage of all deaths that are caused by self-harm is highest in younger adults.

Data from GBD 2015 Mortality and Causes of Death Collaborators. Global, regional, and national life expectancy, all-cause mortality, and cause-specific mortality for 249 causes of death, 1980–2015: A systematic analysis for the Global Burden of Disease Study 2015. *Lancet* 2016; 388:1459–544.

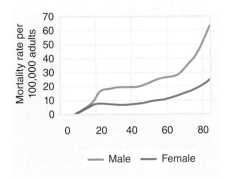

FIGURE 16–12 The rate of deaths from self-harm is highest in older adults.

Data from GBD 2015 Mortality and Causes of Death Collaborators. Global, regional, and national life expectancy, all-cause mortality, and cause-specific mortality for 249 causes of death, 1980–2015: A systematic analysis for the Global Burden of Disease Study 2015. *Lancet* 2016;388:1459–544.

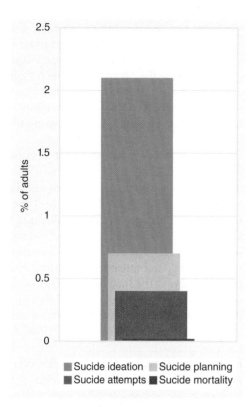

FIGURE 16–13 Percentage of adults reporting suicidal ideation, planning, and attempts in a 1-year period.

Data from Borges G, Nock MK, Haro Abad JM, Hwant I, Sampson NA, Alonso J, et al. Twelve month prevalence of and risk factors for suicide attempts in the WHO World Mental Health Surveys. *J Clin Psychiatry* 2010; 71:1617–28.

Many types of mental health disorders are associated with an increased risk of suicide, including schizophrenia, depressive disorders, bipolar disorder, some types of anxiety disorders, and substance use disorders.[63] However, most people with mental illnesses do not engage in self-harm, and suicide is not the leading cause of the increased risk of premature death among people with mental health disorders.[65] Instead, mental illnesses lead to reduced use of preventive health services (such as vaccination and cancer screening), poorer management of other chronic health conditions (such as hypertension and diabetes), and the adoption of unhealthy behaviors (such as tobacco use and physical inactivity), and those risk factors increase the

risk of premature mortality.[66] Access to comprehensive health services, not just access to emergency psychiatric care, is required to reduce the rate of preventable mortality among people with mental health disorders and others who may be contemplating suicide.

▶ 16.9 Autism and Neurodevelopmental Disorders

Mental illnesses are often grouped with developmental disorders and neurological disorders under a broader umbrella of neuropsychiatric disorders. **Neurodevelopmental disorders** are neurological and developmental disorders that present in childhood, and they require early intervention for the best outcomes. In the DSM-5, the neurodevelopmental disorder category includes intellectual disabilities, communication disorders, autism spectrum disorder, attention-deficit/hyperactivity disorder (ADHD), specific learning disorders, motor disorders, and other early-onset conditions.[30] The most common childhood mental and developmental disorders are anxiety disorders, ADHD, conduct disorder, autism, and intellectual disabilities.[67]

Early intervention for neurodevelopmental disorders is helpful for improving health, behavior, school achievement, and other factors related to productivity and quality of life.[68] For example, CBT can successfully treat anxiety disorders in children,[69] and medications can be effective for managing ADHD.[70] **Autism** is a lifelong neurodevelopmental disorder that begins in early childhood and causes mild to severe challenges with social communication and other functions.[71] Autism spectrum disorders affect about 1 in 130 people worldwide, and this rate appears to be fairly consistent across regions.[72] Autism has become a higher global health priority as the prevalence has increased while the risk factors for autism and the causes of the rising diagnosis rates remain unidentified.[73] Early intervention can improve cognitive and language skills as well as behavior among children with autism spectrum disorders.[74]

▶ ## 16.10 Dementia and Neurocognitive Disorders

Neurocognitive disorders are neurological and cognitive disorders that typically develop in older adulthood. **Dementia** is a chronic syndrome characterized by memory loss, confusion, and other signs of impaired cognitive function. Over time, people with dementia often develop speech and communication difficulties, disorientation to time and place, and mood and behavior changes.[75] As the symptoms of dementia become worse, affected adults may be unable to live independently. About 5%–7% of adults aged 60 years and older have a form of dementia. The prevalence of dementia increases dramatically with age, increasing from less than 1% at age 60 years to more than 10% by age 80 years and more than 25% by age 90 years.[76] **Alzheimer's disease** is the most prevalent form of dementia, accounting for about two-thirds of diagnosed dementia cases.[75] Dementia may also be caused by blocked blood vessels and strokes (vascular dementia), the buildup of alpha-synuclein proteins in the brain (Lewy body dementia), and other pathologic processes. Approximately 35 million people worldwide had dementia in 2010, and this number is expected to nearly double to 65 million people by 2030.[76] However, many people with dementia remain undiagnosed. Among those who are diagnosed, many are not receiving care or are receiving inadequate health care and social support.[77]

Not all neurocognitive disorders are related to aging. Some are the result of injuries. **Traumatic brain injury (TBI)** is short- or long-term damage arising from a concussion or other form of intracranial injury sustained during a traffic collision, fall, violent encounter, sporting event, or other cause of head trauma.[78] Severe and moderate TBI can cause death or permanent cognitive impairment.[79] Even mild TBI may cause several months of cognitive deficits.[80]

▶ ## 16.11 Mental Health Care

Many mental illnesses are treatable. Medications can relieve symptoms and prevent relapses, therapy can help people with mental illnesses understand and change their thoughts and behaviors, and social rehabilitation that focuses on practical skills can help people with mental illnesses return to normal activities. A variety of professionals are equipped to offer mental health care. A **psychiatrist** is a physician with advanced training in mental health who is able to prescribe psychiatric medications. A **psychologist** has advanced training in counseling and is able to offer a variety of types of individual and group therapy. Nurses, social workers, and other healthcare and social service professionals may be trained and licensed to offer mental health care. Primary care providers and community service organizations, including religious organizations, also provide services for individuals and families seeking assistance.[81]

Unfortunately, mental health therapies are extremely underused. Considerably fewer than half of adults with severe mental illnesses receive any mental healthcare services, and an even lower proportion of people with mild or moderate mental illnesses receive medical care.[82] Many people do not know that help is available, so they do not seek clinical help. For others, fear of the stigma of being diagnosed with a mental illness prevents them from seeking treatment. Many people who would like mental health assistance do not have access to a mental health specialist. In most low-income countries, there are more than 100,000 people for every one psychiatrist (**FIGURE 16–14**) and there are few beds available for inpatient psychiatric care (**FIGURE 16–15**).[83]

The risk factors for mental illness include living in poverty, experiencing a conflict or disaster, and having a severe physical disease, so the populations that have the greatest need for mental health services often have the least access to them.[84] A mental health package for treatment of depression, bipolar disorder, schizophrenia, and alcoholism with antidepressant, mood-stabilizing, and antipsychotic medications and psychosocial therapy could cost only a few dollars per adult each year in low- and middle-income countries.[85] However, this would be a large portion of the health budget in many low-income countries. The majority of the money allocated to mental health care is spent on long-term inpatient care rather than on more cost-effective interventions like community-based treatment.[86]

The public health actions for improving mental health care include educating the public about mental illness, providing mental health treatment as part of primary health care, and involving communities and families in caring for people with mental illnesses.[87] When families and social groups, employers, and public service providers (including the healthcare, education, and justice systems) are prepared to support people with mental health conditions, most people with mental illnesses are able to actively engage in social events, participate in the economy, and be protected from discrimination and violence.[88]

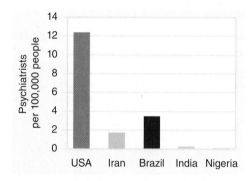

FIGURE 16–14 Psychiatrists per 100,000 people. (Data are not available for all featured countries.)

Data from *Mental health atlas 2014*. Geneva: WHO; 2015.

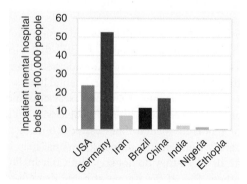

FIGURE 16–15 Inpatient mental hospital beds per 100,000 people.

Data from *Mental health atlas 2014*. Geneva: WHO; 2015.

▶ References

1. Steel Z, Marnane C, Iranpour C, et al. The global prevalence of common mental disorders: A systematic review and meta-analysis 1980–2013. *Int J Epidemiol.* 2014;43:476–93.
2. Bruffaerts R, Vilagut G, Demyttenaere K, et al. Role of common mental and physical disorders in partial disability around the world. *Br J Psychitar.* 2012;200:454–61.
3. Sánchez J, Rosenthal DA, Chan F, Brooks J, Bezyak JL. Relationships between World Health Organization International Classification of Functioning, Disability and Health constructs and participation in adults with severe mental illness. *Rehabil Res Policy Educ.* 2016;30:286–304.
4. Whiteford HA, Degenhardt L, Rehm J, et al. Global burden of disease attributable to mental and substance use disorders: Findings from the Global Burden of Disease Study 2010. *Lancet.* 2013;382:1575–86.
5. GBD 2015 Disease and Injury Incidence and Prevalence Collaborators. Global, regional, and national incidence, prevalence, and years lived with disability for 310 diseases and injuries, 1990–2015: A systematic analysis for the Global Burden of Disease Study 2015. *Lancet.* 2016;388:1545–602.

6. Patel V, Chisholm, Parikh R, et al. Global priorities for addressing the burden of mental, neurological, and substance use disorders (Chapter 1). *Disease control priorities*. 3rd ed. *Mental, neurological, and substance use disorders (Volume 4)*. Washington DC: IBRD/World Bank; 2015.

7. Hyman S, Parikh R, Collins PY, Patel V. Adult mental disorders (Chapter 4). *Disease control priorities*. 3rd ed. *Mental, neurological, and substance use disorders (Volume 4)*. Washington DC: IBRD/World Bank; 2015.

8. Collins PY, Patel V, Joestl SS, March D, Insel TR, Daar AS. Grand challenges in global mental health. *Nature*. 2011;475:27–30.

9. United Nations. *Transforming our world: The 2030 Agenda for Sustainable Development*. New York: UN; 2015.

10. Whiteford HA, Ferrari AJ, Degenhardt L, Feigin V, Vos T. Global burden of mental, neurological, and substance use disorders: An analysis from the Global Burden of Disease Study 2010 (Chapter 2). *Disease control priorities*. 3rd ed. *Mental, neurological, and substance use disorders (Volume 4)*. Washington DC: IBRD/World Bank; 2015.

11. *WHO resource book on mental health, human rights and legislation*. Geneva: WHO; 2005.

12. *Mental health and development: Targeting people with mental health conditions as a vulnerable group*. Geneva: WHO; 2010.

13. Becker AE, Kleinman A. Mental health and the global agenda. *New Engl J Med*. 2013;369:66–73.

14. Tandon R, Gaebel W, Barch DM, et al. Definition and description of schizophrenia in the DSM-5. *Schizophr Res*. 2013;150:3–10.

15. McGrath J, Saha S, Chant D, Welham J. Schizophrenia: A concise overview of incidence, prevalence, and mortality. *Epidemiol Rev*. 2008;30:67–76.

16. Rajji TK, Ismail Z, Mulsant BH. Age at onset and cognition in schizophrenia: Meta-analysis. *Br J Psychiatry*. 2009;195:286–93.

17. de Jesus MJ, Razzouk D, Thara R, Eaton J, Thornicroft G. Packages of care for schizophrenia in low- and middle-income countries. *PLoS Med*. 2009;6:e1000165.

18. Rössler W, Salize HJ, van Os J, Riecher-Rössler A. Size of burden of schizophrenia and psychotic disorders. *Eur Neuropsychopharmacol*. 2005;15:399–409.

19. Lora A, Kohn R, Levav I, McBain R, Morris J, Saxena S. Service availability and utilization and treatment gap for schizophrenic disorders: A survey in 50 low- and middle-income countries. *Bull World Health Organ*. 2012;90:47–54B.

20. Gerlinger G, Hauser M, De Hert M, Lacluyse K, Wampers M, Correll CU. Personal stigma in schizophrenia spectrum disorders: A systematic review of prevalence rates, correlates, impact and interventions. *World Psychiatry*. 2013;12:155–64.

21. Corrigan PW, Morris SB, Michaels PJ, Rafacz JD, Rüsch N. Challenging the public stigma of mental illness: A meta-analysis of outcome studies. *Psychiatr Serv*. 2012;63:963–73.

22. Phillips ML, Kupfer DJ. Bipolar disorder diagnosis: Challenges and future directions. *Lancet*. 2013;381:1663–71.

23. Geddes JR, Mmiklowitz DJ. Treatment of bipolar disorder. *Lancet*. 2013;381:1672–82.

24. Merikangas KR, Jin R, He JP, et al. Prevalence and correlates of bipolar spectrum disorder in the World Mental Health Survey initiative. *Arch Gen Psychiatry*. 2011;68:241–51.

25. Hawke LD, Parikh SV, Michalak EE. Stigma and bipolar disorder: A review of the literature. *J Affect Disord*. 2013;150:181–91.

26. *Depression: What you need to know*. Bethesda, MD: National Institute of Mental Health; 2015.

27. Ferrari AJ, Somerville AJ, Baxter AJ, et al. Global variation in the prevalence and incidence of major depressive disorder: A systematic review of the epidemiological literature. *Psychol Med*. 2013;43:471–81.

28. Hölzel L, Härter M, Reese C, Kriston L. Risk factors for chronic depression: A systematic review. *J Affect Disord*. 2011;129:1–13.

29. Ferrari AJ, Charlson FJ, Norman RE, et al. Burden of depressive disorders by country, sex, age, and year: Findings from the Global Burden of Disease Study 2010. *PLoS Med*. 2013;10:e1001547.

30. *Diagnostic and statistical manual of mental disorders (DSM-5®)*. 5th ed. Arlington, VA: American Psychiatric Association (APA) Publishing; 2013.

31. Kessler RC, Bromet EJ. The epidemiology of depression across cultures. *Annu Rev Public Health*. 2013;34:119–38.

32. Kohrt BA, Rasmussen A, Kaiser BN, et al. Cultural concepts of distress and psychiatric disorders: Literature review and research recommendations for global mental health epidemiology. *Int J Epidemiol*. 2014;43:365–406.

33. Simon GE, Goldberg DP, Von Korff M, Ustün TB. Understanding cross-national differences in depression prevalence. *Psychol Med*. 2002;32:585–94.

34. Patel V, Simon G, Chowdhary N, Kaaya S, Araya R. Packages of care for depression in low- and middle-income countries. *PLoS Med*. 2009;6:e1000159.

35. *WHO model list of essential medicines (19th list)*. Geneva: WHO; 2015.

36. Andrade LH, Alonso J, Mneimneh Z, et al. Barriers to mental health treatment: Results from the WHO World Mental Health (WMH) surveys. *Psychol Med*. 2014;44:1303–17.

37. Moussavi S, Chatterji S, Verdes E, Tandon A, Patel V, Ustun B. Depression, chronic diseases, and decrements in health: Results from the World Health Surveys. *Lancet.* 2007;370:851–8.

38. Patel G, Fancher TL. In the clinic: Generalized anxiety disorder. *Ann Intern Med.* 2013;159:ITC6.

39. Craske MG, Kircanski K, Epstein A, et al. Panic disorder: A review of DSM-IV panic disorder and proposals for DSM-V. *Depress Anxiety.* 2010;27:93–112.

40. Baxter AJ, Scott KM, Vos T, Whiteford HA. Global prevalence of anxiety disorders: A systematic review and meta-regression. *Psychol Med.* 2013;43:897–910.

41. Baxter AJ, Vos T, Scott KM, Ferrari AJ, Whiteford HA. The global burden of anxiety disorders in 2010. *Psychol Med.* 2014;44:2363–74.

42. O'Brien C. Addiction and dependence in DSM-V. *Addiction.* 2011;106:866–7.

43. Alavi SS, Ferdosi M, Jannatifard F, Eslami M, Alaghemandan H, Setare M. Behavioral addiction versus substance addiction: Correspondence of psychiatric and psychological views. *Int J Prev Med.* 2012;3:290–4.

44. *Public policy statement: Definition of addiction.* Chevy Chase, MD: American Society of Addiction Medicine (ASAM); 2011.

45. Medina-Mora M, Monteiro M, Room R, et al. Alcohol use and alcohol use disorders (Chapter 7). *Disease control priorities.* 3rd ed. *Mental, neurological, and substance use disorders (Volume 4).* Washington DC: IBRD/World Bank; 2015.

46. *Global status report on alcohol and health 2014.* Geneva: World Health Organization; 2014.

47. Rehm J, Mathers C, Popova S, Thavorncharoensap M, Teerawattananon Y, Patra J. Global burden of disease and injury and economic cost attributable to alcohol use and alcohol use disorders. *Lancet.* 2009;373:2223–33.

48. Benegal V, Chand PK, Obot IS. Packages of care for alcohol use disorders in low- and middle-income countries. *PLoS Med.* 2009;6:e100170.

49. Degenhardt L, Hall W. Extent of illicit drug use and dependence, and their contribution to the global burden of disease. *Lancet.* 2012;379:55–70.

50. Degenhardt L, Stockings E, Strang J, Marsden J, Hall WD. Illicit drug dependence (Chapter 6). *Disease control priorities.* 3rd ed. *Mental, neurological, and substance use disorders (Volume 4).* Washington DC: IBRD/World Bank; 2015.

51. *World drug report 2016.* Vienna: United Nations Office on Drugs and Crime (UNODC); 2016.

52. *ATLAS on substance use: Resources for the prevention and treatment of substance use disorders.* Geneva: WHO; 2010.

53. *Facing addition in America: The Surgeon General's report on alcohol, drugs, and health.* Washington

DC: U.S. Department of Health & Human Services (HHS); 2016.

54. Soomro GM. Obsessive compulsive disorder. *BMJ Clin Evid.* 2012;2012:1004.

55. Benjet C, Bromet E, Karam EG, et al. The epidemiology of traumatic event exposure worldwide: Results from the World Mental Health Survey Consortium. *Psychol Med.* 2016;46:327–43.

56. Yehuda R. Post-traumatic stress disorder. *N Engl J Med.* 2002;346:108–14.

57. Smink FRE, van Hoeken D, Hoek HW. Epidemiology of eating disorders: Incidence, prevalence and mortality rates. *Curr Psychiatry Rep.* 2012;14:406–14.

58. Kessler RC, Berglund PA, Chiu WT, et al. The prevalence and correlates of binge eating disorder in the WHO World Mental Health surveys. *Biol Psychiatry.* 2013;73:904–14.

59. *Preventing suicide: A global imperative.* Geneva: WHO; 2014.

60. GBD 2015 Mortality and Causes of Death Collaborators. Global, regional, and national life expectancy, all-cause mortality, and cause-specific mortality for 249 causes of death, 1980–2015: A systematic analysis for the Global Burden of Disease Study 2015. *Lancet.* 2016;388:1459–544.

61. *World Health Statistics 2016.* Geneva: WHO; 2016.

62. Shah A. The relationship between suicide rates and age: An analysis of multinational data from the World Health Organization. *Int Psychogeriatr.* 2007;19:1141–52.

63. Borges G, Nock MK, Haro Abad JM, et al. Twelve month prevalence of and risk factors for suicide attempts in the WHO World Mental Health surveys. *J Clin Psychiatry.* 2010;71:1617–28.

64. Vijayakumar L, Phillips MR, Silverman MM, Gunnell D, Carli V. Suicide (Chapter 9). *Disease control priorities.* 3rd ed. *Mental, neurological, and substance use disorders (Volume 4).* Washington DC: IBRD/World Bank; 2015.

65. Charlson FJ, Baxter AJ, Dua T, Degenhardt L, Whiteford HA, Vos T. Excess mortality from mental, neurological, and substance use disorders in the Global Burden of Disease Study 2010 (Chapter 3). *Disease control priorities.* 3rd ed. *Mental, neurological, and substance use disorders (Volume 4).* Washington DC: IBRD/World Bank; 2015.

66. Walker ER, McGee RE, Druss BG. Mortality in mental disorders and global disease burden implications: A systematic review and meta-analysis. *JAMA Psychiatry.* 2015;72:334–41.

67. Scott JG, Mihalopoulos C, Erskine HE, Roberts J, Rahman A. Childhood mental and developmental disorders (Chapter 8). *Disease control priorities.* 3rd ed. *Mental, neurological, and substance use disorders (Volume 4).* Washington DC: IBRD/World Bank; 2015.

68. Kieling C, Baker-Henningham H, Belfer M, et al. Child and adolescent mental health worldwide: Evidence for action. *Lancet.* 2011;378:1515–25.

69. James AC, James G, Cowdrey FA, Soler A, Choke A. Cognitive behavioural therapy for anxiety disorders in children and adolescents. *Cochrane Database Syst Rev.* 2013;(6):CD004690.

70. Thapar A, Cooper M. Attention deficit hyperactivity disorder. *Lancet.* 2016;387:1240–50.

71. Constantino JN, Charman T. Diagnosis of autism spectrum disorder: Reconciling the syndrome, its diverse origins, and variation in expression. *Lancet Neurol.* 2016;15:279–91.

72. Baxter AJ, Brugha TS, Erskine HE, Scheurer RW, Vos T, Scott JG. The epidemiology and global burden of autism spectrum disorders. *Psychol Med.* 2015;45:601–13.

73. Elsabbagh M, Divan G, Koh YJ, et al. Global prevalence of autism and other pervasive developmental disorders. *Autism Res.* 2012;5:160–79.

74. Warren Z, McPheeters ML, Sathe N, Foss-Feig JH, Glasser A, Veenstra-Vanderweele J. A systematic review of early intensive intervention for autism spectrum disorders. *Pediatrics.* 2011;127:e1303–11.

75. *Dementia: A public health priority.* Geneva: WHO; 2012.

76. Prince M, Bryce R, Albanese E, Wimo A, Ribeiro W, Ferri CP. The global prevalence of dementia: A systematic review and metaanalysis. *Alzheimers Dement.* 2013;9:65–75.

77. *World Alzheimer report 2016: Improving healthcare for people living with dementia.* London: Alzheimer's Disease International; 2016.

78. Hyder AA, Wunderlich CA, Puvanachandra P, Gururaj G, Kobusingye OC. The impact of traumatic brain injuries: A global perspective. *NeuroRehabilitation.* 2007;22:341–53.

79. Maas AI, Stocchetti N, Bullock R. Moderate and severe traumatic brain injury in adults. *Lancet Neurol.* 2008;7:728–41.

80. Carroll LJ, Cassidy JD, Cancelliere C, et al. Systematic review of the prognosis after mild traumatic brain injury in adults: Cognitive, psychiatric, and mortality outcomes: Results of the International Collaboration on Mild Traumatic Brain Injury Prognosis. *Arch Phys Med Rehabil.* 2014;94(3 Suppl):S152–73.

81. Shidhaye R, Lund C, Chishold D. Health care platform interventions (Chapter 11). *Disease control priorities.* 3rd ed. *Mental, neurological, and substance use disorders (Volume 4).* Washington DC: IBRD/World Bank; 2015.

82. Wang PS, Aguilar-Gaxiola S, Alonsa J, et al. Use of mental health services for anxiety, mood, and substance disorders in 17 countries in the WHO world mental health surveys. *Lancet.* 2007;370:841–850.

83. *Mental health atlas 2014.* Geneva: WHO; 2015.

84. *Mental Health Action Plan 2013–2020.* Geneva: WHO; 2013.

85. Chisholm D, Lund C, Saxena S. Cost of scaling up mental healthcare in low- and middle-income countries. *Br J Psychiatry.* 2007;191:528–535.

86. Levin C, Chisholm D. Cost-effectiveness and affordability of interventions, policies, and platforms for the prevention and treatment of mental, neurological, and substance use disorders (Chapter 12). *Disease control priorities.* 3rd ed. *Mental, neurological, and substance use disorders (Volume 4).* Washington DC: IBRD/World Bank; 2015.

87. Petersen I, Evans-Lacko S, Semrau M, et al. Population and community platform interventions (Chapter 10). *Disease control priorities.* 3rd ed. *Mental, neurological, and substance use disorders (Volume 4).* Washington DC: IBRD/World Bank; 2015.

88. Herrman H, Saxena S, Moddie R, editors. *Promoting mental health: Concepts, emerging evidence, practice: Summary report.* Geneva: WHO; 2004.

CHAPTER 17

Injuries

Road traffic injuries, violence, and other unintentional and intentional injuries are frequent causes of death and disability across the lifespan. The particular risks vary by age and sex. Children have an elevated risk of drowning and abuse, women are at risk from burns and gender-based violence, older adults are at risk from falls, and young men have a substantial risk of injury from occupational and recreational exposures. Most of these injuries are preventable.

▶ 17.1 Injuries and Global Health

An **injury** is physical damage to the body inflicted by an external force. An injury may take the form of trauma to the brain or spinal cord, a fracture of a bone, a strain or sprain of a joint, a deep gash that tears through the skin, damage to internal organs, or another type of wound. Mild injuries may cause a few days or weeks of pain and activity limitations. Moderate and severe trauma may cause long-term disability or death. Globally, about 1 in 12 deaths each year is due to an injury (**FIGURE 17–1**).[1] Nonfatal injuries can cause permanent disability, such as cognitive impairment from head trauma, paralysis from spinal trauma, limb amputations from crush wounds, joint contractures from burns, and severe mobility limitations from poorly healed fractures and joint injuries.

The words "injury" and "accident" are not synonyms. An **accident** is an unfortunate event that happens by chance. The word accident implies that nothing could have been done to prevent the misfortune. But most injuries are not due to bad luck. Most injuries could have been prevented with safety measures. An **unintentional injury** is an unplanned injury that happens very quickly, like a collision between motor vehicles, a fall off a ladder, or a burn from a spilled pot of boiling water.[2] Unintentional injuries can be prevented with the use of safety belts and child car seats in motor vehicles, helmets for cyclists, designated drivers who have not consumed alcohol, flame-resistant clothing, smoke detectors, fencing around bodies of water, swimming lessons, protective eyewear, safety harnesses when working at dangerous heights, locked storage of weapons and ammunition, and hundreds of other preventive safety measures that can be implemented by individuals, households, workplaces, and communities.[3] An **intentional injury** is a purposefully inflicted physical trauma. Intentional injuries can be prevented by addressing the psychological factors leading to self-harm and implementing interventions that reduce violence.[4]

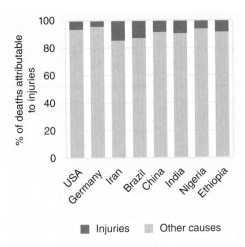

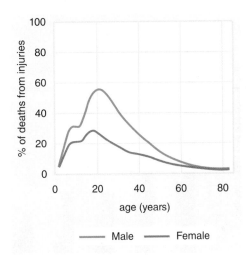

FIGURE 17-1 About 1 in 12 deaths is due to injuries.
Data from GBD 2015 Mortality and Causes of Death Collaborators. Global, regional, and national life expectancy, all-cause mortality, and cause-specific mortality for 249 causes of death, 1980–2015: A systematic analysis for the Global Burden of Disease Study 2015. *Lancet* 2016;388:1459–544.

FIGURE 17-2 The percentage of deaths from injuries peaks among adolescents and young adults.
Data from GBD Mortality and Causes of Death Collaborators. Global, regional, and national life expectancy, all-cause mortality, and cause-specific mortality for 249 causes of death, 1980–2015: A systematic analysis for the Global Burden of Disease Study 2015. *Lancet* 2016; 388:1459–544.

Young people and males bear a disproportionate burden from injuries. The percentage of deaths that are due to injuries (rather than infections, noncommunicable diseases, or other causes) peaks in adolescence and young adulthood for both males and females (**FIGURE 17-2**).[1] However, males have higher injury rates than females. Males are more likely to work in hazardous occupations, participate in dangerous recreational activities, spend time on the road, use alcohol, and be involved in fighting and armed conflict.[5] The mortality rate per 100,000 males is more than double the rate in females, and this increased rate of death among males is observed across most age groups as well as many types of injury, including transportation-related injuries, self-harm, falls, interpersonal violence, drowning, and exposure to mechanical forces (**FIGURE 17-3**).[1] Males also have a greater burden than females from disabilities caused by nonfatal injuries (**FIGURE 17-4**).[6]

People residing in low-income areas are more likely than people in high-income areas to live, work, and go to school in unsafe environments. Unsafe environments create an increased risk of injury.[7] Exposure to poisons, fire, extreme weather, and physical trauma are more common in places where there is limited access to safe waste disposal, food must be prepared over a fire, residential structures are not built to withstand earthquakes and other natural disasters, and enforcement of occupational and road safety laws is minimal. The impairment caused by injuries may also be

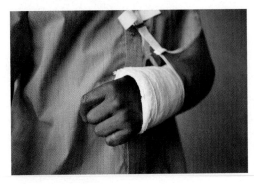

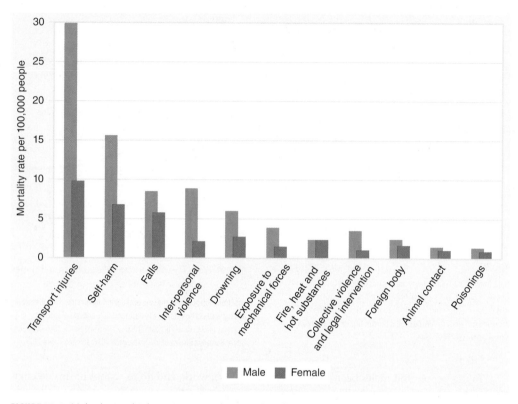

FIGURE 17–3 Males have a higher injury mortality rate than females.

Data from GBD Mortality and Causes of Death Collaborators. Global, regional, and national life expectancy, all-cause mortality, and cause-specific mortality for 249 causes of death, 1980–2015: A systematic analysis for the Global Burden of Disease Study 2015. *Lancet* 2016; 388:1459–544.

more severe and lasting when injured people are unable to access advanced medical, surgical, and rehabilitation services.

Injuries have grown in prominence on the global health agenda in recent years.[8] Several targets within the Sustainable Development Goals (SDGs) aim to reduce the burden from preventable injuries (**FIGURE 17–5**).[9] One ambitious target aims to "halve the number of global deaths and injuries from road traffic accidents" (SDG 3.6) within 5 years (that is, by 2020). SDG 16, which focuses on peace, has an aim of "significantly reducing all forms of violence and related death rates everywhere" (SDG 16.1),

including those related to intentional homicide (SDG 16.1.1), conflict (SDG 16.1.2), and physical, psychological, and sexual violence (SDG 16.1.3). A diversity of other targets aim to eliminate violence against women and girls, including eliminating trafficking and exploitation (SDG 5.2), ending early and forced marriage and female genital mutilation (SDG 5.3), and ensuring access to sexual and reproductive health services (SDG 5.6). Achieving these targets will require increased access to safety tools, to health education that promotes risk-reduction behaviors, and to policy changes that protect people of all ages from violence.

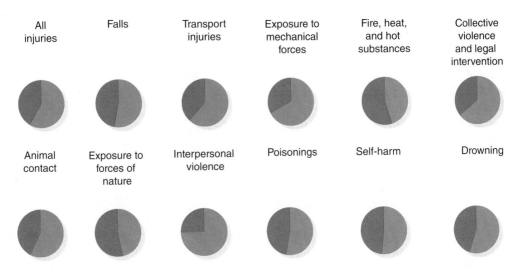

FIGURE 17-4 Males account for a higher percentage of injury-related years lived with disability (YLDs) than females.

Data from GBD Disease and Injury Incidence and Prevalence Collaborators. Global, regional, and national incidence, prevalence, and years lived with disability for 310 diseases and injuries, 1980–2015: A systematic analysis for the Global Burden of Disease Study 2015. *Lancet* 2016; 388:1545–602.

1.5.1	
11.5.1	Number of deaths, missing persons, and persons affected by disaster per 100,000 people
13.1.2	
3.4.2	Suicide mortality rate
3.6.1	Number of road traffic fatal injury deaths (within 30 days of the collision) per 100,000 population
3.9.3	Mortality rate attributable to unintentional poisoning
8.8.1	Frequency rate of fatal and nonfatal occupational injuries
16.1.1	Number of victims of intentional homicide per 100,000 population
16.1.2	Conflict-related deaths per 100,000 population
16.1.3	Proportion of the population subjected to physical, sexual, or psychological violence in the previous 12 months

FIGURE 17-5 Examples of Sustainable Development Goals indicators related to injuries and violence.

Data from United Nations Economic and Social Council. *Report of the Inter-Agency and Expert Group on Sustainable Development Goal Indicators* (E/CN.3/2016/2/Rev.1). New York: UN; 2016.

▶ 17.2 Transport Injuries

About one in three injury deaths among males and one in four injury deaths among females worldwide are due to transportation-related traumas (**FIGURE 17–6**).[1] Nearly all of these transport injuries are **road traffic injuries (RTIs)**, injuries sustained in collisions involving at least one moving motor vehicle (as opposed to injuries sustained when an individual falls off a bicycle). Although the number of cars per person is higher in high-income countries than in low-income countries (**FIGURE 17–7**), the mortality rate from road traffic injuries is higher in middle-income and low-income countries than in high-income countries (**FIGURE 17–8**).[10] This is partly because most vehicle collisions in high-income countries involve two motor vehicles crashing together, while in lower-income countries, the victims of a collision are often motorcyclists or pedestrians who are struck by a car or truck (**FIGURE 17–9**).[10] The difference in mortality rates is exacerbated by people in low- and middle-income

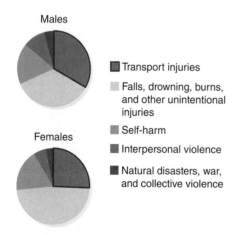

FIGURE 17–6 Transportation-related deaths account for a large percentage of all deaths from injuries.

Data from GBD Mortality and Causes of Death Collaborators. Global, regional, and national life expectancy, all-cause mortality, and cause-specific mortality for 249 causes of death, 1980–2015: A systematic analysis for the Global Burden of Disease Study 2015. *Lancet* 2016; 388:1459–544.

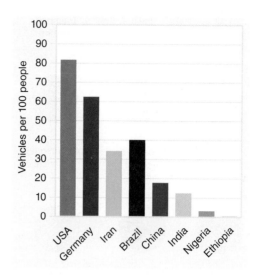

FIGURE 17–7 Number of registered vehicles per 100 people.

Data from *Global status report on road safety 2015*. Geneva: WHO; 2015.

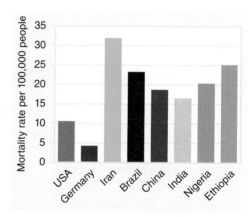

FIGURE 17–8 Road traffic mortality rate per 100,000 population.

Data from *Global status report on road safety 2015*. Geneva: WHO; 2015.

countries having less access to lifesaving medical and surgical care (**FIGURE 17–10**).[11]

A diversity of laws are recommended for reducing road traffic injuries.[10] Speed limits can be lowered and enforced, such as limiting urban speed limits to 50 kilometers per hour (30 miles per hour) for local streets that are not highways. Motorcycle helmets can be mandated for drivers and passengers.

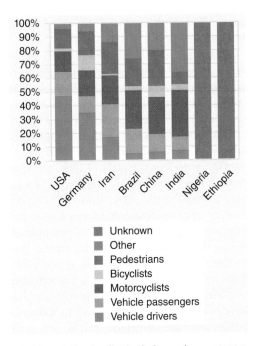

Legend:
- Unknown
- Other
- Pedestrians
- Bicyclists
- Motorcyclists
- Vehicle passengers
- Vehicle drivers

FIGURE 17–9 Road traffic deaths by road user category.
Data from *Global status report on road safety 2015*. Geneva: WHO; 2015.

Seat belts can be required for all car drivers and passengers. The use of child car seats or other restraints for infants and small children can be mandated, and children can be restricted from sitting in the front seats of vehicles. The legal blood alcohol limit can be reduced to 0.05 g/dL or less, with a zero-tolerance policy for any alcohol among young and inexperienced drivers and for commercial drivers who are operating heavy trucks. Restrictions can be set for driving under the influence of any substances that might cause impairment, including prescription medications. Distracted driving can be limited by banning texting and other mobile phone activities while driving. Additionally, governments can mandate vehicle safety standards, build safer roads with good markings and signage, provide sidewalks and bike lanes to keep pedestrians and cyclists away from car and truck traffic, and promote enforcement of safety laws. These interventions can be very cost-effective.[12] A basic package of road safety

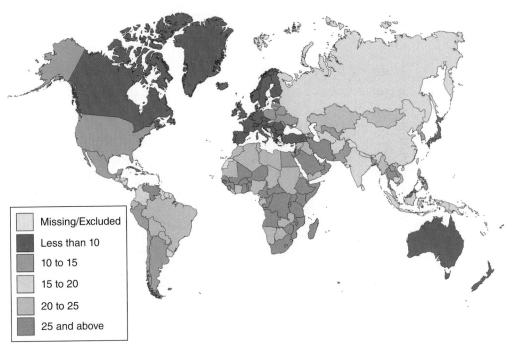

Legend:
- Missing/Excluded
- Less than 10
- 10 to 15
- 15 to 20
- 20 to 25
- 25 and above

FIGURE 17–10 Road traffic mortality rate per 100,000 population (2013).
Data from *World health statistics 2017*. Geneva: WHO; 2017.

interventions—enforcement of speed limits, drunk driving laws, seatbelt use in cars, and helmet use by all motorcyclists and child bicyclists—could cost considerably less than a dollar per person per year in Africa and Southeast Asia.[13]

▶ 17.3 Falls

A **fall** is an event that causes a person to land on the ground or floor. Some falls start from a great height, such as a fall from scaffolding or a tall ladder. Some falls begin with the individual in a standing or sitting position. For children, falls may occur as a result of climbing on or rolling off furniture, playing on outdoor structures, tumbling out a window, or other activities.[3] These types of falls might cause concussions, fractures, and other potentially serious trauma, but they are rarely fatal. By contrast, falls in adults frequently start a trajectory that leads to death.[14] The percentage of deaths attributable to falls peaks in childhood, but the rate of death

from falls is highest among the oldest adults (**FIGURE 17-11**).[1]

Falls in older adults most often occur among people who have existing problems with balance, strength, and gait as well as comorbidities that increase the risk of a fall, such as neurological conditions, low vision, cardiovascular diseases, arthritis, and osteoporosis.[15] The fall may cause soft tissue damage as well as fractures of hips, arms, or other bones. Hip fractures may require surgery to stabilize the pelvis followed by weeks or months of confinement to a bed, and that extended time reclining makes pneumonia, bedsores (infected skin wounds), strokes due to deep vein thromboses, and other problems more likely in addition to exacerbating weakness and frailty.[16] The interventions that have been shown to be effective in reducing falls in older adults include exercise programs focused on strength and balance training; treatment of health conditions that increase the risk of falls; and removal of hazards in the home, such as throw rugs, unstable furniture, and poor lighting.[17]

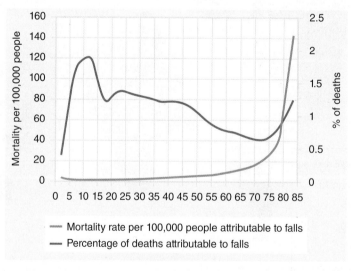

— Mortality rate per 100,000 people attributable to falls
— Percentage of deaths attributable to falls

FIGURE 17-11 The mortality rate from falls increases dramatically in older adulthood.

Data from GBD Mortality and Causes of Death Collaborators. Global, regional, and national life expectancy, all-cause mortality, and cause-specific mortality for 249 causes of death, 1980–2015: A systematic analysis for the Global Burden of Disease Study 2015. *Lancet* 2016; 388:1459–544.

▶ 17.4 Drowning

Drowning is the process of experiencing respiratory impairment due to being submerged or immersed in water or another liquid.[18] Drowning can occur in a large body of water like an ocean, lake, or river; in a smaller body of water like a swimming pool, pond, or irrigation ditch; and even in a small water container, such as a bathtub or bucket. Drowning often results in death, although it is possible to resuscitate some victims who have been under water for only a few minutes and are still alive when rescue attempts are initiated.[19]

The percentage of deaths due to drowning peaks in childhood, and there is a U-shaped curve for the mortality rate from drowning, with young children and older adults both having higher drowning mortality rates (**FIGURE 17–12**).[1] Toddlers can easily drown in shallow water if they trip and cannot stand up, and they can topple head-first into small wash buckets and be unable to remove themselves before they suffocate.[20] Alcohol consumption is a contributor to many cases of drowning in adults, since alcohol makes people more likely to swim alone or in dangerous settings, less likely to use floatation devices, and more likely to capsize a boat.[21] Older adults may have health issues like neurological or cardiovascular disorders that increase the likelihood of falling into water, losing consciousness while bathing, or being unable to safely exit a body of water.[22]

Key risk factors for drowning include a lack of physical barriers between people and bodies of water, lack of close supervision of infants and young children, lack of safe places to cross rivers and other bodies of water, poor swimming skills, alcohol use when near water, lack of safety measures for boats and other vessels, floods from extreme weather, and lack of training in safe rescue and resuscitation.[23] Key actions to reduce the risk of drowning include installing barriers to limit access to dangerous waters, such as covering drinking water barrels and fencing swimming pools; offering swimming and water safety lessons; enforcing boating and ferry regulations, such as limits to the numbers of passengers per vessel and

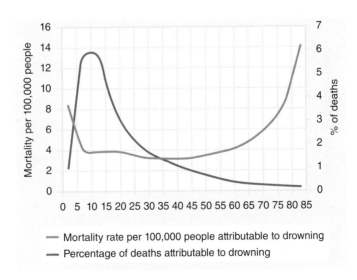

— Mortality rate per 100,000 people attributable to drowning
— Percentage of deaths attributable to drowning

FIGURE 17–12 The percentage of deaths attributable to drowning is highest in childhood.

Data from GBD Mortality and Causes of Death Collaborators. Global, regional, and national life expectancy, all-cause mortality, and cause-specific mortality for 249 causes of death, 1980–2015: A systematic analysis for the Global Burden of Disease Study 2015. *Lancet* 2016; 388:1459–544.

mandates to have personal floatation devices on board for all passengers; and preparing people to survive floods by initiating early warning systems and discouraging unsafe behaviors like driving across flooded streets.[23]

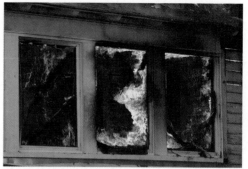

▶ 17.5 Burns

A **burn** is an injury to skin or deeper tissues that is caused by contact with fire, boiling water, or other very hot substances or, less often, by radiation, electricity, friction, extreme cold, and some types of chemicals. Burns are classified into three levels of severity. First-degree burns cause redness and pain but do not blister. Second-degree burns that penetrate through some layers of skin often cause painful blisters. Third-degree burns extend through all the layers of skin, causing extensive and possibly fatal damage. Burns that are severe, burns that cover a sizeable proportion of the body's surface area, burns on the face or hands or other critical areas, and other serious

burn injuries often require lengthy hospitalizations.[24] Initial care focuses on managing fluid loss and preventing infection. Skin grafts, amputations, and other advanced wound care techniques may be necessary to prevent death, disability, and disfigurement. Later, contractures (tightened skin that restricts the movement of a joint) and other types of scars may need to be surgically corrected.

The percentage of deaths that are attributable to burns peaks in early adulthood (**FIGURE 17–13**).[1] In lower-income

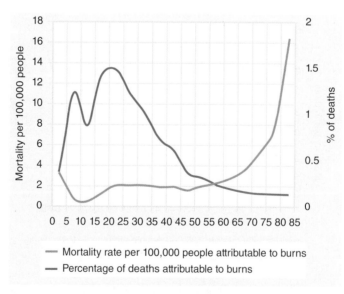

— Mortality rate per 100,000 people attributable to burns
— Percentage of deaths attributable to burns

FIGURE 17–13 The percentage of deaths attributable to burns is highest in early adulthood.

Data from GBD Mortality and Causes of Death Collaborators. Global, regional, and national life expectancy, all-cause mortality, and cause-specific mortality for 249 causes of death, 1980–2015: A systematic analysis for the Global Burden of Disease Study 2015. *Lancet* 2016; 388:1459–544.

countries, house fires are often caused by kerosene lamps or stoves tipping over, and many women and the toddlers they care for suffer from burns sustained when cooking over open fires. Lamps and stoves that are designed to be difficult to tip over can reduce the risk of fires and scalds.[25] In higher-income and urban areas, effective strategies for reducing burns include smoke alarms, devices that limit the temperature of hot water in the home, making children's sleepwear out of fire-resistant fabrics, safely wiring the electrical systems in buildings, installing sprinklers in buildings, making child-resistant cigarette lighters, and making fireworks safer.[25]

▶ 17.6 Other Unintentional Injuries

In addition to transportation injuries, falls, drowning, and burns, unintentional injuries are caused by exposure to mechanical forces, such as crush injuries from industrial and agricultural tools, equipment, and machinery; injuries from foreign bodies, such as aspiration of an object that causes choking or ingestion of an object that causes blockages in the digestive tract; animal attacks, most often from dogs but also from snakes and other venomous and nonvenomous animals; poisonings, often related to occupational use of pesticides; and exposure to extreme environmental heat and cold. Occupational, environmental, and behavioral prevention strategies must be tailored to the particular risks at a site. For example, some snake bites can be prevented by keeping the ground around homes clear of vegetation, poisonings at work can be reduced with restricted use of dangerous substances and mandated use of personal protective equipment, and poisonings at home can be reduced by storing cleaning products and other chemicals in places that cannot be accessed by small children.[26]

▶ 17.7 Intentional Injuries

Most injuries are unintentional, but some injures are the result of intentional self-harm or deliberate harm by others, including about one in four injury deaths (**FIGURE 17-14**).[1] **Violence** is the use of force or power to threaten or inflict physical, sexual, and/or psychological harm on another person.[27] Violence is associated with physical injuries as well as an increased risk of depression, anxiety, post-traumatic stress disorder, substance abuse, suicidal thinking, and adoption of risky behaviors.[28]

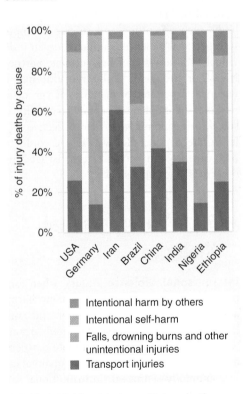

FIGURE 17-14 Most injuries and injury deaths are unintentional, but some are the result of intentional self-harm or harm by others.

Data from GBD Mortality and Causes of Death Collaborators. Global, regional, and national life expectancy, all-cause mortality, and cause-specific mortality for 249 causes of death, 1980–2015: A systematic analysis for the Global Burden of Disease Study 2015. *Lancet* 2016; 388:1459–544.

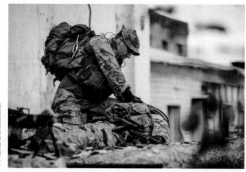

There are three main categories of violence: self-directed violence, interpersonal violence, and collective violence.[27] **Self-directed violence** is physical trauma inflicted by an individual on his or her own body, such as cutting and suicide attempts. Interpersonal violence is inflicted on an individual by a family member, intimate partner, friend, or stranger.[29] **Collective violence** is violence perpetrated by members of a group as part of a shared plan to accomplish a political, social, or economic goal. The collective violence category includes war, armed conflicts, mob violence, gang violence, terrorist acts, and other acts of group violence.[30]

▶ 17.8 Interpersonal Violence

Interpersonal violence occurs when one person threatens to harm or actually harms another individual through power and control.[31] Interpersonal violence often occurs within families or between intimate partners, but some assaults are inflicted by acquaintances in community settings or in institutional settings, such as schools or workplaces, and some are inflicted by strangers engaging in random acts of violence.[27] Interpersonal violence can occur across the lifespan, from child maltreatment and youth violence to elder abuse. A different set of prevention activities have been shown to be helpful for each stage of life.

Child abuse and maltreatment may take the form of physical abuse (including physical punishments, such as hitting and beating a child), sexual abuse, emotional and psychological abuse, or neglect.[32] A global partnership aiming to end violence against children identified seven key strategies for protecting children that can be summarized by the acronym INSPIRE: Implement and enforce laws that ban corporal punishment of children and criminalize sexual abuse and exploitation; change societal Norms and values to create a culture of equity and community involvement in child protection; create Safe environments; provide Parent and caregiver support, including parenting education and home visits by nurses; strengthen Income and economic security to reduce the stresses of poverty on families; launch and maintain Response and support services for treating injuries, investigating and addressing possible cases of abuse, and providing social welfare services to families with vulnerable children; and implement Education and life skills training to enhance children's ability to recognize and report abuse and neglect.[33]

Youth violence often involves interpersonal conflict between an adolescent or young adult aggressor and another person of a similar age.[34] The risk factors for involvement in youth violence include being male, being a school dropout (or delinquent) or performing poorly in school, lacking social connectedness, using alcohol and drugs, living in a low-income household, and having a history of child abuse and exposure to violence.[35] The key strategies to reduce youth violence include anger management and conflict resolution training, school-based bullying prevention programs, counseling for young people already involved in violence, and community-based strategies that reduce poverty and crime.[35] Reducing the harmful use of alcohol and restricting access to guns, knives, and other weapons is also helpful for reducing injuries from violence among young people.[4]

Most abuse of older adults with cognitive and physical impairments (and adults of other ages who have disabilities) is inflicted by a family member or caregiver. Physical abuse may include assaults, the use of physical restraints or unnecessary medications to control the individual, malnutrition and dehydration due to withholding food and water, poor attention to hygiene and cleanliness, untreated medical conditions, and isolation.[27] Other forms of abuse may involve emotional abuse, sexual abuse, and financial abuse, such as withdrawing the adult's money from banks, changing wills, or confiscating property. Strategies for preventing these types of abuse and mistreatment include caregiver support, professional standards for residential care facilities, information campaigns for the public and for care professionals, and the availability of adult protective services.[27]

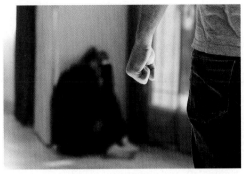

© sdecoret/Shutterstock

▶ 17.9 Gender-Based Violence

Gender-based violence (GBV) is physical, emotional, and/or sexual abuse inflicted on an individual because of that individual's gender. GBV usually involves victimization of females.[36] Females may have little power over their own bodies both because of gender norms that give men authority over women and because women tend to be smaller and physically weaker than men. Transgender people also have a very high likelihood of experiencing GBV.[37]

Violence against females may occur at any stage of their lives.[36] Pregnancies with female fetuses may be terminated by sex-selective abortions. Infant daughters may be killed by families with a cultural preference for sons. Young girls may be subjected to **female genital mutilation (FGM)**, also called female genital cutting, which is the partial or complete removal of the external female genitalia of an infant or child. Women who had this procedure

when they were children have significantly increased risks of urinary tract and reproductive tract infections, menstrual problems, sexual dysfunction, and obstetric complications.[38] FGM remains common among some populations in parts of Africa and the Middle East as well as among people in other countries with heritage from those regions.[39] Girls also may be forced into early marriages or into pornography, prostitution, and trafficking.[40] Adolescents and adult women may be subjected to dating, courtship, and marriage violence, including coerced sex and rape, and they may experience sexual harassment, forced pregnancies, trafficking, and acts of violence like "honor killings" and acid throwing.[40] The health consequences of GBV may include psychological trauma, serious injuries (including injuries to fetuses when pregnant women are attacked), infections with HIV and other pathogens, and death.

A very common form of GBV is **intimate partner violence (IPV)**, physical or sexual violence perpetrated by a current or former spouse or partner, such as being slapped, hit, kicked, choked, or beaten; being threatened with a weapon or injured by one; or being forced to have sexual intercourse or perform other sexual acts.[41] About one in three women worldwide has experienced physical IPV, sexual IPV, and/or non-partner sexual assault.[41] Reducing intimate partner and sexual violence requires individual behavior changes but is also dependent on social and cultural shifts in thinking about gender equity and healthy relationships.[28] This requires changing the attitudes of both men and women. Many women continue to believe that a man has good reason to beat his wife if she does not complete the housework, disobeys her husband, is unfaithful, or if the husband suspects infidelity, and many women believe it is not acceptable for a woman to refuse sex with her husband even if she does not want to have sex, her partner is drunk or mistreating her, or she is sick.[42] The most successful interventions to reduce IPV and other forms of GBV—including FGM, child marriage, and non-partner sexual assault—engage diverse stakeholders in activities that change the attitudes and behaviors of boys, girls, men, and women.[43]

▶ References

1. GBD 2015 Mortality and Causes of Death Collaborators. Global, regional, and national life expectancy, all-cause mortality, and cause-specific mortality for 249 causes of death, 1980–2015: A systematic analysis for the Global Burden of Disease Study 2015. *Lancet.* 2016;388:1459–544.

2. Norton R, Ahuja R, Hoe CH, et al. Non-transport unintentional injury (Chapter 4). *Disease control priorities.* 3rd ed. *Injury prevention and environmental health (Volume 7).* Washington DC: IBRD/World Bank; 2017.

3. *World report on child injury prevention.* Geneva: WHO/UNICEF; 2008.

4. *Violence prevention: The evidence.* Geneva: WHO; 2010.

5. Courtenay WH. Behavioral factors associated with disease, injury, and death among men: Evidence and implications for prevention. *J Men's Stud.* 2000;9:81–142.

6. GBD 2015 Disease and Injury Incidence and Prevalence Collaborators. Global, regional, and national incidence, prevalence, and years lived with disability for 310 diseases and injuries, 1980–2015: A systematic analysis for the Global Burden of Disease Study 2015. *Lancet.* 2016;388:1545–602.

7. Laflamme L, Burrows S, Hasselberg M. *Socioeconomic differences in injury risks: A review of findings and a discussion of potential countermeasures.* Copenhagen: WHO-EURO; 2009.

8. Mock C, Kobusingye O, Nugent R, Smith KR. Injury prevention and environmental health: Key messages from the volume (Chapter 1). *Disease control priorities.* 3rd ed. *Injury prevention and environmental health (Volume 7).* Washington DC: IBRD/World Bank; 2017.

9. United Nations. *Transforming our world: The 2030 Agenda for Sustainable Development.* New York: UN; 2015.

10. *Global status report on road safety 2015.* Geneva: WHO; 2015.

11. Sharma BR. Road traffic injuries: A major global public health crisis. *Public Health* 2008;122:1399–1406.

12. Bachani A, Peden M, Gururaj G, Norton R, Hyder A. Road traffic injuries (Chapter 3). *Disease control priorities.* 3rd ed. *Injury prevention and environmental health (Volume 7).* Washington DC: IBRD/World Bank; 2017.

13. Chisholm D, Naci H, Hyder AA, Tran NT, Peden M. Cost effectiveness of strategies to combat road traffic injuries in sub-Saharan Africa and South East Asia: Mathematical modeling study. *BMJ.* 2012;344:e612.

14. Kannus P, Sievänen H, Palvanen M, Järvinen T, Parkkari J. Prevention of falls and consequent injuries in elderly people. *Lancet.* 2005;366:1885–93.

15. Ambrose AF, Paul G, Hausdorff JM. Risk factors for falls among older adults: A review of the literature. *Maturitas.* 2013;75:51–61.

16. Beaupre LA, Jones CA, Saunders LD, Johnston DWC, Buckingham J, Majumdar SR. Best practices for elderly hip fracture patients: A systematic overview of the evidence. *J Gen Intern Med.* 2005;20:1019–25.

17. Gillespie LD, Robertson MC, Gillespie WJ, et al. Interventions for preventing falls in older people living in the community. *Cochrane Database Syst Rev.* 2012;12(9):CD007146.

18. van Beeck EF, Branche CM, Szpilman D, Modell JH, Bierens JJLM. A new definition of drowning: Towards documentation and prevention of a global public health problem. *Bull World Health Organ.* 2005;83:853–6.

19. Szpilman D, Bierens JJLM, Handley AJ, Orlowski JP. Drowning. *N Engl J Med.* 2012;366:2102–10.

20. Jumbelic MI, Chambliss M. Accidental toddler drowning in 5-gallon buckets. *JAMA.* 1990;263:1952–3.

21. Hingson R, Howland J, Alcohol and non-traffic unintended injuries. *Addiction.* 1993;88:877–83.

22. Lin CY, Wang YF, Lu TH, Kawach I. Unintentional drowning mortality, by age and body of water: An analysis of 60 countries. *Inj Prev.* 2015;21:e43–50.

23. *Global report on drowning: Preventing a leading killer.* Geneva: WHO; 2014.

24. Orgill DP. Excision and skin grafting of thermal burns. *N Engl J Med.* 2009;360:893–901.

25. *Burn prevention: Success stories and lessons learned.* Geneva: WHO; 2011.

26. Prüss-Ustün A, Wolf J, Corvalán C, Bos R, Neira M. *Preventing disease through healthy environments: A global assessment of the burden of disease from environmental risks.* Geneva: WHO; 2016.

27. Krug EG, Dahlberg LL, Mercy JA, Zwi AB, Lozano R. *World report on violence and health.* Geneva: WHO; 2002.

28. *Global status report on violence prevention 2014.* Geneva: WHO; 2014.

29. Mercy J, Hillis S, Butchart A, et al. Interpersonal violence: Global impact and paths to prevention (Chapter 5). *Disease control priorities.* 3rd ed. *Injury prevention and environmental health (Volume 7).* Washington DC: IBRD/World Bank; 2017.

30. *Injury: A leading cause of the global burden of disease, 2000.* Geneva: WHO; 2002.

31. Waters H, Hyder A, Rajkotia Y, Basu S, Rehwinkel JA, Butchart A. *The economic dimensions of interpersonal violence.* Geneva: WHO; 2004.

32. *Preventing child maltreatment: A guide to taking action and generating evidence.* Geneva: WHO/International Society for Prevention of Child Abuse and Neglect (ISPCAN); 2006.

33. *INSPIRE: Seven strategies for ending violence against children.* Geneva: WHO; 2016.

34. *Hidden in plain sight: A statistical analysis of violence against children.* New York: UNICEF; 2014.

35. *Preventing youth violence: An overview of the evidence.* Geneva: WHO; 2015.

36. Watts C, Zimmerman C. Violence against women: Global scope and magnitude. *Lancet.* 2002;359:1232-7.

37. Reisner SL, Poteat T, Keatley J, et al. Global health burden and needs of transgender populations: A review. *Lancet.* 2016;388:422–36.

38. Berg RC, Underland V, Odgaard-Jensen J, Fretheim A, Vist GE. Effects of female genital cutting on physical health outcomes: A systematic review and meta-analysis. *BMJ Open.* 2014;4:e006316.

39. *Female genital mutilation/cutting: A statistical overview and exploration of the dynamics of change.* New York: UNICEF; 2013.

40. *Global plan of action to strengthen the role of the health system within a national multisectoral response to address interpersonal violence, in particular against women and girls, and against children.* Geneva: WHO; 2016.

41. García-Moreno C, Pallitto C, Devries K, Stöckl H, Watts C, Abrahams N. *Global and regional estimates of violence against women.* Geneva: WHO; 2013.

42. García-Moreno C, Jansen HAFM, Ellsberg M, Heise L, Watts C. *WHO multi-country study on women's health and domestic violence against women: Initial results on prevalence, health outcomes and women's responses.* Geneva: WHO; 2005.

43. Ellsburg M, Arango DJ, Morton M, et al. Prevention of violence against women and girls: What does the evidence say? *Lancet* 2015; 385:1555–66.

CHAPTER 18

Promoting Neonatal, Infant, Child, and Adolescent Health

Child survival rates increased significantly over the past 25 years, but they did not reach the targets spelled out in the Millennium Development Goals. Intensified efforts to improve neonatal, infant, and child survival will be required to meet the Sustainable Development Goals by 2030. Expanding access to early childhood development interventions, school health and safety programs, and adolescent health services will help children thrive as they transition into healthy adulthood.

▶ 18.1 Progress in Child Survival

One of the greatest success stories in global health is the steady reduction in child mortality that has been achieved in recent decades. The **under-5 mortality rate** (U5MR), the number of children who die before their fifth birthdays per 1000 live births, significantly improved between 1950 and the present (**FIGURE 18–1**). The **infant mortality rate** (IMR), the number of deaths of infants per 1000 live births, has also steadily improved (**FIGURE 18–2**).[1] In just the 25 years from 1990 to 2015, the under-5 child mortality rate dropped by more than 50%, from 12.7 million deaths in 1990 to 5.9 million under-5 child deaths worldwide in 2015 (**FIGURE 18–3**).[2] The improvements were observed in all age groups for young children. The number of deaths in the first month after birth dropped from 5.1 million to 2.7 million over that 25-year period. The number of postneonatal deaths within the first year of life dropped from 8.9 million to 4.5 million.[2] Improvements in neonatal, infant, and under-5 child mortality have occurred in countries of all income levels (**FIGURE 18–4**).[3]

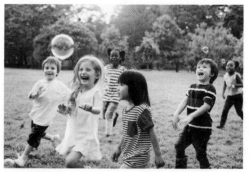

© Rawpixel.com/Shutterstock

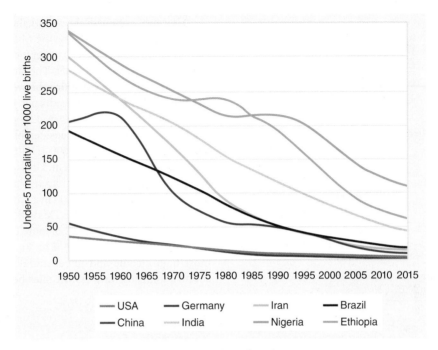

FIGURE 18–1 The under-5 mortality rate has decreased significantly since 1950.

Data from United Nations Department of Economic and Social Affairs. *World population prospects: The 2017 revision*. New York: UN; 2017.

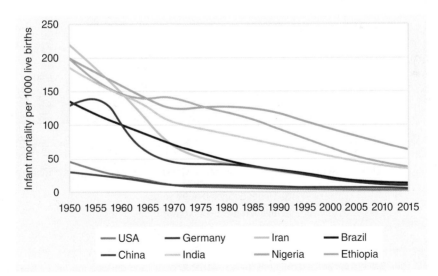

FIGURE 18–2 The infant mortality rate has decreased over time, but large differences by income level remain.

Data from United Nations Department of Economic and Social Affairs. *World population prospects: The 2017 revision*. New York: UN; 2017.

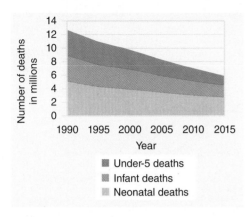

FIGURE 18-3 The number of young children dying each year decreased significantly between 1990 and 2015.

Data from *Committing to child survival: A promise renewed. Progress report 2015.* New York: UNICEF; 2015.

However, even with the remarkable downward trend in child mortality, the Millennium Development Goals (MDGs) target for improving child survival was not met. The aim was to reduce the U5MR by two-thirds between 1990 and 2015 (MDG 4), to 30 deaths per 1000 live births.[4] In 2015, the U5MR was 42.5 per 1000 live births, a rate that was considerably higher than the targeted 30 per 1000 (**FIGURE 18-5**). The Sustainable Development Goals (SDGs) aim to reduce the under-5 child mortality rate to less than 25 deaths per 1000 live births in all countries by 2030 (SDG 3.2).[5] This will require a decrease in the global U5MR of more than 40% between 2015 and 2030 (**FIGURE 18-6**).[4] Because most high-income and upper-middle-income countries already have U5MR rates below this

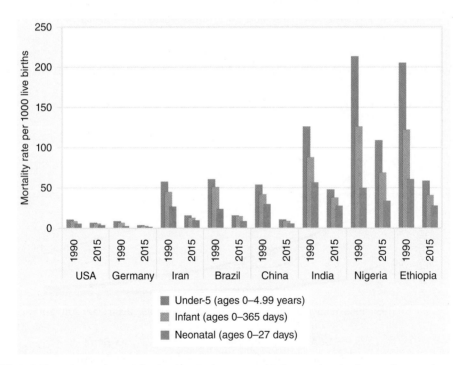

FIGURE 18-4 There were substantial reductions in the neonatal, infant, and under-5 mortality rates between 1990 and 2015.

Data from You D, Hug L, Ejdemyr S, Idele P, Hogan D, Mathers C, Gerland P, New JR, Alkema L; United Nations Inter-agency Group for Child Mortality Estimation (UN IGME). Global, regional, and national levels and trends in under-5 mortality between 1990 and 2015, with scenario-based projections to 2030: A systematic analysis by the UN Inter-agency Group for Child Mortality Estimation. *Lancet* 2015; 386:2275–86.

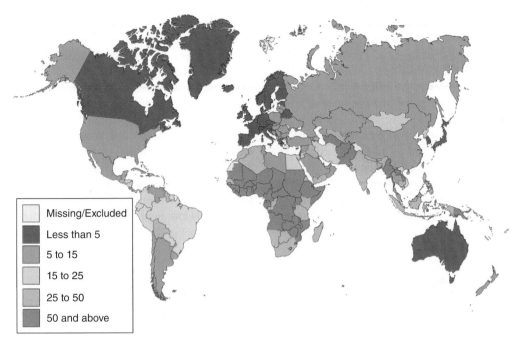

FIGURE 18–5 Under-5 mortality rate per 1000 live births (2015).

Data from UN Inter-Agency Group for Child Mortality Estimation (IGME). *Levels & trends in child mortality report 2015*. New York: UNICEF; 2015.

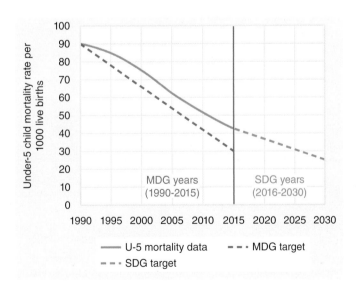

FIGURE 18–6 The MDG target for reducing the under-5 child mortality rate was not met despite significant improvements in survival.

Data from UN Inter-Agency Group for Child Mortality Estimation (IGME). *Levels & trends in child mortality report 2015*. New York: UNICEF; 2015.

threshold, there will still be a gap in child survival between high- and low-income countries even if the U5MR target is met by 2030. It would be technologically possible to achieve a "grand convergence" of health metrics by the year 2030 by reducing the maternal mortality and child mortality rates in low-income countries to the already-low levels in high-income countries, but this ambitious goal would require doubling funding for maternal and child health.[6]

The underlying cause of most child deaths worldwide is poverty.[7] Nearly all child mortality occurs in lower-income countries, where limited access to medical care for newborns, common but usually preventable child infections like diarrhea and pneumonia, and undernutrition continue to cause millions of deaths each year. Most children who die in low-income countries would not have become ill if they lived in high-income countries. If they had become ill in a high-income country rather than a low-income one, most of these children would have survived their illnesses and not died from them. Numerous low-cost interventions are effective at improving infant and child survival, but interventions that address specific health problems need to be accompanied by

1.2.1	Proportion of children living below the national poverty line
2.1.1	Prevalence of undernourishment
2.1.2	Prevalence of food insecurity
2.2.1	Prevalence of stunting among children under 5 years of age
2.2.2	Prevalence of malnutrition (wasting and overweight) among children under 5 years of age
3.2.2	Neonatal mortality rate (deaths per 1000 live births)
3.2.1	Under-5 mortality rate (deaths per 1000 live births)
3.3.3	Incidence of malaria per 1000 persons per year
3.7.2	Adolescent birth rate (aged 10–19 years) per 1000 women in that age group
3.8.1	Coverage of essential health services (including access to essential medicines and vaccines, newborn and child health services, and other services)
4.2.1	Percentage of children under 5 years of age who are developmentally on track in health, learning, and psychosocial well-being
8.7.1	Percentage and number of children aged 5–17 years engaged in child labor
16.2.1	Percentage of children aged 1–17 years who experienced any physical punishment or psychological aggression by caregivers in the last month

FIGURE 18–7 Examples of Sustainable Development Goals targets related to newborn, child, and adolescent health.

Data from United Nations Economic and Social Council. *Report of the Inter-Agency and Expert Group on Sustainable Development Goal Indicators* (E/CN.3/2016/2/Rev.1). New York: UN; 2016.

socioeconomic development to break the cycle of poverty that makes children born into extreme poverty so much more likely to die than children who happen to be born into wealthier families. The successes in decreasing child mortality during the MDG years were achieved, in part, because the MDGs addressed the socioeconomic and environmental conditions that put some children at especially high risk of illness, disability, and death.[8] The SDGs call for continued improvements in poverty reduction, sustainable economic growth, and access to nutrition, education, clean water, sanitation, electricity, employment, safety, peace, and the other tools that will enable more children around the world to enjoy long, healthy, productive lives (**FIGURE 18–7**).[5]

▶ 18.2 Improving Neonatal Survival

Neonatal mortality accounts for an increasing percentage of pediatric deaths. The percentage of deaths before the 15th birthday that occur during the first month after birth increased from about one in three under-15 deaths in 1990 to nearly 40% in 2015 (**FIGURE 18–8**).[9] This increasing proportion is evidence that the mortality rates among neonates have not decreased as quickly as the mortality rates among older infants and children. The SDGs aim to reduce the neonatal mortality rate (NMR) to less than

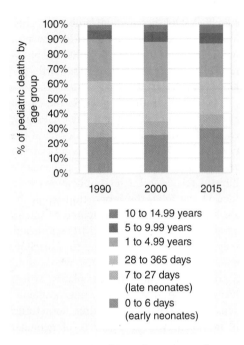

FIGURE 18–8 Neonatal mortality accounts for a large proportion of pediatric deaths (birth to age 15 years) worldwide.

Data from GBD 2015 Child Mortality Collaborators. Global, regional, national, and selected subnational levels of stillbirths, neonatal, infant, and under-5 mortality, 1990–2015: A systematic analysis for the Global Burden of Disease Study 2015. *Lancet* 2016; 388:1725–74.

12 deaths per 1000 live births in all countries by 2030 (SDG 3.2).[4] This will require a decrease in the global NMR of more than 35% between 2015 and 2030 (**FIGURE 18–9**). The *Every Newborn* action plan endorsed by the World Health

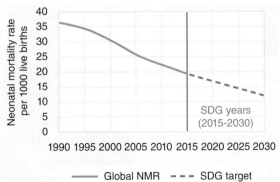

FIGURE 18–9 The Sustainable Development Goals aim to substantially reduce the neonatal mortality rate.

Data from UN Inter-Agency Group for Child Mortality Estimation (IGME). *Levels & trends in child mortality report 2015*. New York: UNICEF; 2015.

Assembly establishes a more ambitious goal, aiming for every country in the world to have an NMR of less than 10 deaths per 1000 live births and a stillbirth rate of less than 10 stillbirths per 1000 total births by 2035.[10]

The risk of death is higher on the day of birth than on any subsequent day.[11] Globally, 15% of all under-5 child deaths occur on the day of birth (**FIGURE 18–10**). This proportion does not include stillbirths. If preventable stillbirths related to birth complications were added to the total, the proportion would be even higher. In some high-income countries that already have very low NMRs, clinicians are aggressive about attempting to resuscitate very low birthweight neonates who would be considered stillbirths in places where advanced technologies are not available. Intensive resuscitation measures sometimes add newborns with a high risk of neonatal death to the denominator of live births, making the NMR look worse, but those actions enable some fragile newborns to take a first breath and possibly live. In lower-income countries where resuscitation tools are not routinely available, currently high NMR rates might be artificially low because they do not include late-term stillbirths in the calculations. In all countries, interventions on the day of birth are critically important for improving the percentage of pregnancies that result in healthy newborns who will survive into healthy childhood.

Just three conditions account for more than four in five newborn deaths: preterm birth, asphyxia and other complications during labor and delivery, and neonatal infections.[10] These major causes of neonatal mortality can be addressed with interventions from preconception through the weeks after birth.[12] Immunizing pregnant women with tetanus toxoid protects their babies from tetanus infection. During the intrapartum period, women and their babies can be saved with actions like giving corticosteroids to women who go into preterm labor in order to prepare the lungs of fetuses to breathe, having skilled attendants care for women during labor and delivery in a clean environment, and managing complications with caesarian sections and other advanced emergency obstetrical procedures. After delivery, newborn resuscitation, prevention of hypothermia, and initiation of breastfeeding keep newborns alive. Neonatal mortality is also reduced by treating maternal infections, such as malaria and syphilis, and by managing maternal health issues, such as diabetes.[13] In addition to preventing mortality, these interventions help reduce the risk of neurodevelopmental impairment and other long-term disabilities in surviving babies.[14]

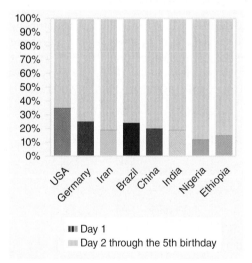

Day 1
Day 2 through the 5th birthday

FIGURE 18–10 A large percentage of under-5 deaths occur on the day of birth.

Data from *Surviving the first day: State of the world's mothers 2013*. London: Save the Children; 2013.

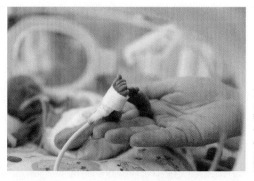

A variety of inexpensive packages of interventions could potentially enable major improvements in neonatal survival.[15] For example, a package of four easy-to-deliver interventions—corticosteroid injections for women in preterm labor, newborn resuscitation devices, chlorhexidine to clean the umbilical cord and prevent infections, and injectable antibiotics to treat newborn sepsis and pneumonia—would cost only a few dollars per baby and could save one million neonates each year.[11] Spending just $1 or $2 more per person each year to increase access to quality antenatal care, assisted labor and delivery, and newborn care in low- and middle-income countries could be enough to reduce neonatal deaths by up to 70% and stillbirths by up to 33%.[15] These types of interventions may also save money in the long term by reducing healthcare costs associated with disability and by increasing economic productivity.[14] The biggest barriers to expanding access to neonatal health programs are not having enough funding, not having enough trained health workers to provide obstetric and neonatal health services, and not having the resources and leadership to manage the logistics of scaling up delivery of quality care.[16] These barriers can be overcome when citizens and communities call for change, when governments choose to prioritize progress on child health, and when partners make commitments to provide support and accountability.[2]

▶ 18.3 Promoting Infant and Child Health

Some of the earliest international health initiatives focused on child health. In the 20th century, several large-scale multinational initiatives improved the lives of millions of children around the world.[17] One of the first efforts heavily promoted by the World Health Organization (WHO) and UNICEF supported **primary health care (PHC)**, a community-based approach to health that employs community health workers and focuses as much on prevention as on cures.[18] PHC became the focus of most international health work following the Alma-Ata Conference of 1978, which developed the goal of achieving "Health for All by 2000" through the reduction of barriers to healthcare access, especially in poor and rural areas.[19] PHC prioritizes prevention of locally common infectious diseases, provision of essential medications and treatments for common diseases and injuries, promotion of nutrition, coordination of health services with traditional health practitioners, and programming for maternal and child health, including immunization and family planning.[20] PHC is a "horizontal" approach to health care that emphasizes routine access to comprehensive primary care, rather than a "vertical" approach that targets selected diseases with specific interventions (like special vaccination days) that are managed outside the public healthcare system.[21]

A hallmark of PHC is regularly scheduled health clinics for children younger than 5 years old in order to monitor child growth and provide recommended immunizations.[22] The Expanded Program on Immunization (EPI) was started in 1974 by WHO to expand the number and types of vaccines routinely given to children. More than four decades later, the program is still supporting the delivery of essential vaccines to children across the globe.[23] When all children, whether sick or healthy, have frequent interactions with the healthcare system through under-5 health clinics, warning signs for potentially life-threatening conditions in relatively healthy children can be detected early and treated. For example, growth monitoring tracks child weight so that caregivers will know if a child has lost weight or is failing to gain weight. Weight loss or stagnation can be a sign of serious illness, and early detection means that a nutritional intervention can be implemented before a health crisis occurs.

GOBI, an initiative started in the 1980s by UNICEF, focused on increasing child survival by promoting four simple interventions: Growth monitoring, Oral rehydration therapy for diarrhea, Breastfeeding, and Immunization.[24] Later, a partnership between UNICEF, WHO, and the World Bank added three community-focused components to the mix—family planning, food production, and female education—creating a program called GOBI/FFF.[25]

Integrated Management of Childhood Illness (IMCI) is a package of simple, affordable, and effective interventions for major childhood illnesses and undernutrition that was first developed by UNICEF and WHO in 1995.[26] The term "integrated" has several layers of meaning.[27] One aspect of integration is an emphasis on the interrelatedness of children's health conditions. A child with malaria is more vulnerable to diarrhea. A child with vitamin A deficiency is more vulnerable to death from measles. Clinicians working under an IMCI framework complete a series of medical assessments on each sick child that allows for diagnosis of underlying conditions in addition to the primary illness. Integration also emphasizes families and communities working together with the staff in various levels of healthcare facilities to care for sick children.

IMCI aims to improve family and community health practices as well as the case management skills of healthcare staff. To advance this goal, IMCI provides home healthcare guidelines for families with young children and evidence-based decision charts for clinicians to use when assessing children and treating common illnesses.[28] For example, the family of a child with diarrhea should know how to prepare oral rehydration therapy correctly and know what symptoms require the child to be taken to the local clinic or hospital. The local clinic should support community health education programs, provide care for advanced cases of dehydration, and make referrals for hospital-based treatment, if necessary. In places where malaria is common, parents should know how to use bednets to prevent mosquito bites and how to recognize fevers and other symptoms of malaria. The local clinic should support those community health education efforts, treat cases of malaria that do occur, and make referrals for advanced treatment when it is needed. IMCI clinical guidelines, which focus on management of serious childhood diseases at healthcare facilities, are often paired with **Integrated Community Case Management (iCCM)** guidelines that provide community health workers with algorithms for treating uncomplicated childhood infections in homes.[29]

Each of these historic international child health programs contributed to significant improvements in global child health metrics, but infant and child health statistics show that there is still a great deal of work to be done. In order to ensure that as many children as possible have a healthy start in life, it is important to further improve access to safe drinking water and nutritional foods, educate parents about infectious disease prevention, promote breastfeeding, increase access to essential medications and immunizations, and implement other important public health measures. As of 2015, The Partnership for Maternal, Newborn & Child Health, which was launched in 2005, had more than 725 partner groups representing a diversity of sectors.[30] The ministries of health and collaborating agencies in low- and middle-income countries have expanded access to antibiotics, clean water, antimalarial medications, and other tools for preventing and treating pneumonia, diarrhea, malaria, and other potentially fatal infectious diseases in urban and rural areas within their own borders. Gavi and other organizations have expanded access to vaccines that protect against measles and other life-threatening infections. UNICEF and numerous other multinational groups have promoted breastfeeding, distributed micronutrients to children, supported agricultural development, and taken other actions to prevent infant and child malnutrition. Other United Nations agencies, partner governments, clinical professional associations, nongovernmental organizations, private sector companies, academic institutes, foundations and other donors, and countless others are working at the local, national, regional, and global levels to reduce infant and child mortality and promote health and well-being in the early years.

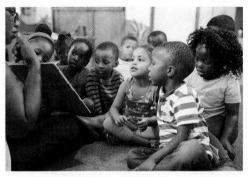

▶ 18.4 Promoting Early Childhood Development

Global child health in the 21st century is about helping babies and children thrive rather than merely investing in keeping kids alive.[31] Access to nutrition, health services, and social interaction with parents and other caregivers in the first months and years of life is critical not only for health but for preparing young children for success in school and, later on, for healthy and productive adulthood.[32] Economic evaluations show that a diversity of health and nutritional, environmental, educational, social, and economic interventions for young children and their families yield long-term benefits not only for those individuals but also for their families, communities, and nations.[33]

Early childhood development (ECD) interventions target the physical, cognitive, emotional, and social development of infants and children.[34] The ECD process begins during the first 1000 days, the time period encompassing the approximately one thousand days from conception through the second birthday.[35] Adequate maternal access to micronutrients and calories during pregnancy has a beneficial impact on fetal development, and assisted delivery helps reduce the risk of brain damage from birth trauma. During the first 2 years after birth, cognitive development, language acquisition, motor skills, and socio-emotional development are facilitated by psychosocial stimulation from parents and other caregivers that promotes mental development; by nutritious food that allows for health, growth,

physical activity, and brain development; and by a clean and safe environment that protects children from infectious diseases and violence.[36] ECD continues through the preschool years as children gain the self-regulation and learning skills necessary for success in a primary school classroom.[37] One of the SDGs aims to "ensure that all girls and boys have access to quality early childhood development, care, and pre-primary education, so that they are ready for primary education" (SDG 4.2).[5] Achieving this goal will require cooperation across the health, education, social service, and economic development sectors.[38]

▶ 18.5 Children with Special Needs

A disability is not defined merely as a physical, cognitive, sensory, or other impairment (or a combination of impairments). A disability is also a function of the social context and environment in which a person with an impairment lives, learns, and works. Consider the example of hearing loss. Some children who grow up Deaf are part of a vibrant community with a shared language (a local form of sign language) and culture, especially if they are born into a Deaf family. (The use of the capitalized term Deaf is used to indicate Deaf culture and identity.) For these individuals, deafness is not considered to be a disability.[39] But some people who grow up deaf or hard of hearing never have the opportunity to learn a language,

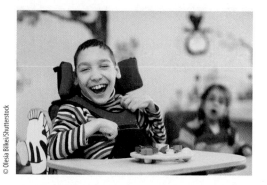

attend school, or be fully involved in the lives of their families and communities. In that environment, being deaf is a disability because it causes activity limitations and participation restrictions. Many children with various types of special needs have difficulty accessing health and educational services, especially when they live in low- and middle-income countries. Those barriers can have negative consequences that persist for a lifetime.[40]

Children with special needs have the healthiest life trajectories when they are able to access interventions early in life.[41] For example, babies with cleft lip or cleft palate, which occurs when the upper lip or the roof of the mouth is unclosed, may require surgery to be able to suck properly and receive adequate nutrition. Children born with cerebral palsy and other mobility disabilities can develop their motor skills to their highest potential when they have physical therapy and the use of braces, crutches, and walkers at an early age. Children with developmental disabilities may benefit from various types of physical, occupational, communication, and other therapies early in life.[42] Unfortunately, many parents do not have the resources or ability to have their children start therapy at an early age, do not know what therapy to provide at home for their children, and are not able to help their children with special needs access education.[43] Increasing access to support services, rehabilitation, and assistive technologies by children with special needs is both a public health priority and a human rights issue.[44]

▶ 18.6 Health Promotion for Older Children

Most of the attention on health in pediatric populations is devoted to under-5 children because the youngest age groups have the highest mortality rates. Although the mortality rate for older children and adolescents is low, health education interventions during these age periods can be valuable for keeping older children safe and also for preparing them for active and healthy adulthood.[45] Many of the health interventions for school-aged children are delivered at primary schools.[46] For example, one of the major contributors to reduced health status in middle childhood and early adolescence is iron deficiency anemia, which is often caused by a combination of rapid growth, inadequate dietary intake of iron, and malaria and hookworm infections. School-based feeding and deworming programs for primary school children are effective in improving school attendance, child health and development, and learning.[47] School health programs also provide health and hygiene education and support for activities related to infection prevention, nutrition, physical fitness, mental health and well-being, injury prevention and safety awareness, medical and dental care, and healthy relationships and bullying prevention.[48]

Initiatives to support the rights of children also contribute to protecting their health and enabling them to flourish. In 1989,

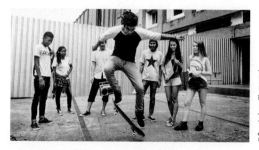

the General Assembly of the United Nations adopted the Convention on the Rights of the Child, which declares that the rights of the child include an adequate standard of living, freedom from all forms of exploitation, protection from all forms of violence, access to education and appropriate information, the right to be heard, and the right to rest, leisure, and play.[49] Acknowledging the right of every child in the world to these protections is a start, but this recognition must be acted on to be meaningful. Millions of children are still hungry, abused, exposed to war and other forms of violence, unable to attend school, and otherwise being denied their human rights.[50] Girls are especially vulnerable to abuse and neglect. When a family has limited resources, girls may face discrimination within the family due to preferential treatment of sons. Daughters may not be allowed to attend school and may be forced into early marriage.[51] In 1995, the United Nations adopted the Beijing Declaration that affirms several strategic objectives for promoting the rights of the "girl-child," including eliminating educational discrimination, the exploitation of child laborers, and violence against children. Although some improvements have been achieved, such as increasing school enrollment, significant inequalities between boys and girls remain in many regions of the world. Those inequalities can have significant adverse health effects for girls and young women.[52]

▶ 18.7 Health Promotion for Adolescents

Adolescence is a time characterized by rapid physical, sexual, neurological, psychological, and social development.[53] This developmental stage may begin at around 10 years of age (especially for girls) and extend until around 19 years of age (especially for

boys).[54] As children age into the adolescent stage, the proportion of deaths attributable to infections decreases as the proportion of deaths from injuries increases and adolescent females begin to experience the risks associated with pregnancy (**FIGURE 18–11**).[9] The distribution of years lived with disability (YLDs) attributable to various conditions shifts from younger children having a substantial burden of disability from infections, iron deficiency anemia, and asthma to adolescents having a high burden from depression, anxiety, back pain, and headaches (**FIGURE 18–12**).[55] In some regions, the rate of teen pregnancy is high due to limited access to reproductive health services and to other cultural and economic factors (**FIGURE 18–13**). Maternal mortality is a significant contributor to deaths among young women in many of the places where teen pregnancy is common.[56]

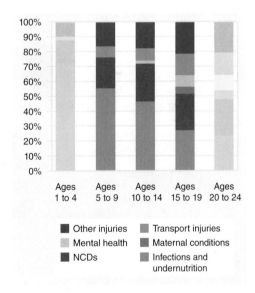

FIGURE 18–11 Infectious diseases and injuries are common preventable causes of child and adolescent mortality.

Data from GBD 2015 Child Mortality Collaborators. Global, regional, national, and selected subnational levels of stillbirths, neonatal, infant, and under-5 mortality, 1990–2015: A systematic analysis for the Global Burden of Disease Study 2015. *Lancet* 2016; 388:1725–74.

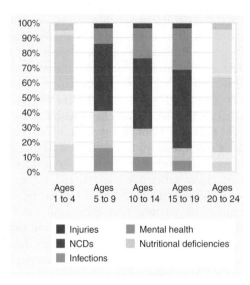

FIGURE 18-12 A diversity of conditions contribute to the years lived with disability (YLDs) among children and adolescents.

Data from GBD Disease and Injury Incidence and Prevalence Collaborators. Global, regional, and national incidence, prevalence, and years lived with disability for 310 diseases and injuries, 1990–2015: A systematic analysis for the Global Burden of Disease Study 2015. *Lancet* 2016; 388:1545–602.

Adolescent health interventions focus on the immediate needs of youth and also on setting the foundation necessary for those young people to become healthy adults.[57] The goal is to address risk factors and to identify and promote protective factors that will prevent health problems emerging later on.[58] The highest-impact health interventions for adolescents include programs for mental health (including prevention of suicide, alcohol abuse, and drug abuse), injury prevention (including prevention of violence), and reproductive health (including access to tools for preventing pregnancy, HIV, and other sexually transmitted infections), as well as interventions that promote nutritious diets, physical activity, tobacco-free living, and other aspects of healthy adult lifestyles.[59] Addressing broader concerns, such as youth unemployment, limited access to advanced education and vocational training, and unhealthy and violent environments, also promotes improved physical, mental, and social health among adolescents.[60]

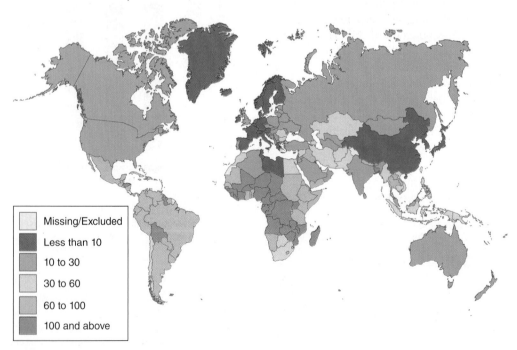

FIGURE 18-13 Birth rate per 1000 females aged 15–19 years (2005–2014).

Data from *World health statistics 2017.* Geneva: WHO; 2017.

References

1. UN Department of Economic and Social Affairs. *World population prospects: The 2015 revision.* New York: UN; 2015.
2. *Committing to child survival: A promise renewed. Progress report 2015.* New York: UNICEF; 2015.
3. You D, Hug L, Ejdemyr S, et al. Global, regional, and national levels and trends in under-5 mortality between 1990 and 2015, with scenario-based projections to 2030: A systematic analysis by the UN Inter-agency Group for Child Mortality Estimation. *Lancet.* 2015;386:2275–86.
4. UN Inter-agency Group for Child Mortality Estimation (IGME). *Levels & trends in child mortality report 2015.* New York: UNICEF; 2015.
5. United Nations. *Transforming our world: The 2030 Agenda for Sustainable Development.* New York: UN; 2015.
6. Jamison DT, Summers LH, Alleyne G, et al. Global health 2035: A world converging within a generation. *Lancet.* 2013;382:1898–955.
7. *The state of the world's children 2016: A fair chance for every child.* New York: UNICEF; 2016.
8. *Progress for children: Beyond averages: Learning from the MDGs.* New York: UNICEF; 2015.
9. GBD 2015 Child Mortality Collaborators. Global, regional, national, and selected subnational levels of stillbirths, neonatal, infant, and under-5 mortality, 1990–2015: A systematic analysis for the Global Burden of Disease Study 2015. *Lancet.* 2016;388:1725–74.
10. *Every Newborn: An action plan to end preventable deaths.* Geneva: WHO/UNICEF; 2014.
11. *Surviving the first day: State of the world's mothers 2013.* London: Save the Children; 2013.
12. Darmstadt GL, Bhutta ZA, Cousens S, et al. Evidence-based, cost-effective interventions: How many newborn babies can we save? *Lancet.* 2005;365:977–85.
13. Gülmezoglu AM, Lawrie TA, Hezelgrave N, et al. Interventions to reduce maternal and newborn morbidity and mortality (Chapter 7). *Disease control priorities.* 3rd ed. *Reproductive, maternal, newborn, and child health (Volume 2).* Washington DC: IBRD/World Bank; 2016.
14. Lawn JE, Blencowe H, Oza S, et al. Every Newborn: Progress, priorities, and potential beyond survival. *Lancet.* 2014;384:189–205.
15. Bhutta ZA, Das JK, Bahl R, et al. Can available interventions end preventable deaths in mothers, newborn babies, and stillbirths, and at what cost? *Lancet.* 2014;384:347–70.
16. Dickson KE, Simen-Kapeu A, Kinney MV, et al. Health-systems bottlenecks and strategies to accelerate scale-up in countries. *Lancet.* 2014;384:438–54.
17. Claeson M, Waldman RJ. The evolution of child health programmes in developing countries: From targeting diseases to targeting people. *Bull World Health Organ.* 2000;78:1234–45.
18. Cueto M. The origins of primary health care and selective primary health care. *Am J Public Health.* 2004;94:1864–74.
19. Hall JJ, Taylor R. Health for all beyond 2000: The demise of the Alma-Ata Declaration and primary health care in developing countries. *Med J Aust.* 2003;178:17–20.
20. Walley J, Lawn JE, Tinker A, et al. Primary health care: Making Alma-Ata a reality. *Lancet.* 2008;372:1001–7.
21. Msuya J. *Horizontal and vertical delivery of health services: What are the trade offs?* Washington DC: World Bank; 2004.
22. Rifkin SB, Walt G. Why health improves: Defining the issues concerning 'comprehensive primary health care' and 'selective primary health care.' *Soc Sci Med.* 1986;23:559–66.
23. *WHO's vision and mission: Immunization and vaccines 2015–2030.* Geneva: WHO; 2015.
24. Schuftan C. The child survival revolution. *Fam Pract.* 1990;7:329–32.
25. Cash R, Keusch GT, Lamstein J, editors. *Child health and survival: The UNICEF GOBI-FFF Program.* London: Croom Helm; 1987.
26. Lambrechts T, Bryce J, Orinda V. Integrated management of childhood illness: A summary of first experiences. *Bull World Health Organ.* 1999;77:582–94.
27. Costello AM, Dalglish SL; Strategic Review Study Team. *Towards a grant convergence for child survival and health: A strategic review of options for the future building on lessons learnt from IMNCI.* Geneva: WHO; 2016.
28. *Child health in the community: "Community IMCI" briefing package for facilitators.* Geneva: WHO; 2004.
29. *WHO/UNICEF joint statement: Integrated Community Case Management (iCCM).* New York: UNICEF; 2012.
30. *The Partnership for Maternal, Newborn & Child Health (in support of Every Woman Every Child): 2015 annual report.* Geneva: PMNCH; 2015.
31. Black MM, Walker SP, Fernald LCH, et al. Early childhood development coming of age: Science through the life course. *Lancet.* 2017;389:77–90.
32. *The Global Strategy for Women's, Children's and Adolescents' Health (2016–2030).* New York: Every Woman Every Child (EWEC); 2015.
33. Denboba AD, Sayre RK, Wodon QT, Elder LK, Rawlings LB, Lombardi J. *Stepping up early childhood development: Investing in young children for high returns.* Washington DC: World Bank; 2014.

34. Britto PR, Lye SJ, Proulx K, et al. Nurturing care: Promoting early childhood development. *Lancet.* 2017;389:91–102.

35. Alderman H, Behrman J, Glewwe P, Fernald L, Walker S. Child physical, cognitive, and socio-emotional development (Chapter 7). *Disease control priorities.* 3rd ed. *Child and adolescent health and development (Volume 8).* Washington DC: IBRD/World Bank; 2017.

36. Aboud FE, Yousafzai AK. Very early childhood development (Chapter 13). *Disease control priorities.* 3rd ed. *Reproductive, maternal, newborn, and child health (Volume 2).* Washington DC: IBRD/World Bank; 2016.

37. Anderson LM, Shinn C, Fullilove MT, et al. The effectiveness of early childhood development programs: A systematic review. *Am J Prev Med.* 2003;24(Suppl 3):32–46.

38. Richter LM, Daelmans B, Lombardi J, et al. Investing in the foundation of sustainable development: Pathways to scale up for early childhood development. *Lancet.* 2017;389:103–18.

39. Jones M. Deafness as culture: A psychosocial perspective. *Disability Stud Q.* 2002;22:51–60.

40. Graham N, Schultz L, Mitra S. Mont D. Children with disabilities (Chapter 17). *Disease control priorities.* 3rd ed. *Child and adolescent health and development (Volume 8).* Washington DC: IBRD/World Bank; 2017.

41. *Early childhood development and disability: A discussion paper.* Geneva: WHO/UNICEF; 2012.

42. *Disabled village children: A guide for community health workers, rehabilitation workers, and families.* Palo Alto CA: Hesperian; 2009.

43. *World report on disability 2011.* Geneva: WHO; 2011.

44. *WHO Global Disability Action Plan 2014–2012: Better health for all people with disability.* Geneva: WHO; 2014.

45. Hill K, Zimmerman L, Jamison D. Mortality at ages 5 to 19: Levels and trends, 1990 to 2010 (Chapter 2). *Disease control priorities.* 3rd ed. *Child and adolescent health and development (Volume 8).* Washington DC: IBRD/World Bank; 2017.

46. Bundy D, Horton S. Interventions during the life course, ages 5 to 19 years: Conceptual framework (Chapter 6). *Disease control priorities.* 3rd ed. *Child and adolescent health and development (Volume 8).* Washington DC: IBRD/World Bank; 2017.

47. Bundy D, Appleby L, Bradley M, et al. Deworming (Chapter 13). *Disease control priorities.* 3rd ed. *Child and adolescent health and development (Volume 8).* Washington DC: IBRD/World Bank; 2017.

48. Bundy D, Schultz L, Sarr B. Platforms to reach school-age children (Chapter 20). *Disease control priorities.* 3rd ed. *Child and adolescent health and development (Volume 8).* Washington DC: IBRD/World Bank; 2017.

49. *Convention on the Rights of the Child.* New York: United Nations; 1989.

50. Hammarberg T. The UN Convention on the Rights of the Child, and how to make it work. *Human Rights Q.* 1990;12:97–105.

51. Ferrant G, Nowacka K, Thim A. *Living up to Beijing's vision of gender equality: Social norms and transformative change.* Paris: OECD; 2015.

52. *The Beijing Declaration and Platform for Action Turns 20.* New York: UN Women; 2015.

53. Viner R, Allen NB, Patton G. Puberty, developmental processes, and health interventions (Chapter 9). *Disease control priorities.* 3rd ed. *Child and adolescent health and development (Volume 8).* Washington DC: IBRD/World Bank; 2017.

54. *Health for the world's adolescents: A second chance in the second decade.* Geneva: WHO; 2014.

55. GBD 2015 Disease and Injury Incidence and Prevalence Collaborators. Global, regional, and national incidence, prevalence, and years lived with disability for 310 diseases and injuries, 1990–2015: A systematic analysis for the Global Burden of Disease Study 2015. *Lancet.* 2016;388:1545–602.

56. UN Department of Economic and Social Affairs. *World population monitoring: Adolescents and youth.* New York: UN; 2012.

57. Sawyer SM, Afifi RA, Bearinger LH, et al. Adolescence: A foundation for future health. *Lancet.* 2012;379:1630–40.

58. Catalano FR, Fagan AA, Gavin LE, et al. Worldwide application of prevention science in adolescent health. *Lancet.* 2012;379:1653–64.

59. Patton GC, Sawyer SM, Santelli JS, et al. Our future: A *Lancet* commission on adolescent health and wellbeing. *Lancet.* 2016;387:2423–78.

60. Viner RM, Ozer EM, Denny S, et al. Adolescence and the social determinants of health. *Lancet.* 2012;379:1641–52.

CHAPTER 19

Promoting Healthy Adulthood and Aging

A fundamental goal of global health is to enable as many people as possible to maintain their health well into old age. The number of older adults around the world is increasing at a rapid rate. Many of those individuals will develop chronic diseases and disabilities that eventually will limit their independence. Young and middle-aged adults have the opportunity to take actions that lower their risk of premature death and lengthy periods of disability. Communities and nations can implement socioeconomic, environmental, and health policies that will improve the quality of life for people across the life span.

▶ 19.1 Aging and Global Health

The world population is aging rapidly as more children survive to adulthood and more adults survive to very old age.[1] Preventive interventions (such as reduced tobacco use), medical therapies (such as the availability of medications for common cardiovascular conditions), and other health promotion and disease prevention initiatives are allowing adults in countries across the income spectrum to live to older ages.[2] While the life expectancies at birth are quite different in high-income and low-income countries, the life expectancies for adults are more similar. Even in many low-income countries, the typical 50-year-old can expect to celebrate his or her 75th birthday and the typical 70-year-old can

expect to celebrate his or her 80th birthday (FIGURE 19–1).[3] The number of people worldwide who are 60 years old or older is expected to increase from about 900 million in 2015 to 1.4 billion in 2030 and more than 2 billion by 2050.[4] The number of people who are 80 years old or older is expected to rise from about 125 million in 2015 to 200 million in 2030 and more than 430 million by 2050 (FIGURE 19–2).

The **mortality transition** describes decreases in the rates of death for age groups across the life span. When the mortality rate is lower, life expectancies increase. The fertility transition describes a decrease in the population birth rate as the average woman delivers fewer children. When these two components of the demographic transition occur together—when both death rates and birth rates decrease—the number of older adults grows at a faster rate than the number of children.[5] During this

425

	USA	Germany	Iran	Brazil	China	India	Nigeria	Ethiopia
At least half of **newborns** will live until age…	79.6	81.3	76.2	75.8	76.5	68.9	54.1	66.0
At least half of **5-year-old children** will live to age…	80.1	81.5	77.3	77.0	77.4	72.1	60.2	69.8
At least half of **15-year-old adolescents** will live to age…	80.2	81.5	77.4	77.2	77.6	72.5	62.6	70.8
At least half of **50-year-old adults** will live to age…	82.2	82.7	79.0	80.4	78.9	75.9	71.2	76.0
At least half of **70-year-old adults** will live to age…	86.1	85.8	82.1	85.1	82.5	81.7	78.2	81.4
At least half of **85-year-old adults** will live to age…	91.8	91.2	89.8	92.3	90.4	90.6	88.0	89.6

FIGURE 19–1 Life expectancies at birth are highest in high-income countries, but the conditional life expectancies for older adults are similar across countries (2015).

Data from United Nations Department of Economic and Social Affairs. *World population prospects: The 2017 revision*. New York: UN; 2017.

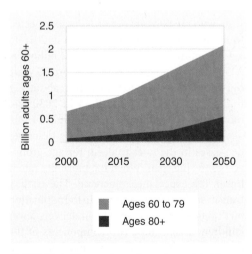

FIGURE 19–2 The number of people worldwide who are aged 60 years and older will increase in the coming decades.

Data from United Nations Department of Economic and Social Affairs. *World population ageing 2015*. New York: UN; 2015.

aging transition, the percentage of the population represented by older adults increases and the percentage of children shrinks, even in places where the number of children is rising as part of overall population growth. An increase in the percentage of older adults in the population is projected to occur over the coming decades in countries of all income levels (**FIGURE 19–3**).[4] Globally, the percentage of the total population that is 60 years old or older will more than double between 2000 and 2050, rising from 10% in 2000 to about 21.3% by 2050.[3] The percentage of world's people who are aged 80 years or older will nearly triple during that time span, increasing from about 1.2% in 2000 to 4.3% in 2050 (**FIGURE 19–4**).

The ultimate goal of public health is to enable as many people as possible to enjoy long, healthy lives. Increases in longevity are only a partial success when those

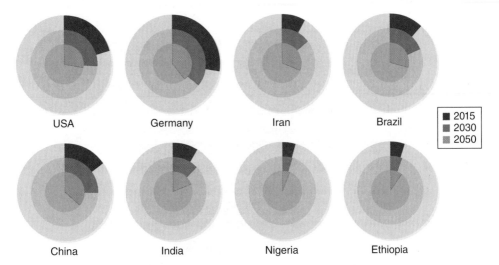

FIGURE 19–3 The percentage of the population that is aged 60 years and older is projected to increase in every country.

Data from United Nations Department of Economic and Social Affairs. *World population ageing 2015*. New York: UN; 2015.

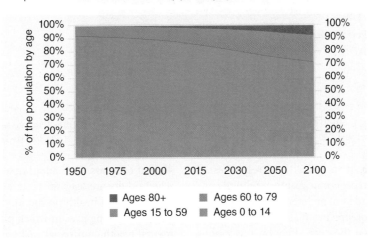

FIGURE 19–4 The percentage of the global population that is aged 60 years and older is increasing rapidly.

Data from United Nations Department of Economic and Social Affairs. *World population prospects: The 2017 revision*. New York: UN; 2017.

additional years of life are not healthy ones. At present, the typical older adult experiences about 10 years of disability prior to death (**FIGURE 19–5**).[6] Many older adults require several years of assistance with routine activities of daily living. Eldercare is expensive for the families who provide the bulk of the caregiving. The economic productivity of households and nations is reduced when women and men take time away from other types of labor to

care for aging family members.[7] However, the emerging challenges associated with aging can be considered welcome ones because they are the result of the excellent progress that has been made on enabling more people worldwide to live longer lives. Creative solutions will be required to address the resource needs of growing older adult populations, including the strain that managing age-related health problems will place on health systems. Each community and

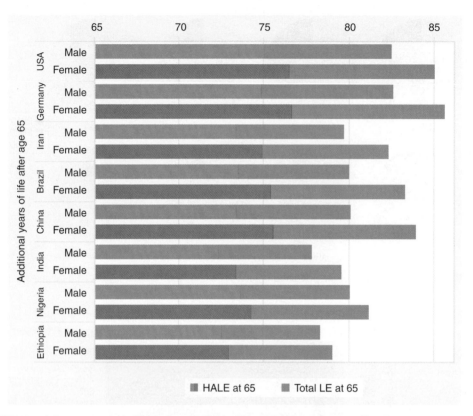

FIGURE 19–5 Life expectancy (additional years of life) and healthy life expectancy (HALE) at age 65 years.

Data from GBD 2015 DALYs and HALE Collaborators. Global, regional, and national disability-adjusted life years (DALYs) for 315 diseases and injuries and healthy life expectancy (HALE), 1990–2015: A systematic analysis for the Global Burden of Disease Study 2015. *Lancet* 2016; 388:1603–58.

nation will need to tailor their responses to aging based on economic realities, cultural considerations, and local preferences. Policymakers will be best equipped to make these important decisions when they can draw on the lessons learned by others from across the globe.

▶ 19.2 Health Promotion in Early and Middle Adulthood

Adulthood is often divided into three developmental stages.[8] Early adulthood extends roughly from ages 20 to 39 years. Middle adulthood encompasses the time between about ages 40 and 64 years. Late adulthood is the period when adults are ages 65 years and older. The overall goal of health promotion among adults is to enable long lives in which physical health, mental health, and social well-being are maintained. For early and middle adulthood, this translates into three key aims: reducing mortality to as close to zero as possible, since any death of a young or middle-aged adult is considered to be premature; reducing disability so that as many men and women as possible are leading productive, independent, and pain-free lives; and addressing the modifiable risk factors that are likely to cause disability and premature death at any point in the adult life course.

Injuries are the most common cause of death in early adulthood, and more young adults die from infections than from

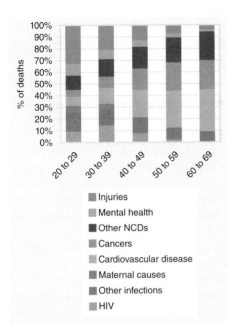

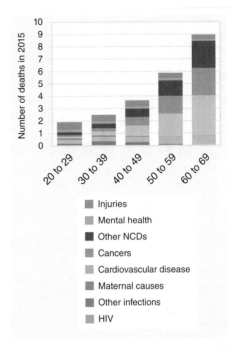

FIGURE 19–6 As adults age, the likelihood of death from a noncommunicable disease increases.

Data from GBD Mortality and Causes of Death Collaborators. Global, regional, and national life expectancy, all-cause mortality, and cause-specific mortality for 249 causes of death, 1990–2015: A systematic analysis for the Global Burden of Disease Study 2015. *Lancet* 2016; 388:1459–544.

FIGURE 19–7 The annual number of deaths of older adults is greater than the number of deaths of younger adults.

Data from GBD Mortality and Causes of Death Collaborators. Global, regional, and national life expectancy, all-cause mortality, and cause-specific mortality for 249 causes of death, 1990–2015: A systematic analysis for the Global Burden of Disease Study 2015. *Lancet* 2016; 388:1459–544.

noncommunicable diseases (NCDs).[9] By middle adulthood, the majority of deaths are attributable to NCDs (**FIGURE 19–6**). The number of deaths worldwide each year from infections and injuries remains relatively similar across adult age groups, but the relative proportion of deaths from non-NCD conditions shrinks as the number of deaths from NCDs expands dramatically with aging (**FIGURE 19–7**).

There is considerable variation by country in the distribution of causes of deaths among adults in the typical reproductive ages (roughly 15–49 years), with infectious disease deaths common in low-income countries and rare in high-income countries (**FIGURE 19–8**).[9] Mortality reduction interventions for early adults need to be tailored to the target population. Injury prevention is among the top priorities in most high-income countries. Infection control is a leading priority in most low-income countries. For middle-aged adults, prevention

and management of cardiovascular disease and other NCDs constitute an important mortality prevention strategy in most countries.

The causes of disability in the various stages of adulthood are quite different from the causes of death. In early adulthood, mental health disorders (especially depression) are the most common cause of years lived with disability (YLDs).[10] In middle adulthood, musculoskeletal disorders (mostly lower back pain) are the most common cause of YLDs. In older adulthood, sense organ disorders (primarily hearing loss) become prominent (**FIGURE 19–9**). Mental health and musculoskeletal disorders are common causes of lost productivity among reproductive-age adults in all countries (**FIGURE 19–10**).[10] Addressing these issues requires increased access to and utilization of health services, including

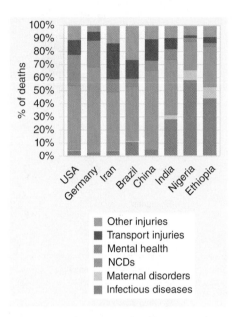

Other injuries
Transport injuries
Mental health
NCDs
Maternal disorders
Infectious diseases

FIGURE 19–8 There is considerable variation by country in the distribution of causes of death among adults of typical reproductive ages (15–49 years).

Data from GBD Mortality and Causes of Death Collaborators. Global, regional, and national life expectancy, all-cause mortality, and cause-specific mortality for 249 causes of death, 1990–2015: A systematic analysis for the Global Burden of Disease Study 2015. *Lancet* 2016; 388:1459–544.

counseling for mental health conditions, medications for pain management, and assistive devices, such as hearing aids.

Early and middle adulthood are also opportune times for taking steps to prevent disability in older adulthood. The cohort of young adults who had their 25th birthdays in 2015 will celebrate their 60th birthdays in 2050. The most cost-efficient way to improve the health status of those future older adults while reducing the burden that their health problems will place on households and national economies is for today's young adults to take steps to prevent or delay the onset of NCDs.[11] Key behavior changes include avoiding unsafe sex, the harmful use of alcohol, and all tobacco use; using medications and other approaches to maintain a low blood pressure, healthy blood sugar levels, and low cholesterol levels; maintaining a healthy weight, eating a nutritious diet, and

engaging in routine physical activity; and taking steps to minimize the risks of injury from occupational and recreational exposures.[12]

▸ 19.3 Health Promotion for Older Adults

Many older adults live active and independent lives. However, most will at some point develop a cardiovascular disease, a chronic respiratory disease, a musculoskeletal condition like arthritis, a neuropsychiatric condition such as dementia or depression, a sensory impairment like hearing or vision loss, or several of these chronic conditions at the same time, and these conditions may limit their independence. The number of years an individual adult lives without disability is a function of a lifetime of health-related behaviors in addition to being influenced by personal characteristics like genetics and psychosocial factors.[13] The most successful interventions for promoting longevity and postponing age-related disability are ones that encourage younger people to adopt active lifestyles and take other steps to protect their health as they age. Once older adults develop chronic conditions, rehabilitation and other interventions can slow the decline in function and ensure that all basic needs are met.[14]

The quality of life of older adults can be improved with tools that support autonomy, mobility, and social connections. These include affordable preventive and therapeutic healthcare services, including medications for managing chronic health problems and controlling pain; safe, comfortable, and accessible home and community environments; and strong family and social support.[13] As more assistance with activities of daily living becomes required, the goals for individual care shift from supporting independence toward enabling dignity and comfort for older adults as they experience the final stage of the life course.[15] A good death is one in which the dying individual is not merely

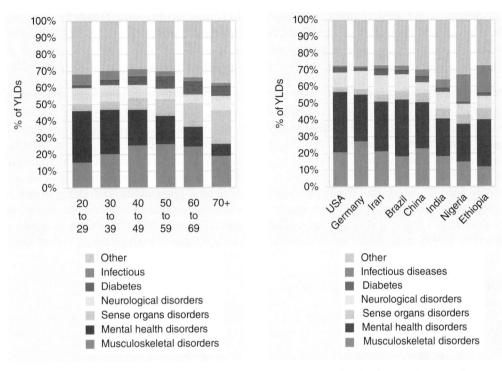

FIGURE 19–9 Mental health and musculoskeletal disorders contribute the largest proportion of years lived with disability (YLDs) among younger adults.

Data from GBD Disease and Injury Incidence and Prevalence Collaborators. Global, regional, and national incidence, prevalence, and years lived with disability for 310 diseases and injuries, 1990–2015: A systematic analysis for the Global Burden of Disease Study 2015. *Lancet* 2016; 388:1545–602.

FIGURE 19–10 The distribution of causes of disability among adults of typical reproductive ages (15–49 years) is similar across countries.

Data from GBD Disease and Injury Incidence and Prevalence Collaborators. Global, regional, and national incidence, prevalence, and years lived with disability for 310 diseases and injuries, 1990–2015: A systematic analysis for the Global Burden of Disease Study 2015. *Lancet* 2016; 388:1545–602.

avoiding suffering but is encircled by social, spiritual, and other types of support during the final weeks of life.[16]

▶ 19.4 Caring for Aging Populations

Many older people contribute to their families and communities by taking care of their grandchildren, providing mentorship and guidance for younger employees, connecting younger generations to their cultural heritage, and sharing the wisdom gained from decades of life experience. However, most older adults will eventually encounter challenges that limit their ability to live independently. Living with family members when assistance with activities of daily living becomes necessary is often the preference of both older people and their families. In most of the world, eldercare is provided by spouses, children, and other family members, and institutionalization of older people is uncommon. However, decreasing fertility rates in many parts of the world mean that there are fewer young people to care for older family members. The increasing proportion of women who work outside the home also limits the number of people available to provide in-home care. An increasing proportion of older adults in a population puts stress on healthcare systems as well as on caregivers.

Several social support ratios calculated from demographic data are used as indicators of population aging. These population characteristics help social service providers and policymakers to understand the current needs of the populations they serve and create plans that will help their populations prepare for the future. The **dependency ratio** quantifies the number of dependent children and older people for every young or middle-aged adult (typically defined as people aged 15–64 years). The dependency ratio is increasing in high-income countries as a result of aging and it is decreasing (for now) in low-income countries because of decreasing fertility rates (**FIGURE 19–11**).[3] The **elderly support ratio** (also called the old-age dependency ratio) is usually defined as the number of people aged 65 years and older for every person aged 15–64 years in a population. (Because many older women and men remain active and economically independent, alternate measurements of the elderly support ratio may include only dependent older people.) Populations with relatively few working adults for each older adult are more aged populations. The **aging index** is usually calculated as the number of people aged 65 years or older for every 100 children younger than 15 years of age. A higher aging

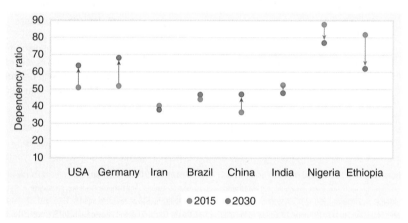

FIGURE 19–11 The dependency ratio (the number of people aged 0–14 years and 65+ years per 100 people aged 15–64 years) is expected to increase in high-income countries and decrease in low-income countries.

Data from United Nations Department of Economic and Social Affairs. *World population prospects: the 2017 revision*. New York: UN; 2017.

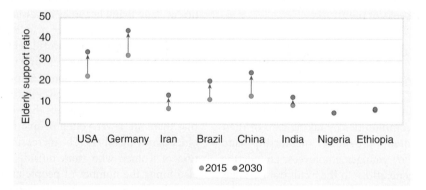

FIGURE 19–12 The elderly support ratio (the number of people aged 65+ years per 100 people aged 15–64 years) is expected to increase.

Data from United Nations Department of Economic and Social Affairs. *World population prospects: The 2017 revision*. New York: UN; 2017.

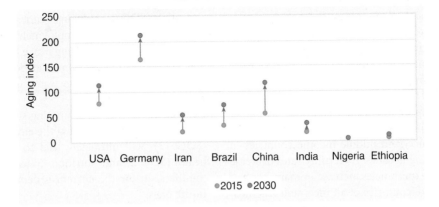

FIGURE 19–13 The aging index (the number of people aged 65+ years per 100 people aged 0–14 years) is expected to increase.

Data from United Nations Department of Economic and Social Affairs. *World population prospects: The 2015 revision*. New York: UN; 2015.

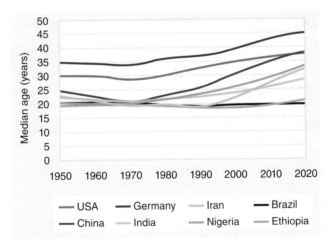

FIGURE 19–14 The median age of the population has increased in most high- and middle-income countries.

Data from United Nations Department of Economic and Social Affairs. *World population prospects: The 2017 revision*. New York: UN; 2017.

index indicates a more aged population. The elderly support ratio (**FIGURE 19–12**) and the aging index (**FIGURE 19–13**) are increasing in high-income and middle-income countries.[3] In most countries, trends for all three indices and a rapidly rising median population age (that is, the age of the middle person in the population if everyone in the country is ordered from youngest to oldest) (**FIGURE 19–14**) point toward a future with greater demands for eldercare.

Few countries are prepared to support a rapidly increasing number of older people with chronic illnesses and disabilities.[17] In high-income countries, the growing proportion of older adults is already creating significant challenges for aging adults, caregivers, health systems, and national pension systems. The national pension programs of many industrialized countries, especially in Europe, might be on the pathway to collapse because there may not be enough young workers paying into the programs to support retirees adequately.[18] The retirement age is being increased and retirement benefits are being cut. In industrializing countries where retirement accounts and pension plans are not the norm, aging is also expected to become a major social issue. The migration of rural young people to cities means that adult children often live far from their aging parents and cannot provide daily care, and few families have the resources to hire caregivers or nursing assistants.[19] The ability to care for older people will become a significant concern in middle-income countries in the coming decades. As fertility rates decrease and life expectancies increase in many parts of the world, countries of all income levels must prepare to support a growing population of older adults.[20] Communities must prepare to support the physical needs and psychosocial well-being of older adults,[21] and primary health providers must prepare to provide care coordination for older adults managing multiple chronic diseases.[11]

▶ 19.5 Health Promotion Across the Life Span

The Sustainable Development Goals (SDGs) focused on health aim to "ensure healthy lives and promote well-being for all at all ages" (SDG 3).[22] Many global health interventions are focused on one age group, but the interventions with the greatest impact are often those that yield benefits for all age groups, such as ones that improve socioeconomic and environmental conditions for entire communities.[23] For example, clean indoor and outdoor air protects the developing lungs of young children and also reduces the risk of cardiovascular and lung disease in older adults;[24] clean water prevents diarrheal diseases in people of all ages;[25] and economic development and increased access to health services benefit young and old alike.[26] One of the foundational premises of the SDGs is that economic development, environmental sustainability, and improved health are intertwined. Progress on socioeconomic goals, such as ending poverty (SDG 1), improving the quality of

education (SDG 4), reducing gender inequalities (SDG 5), expanding employment opportunities (SDG 8), and fostering peace (SDG 16), and progress on environmental goals, such as ensuring access to clean water and sanitation (SDG 6), increasing access to affordable clean energy (SDG 7), promoting sustainability (SDG 12), and protecting the environment (SDG 13), will ultimately lead to improved health (SDG 3) and nutrition (SDG 2) across the life span for the current generations and future ones.[27]

▶ References

1. Lutz W, Sanderson W, Scherbov S. The coming acceleration of global population ageing. *Nature.* 2008;451:716–9.
2. Mathers CD, Stevens GA, Boerma T, White RA, Tobias MI. Causes of international increases in older age life expectancy. *Lancet.* 2015;385:540–8.
3. UN Department of Economic and Social Affairs. *World population prospects: The 2017 revision.* New York: UN; 2017.
4. UN Department of Economic and Social Affairs. *World population ageing 2015.* New York: UN; 2015.
5. Lee R. The demographic transition: Three centuries of fundamental change. *J Econ Persp.* 2003;14: 167–90.
6. GBD 2015 DALYs and HALE Collaborators. Global, regional, and national disability-adjusted life years (DALYs) for 315 diseases and injuries and healthy life expectancy (HALE), 1990–2015: A systematic analysis for the Global Burden of Disease Study 2015. *Lancet.* 2016;388:1603–58.
7. Bloom DE, Chatterji S, Kowal P, et al. Macroeconomic implications of population ageing and selected policy responses. *Lancet.* 2015;385:649–57.
8. Levinson DJ. A conception of adult development. *Am Psychol.* 1986;41:3–13.
9. GBD 2015 Mortality and Causes of Death Collaborators. Global, regional, and national life expectancy, all-cause mortality, and cause-specific mortality for 249 causes of death, 1990–2015: A systematic analysis for the Global Burden of Disease Study 2015. *Lancet.* 2016;388:1459–544.
10. GBD 2015 Disease and Injury Incidence and Prevalence Collaborators. Global, regional, and national incidence, prevalence, and years lived with disability for 310 diseases and injuries, 1990–2015: A systematic analysis for the Global Burden of Disease Study 2015. *Lancet.* 2016;388:1545–602.

11. Prince MJ, Wu F, Guo Y, et al. The burden of disease in older people and implications for health policy and practice. *Lancet.* 2015;385:549–62.

12. GBD 2015 Risk Factor Collaborators. Global, regional, and national comparative risk assessment of 79 behavioural, environmental and occupational, and metabolic risks or clusters of risks, 1990–2015: A systematic analysis for the Global Burden of Disease Study 2015. *Lancet.* 2016;388:1545–602.

13. *Active ageing: A policy framework.* Geneva: WHO; 2002.

14. *World report on ageing and health.* Geneva: WHO; 2015.

15. *WHO global strategy on people-centered and integrated health services: Interim report.* Geneva: WHO; 2015.

16. Emanuel EJ, Emanuel LL. The promise of a good death. *Lancet.* 1998;351(Suppl 2):S21–9.

17. *Multisectoral action for a life course approach to healthy ageing: draft global strategy and plan of action on ageing and health: Report by the Secretariat (A69/17).* Geneva: World Health Assembly; 2016.

18. Foster L, Walker A. Active and successful aging: A European policy perspective. *Gerontologist.* 2015; 55:83–90.

19. Silverstein M, Giarrusso R. Aging and family life: A decade review. *J Marriage Fam.* 2010;72:1039–58.

20. *Why population aging matters: A global perspective.* Washington DC: U.S. Department of State and U.S. National Institute on Aging; 2007.

21. Steptoe A, Deaton A, Stone AA. Subjective wellbeing, health, and ageing. *Lancet.* 2015;385:640–8.

22. United Nations. *Transforming our world: The 2030 Agenda for Sustainable Development.* New York: UN; 2015.

23. Frieden TR. A framework for public health action: The health impact pyramid. *Am J Public Health.* 2010;100:590–5.

24. *Burden of disease from the joint effects of household and ambient air pollution for 2012.* Geneva: WHO; 2014.

25. Prüss-Üstün A, Bos R, Gore F, Bartram J. *Safe water, better health: costs, benefits and sustainability of interventions to protect and promote health.* Geneva: WHO; 2008.

26. *Closing the gap in a generation: Health equity through action on the social determinants of health: Final report of the Commission on Social Determinants of Health.* Geneva: WHO; 2008.

27. *World health statistics 2016: Monitoring health for the SDGs.* Geneva: WHO; 2016.

CHAPTER 20

Global Health Careers

Global health is a multidisciplinary field that draws on knowledge of the sciences and social sciences, skills in a diversity of clinical and nonclinical practice areas, and aptitudes in cross-cultural communication, interprofessionalism, and other soft skills. There are many educational tracks and career pathways that can prepare people to make the world a healthier home for current and future generations.

▶ 20.1 Career Pathways in Global Health

There are many pathways to a career in global health. A diversity of professionals are involved in delivering health-related services to individuals and communities: physicians and surgeons, nurses, dentists, psychologists, therapists, emergency medical technicians, and clinicians with expertise in other practice areas as well as public health workers, social workers, emergency management professionals, program administrators, project managers, and many others. These practitioners and their colleagues may work in or near their home communities to improve access to quality medical, psychological, and other health-related services, or they may work in distant locations to support the goals of global public health partnerships. Health sector experts often work alongside people with expertise in other aspects of international and community development to support socioeconomic progress and environmental health. Another set of global health professionals works on the financing, management, and administration of global

health policies and plans. These specialists apply their expertise in public policy, business, communication, law, and other professional practice areas to work at government agencies, foundations and other nonprofit organizations, for-profit corporations, and other groups. Many of the people who serve in leadership roles in global health today were leaders in other fields before choosing to apply their talents to global health issues.

Global health also overlaps with many lines of work that are not specifically focused on financing and implementing global health interventions. Scientists working at scales from the molecular level to the ecosystem level and beyond are making discoveries that will inform future global health activities. Engineers are inventing new tools for global health. Social scientists are providing insights about human and organizational behaviors and social systems. Policymakers in many fields are becoming more aware of the links between health and all other policy areas, and they are incorporating health promotion strategies into their recommendations.[1] Work that advances any of the Sustainable Development Goals (SDGs) can be considered to be promoting global health advancement. By this standard, anyone working in education, social work, politics, economic development, international relations, security, or other socio-political fields; in technology, agriculture, energy, transportation, sanitation, or other environmental resource sectors; or in nearly any other area might be contributing to global health.[2]

▶ # 20.2 Global Health Education

The diversity of professional pathways within global health means that there are many educational tracks that can lead to a global health career. Global health is a **multidisciplinary** field in which people from diverse areas of academic study pool their expertise to solve challenging problems. No particular undergraduate major or graduate program is necessary for entering or advancing in the global health workforce. However, all global health professionals are expected to be knowledgeable about the global burden of disease, the effects of globalization on health and health care, and the social and environmental determinants of health (**FIGURE 20–1**).[3]

The Council on Education for Public Health (CEPH), which accredits public health educational programs, has identified several

Domain		Competency
Global burden of disease	1a	Describe the major causes of morbidity and mortality around the world, and how the risk for disease varies with regions.
	1b	Describe major public health efforts to reduce disparities in global health.
	1c	Validate the health status of populations using available data.
Globalization of health and health care	2a	Describe different national models or health systems for provision of health care and their respective effects on health and healthcare expenditure.
	2b	Describe how global trends in healthcare practice, commerce and culture, multinational agreements, and multinational organizations contribute to the quality and availability of health and health care locally and internationally.
	2c	Describe how travel and trade contribute to the spread of communicable and chronic diseases.
	2d	Describe general trends and influences in the global availability and movement of healthcare workers.
Social and environmental determinants of health	3a	Describe how cultural context influences perceptions of health and disease.
	3b	List major social and economic determinants of health and their effects on the access to and the quality of health services and on differences in morbidity and mortality between and within countries.
	3c	Describe the relationship between access to and quality of water, sanitation, food, and air on individual and population health.

FIGURE 20–1 Key global health knowledge domains from the Consortium of Universities for Global Health.

Reproduced from Jogerst K, Callender B, Adams V, Evert J, Fields E, Hall T, Olsen J, Rowthorn V, Rudy S, Shen J, Simon L, Torres H, Velji A, Wilson LL. Identifying interprofessional global health competencies for 21st-century health professionals. *Ann Global Health* 2015; 81:239–47. Reprinted with permission from Elsevier and authors.

competencies that are prerequisites for graduate education in public health (**FIGURE 20–2**).[4] All of these general public health knowledge areas are also relevant to future global health professionals. They also highlight how coursework across a variety of disciplines—health-specific courses plus courses in statistics, environmental science, biology, psychology, sociology, political science, and economics—is valuable for students aspiring to work in the global health arena. For example, a course on **medical anthropology** will provide an understanding of the global diversity of perspectives on health, disease, illness, sickness, and healing, and a course on **public policy** will explain the processes for developing, implementing, funding, enforcing, administering, and evaluating laws, regulations, policies, and government-sponsored programs.

A **liberal arts** education—that is, a program of study that includes exposure to the humanities, social sciences, and sciences—is a good foundation for understanding the social-behavioral and biological-environmental contributors to health and disease. (The general education requirements at most colleges and universities in the United States provide broad exposure to the liberal arts that complements focused studies in a particular major or concentration area.) However, there is no particular checklist of courses that must be taken to be on track for a global health career. Studies within a particular major or during advanced professional training can be supplemented with electives that fill gaps in knowledge and enhance skills in the particular area of expertise that the learner intends to apply to global health work.

Profession and Science of Public Health	Factors Related to Human Health
Explain public health history, philosophy, and values.	Explain the effects of environmental factors on a population's health.
Identify the core functions and essential services of public health.	Explain the biological and genetic factors that affect a population's health.
Explain the role of quantitative and qualitative methods and sciences in describing and assessing a population's health.	Explain the behavioral and psychological factors that affect a population's health.
List major causes and trends of morbidity and mortality in populations.	Explain the social, political, and economic determinants of health and how they contribute to population health and health inequities.
Discuss the science of prevention in population health.	Explain how globalization affects the global burden of disease.
Explain the critical importance of evidence in advancing public health knowledge.	Explain an ecological perspective on the connections among human health, animal health, and ecosystem health.

FIGURE 20–2 Foundational public health knowledge identified by the Council on Education for Public Health.

Data from *Accreditation criteria: Schools of public health and public health programs.* Silver Spring MD: Council on Education for Public Health (CEPH); 2016.

One of the SDG targets calls for steps to "ensure that all learners acquire the knowledge and skills needed to promote sustainable development, including, among others, through education for sustainable development and sustainable lifestyles, human rights, gender equality, promotion of a culture of peace and non-violence, global citizenship, and appreciation of cultural diversity and of culture's contribution to sustainable development" (SDG 4.7).[5] These educational goals apply to all levels of the educational system, from primary school through advanced degrees, and they also align with the diversity of areas in which global health professionals must develop competencies.

Successful global health careers are built on both technical aptitudes and on **soft skills**, the personal, social, emotional, and communication skills that equip people to productively contribute to and lead work teams and other collaborative activities. One of the soft skills valued in global health is **interprofessionalism**, the ability to work with and communicate well with colleagues in different clinical and nonclinical practice areas in order to achieve a shared goal. Global health also values compassion, empathy, and a sense of solidarity with other human beings, whether those people live next door or on the other side of the planet.[6] Soft skills that are valued across work sectors include communication, courtesy, flexibility, integrity, positive attitude, professionalism, responsibility, social skills, teamwork, and work ethic.[7] For global health careers, aptitudes in capacity strengthening; collaboration, partnering, and communication; ethical reasoning and professional practices; health equity and social justice; program management; sociocultural and political awareness; and strategic analysis have been identified as critical both by the Association of Schools and Programs of Public Health (ASPPH),[8] which is the organization for institutions with public health programs accredited by CEPH,[9] and by the Consortium of Universities for Global Health (CUGH), which is a professional network for medical schools and other academic health programs.[3]

▶ 20.3 Experiential Learning in Global Health

Being proficient in any professional discipline requires a mix of knowledge, skills, and abilities (KSAs). After foundational knowledge in a field has been acquired, skills and abilities can be developed through applied learning experiences. In global health, the typical options for gaining experience include service-learning courses, study abroad (including international clinical electives), internships, and volunteering with diverse local populations or in international settings.[10] Fellowships and other designated career development programs may provide additional opportunities for structured learning experiences. Employees (and volunteers) at any stage of their careers can seek mentorship and complete continuing education activities that expand their skill sets and competencies.

The best experiential learning opportunities in global health are ones that are equally beneficial to the learner, the host organization, and the host community.[11] This requires mutual respect and assurances that none of the parties will be exploited, undermined, or harmed.[12] For example, mutual respect means that volunteers should not engage in practices that are beyond the scope of their abilities. A student without hands-on medical training at home should not provide clinical care in a foreign country, and a student without supervised counseling experience at home should not provide mental health care in a foreign country. **Voluntourism**, or volunteer tourism, is travel for the purpose of volunteering, and it usually combines vacation with international service.[13] Short-term volunteer experiences offer little time to build relationships with local partners, so the participants must be especially sensitive to local norms and committed to supporting local practitioners and their trainees rather than displacing them or competing with them.[14]

One of the goals of experiential learning is to gain **cultural competency**, the ability to communicate effectively with people from different cultures and backgrounds.[15] Cross-cultural communication is about much more than language skills. Cultural competency encompasses awareness of one's own cultural rules and biases, knowledge about other cultures, skills in verbal and nonverbal communication, and characteristics like empathy, curiosity, and openness that enable effective communication.[16] These skills are valuable not only for working on multidisciplinary international teams but also for enhancing practice within one's home community and workplace.

▶ 20.4 Global Health Matters

As global health has matured as a field of study, research, and application, several activities have emerged as important global health functions, including protecting the world from dangerous infectious diseases, saving the lives of children and their mothers, and promoting global security and economic growth by finding cost-efficient solutions for expensive health issues (**FIGURE 20–3**).[17] Global health interventions could make unparalleled improvements in the lives of billions of people during the 21st century by promoting health, preventing disease and disability, improving health standards, reducing health disparities, tackling the health and security problems associated with extreme poverty, and bringing together people from across the world as equals to address shared challenges.

A brief summary of the core messages of *Introduction to Global Health* highlights the many reasons why global health matters and why careers and volunteer work that contribute to global health can be very meaningful. Global health is a dynamic field, and health interventions are effective in preventing adverse health outcomes and promoting

transitions toward improved population health (Chapter 1). International trade and other globalization processes have increased the risk of pandemics while also creating opportunities to work together to address shared concerns and enhance security.

The SDGs provide a global framework for prioritizing investments in poverty reduction and other outcomes that will reduce global health disparities and promote global security. Health metrics are a tool for evaluating population health needs, selecting cost-effective health interventions, and tracking progress toward achieving goals (Chapter 2). Improvements in economics, education, employment opportunities, equity, and governance yield benefits for population health (Chapter 3). Improvements in access to clean drinking water, toilets, clean energy, unpolluted air, safe jobs, and planned cities, and the adoption of sustainable practices, enable healthier human living and a healthier planet (Chapter 4). Health and human rights are inextricably connected, and populations are healthier when everyone has access to the tools for health (Chapter 5). Personal and public health activities are financed by a diversity of governmental, private, and corporate entities (Chapter 6), and global health interventions are implemented by people working for governmental and intergovernmental agencies, nonprofit organizations, and for-profit corporations who apply their expertise to solving complex challenges (Chapter 7). A wide range of educational and professional pathways can lead to a career in global health.

A diverse set of health conditions can be considered to fall under the umbrella of global health, including HIV, tuberculosis, and antimicrobial resistance (Chapter 8); diarrheal diseases, pneumonia, influenza, and vaccine-preventable infections (Chapter 9); malaria, other vectorborne diseases, and emerging infectious diseases (Chapter 10); reproductive and sexual health (Chapter 11); undernutrition, overnutrition, and food safety (Chapter 12); cancer (Chapter 13);

Priority Area		Recommendation
Secure against global threats	Achieve global health security	Improve international emergency response coordination.
		Combat antimicrobial resistance.
		Build public health capacity in low- and middle-income countries.
	Address continuous threats	Envision the next generation of the President's Emergency Plan for AIDS Relief (PEPFAR).
		Confront the threat of tuberculosis.
		Sustain progress toward malaria elimination.
Enhance productivity and economic growth	Invest in women's and children's health	Improve survival in women and children.
		Ensure healthy and productive lives for women and children.
	Promote cardiovascular health and prevent cancer	Promote cardiovascular health and prevent cancer.
Maximize returns on investments	Catalyze innovation	Accelerate the development of medical products.
		Improve digital health infrastructure.
	Smart financing strategies	Transition investments toward global public goods.
		Optimize resources through smart financing.
	Global health leadership	Commit to continued global health leadership.

FIGURE 20–3 Recommended actions from the National Academies of Sciences, Engineering, and Medicine's Committee on Global Health and the Future of the United States.

Data from National Academies of Sciences, Engineering, and Medicine. *Global health and the future role of the United States*. Washington: The National Academies Press; 2017.

cardiovascular diseases (Chapter 14); chronic respiratory diseases and diabetes (Chapter 15); mental health and substance use disorders (Chapter 16); and injuries (Chapter 17). While the health profiles of low-income and high-income populations can be quite different when comparing countries or comparing sub-populations within the same country, there are also many shared socioeconomic, environmental, and health concerns.[18] Opportunities to improve the health status of individuals, communities, and the world exist throughout the life span, from the prenatal period (Chapter 18) through older adulthood (Chapter 19). Everyone can be involved in making communities all over the world healthier places for current and future generations.

▶ References

1. *Health in All Policies (HiAP): Framework for country action.* Geneva: WHO; 2014.

2. Hughes BB, Kuhn R, Peterson CM, Rothman DS, Solórzano JR. *Patterns of potential human progress (volume 3). Improving global health: Forecasting the next 50 years.* Denver: Pardee Center for International Futures; 2011.

3. Jogerst K, Callender B, Adams V, et al. Identifying interprofessional global health competencies for 21st-century health professionals. *Ann Global Health.* 2015;81:239–47.

4. *Accreditation criteria: Schools of public health and public health programs.* Silver Spring MD: Council on Education for Public Health (CEPH); 2016.

5. United Nations. *Transforming our world: The 2030 Agenda for Sustainable Development.* New York: UN; 2015.

6. Benatar SR, Daar AS, Singer PA. Global health ethics: The rationale for mutual caring. *Int Affairs.* 2003;79:107–38.

7. Robles MM. Executive perceptions of the top 10 soft skills needed in today's workplace. *Bus Commun Q.* 2012;75:453–65.

8. *Global health competency model (final version 1.1).* Washington DC: ASPPH; 2011.

9. Calhoun JG, Spencer HC, Buekens P. Competencies for global health graduate education. *Infect Dis Clin North Am.* 2011;25:575–92.

10. Arya AN, Evert J, eds. *Global health experiential education: From theory to practice.* New York: Routledge; 2018.

11. Stone GS, Olson KR. The ethics of medical volunteerism. *Med Clin North Am.* 2016;100:237–46.

12. Melby MK, Loh LC, Evert J, Prater C, Lin H, Khan OA. Beyond medical "missions" to impact-drive short-term experiences in global health (STEGHs): Ethical principles to optimize community benefit and learner experience. *Acad Med.* 2016;91:633–8.

13. Lasker JN. *Hoping to help: The promises and pitfalls of global health volunteering.* Ithaca NY: Cornell University Press; 2016.

14. Loh LC, Cherniak W, Dreifuss BA, Dacso MM, Lin HC, Evert J. Short term global health experiences and local partnership models: A framework. *Global Health.* 2015;11:50.

15. Napier AD, Ancarno C, Butler B, et al. Culture and health. *Lancet.* 2014;384:1607–39.

16. *Intercultural knowledge and competence VALUE rubric.* Washington DC: Association of American Colleges and Universities (AAC&U); 2009.

17. *Global health and the future role of the United States.* Washington DC: The National Academies Press; 2017.

18. Frenk J, Gómez-Dantés O, Moon S. From sovereignty to solidarity: A renewed concept of global health for an era of complex interdependence. *Lancet.* 2014;383:94–7.

Glossary

abortion the termination or loss of a pregnancy

abstinence refraining from sexual intercourse and other types of genital contact

abstract a one-paragraph summary of the methods, results, and conclusions of a scientific investigation

accident an unfortunate event that happens by chance

acculturation the complex process of adopting the practices, traditions, values, and identity of a new community after migrating

active immunity protection against infectious diseases that occurs when the body's immune system produces antibodies against a specific infectious agent

active management of the third stage of labor (AMTSL) prevention of postpartum hemorrhage through injections of oxytocin, controlled cord traction, and uterine massage

active surveillance the process of public health officials contacting healthcare providers to ask about how often they are diagnosing particular types of disease

active TB the symptomatic, contagious form of tuberculosis

activities of daily living (ADLs) routine daily self-care functions

acute respiratory infection (ARI) a short-term infection of the respiratory tract that typically has a rapid onset and resolves without becoming a chronic infection

addiction a cognitive and neurological condition characterized by adverse behaviors related to physical or psychological dependence

adjuvant an ingredient added to some types of vaccines to boost the body's immune response to the vaccine

adolescence a period from about age 10 to 19 years that is characterized by rapid physical, sexual, neurological, psychological, and social development

adverse event adverse reactions and other medical events that occur after an individual receives a vaccination or medication but which appear to be coincidental rather than being a result of the medical exposure

adverse reaction a side effect of a medication or vaccination

advocacy the process of increasing awareness of a specific cause in order to influence policy and resource allocation decisions related to that issue

***Aedes* mosquitoes** a genus of mosquito that thrives in urban areas

aging index the number of people aged 65 years or older for every 100 children younger than 15 years old

aging transition the health transition characterized by the percentage of the population represented by older adults increasing and the percentage of children decreasing

AIDS the acquired immunodeficiency syndrome that occurs as a result of the destruction of immune system cells by the HIV virus

airborne transmission the acquisition through inhalation of pathogens that have been aerosolized or suspended as droplets in the air

allele a version of a gene

allergy an immune dysfunction in which the body is hypersensitive to foreign substances that are usually not harmful

Alzheimer's disease the most prevalent form of dementia

ambient air pollution the presence of harmful chemicals or other substances in outdoor air at concentrations above the thresholds established for human safety

amino acid organic compounds that contain carbon, hydrogen, oxygen, and nitrogen, and are the base units for proteins

anemia a deficiency of red blood cells or hemoglobin that causes fatigue

angina chest pain or tightness caused by the heart muscle not getting an adequate supply of oxygen

angiogenesis the formation of new blood vessels that nourish a new cancerous tumor

angioplasty a procedure that physically opens and unclogs a blocked artery

Anopheles **mosquitoes** the genus of mosquitoes that spread malaria

anorexia a lack of appetite

anorexia nervosa an eating disorder characterized by a person having a distorted body image and feeling fat even when emaciated

antenatal care routine preventive healthcare consultations during pregnancy that allow clinicians to identify and address potential health problems in a woman or fetus

anthrax an infection with *Bacillus anthracis*

anthropometry the measurement of the human body

anthroponosis an infectious disease that usually occurs only in humans

antibody a protein produced by the human body (by B lymphocytes) in response to the presence of antigens

antigen a foreign substance in the body that triggers an immune response

antigenic drift a mutation to an influenza virus that occurs when small genetic mutations bring about small changes in the surface antigens of the virus

antigenic shift a mutation to an influenza virus that occurs when two very different influenza types of influenza A viruses attack the same cell and the genetic material from both recombines to form a new strain of influenza

antimicrobial resistance (AMR) a change in a pathogen that makes a particular type of drug (or drugs) ineffective against the pathogen

antiretroviral (ARV) medications for viral infections that suppress the viral count and slow the progression of symptoms

antiretroviral therapy (ART) combinations of three or more different types of medication that are taken together to combat HIV

aortic aneurysm a bulge in the aorta that can rupture and cause a rapid death from internal bleeding

apnea long pauses in breathing

apoptosis a process of programmed cell death

appropriate technology affordable and environmentally sustainable technology that can be locally operated and maintained

arbovirus an arthropod-borne virus

arsenicosis chronic arsenic poisoning from being exposed to contaminated water over a long period of time

artemisinin-based combination therapy (ACT) malaria treatment that combines at least two different antimalarial drugs, one of which is an artemisinin-based drug

arthropod an insect or an arachnid (a spider, tick, or mite)

ascariasis the disease caused by the intestinal roundworms that have parasitized more people than any other helminth

assisted reproductive technologies fertility treatments that handle eggs or embryos

assistive device a tool than helps with the performance of a task

asthma a chronic, but reversible, inflammation of the airways that causes episodes of wheezing (especially when exhaling), coughing, chest tightness, and shortness of breath

asylum seeker an involuntary migrant who asks for protection from a host country after arriving in that country rather than waiting for a refugee application to be processed prior to traveling

atherosclerosis the thickening and hardening of the walls of the arteries that carry oxygen-rich blood from the heart to the rest of the body

atrial fibrillation an arrhythmia in which the atria (the upper chambers of the heart) quiver fast and irregularly rather than contracting and relaxing at a regular beat

autism a lifelong neurodevelopmental disorder that begins in early childhood and causes challenges with social communication and other functions

autoimmune disorder a disease that occurs when the body has difficulty distinguishing between "self" and "non-self" and begins to attack its own cells

autosomal gene a gene that is not located on the sex chromosome and is therefore not sex-linked

bacterium a microscopic single-celled prokary-otic organism

BCG (Bacillus Calmette-Guérin) a tuberculosis vaccine that is used in many countries to confer some protection against TB disease in children

behavior change the process of adopting healthier habits and maintaining those new practices

behavioral risk factor a behavior that can be adopted, stopped, or changed in order to reduce the risk of disease

benign a tumor that is not composed of cancer cells

benign prostatic hyperplasia (BPH) an enlargement of the prostate gland that may cause difficulty with urination and with sexual performance

beriberi thiamine deficiency that causes weakness and heart arrhythmias

bilateral aid money given from the government of a higher-income country to the government of a lower-income country

Bill & Melinda Gates Foundation the largest private foundation in the world

binge-eating disorder an eating disorder characterized by repeated incidents of consuming large quantities of food without subsequent purging

bioavailability the proportion of the nutrient consumed that is able to be absorbed and used by the body

biodiversity the presence of a wide variety of plant and animal species within a particular environment

biomass fuel from organic materials like wood, vegetation, or animal waste

biopsy a small sample of cells or tissues collected through an incision or with a needle so that the specimen can be examined for the presence or absence of cancer

biostatistics the science of analyzing health data and interpreting the results so that they can be applied to solving public health problems

bioterrorism the deliberate release of pathogens, chemicals, or other agents that can cause illness and possibly death of people, animals, or plants

bipolar disorder a depressive disorder characterized by alternating periods of depression and mania or hypomania

birth asphyxia a birth complication that occurs when a newborn fails to take a first breath immediately after delivery and is therefore deprived of oxygen

birth rate the annual number of births in a population per 1000 total people in that population (or other units)

birth spacing waiting until at least two years after the birth of one child before conceiving the next child

bladder cancer cancer of the urinary bladder

blindness having no light perception or vision that even with corrective lenses is no better than 20/400 in the best eye

body mass index (BMI) a measure of body composition calculated by taking weight in kilograms and dividing it by the square of the height in meters

brain drain the migration of healthcare professionals trained in low- and middle-income countries to higher paying jobs in high-income countries

breast cancer cancer of the breast in females or males

bronchitis inflammation of the bronchi that is characterized by a productive cough, narrowing of the airways, and excess mucus production

bulimia nervosa an eating disorder characterized by frequent binge-purge cycles

burden of disease the adverse impact of a particular health condition (or group of conditions) on a population

burn an injury to skin or deeper tissues that is caused by contact with fire, boiling water, or other very hot substances or, less often, by radiation, electricity, friction, extreme cold, and some types of chemicals

Buruli ulcer an infection with *Mycobacterium ulcerans* that causes disfiguring lesions

bypass surgery a surgical procedure that uses a healthy blood vessel from another part of the body to restore blood flow to the heart muscle by bypassing the damaged area

cesarean section the surgical delivery of a neonate through an incision in the mother's abdomen and uterus

calcium a mineral used by the body for strengthening bones and teeth in addition to playing critical roles in muscle and nerve function

calorie a unit based on the amount of energy required to raise the temperature of 1 gram of water by 1 degree Celsius

cancer a disease that occurs when abnormal cells begin to reproduce uncontrollably, often invading nearby tissues and then spreading to other parts of the body

candidiasis an overgrowth of the fungus *Candida*

carbohydrate chain of sugars

carcinogen a substance that can cause genetic mutations that lead to cancer

carcinoma a cancer that forms in epithelial tissues that line the inside or outside of the body

cardiomyopathy a disease of the heart muscles that causes the heart to enlarge and become weaker

cardiovascular disease (CVD) a disorder of the heart or blood vessels

caries holes (cavities) in the teeth that are created by demineralization and decay

carrier a person with a persistent contagious infection who does not have symptoms of the disease but can pass the infectious agent on to others

carrying capacity the maximum human population the Earth can sustain

case detection rate (CDR) the proportion of people with a disease who are diagnosed as having that disease

case fatality rate (CFR) the percentage of people with a disease who die from that disease

cataracts clouding of the lenses of the eye that makes vision fuzzy

catastrophe a critical incident that overwhelms the local humanitarian response network and requires extensive outside assistance

causal factor an exposure that has been scientifically tested and shown to occur before the disease outcome and to contribute directly to its occurrence

CD4 cells lymphocytes that have a CD4 glycoprotein on their surfaces

Centers for Disease Control and Prevention (CDC) the lead health protection agency in the United States, which responds to outbreaks and other public health emergencies as one of its many functions

cerebral malaria malaria infections that cause seizures and coma

cerebral palsy a neuromuscular disorder that may result from birth trauma and is characterized by permanent difficulties with movement, balance, and posture

cervical cancer cancer of the uterine cervix

cestode a tapeworm consisting of a mouthpiece (scolex) and numerous segments

Chagas disease an infection with *Trypanosoma cruzi* parasites that is spread by "kissing bugs" in parts of the Americas and can cause chronic damage to the heart and digestive tract

chemotherapy the treatment of disease using chemical substances

chikungunya a mosquito-borne viral infection that can cause chronic arthritis

child labor a violation of child rights that occurs when a child has an excessive workload, unsafe work conditions, or extreme work intensity that may harm the child's physical health, mental health, or moral development

child sponsorship a charitable donation model in which a donor selects a child to sponsor and then receives regular updates about that particular child in exchange for continued monthly contributions to the host organization

chlamydia a sexually transmitted infection caused by *Chlamydia trachomatis*

cholera an infection with *Vibrio cholerae* bacteria that causes large volumes of severe watery diarrhea to be secreted into the small intestine

cholesterol a waxy lipid (fat) that is a major component of the plaque that causes atherosclerosis

chronic kidney disease (CKD) a progressive loss of kidney function characterized by a reduced glomerular filtration rate (GFR) and increased urinary albumin levels

chronic obstructive pulmonary disease (COPD) a chronic, progressive disease that limits airflow and causes shortness of breath and productive coughing

chronic respiratory diseases (CRDs) long-term noncommunicable diseases of the airway, bronchi, and lungs

circumcision the surgical removal of the foreskin of the penis

cirrhosis irreversible scarring of the liver that impedes the flow of blood through the liver and prevents the liver from functioning normally

cisgender a person with a gender identity that aligns with the sex assigned to that person at birth

climate change a long-term shift in weather patterns and average temperatures

clinical trial a research study that evaluates the safety and effectiveness of a health intervention

Codex Alimentarius international food standards compiled by scientific panels hosted by the United Nations

cognitive behavioral therapy (CBT) a form of talk therapy in which a therapist helps an individual understand his or her thoughts, feelings, and behaviors and identify actions that can be taken to correct problems

co-insurance a percentage of the costs of healthcare services that is paid out-of-pocket by an insured patient

collective violence violence perpetrated by members of a group as part of a shared plan to accomplish a political, social, or economic goal

colorectal cancer cancer in the end of the large intestine or in the rectum

colostrum the milk produced in the first days after giving birth

community development a process through which community members identify their own development priorities and take action to achieve them

community-led total sanitation (CLTS) programs implemented to encourage toilet use in places where residents are accustomed to open defecation and have not yet adopted new sanitation behaviors

complementary foods foods introduced into an infant's diet while continuing to breastfeed the infant

complementary proteins protein-containing foods that do not contain all the essential amino acids alone, but do contain all of the essential amino acids when consumed together

complete protein a protein that contains all of the essential amino acids

complex humanitarian emergency a situation that occurs when civil conflict or war causes mass migration of civilian populations, food insecurity, and long-term public health concerns

condom a physical barrier used to prevent sperm from coming into contact with an egg after sexual contact

contact tracing the process of identifying the primary contacts of infected individuals as well as, perhaps, the contacts of those primary contacts, so that they can be tested and monitored

continued feeding the process of encouraging children with diarrhea to eat the same foods that they normally consume and continuing to breastfeed infants and young children with diarrhea as usual during their illness

contraception the intentional prevention of pregnancy

contraindication a condition that makes it unsafe for an individual to receive a particular vaccine, medication, device, procedure, or other medical intervention

control the process of using public health interventions to reduce the incidence or prevalence of a condition to a substantially lower level within a community or a larger geopolitical area

copay a fixed fee that is paid out-of-pocket by an insured patient when receiving routine health services

coronary artery disease (CAD) a condition that occurs when atherosclerosis of the arteries that provide blood to the heart reduces blood flow to the heart muscle

corporate social responsibility (CSR) the positive social and environmental actions a company voluntarily supports

corruption politically powerful people abusing their positions for personal gain

cost-effectiveness analysis (CEA) an economic analysis that compares the health gains from an intervention to the financial costs of that intervention

counterfeit an illegal product that is marketed deceptively

cretinism brain damage and stunted growth caused by a lack of maternal iodine during fetal development

crisis a critical incident that can easily be addressed with local humanitarian resources

cryptosporidiosis a waterborne protozoal disease caused by species of *Cryptosporidium*

cultural competency the ability to communicate effectively with people from different cultures and backgrounds

culture a way of living, believing, behaving, communicating, and understanding the world that is shared by members of a social unit

cycle of infection a description of how an infectious agent passes between different species

cysticercosis the disease caused by *Taenia solium* tapeworms forming cysts in muscle tissue or other parts of the body

DDT (dichloro-diphenyl-trichloroethane) a long-lasting insecticide that is used for indoor residual spraying as part of malaria control programs

death rate the annual number of all-cause or cause-specific deaths per 1000 people in a population (or other units)

deductible the amount that an insured person must spend out-of-pocket on health care each year (in addition to premiums) before the insurance company begins paying for health services

DEET (*N,N*-diethyl-*m*-toluamide) a chemical that is an effective insect repellent

default rate the proportion of people who are diagnosed with an infectious disease and begin treatment but do not complete the full course of treatment

definitive host the animal host in which a parasite reaches sexual maturity and reproduces

dehydration the excessive loss of water from the body

deliverable a product, service, or other result of a project

delusion false beliefs that are irrational but seem very real to the person experiencing them

dementia a chronic syndrome characterized by memory loss, confusion, and other signs of impaired cognitive function

demographic transition the changes in population composition that accompany the shift toward lower birth and death rates that often occurs as populations move from being lower-income economies toward being middle-income and then higher-income economies

demography the study of the size and composition of human populations

dengue a mosquito-borne viral infection that causes severe pain and a risk of hemorrhagic fever

dependency ratio the number of dependent children and older people for every person of working age (often defined as people aged 15–64 years)

depressive disorder a mental health disorder characterized by sadness, hopelessness, loss of interest in usual activities, fatigue, poor concentration, and other negative thoughts, feelings, and physical symptoms that interfere with normal daily activities

development a long-term process of improving the socioeconomic and environmental conditions that are associated with reduced population health status

development assistance for health (DAH) official development assistance designated for health activities

diagnostic accuracy the proportion of people who receive a test who are true positives or true negatives

dialysis the process of using a machine to filter the blood

diarrhea loose or liquid feces and an increased frequency of defecation

diastolic blood pressure the pressure in the blood vessels when the heart is at rest in between beats

diphtheria a vaccine-preventable bacterial infection that can cause fatal airway obstruction

diplomacy the process of negotiating agreements between countries, resolving disputes without conflict, and navigating other aspects of international relations

disability a restriction in activity and participation that results from an impairment and a social and environmental context

disability-adjusted life year (DALY) a quantitative estimate of the total burden of disease in a population from both premature deaths (YLLs) and disability (YLDs)

disaster a critical incident in which the need for assistance exceeds local humanitarian capacity

discrimination actions taken against an individual because of that person's membership in a sociocultural group

disease the presence of symptoms or illness

distributive justice the ethical principle that needed resources in a population should be fairly allocated

Doctors Without Borders the name used in the United States for the international humanitarian organization Médecins Sans Frontières (MSF)

dominant an allele that a person will be expressed if it is inherited from one or both parents

DOTS (directly observed therapy, short-course) the protocol recommended by the World Health Organization for treatment of tuberculosis

dracunculiasis the disease caused by meter-long *Dracunculus medinesis* worms slowly evacuating themselves from the human body over several weeks

drowning the process of experiencing respiratory impairment due to being submerged or immersed in water or another liquid

dysentery bloody diarrhea

early breastfeeding breastfeeding within the first hours after giving birth

early childhood development (ECD) the physical, cognitive, emotional, and social development that occurs during the 1000 days from conception through the second birthday

Ebola a viral hemorrhagic fever transmitted via contact with the body fluids of infected individuals

echinococcocis the disease caused by human infestation by the tapeworm *Echinocococcus granulosus*

ecological footprint a measure of how much burden human consumption places on the biosphere

ecotoxicology the study of the impact of toxic exposures on populations, communities, and ecosystems

ectopic pregnancy a medical emergency caused by a fertilized egg implanting in the fallopian tubes or another location outside the uterus

edema fluid retention in extracellular spaces that causes swelling of the tissues in the arms, legs, and face

edentulism the loss of most or all of one's teeth

effectiveness a measure of the success of an intervention under real-world conditions

efficiency an evaluation of the cost-effectiveness of an intervention that is based on both its effectiveness and resource considerations

elderly support ratio the number of people aged 65 years and older for every person aged 15–64 years in a population

elephantiasis chronic lymphedema that causes the skin of an affected limb to thicken and develop a coarse texture

elimination the process of using public health interventions to remove an infectious disease from a community or a larger geopolitical area

emergency a critical incident that stresses local humanitarian resources but can still be managed locally

emergency management the process of overseeing all resources and responsibilities related to emergencies and disasters, including prevention, preparedness, response, and recovery

emergency obstetric and newborn care (EmONC) a core set of actions that can save the lives of women and neonates during the perinatal period

emerging infectious disease (EID) diseases caused by a new pathogen beginning to affect human populations or an existing pathogen changing the kind of disease it causes

emphysema a disease that occurs when the alveoli (the tiny air sacs in the lungs) lose elasticity and become distended or destroyed

encephalitis an acute inflammation of the brain

endemic an adverse health condition that is always present in a particular population

endometriosis a condition in which some of the tissue that lines the uterus is located on the ovaries or in other parts of the abdominal cavity

endowment a large donation made to a nonprofit organization so that the funds can be invested and the interest from the investment can be used to support the operation of the charity

enrichment the process of adding nutrients lost during handling, processing, or storage back to food products

enteric infections of the intestinal tract

environmental health the study of the connections between human health and environmental exposures, such as air quality, water quality, and waste

epidemic an epidemiological event characterized by a disease occurring more often than usual and causing more than a few sporadic occurrences of disease

epidemiologic transition (epidemiological transition) the health transition characterized by a shift from infectious diseases to chronic non-communicable diseases being the primary cause of deaths and disability in a population

epidemiology the study of the distribution of health problems in populations, the risk factors for developing those conditions, and the effectiveness of interventions to address concerns

epigenetics the differential expression of genetic code through activation or inactivation of genes

epilepsy a chronic seizure disorder characterized by episodes of excessive and abnormal electrical activity in the brain

eradication the process of using public health interventions to eliminate an infectious disease globally, so that there is no risk of natural infection or disease anywhere in the world

esophageal cancer cancer of the esophagus

essential amino acid an amino acid that cannot be produced by the human body and must be acquired from food

essential medication a drug that has been identified as a high priority for a country's health system to have in stock at all times because it is a cost-effective treatment for a common health issue

Essential Support Functions (ESF) critical service areas that require immediate attention after a disaster

ethnicity social groupings based on many dimensions of cultural heritage, nationality, language, religion, tribal affiliation, and other factors

etiology the study of the causes of disease

evaluation an assessment of how well a project, program, or policy has met its goals

exclusive breastfeeding breastmilk is the only substance the baby consumes

Expanded Program on Immunization (EPI) a program started in 1974 by WHO to expand the number and types of vaccines routinely given to children

expatriate a person who is temporarily living in another country and intends to return to his or her home country

extinction the process of destroying all laboratory specimens of an eradicated pathogen, so that there is no possibility of the pathogen reentering the human population

extreme poverty surviving on less income than an international poverty line, typically set at an income of less than \$1 or \$2 per person per day

faith-based organization (FBO) a nongovernmental organization sponsored by a religious or religiously affiliated entity

falciparum malaria an infection with *Plasmodium falciparum*, the species of *Plasmodium* that typically causes the most severe symptoms

fall an event that causes a person to land on the ground or floor

family planning a process by which women and men make informed decisions about how many children they want to have, how many years apart they want those pregnancies to be, and the actions they will take to achieve these goals

famine widespread hunger occurring when a large proportion of a population has very low food security for an extended period of time

fat a lipid of animal origin like butter or lard that is solid at room temperature

fat-soluble vitamin a vitamin that is able to be stored in body tissues

fecal-oral transmission ingestion by a person of products contaminated with fecal matter from animals or humans

female genital mutilation (FGM) the partial or complete removal of the external female genitalia of an infant or child

fertility a woman's total number of births, including live births and stillbirths

fertility rate the average number of children a woman gives birth to during her childbearing years

fertility transition the health transition characterized by a reduction in the average number of offspring the typical female gives birth to

fiber a nondigestible complex carbohydrate found in unprocessed plant-based foods

fibroids benign tumors in the uterus that can cause heavy bleeding and pelvic pain

financing the provision of money for a particular activity and the management of that investment

fluoride a mineral that is essential for the development of strong teeth and bones

folate a B vitamin that is critical for growth, red blood cell production, and fetal development

folic acid a synthetic form of folate that can be added to foods or supplements

fomite an inanimate object or surface that has been contaminated with infectious agents

food intoxication illness caused when ingested bacteria produce toxins in the body

food security security that exists when members of a household or community reliably have access to enough food to be healthy, active, and productive

food system the entire process of growing or producing food, processing and packaging food, distributing and selling food (which may require transportation and storage), and preparing and consuming food

foreign direct investment (FDI) a business investment made by a corporation or an individual in another country

foreign policy the strategies and approaches a country uses to engage with other nations while protecting its own interests

fortification the process of adding micronutrients not naturally present in a food's ingredients to a food product

foundation a charitable trust that gives grants to other nonprofit organizations

Framework Convention on Climate Change (FCCC) an international environmental treaty that seeks to reduce greenhouse gas emissions

Framework Convention on Tobacco Control (FCTC) the world's first global health treaty negotiated through the World Health Organization (WHO), which aims to significantly reduce the global prevalence of tobacco use

functional literacy the ability to understand written words well enough to complete normal daily tasks

fungus a eukaryotic organism, such as mold or yeast

Gavi a global partnership formerly known as the Global Alliance for Vaccines and Immunization that works with lower-income countries to identify vaccine priorities and then procure and distribute the vaccines

gender social, cultural, and psychological aspects of being male or female

gender identity an individual's sense of maleness or femaleness

gender roles how a culture believes men and women should behave

gender-based violence physical, emotional, and sexual abuse inflicted on an individual because of that individual's gender

generalized anxiety disorder an anxiety disorder characterized by persistent excessive worrying about numerous concerns

generic drug a medicine with the same active ingredient as a brand-name drug that usually costs less than the brand-name version

genetics the study of genes, genetic variation, and heredity, the passing of genes from parents to their biological offspring

genotype the set of alleles a person inherits for a particular gene

gestational diabetes elevated blood sugar that is first diagnosed during pregnancy and typically resolves after delivery

giardiasis a waterborne protozoal disease caused by species of *Giardia* that can cause persistent diarrhea

Gini Index a measure of the inequality in the distribution of incomes within a particular country

glaucoma elevated pressure within the eyeball that causes loss of peripheral vision

Global Burden of Disease (GBD) a massive collaborative effort to quantify the epidemiologic profiles of every country in the world that was initiated by the World Health Organization in the 1990s and is now housed at the Institute for Health Metrics and Evaluation (IHME) in Seattle

Global Fund (The Global Fund to Fight AIDS, Tuberculosis and Malaria) a large global health partnership founded in 2002 that uses funds from the governments of high-income countries and other partner organizations to support infectious disease control initiatives in low- and middle-income countries

global health collaborative actions taken to identify and address transnational concerns about the exposures and diseases that adversely affect human populations

global health security public health interventions implemented by governmental and military personnel and other stakeholders to protect populations from threats to health and safety

Global Hunger Index (GHI) a metric that combines statistics about nutrition in under-5 children and the total population to evaluate population malnutrition

global warming a gradual increase in the temperature of Earth's atmosphere

globalization the process of countries around the world becoming more integrated and interdependent across economic, political, cultural, and other domains

GOBI an initiative started in the 1980s by UNICEF that focused on increasing child survival by promoting growth monitoring, oral rehydration therapy for diarrhea, breastfeeding, and immunization

goiter a swollen neck resulting from an enlarged thyroid gland

gonorrhea a sexually transmitted infection caused by *Neisseria gonorrhoeae*

gout a painful swelling of a joint, usually the joint at the base of the big toe, due to elevated levels of uric acid in the blood

governance the processes and structures that enable governments to set policies, provide services, and protect human rights

grant a gift of money that does not have to be repaid

gravidity a woman's total number of pregnancies

greenhouse gas a gas in the atmosphere that traps heat and causes surface temperatures to increase

gross domestic product (GDP) the total amount of goods and services produced in one country by domestic- and foreign-owned companies

gross national income (GNI) the total income from the selling of goods and services produced in one country, including consumer spending, government spending, investments, and exports

gross national product (GNP) the total amount of goods and services produced by one country's companies in that country and by companies owned by that country but operating in other countries

guinea worm disease the disease caused by meter-long *Dracunculus medinesis* worms slowly evacuating themselves from the human body over several weeks

hallucination sensory distortions that cause the affected person to hear, see, feel, smell, or taste something that is not present

health a state of complete physical, mental, and social well-being, and not merely the absence of disease or infirmity

health belief model the theory that individual behavior change is a function of personal perceptions of the severity of the disease, beliefs about personal susceptibility to the disease, and beliefs about the likely benefits from adopting healthier behaviors as well as perceptions about the barriers to action and the self-efficacy to enact change

health diplomacy the use of health projects as part of meeting foreign policy goals

health disparity an avoidable difference in health status between population groups

health information system (HIS) a system that collects, analyzes, and disseminates information about health systems performance

health literacy the ability to access, understand, and apply health information

health promotion an applied social science that encourages individuals and communities to take steps to improve their own health

health system the people, facilities, products, resources, and organizational structures that deliver health services to a population

health transition a shift in the health status of a population that usually occurs in conjunction with socioeconomic development

healthcare-associated infection (HAI) an infection that is contracted while receiving care in a hospital, nursing or rehabilitation center, or other medical facility

healthy life expectancy (HALE) the median number of additional years an individual in a population can expect to live without disability

heart failure a chronic condition in which the heart is not able to pump enough blood to meet the body's need for oxygen

helminth an endoparasitic worm that lives inside the body of its host

hemoglobin a molecule made from iron that holds the oxygen inside red blood cells

hemorrhagic stroke a stroke that occurs when a blood vessel ruptures and causes bleeding in the brain

hepatitis inflammation of the liver

hepatitis A a vaccine-preventable viral infection spread through contaminated food and water that can cause weeks of severe illness associated with liver inflammation

hepatitis B a vaccine-preventable viral infection spread through blood and other body fluids that can cause chronic liver disease

hepatitis C a viral infection spread through injecting drug use and other routes that can cause chronic liver disease

hepatitis E a viral infection spread through contaminated water that can cause acute liver failure in pregnant women

herd immunity a theory that says that reducing the proportion of a population that is susceptible to an infection protects the whole population

herpes an infection caused by a herpesvirus

Hib (*Haemophilus influenzae* type B) a bacterial infection with *Haemophilus influenzae* type b (Hib) that can cause severe pneumonia

highly active antiretroviral therapy (HAART) combinations of three or more different types of drugs that are taken together to combat HIV

highly pathogenic avian influenza (HPAI) a strain of influenza that causes serious disease and high case fatality rates in affected birds

high-risk screening screening that targets people who are known to have an elevated risk of a disease

HIV human immunodeficiency virus (HIV)

hookworm an intestinal worm infection that is acquired by walking barefooted through contaminated soil and can lead to anemia

horizontal program a program that strengthens an existing health system so that it can deliver additional health services

household air pollution the presence of harmful chemicals or other substances in indoor air at concentrations above the thresholds established for human safety

Human Development Index (HDI) an estimate of national development based on composite data on longevity, education, and income

human papillomavirus (HPV) a virus that causes a large proportion of cervical cancer cases

human rights entitlements that are due to every person simply because that person is human

human security freedom from fear and want

hydatid cyst disease a life-threatening condition that occurs when tapeworm larvae cause large cysts in the human liver and lungs

hydrocele lymphedema of the scrotum

hygiene the practice of maintaining cleanliness in order to prevent disease

hyperemesis gravidarum severe nausea and vomiting during early pregnancy that causes dehydration and significant weight loss

hypertension high blood pressure, typically defined as having a systolic blood pressure of 140 mm Hg or higher or a diastolic blood pressure of 90 or higher

hypoxia an inadequate supply of oxygen in body tissues

illness how a person perceives his or her own experience of having an adverse health condition

immigrant a person who has settled in a new country and intends to stay there permanently

immunization the process of a person's immune system developing immunity against a particular infection

impairment a difference or limitation in an anatomical structure, mental or sensory function, or physiological function that constrains the capacity of an individual to do a task or action

in vitro fertilization a type of assistant reproductive technology in which a woman's eggs are extracted from her ovaries, fertilized with sperm in a laboratory setting, and then the resulting embryos are transferred to the uterus

inactivated vaccine a vaccine that contains a killed bacterium or an inactive virus that has been rendered harmless by heat, chemicals, or radiation

incidence the number of new cases of a disease occurring in a population during a time period divided by the total number of people at risk for that disease in that time period

Incident Command System (ICS) an organizational structure used in the United States to provide a clear chain of command for people who respond to an emergency

income the amount of take-home pay earned by household members in a time period

indigenous population population groups that have maintained unique cultural traditions for many generations after the colonization or domination of their traditional homeland by another group

indoor air pollution the presence of harmful chemicals or other substances in household air at concentrations above the thresholds established for human safety

indoor residual spraying (IRS) the application of long-lasting insecticides to walls and other surfaces where mosquitoes might rest, so that mosquitoes that land on those surfaces during the following 6 months or longer will absorb a lethal dose of the insecticidal chemical

induced abortion a chemically or surgically terminated pregnancy

industrial hygiene the process of assessing and mitigating workplace hazards

inequality an avoidable difference in health status between population groups

inequity a health inequality is considered to be unfair and unjust

infant a baby between birth and the first birthday

infant mortality rate (IMR) the number of infants who die before their first birthdays per 1000 live births

infection an infectious agent reproducing inside a person

infectivity the capacity of an infectious agent to cause infection in a susceptible host exposed to the agent

infertility the inability to become pregnant when sexually active and not using contraception or the inability to maintain a pregnancy through to a live birth

influenza a highly contagious respiratory viral infection

influenza-like illness (ILI) that status assigned to people with suspected influenza who have not tested positive for the virus

injecting drug user (IDU) a person who injects illicit drugs for nonmedical use

injury physical damage to the body inflicted by an external force

insecticide-treated net (ITN) a mesh sheet dipped in insecticides and then hung over a bed so that it provides a barrier between sleeping humans and mosquitoes while also killing any mosquitoes that land on it

instrumental activities of daily living (IADLs) the functions required for independent living

insulin a hormone produced by the pancreas that helps the body to maintain a relatively constant level of glucose (sugar) in the bloodstream so that cells have a relatively constant supply of energy

insurance a risk management strategy that protects purchasers against major financial losses

Integrated Community Case Management (iCCM) a strategy that provides community health workers with algorithms for treating uncomplicated childhood infections in homes

Integrated Management of Childhood Illness (IMCI) a package of cost-effective home, community, and clinical interventions for major childhood illnesses and undernutrition that was first developed by UNICEF and WHO in 1995

intentional injury purposefully inflicted physical trauma

Intergovernmental Panel on Climate Change (IPCC) a scientific board that reviews and synthesizes scientific data about climate and weather under the auspices of the United Nations

intermediate host an animal host in which an immature parasite, a larva, develops but does not reach sexual maturity

intermittent preventive treatment (IPT) the use of preventive chemotherapy with anti-malarial medications in vulnerable people so that they maintain therapeutic drug levels in their blood during times of high risk for malaria

internally displaced person (IDP) a person who fled his or her home community because of civil war, famine, natural disaster, or another crisis, but did not cross into another country

International Code of Marketing of Breast-milk Substitutes an international agreement that prevents problematic marketing of infant formula

international cooperation financial assistance, technical support, capacity building, and other development actions implemented by a donor country in a recipient country as part of a foreign policy strategy

international health initiatives targeted toward addressing poverty-related health conditions in lower-income areas

International Health Regulations (IHR) a global health security agreement between all of the members of the United Nations that mandates reporting of outbreaks of infectious diseases of potential international concern and strengthening of public health surveillance systems

International Monetary Fund (IMF) a multi-lateral organization that provides a structure for international monetary policy and makes loans to countries that would otherwise not be able to make payments on their other international loans

international NGO (INGO) a nongovernmental organization with a diverse portfolio of projects implemented in numerous countries

interpersonal violence violence that occurs when one person threatens to harm or actually harms another individual through power and control

interprofessionalism the ability to work and communicate well with colleagues in different practice areas in order to achieve a shared goal

intervention a strategic action intended to improve individual and population health status

intimate partner violence (IPV) physical or sexual violence by a current or former spouse or partner

intrauterine device (IUD) a device that prevents fertilization of eggs by creating a uterine environment that is unfavorable to sperm

iodine an element that is critical for regulating metabolism

iodine deficiency disorders (IDD) impaired cognitive function caused by iodine deficiency

IPT in pregnancy (IPTp) the use of preventive chemotherapy with anti-malarial medications in pregnant women so that they maintain therapeutic drug levels in their blood

iron a mineral the body uses to make the red blood cells that carry oxygen from the lungs to the rest of the cells in the body

iron deficiency anemia (IDA) anemia resulting from inadequate iron intake

ischemia reduced blood supply

ischemic heart disease (IHD) a condition that occurs when atherosclerosis of the arteries that provide blood to the heart reduces blood flow to the heart muscle

ischemic stroke a stroke that occurs when a blocked blood vessel cuts off blood flow to a portion of the brain

isolation the separation of people who have tested positive for a contagious infection from healthy people who are susceptible to the infection

Japanese encephalitis a vaccine-preventable mosquito-borne viral infection that causes outbreaks of encephalitis in Asia and Oceania

jaundice a yellowing of the skin and sclera (the whites of the eyes) due to the build-up of bilirubin levels in the blood

KAP (knowledge, attitudes, and practices) a model that emphasizes the importance of health education for promoting behavior change

kidney cancer cancer in a kidney

kwashiorkor a condition in which a child develops edema and has poor growth as a result of insufficient protein in the diet

landmine a buried explosive device

latent TB infection (LTBI) a latent phase of tuberculosis infection when the bacterium is present within the host but the infected individual does not feel sick and is not contagious

leishmaniasis an infection with protozoa from various species of the *Leishmania* genus that can cause disfigurement and death

leprosy a chronic infection with *Mycobacterium leprae* that causes skin lesions and nerve damage and is more formally known as Hansen's disease

leukemia a blood cancer that begins in the bone marrow where blood is produced by the body

liberal arts the humanities, social sciences, and sciences

life expectancy the median expected age at death among people of a particular age in a population

lifestyle diseases noncommunicable diseases that are associated with health-related behaviors, such as unhealthy diets, sedentariness, tobacco use, and heavy alcohol consumption

lipid a fatty acid, which is a carbohydrate chain with other chemical groups at the ends of the chain

literacy the ability to read and write and apply those communication skills

live attenuated vaccine a vaccine that contains a pathogen that has been weakened with various laboratory techniques

liver cancer cancer of the liver

loan borrowed money that must be repaid with interest

logistics the process of coordinating complex operations, especially the movement of supplies and equipment

long-lasting insecticidal net (LLIN) an insecticide-treated net that has been impregnated with a pesticide that remains effective for 2 years or longer before requiring retreatment

low-and middle-income countries (LMICs) countries that are not high-income countries

low birthweight (LBW) a birthweight of less than 5.5 pounds (2500 grams)

low vision not being able to see better than 20/60 in the best eye even when using glasses or corrective lenses

lower respiratory infection (LRI) an acute respiratory infection of the bronchi and lungs, such as infectious bronchitis and pneumonia

lung cancer the most common cause of cancer death worldwide

lupus an autoimmune disorder most recognized by the butterfly rash that it causes on the face, but which also causes swollen joints and adversely affects numerous other body systems

lymphatic filariasis a mosquito-borne helminth infection that can cause elephantiasis

lymphedema the swelling (edema) of body parts due to retained lymph fluid in the tissues

lymphoma an immune system cancer that starts in the lymph nodes and is associated with some types of chronic infections

macronutrient nutrients such as carbohydrates, protein, and fats and oils that are required to be consumed in relatively large quantities because they provide energy

macular degeneration loss of central vision that occurs when a portion of the retina deteriorates

malaria a parasitic infection with protozoa from the *Plasmodium* species

malarial anemia the destruction of so many red blood cells by malaria-causing parasites that the body cannot adequately transport oxygen through the bloodstream

malignant a tumor that is composed of cancer cells

mammography an X-ray of the breast

marasmus a condition in which a child becomes emaciated, weak, and lethargic because of long-term calorie deprivation

mass drug administration (MDA) the distribution of safe medications to large population groups at regular time intervals as part of strategies for preventing and controlling infectious diseases

maternal and child health (MCH) programs that promote health for pregnant women, newborns, infants, children, and adolescents

maternal mortality death of women from pregnancy-related causes during pregnancy, childbirth, or the six weeks after delivery

maternal mortality rate (MMR) the number of women who die of pregnancy-related causes per 100,000 live births

MDR-TB a multidrug-resistant tuberculosis strain that does not respond to two of standard antibiotic therapies, rifampicin and isoniazid

measles a very contagious vaccine-preventable viral infection that causes red spots all over the body and can be fatal

Médecins Sans Frontières (MSF) a private humanitarian organization that provides medical care to people harmed by violence and advocates for human rights

Medicaid a federal program in the United States that provides funding to states to support state-sponsored health coverage for very low-income citizens

medical anthropology an area within anthropology that seeks to understand the diversity of global perspectives on health, disease, illness, sickness, medicine, and healing

Medicare the federal health funding system in the United States that provides coverage for people aged 65 years and older as well as some younger people with serious permanent disabilities

medicine the practice of preventing, diagnosing, and treating health problems in individuals and families

megacity a metropolitan area with 10 million or more inhabitants

melanoma cancer that originates in pigmented melanocytes in the skin

meningitis an inflammation of the meninges, the membranes that cover the brain and spinal cord

meningococcus meningitis caused by infection with the bacterium *Neisseria meningitidis*

metabolism the rate at which a person's body uses energy

metastasis a secondary cancerous tumor at a new site

miasma foul-smelling gases produced by poorly managed waste that were thought to cause disease prior to the discovery of germs

microcephaly an abnormally small head that is a sign of aberrant brain development

micronutrient a nutrient that the body requires in small amounts, such as a vitamin or mineral

mid upper arm circumference (MUAC) a measure of arm circumference-for-age that is used as an indicator of wasting in a child

migraine a recurrent severe headache that is often accompanied by nausea, vomiting, and sensitivity to light and sound

migrant a person who has moved across an international border and has taken up residence in the new country

Millennium Development Goals (MDGs) a set of eight goals established by the member countries of the United Nations that aimed to significantly reduce global poverty by 2015

mineral inorganic chemical elements

Ministry of Health the term used in most countries to describe the lead governmental health agency

miscarriage the spontaneous loss of a pregnancy prior to the fetal age of viability

mitigation the process of implementing preemptive measures to protect people and property from hazards

modifiable risk factor a risk factor for a disease that can be avoided or mitigated

monitoring ongoing assessment of a project or program to track progress toward achieving predefined targets

monitoring and evaluation (M&E) the systematic collection of information about an ongoing intervention (process evaluation) and the determination of whether the intervention achieved its objectives (impact evaluation)

monogenic disorder a genetic disorder that results from a child inheriting a single disease-causing gene from one or both parents

morbidity the presence of illness or disease

mortality death

mortality rate the annual number of all-cause or cause-specific deaths per 1000 people in a population (or other units)

mortality transition the health transition characterized by decreases in the rates of death for age groups across the life span

mother-to-child transmission (MTCT) transmission of a pathogen from an infected pregnant woman to her offspring during pregnancy, delivery, or breastfeeding

MRSA methicillin-resistant *Staphylococcus aureus*

MSM a classification that encompasses all men who have sex with men and emphasizes sexual behavior rather than sexual identity

multicausal a causal pathway in which many different risk factors contribute to a disease occurring

multidisciplinary an adjective used to describe activities that bring together people from diverse areas of academic study to work on a shared task

multilateral aid funding pooled from many donor countries

multiple sclerosis a chronic, progressive disease that causes inflammatory demyelination of the sheaths of nerve cells in the central nervous system

mumps a vaccine-preventable viral infection that causes swollen cheeks and can lead to infertility in males

mutation a permanent change in the sequence of bases that make up DNA that occurs after birth in response to exposure to radiation, chemicals, pollutants, or other substances

mycetoma a chronic granulomatous inflammatory disease of the subcutaneous tissue of the foot

myocardial infarction (MI) the death of a portion of the heart muscle due to lack of oxygen that occurs when a coronary blood vessel becomes mostly or fully occluded

National Incidence Management System (NIMS) an emergency response framework in the

United States that specifies how different governmental agencies and nongovernmental organizations work together to respond to a disaster

National Institutes of Health (NIH) the lead health research agency within the U.S. Department of Health and Human Services

natural history of disease the usual time line from initial infection with a particular agent to either recovery or death

negative predictive value (NPV) the proportion of people who test negative for a disease who truly do not have disease

neglected tropical diseases (NTDs) infectious diseases that primarily affect the poorest regions of the world and have not historically been a priority for funding agencies, pharmaceutical companies, or global policymakers

nematode a cylindrically shaped roundworm

neonatal mortality rate (NMR) the number of deaths of neonates per 1000 live births

neonate a newborn within his or her first 28 days (4 weeks) after birth

neoplasm a synonym for cancer that is derived from words meaning "new formation"

neurocognitive disorders neurological and cognitive disorders (such as dementia) that typically develop in older adulthood

neurocysticercosis the disease caused by *Taenia solium* tapeworms invading the human nervous system and causing seizures

neurodevelopmental disorders neurological and development disorders that present in childhood and require early intervention for the best outcomes

niacin a B vitamin that is necessary for skin health and for digestive and nervous system function

noncommunicable diseases (NCDs) conditions that are not contagious, such as heart disease and other cardiovascular diseases, cancers, chronic respiratory diseases, diabetes, and other chronic diseases

nonderogable right a human right that is irrevocable in all circumstances

nongovernmental organization (NGO) a nonprofit organization that is privately managed and receives at least some of its funding from private sources

nonmodifiable risk factor a risk factor for a disease that cannot be changed through health interventions

nonprofit organization (NPO) a mission-driven group that reinvests surplus revenue in the organization rather than distributing extra income to owners or shareholders

norovirus a calicivirus that is the most common cause of severe diarrhea in adults

nosocomial infection an infection that is contracted while receiving care in a hospital, nursing or rehabilitation center, or other medical facility

nutrition the consumption of foods that allow the body to survive, grow, heal, and be healthy and the processing of those nutrients within the body

nutrition transition the health transition characterized by a shift from having undernutrition and nutrient deficiencies as the most prevalent nutritional concerns to having overweight and obesity as the dominant nutritional disorders

obesity a body mass index of 30 or greater

obsessive-compulsive disorder (OCD) a mental health disorder characterized by anxiety-inducing recurrent thoughts (obsessions) and repetitive behaviors intended to reduce distress or prevent bad events (compulsions)

obstetric fistula a hole between the rectum or bladder and the vagina that is caused by obstructed labor and constantly leaks urine or feces

obstetric transition the health transition characterized by a shift from a high maternal mortality rate to a negligible rate

obstructed labor an obstetric complication that occurs when the unborn baby is wedged so tightly into the birth canal that blood flow to surrounding tissues is cut off and the tissues start to die

occupational health an applied field focused on primary prevention of injuries and other work-related health problems

OECD (Organisation for Economic Co-operation and Development) an intergovernmental organization comprised of about three dozen of the world's richest countries

official development assistance (ODA) money given by the government of a high-income country to the government of a low-income country to support socioeconomic development

OIE (World Organisation for Animal Health) an intergovernmental group that is not part of the UN system but works closely with FAO and WHO to control the spread of zoonotic infectious diseases and to promote food safety

oil a lipid of plant origin like corn oil or olive oil that is liquid at room temperature

onchocerciasis a black fly borne helminth infection, also called river blindness, that can cause permanent vision loss

One Health a concept that emphasizes the interconnectedness of human health, animal health, and ecological health

open defecation free (ODF) a community status that is earned when all members are using designated toilet facilities and no one is defecating outside

opportunistic infection (OI) an infection that occurs when the body's immune system is weakened enough to give the infectious agents an opportunity to invade

oral contraceptives birth control pills that prevent ovulation when taken as prescribed, so no eggs are released from the ovaries and a pregnancy cannot occur

oral rehydration salts (ORS) a mixture of sugar, salt, and clean drinking water that replaces lost fluids and restores the balance of electrolytes in the blood

oral rehydration therapy (ORT) drinking enough water to prevent or treat the dehydration caused by diarrhea

osteoarthritis a degenerative disease that slowly causes loss of cartilage in the joints, causing pain, stiffness, and disability

osteomalacia vitamin D deficiency in adults whose bones have stopped growing that causes the bones to become soft and prone to breaking

osteoporosis a loss of bone density that significant increases the risk of fractures of the hip, vertebrae, and other bones in older adults

Ottawa Charter an international agreement sponsored by the World Health Organization and approved at a conference in Canada in 1986 that identified the core health promotions actions as including healthy public policies, supportive environments, strong communities, skilled personnel, and expanded access to preventive health services

outbreak an epidemiological event characterized by at least several people becoming ill from a disease that is not usually present in a population

outdoor air pollution the presence of harmful chemicals or other substances in ambient air at concentrations above the thresholds established for human safety

out-of-pocket (OOP) payments cash disbursements made by patients and their families in order to receive health services

ovarian cancer cancer of the ovary

overnutrition a form of malnutrition caused by excessive intake of calories and nutrients

overpopulation a situation that occurs when a population becomes so large that the amount of food and other environmental resources is insufficient to support all members of the population

overweight a body mass index (BMI) of 25 to 29.9

oxytocin a hormone that strengthens uterine contractions during labor and delivery and then helps control postpartum bleeding

palliative care pain management in people with serious chronic illnesses

pancreatic cancer cancer of the pancreas

pandemic a worldwide epidemic

panic disorder an anxiety disorder characterized by repeated panic attacks that last for several intense minutes and cause a racing heartbeat, dizziness or weakness, and other disturbing symptoms

parasite a eukaryotic organism that survives by living in or on a host organism

parasitemia having parasites in the blood

parenteral the intake of a substance into the body through a route other than the digestive tract

parity a woman's total number of live births

Parkinson's disease a chronic, progressive neurodegenerative disorder characterized by motor symptoms, such as slowed movement (bradykinesia), rigidity or stiffness in an arm or leg or other body part, and tremors when a limb is resting

particulate matter substances that are small enough to remain suspended in the air for long periods of time and can travel deep into the lungs

partner notification the process of a patient diagnosed with a sexually transmitted infection or a public health official communicating with the sexual partners of the diagnosed individual about their need to be tested so that they can receive appropriate treatment

passive immunity temporary protection against infectious diseases that is conferred by antibodies produced by another human or an animal, such and that confer protection to newborns

passive surveillance the compilation of reports of notifiable disease diagnoses from medical laboratories

pasteurization a process of heating foods to kill the bacteria that might be present

patent the exclusive rights for one company to sell a new product for several years before other companies are allowed to produce and sell the product

pathogenicity the capacity of an infectious agent to cause disease in an infected host

peer review the process of a scientific manuscript being evaluated by experts who scrutinize the methodology and the reasonableness of the results prior to a report being published

pellagra niacin deficiency that is characterized by dark, peeling skin that sloughs off the body

pelvic inflammatory disease (PID) an infection in the female reproductive system that can cause pain and lead to scarring and infertility

PEPFAR the U.S. President's Emergency Plan for AIDS Relief, which provides financing for increasing access to antiretroviral therapy and other HIV prevention and treatment services in low- and middle-income countries

perinatal mortality stillbirths and deaths within the first 7 days (1 week) after a live birth

periodontitis a periodontal disease characterized by chronic inflammation of the gums, a condition called gingivitis

peripheral artery disease (PAD) narrowed blood vessels that impair blood circulation and can cause severe leg pain and cramping when walking

person who injects drugs (PWID) a person who injects illicit drugs for nonmedical use

personal protective equipment (PPE) gowns, gloves, facemasks, eye protection, and other barriers that prevent infection

pertussis a vaccine-preventable infection that causes weeks of whooping cough and other severe respiratory symptoms

phenotype the way a particular set of alleles is expressed in physical appearance

physical inactivity the failure to regularly engage in exercise of moderate or vigorous intensity

placenta the organ, also called the afterbirth, that provides oxygen and nutrients to the fetus during fetal development

placenta previa a pregnancy complication in which the placenta covers part or all of the cervix and causes bleeding

placental abruption a pregnancy complication in which the placenta separates from the uterine wall prior to delivery

plan a document that describes the steps that will be taken to achieve strategic goals and implement approved policies

planetary health a field of study that emphasizes the dependence of human health on the Earth and seeks to understand the damage that human actions can impose on ecosystem health

Plasmodium a protozoan that causes malaria in humans

pneumococcus pneumonia caused by infection with *Streptococcus pneumoniae*

pneumoconiosis a restrictive lung disease caused by exposure to various types of occupational hazards

pneumonia a disease that occurs when part of a lung fills with fluid

policy a set of principles and procedures defined by governments or other groups to guide decision-making and resource allocation

polio a vaccine-preventable viral infection that can cause paralysis

pooled risk the assumption that if many low-risk people and a few high-risk people all pay premiums to an insurance system over many years, then there will be a pot of money that can be used to pay for major expenses when they occur

population pyramid a graphic that displays the number of males and females by age group in a population

population-based screening screening that targets large groups of people

positive predictive value (PPV) the proportion of people who test positive for a disease who truly have disease

post-exposure prophylaxis (PEP) the process of taking medications after exposure to a pathogen in order to reduce the likelihood of contracting an infection

postpartum hemorrhage severe bleeding within several hours after giving birth

posttraumatic stress disorder (PTSD) a mental health disorder that occurs after a traumatic incident leads to nightmares or other types of distressing recollections of the event

power the authority to control or influence the actions of others

precaution a condition that might make a vaccine ineffective at producing immunity or might increase the likelihood of an adverse reaction in a particular individual to a vaccine, medication, device, procedure, or other medical intervention

preeclampsia a combination of worsening hypertension in the final months of pregnancy along with the presence of protein in the urine that, if untreated, can progress to seizures and death

pre-exposure prophylaxis (PrEP) the process of taking medications prior to a likely exposure to a pathogen in order to reduce the likelihood of contracting an infection

prejudice a perception about an individual based solely on preconceived notions about a sociocultural group to which that person belongs

premium a monthly fee paid for health insurance

prenatal care routine preventive healthcare consultations during pregnancy that allow clinicians to identify and address potential health problems in a woman or fetus

preterm birth the delivery of a baby before the 37th week of pregnancy

prevalence the number of total existing cases of disease in a population divided by the total number of people in the population

prevention science the study of which preventive health interventions are effective in various populations, how successful the interventions are, and how well they can be scaled up for widespread implementation

preventive chemotherapy the distribution of safe medications to large population groups at regular time intervals as part of strategies for preventing and controlling infectious diseases

primary health care (PHC) a system of community-based health that employs community health workers and focuses as much on prevention as on cures

primary infertility infertility in a woman who has never had a live birth

primary prevention actions that keep an adverse health event from ever occurring

program a portfolio of related projects that together achieve part of an action plan

project a series of coordinated tasks that are completed within a limited time period in order to achieve a specific target

project management the process of initiating, planning, executing, monitoring and controlling, and closing out projects

proportionate mortality rate (PMR) the percentage of all people who died in a population whose death was the result of a particular cause

prostate cancer cancer of the male prostate gland

prosthetic a replacement body part

protein a chain of amino acids

protein energy malnutrition (PEM) a severe form of chronic undernutrition due to dietary deficiencies in protein and overall calories

protozoan a single-celled organism that has animal-like characteristics and often lives in water

psychiatrist a physician with advanced training in mental health care

psychologist a mental health professional with advanced training in counseling

public health the promotion of health and prevention of illnesses, injuries, and premature deaths at the population level

public health emergency of international concern (PHEIC) a declaration that can be made under the 2005 International Health Regulations when an infectious disease outbreak is causing serious illness, is likely to spread to other countries, and requires a coordinated global response

public policy the process by which laws, regulations, policies, and government-sponsored programs are developed, implemented, enforced, funded, administered, and evaluated

public–private partnership (PPP) a long-term collaboration in which the costs, risks, and benefits are shared by governmental and non-governmental entities

purchasing power parity (PPP) methods used to adjust comparative economic metrics based on how many goods, services, and other products can be purchased in various populations with a fixed amount of money

quality-adjusted life year (QALY) a quantitative estimate of the additional duration of life and quality of life conferred to populations by successful public health interventions

quarantine the restriction of freedom of movement for healthy contacts of people with an infectious disease as part of a strategy to contain the spread of contagious diseases

rabies an extremely virulent viral infection of the central nervous system that is spread through the saliva of infected mammals

race superficial categories that group individuals based primarily on physical attributes like skin color

radiation therapy the use of high-energy ionizing radiation to damage the DNA of cancer cells, which causes the cells to stop dividing or die

rapid diagnostic test (RDT) a test that can detect the presence of a pathogen (or markers for a pathogen) in a small drop of blood (or another body fluid) within 15 to 30 minutes

ready to use therapeutic food (RUTF) premade food products that are high in energy and protein for undernourished children

recessive an allele that will only be expressed when a person inherits the allele from both parents

Red Cross (ICRC) a private humanitarian organization officially sanctioned by the Geneva Convention and international law to provide specific humanitarian services during times of war

refugee a person who has been forced to move across an international border because of security concerns like war, civil conflict, political strife, or persecution based on race, tribe, religion, political affiliation, or membership in some other group

rehabilitation the process of restoring, improving, or maintaining the highest level of function possible in order to maximize independence and quality of life

relative poverty living on less than the nationally defined poverty line

relief aid that meets the immediate needs of people who might otherwise not have access to water, food, shelter, emergency medical care, and other urgent necessities

remittances funds transferred by international workers back to family members in their home communities

renewable energy energy derived from a source like wind or solar power that is not depleted when it is used

replacement population a state achieved when the typical women gives birth to 2 children, one to replace her and her partner, rather than having a higher fertility rate that generates population growth

reproductive health health issues related to fertility and infertility, contraception, pregnancy and childbirth, gynecologic and urologic health, and the prevention and treatment of sexually transmitted infections

reproductive rights the freedom of women and their partners to decide how many children they want without interference from governments or other organizations

research the process of systematically investigating a topic in order to discover new insights about the world

reservoir the environmental home for an infectious agent

resilience the ability to resist, survive, adapt to, and recover from adverse events

respiratory syncytial virus (RSV) a common cause of severe pneumonia in preterm infants and other vulnerable babies

rheumatic heart disease an inflammatory condition that causes irreversible damage to the heart and heart valves as a result of an untreated infection with group A *Streptococcus*, like strep throat or scarlet fever

rheumatoid arthritis a chronic inflammatory disease that damages cartilage and bones in many joints

riboflavin a B vitamin that contributes to skin and eye health

rickets vitamin D deficiency in children whose bones are still growing and become weak

Rift Valley fever a mosquito-borne zoonotic viral infection that can cause outbreaks of pregnancy loss in livestock herds

risk factor an exposure or characteristic that increases the likelihood of developing a particular disease

risk transition the health transition characterized by a shift from exposures like undernutrition, unsafe water, and indoor air pollution that increase the risk of childhood infectious diseases causing the greatest preventable morbidity and mortality to exposures like obesity, physical inactivity, and tobacco use that increase the risk of chronic diseases being the most prominent risk factors

road traffic injury (RTI) an injury sustained in a collision involving at least one moving motor vehicle

Roll Back Malaria a global partnership that brings together diverse partners to increase and sustain access to effective malaria prevention and treatment technologies

rotavirus the most common cause of severe diarrhea in infants and young children

rubella a vaccine-preventable viral infection that can cause birth defects when pregnant women contract it

rurality the degree to which a particular location is rural

saccharide the molecular units that form carbohydrates

safe drinking water an adequate supply of affordable clean drinking water in or near the home

SAFE strategy the WHO-recommended trachoma control plan, which combines surgery, antibiotics, facial cleanliness, and environmental improvements

sanitation the safe disposal of human excreta (feces)

sarcoma a cancer that arises from connective tissues like bones or muscles

SARS Severe Acute Respiratory Syndrome, a coronavirus infection that causes its victims to develop severe pneumonia

saturated fatty acid a fatty acid in which no more hydrogen can be added to the molecule because only single bonds exist between its carbon atoms

schistosomiasis an infection with *Schistosoma*, blood flukes that cycle in water between humans and snails, that cause bloody urine and an increased risk of bladder cancer

schizophrenia a mental health disorder characterized by distorted perceptions of reality

screening a type of secondary prevention in which all members of a well-defined group of people are encouraged to be tested for a disease based on evidence that members of the population are at risk for the disease and that early intervention improves health outcomes

scurvy vitamin C deficiency that is characterized by bleeding gums, loose teeth, joint pain, and decreased immune system function

secondary attack rate the proportion of susceptible people exposed to a contagious person who contract the infection

secondary infertility the inability to have additional offspring when attempting to conceive after having given birth to a child

secondary prevention the detection of health problems at an early stage when they have not yet caused significant damage to the body and can be treated more easily

sedentariness sitting for long durations each day

self-directed violence physical trauma inflicted by an individual on his or her own body, such as cutting and suicide attempts

self-efficacy an individual's confidence in his or her ability to successfully complete a difficult task

Sendai Framework a global agreement about disaster risk reduction that aims to significantly reduce the number of deaths and the magnitude of destruction caused by natural disasters

sensitivity the proportion of people who truly have a disease who test positive for the disease

sentinel surveillance the continuous collection and analysis of high-quality data from a limited number of clinics or hospitals so that public health officials will be able to detect changes in health status in the larger population from which the sentinel sites were sampled

sepsis widespread inflammation in the body that is triggered by the chemicals released by the body's immune system in response to an infection and can lead to organ failure, shock, and death

severe acute malnutrition (SAM) a state of extreme malnutrition in a child based on a weight-for-height z-score of below –3

sex the biological classification of people as male or female based on genetics and reproductive anatomy

sexual health the enjoyment of safe, voluntary, and nonviolent sexual experiences

sexual orientation an individual's sexual preferences based on attraction, identity, and behavior

sexually transmitted infection (STI) an infection spread through sexual intercourse or other types of sexual contact

sickle cell disease a genetic disorder that causes some red blood cells to become misshapen in a way that can cause painful blockages in small blood vessels

sickness how a person with poor physical or mental health relates to and is regarded by the community

sign an objective indicator of disease that can be clinically observed, such as a rash, cough, fever, or elevated blood pressure

skilled birth attendant (SBA) an obstetrician or gynecologist, another type of physician, a nurse midwife, a nurse, or skilled clinician who can recognize and treat potential complications during and after labor and delivery

smallpox an eradicated viral disease that caused blisters to form over the body

social cognitive theory the theory that behavior is a function of personal factors, behaviors, and environmental conditions and that behavior change, therefore, is about both inner motivation and environmental realities

social determinants of health the personal factors and community conditions that enable or hinder access to health

social justice the principle that moving toward greater equality is valuable for human flourishing

social marketing the use of marketing strategies to change behaviors in targeted populations

social media electronic communication tools that allow users to generate and share content

socioeconomic position (SEP) an individual's standing in a society based on individual and household income, education, gender, occupation, ethnicity and race, and other characteristics

socioeconomic status (SES) an individual's standing in a society based on individual and household income, education, gender, occupation, ethnicity and race, and other characteristics

soft skills the personal, social, emotional, and communication skills that equip people to successfully contribute to and lead work teams and other collaborative activities

soil-transmitted helminth a nematode infection contracted by contact with soil that contains feces contaminated with worm eggs

specificity the proportion of people who are truly free of a disease who test negative for it

spontaneous abortion the miscarriage of a pregnancy prior to the fetal age of viability

stages of change model the theory that describes individual behavior change as a five-stage process from precontemplation to contemplation, preparation for action, action, and maintenance

standard of health targets that governments set for improving the health of the populations they govern

sterilization the use of medical or surgical procedures to intentionally make it difficult or impossible for a person to reproduce

stigma a term used to describe negative attitudes about members of a population group that often lead to discrimination, social exclusion, and other forms of marginalization

stillbirth the death of a fetus late in pregnancy but prior to delivery

stomach cancer cancer of the stomach

Stop TB Partnership an international collaboration with more than 1500 partner organizations that takes the lead on developing on operationalizing action plans for reducing the global burden from tuberculosis

strategy a big picture plan for how to achieve a major goal

Strep throat an illness caused by Group A *Streptococcus* that, if left untreated, can lead to complications, such as scarlet fever or rheumatic fever, a condition that may cause permanent damage to the valves of the heart

stroke the death of cells in the brain due to lack of oxygen from cerebrovascular disease

stunting a condition in which a child has low height-for-age

suicide the intentional act of ending one's own life

supplementation the process of delivering micronutrients through a pill, tablet, or capsule

supply chain management the process of coordinating all steps from selecting and procuring products through transporting, storing, and delivering them

surgery an operation to confirm whether a disease is present or to remove a tumor or other part of the body

surveillance the process of continually monitoring health events in a population so that emerging public health threats can be detected and appropriate control measures can be implemented quickly

sustainability providing for current human needs without compromising the ability of future generations to meet their needs

Sustainable Development Goals (SDGs) a set of 17 goals established by the member countries of the United Nations at the end of 2015 that aim by 2030 to end poverty, protect the planet, and promote prosperity and peace

symptom a subjective indication of illness that is experienced by an individual but cannot be observed by others

syndrome a collection of signs and symptoms that occur together

syndromic surveillance the process of tracking potential outbreaks or other disease events based on reports of symptoms and other types of data rather than relying solely on counts of laboratory-confirmed diagnoses

syphilis a sexually transmitted infection caused by *Treponema pallidum*

systolic blood pressure the pressure in blood vessels when the heart beats

taeniasis the disease caused by *Taenia solium* tapeworms being present in human intestines

TB disease the symptomatic, contagious form of tuberculosis

teratogen a substance that can cause birth defects

tertiary prevention interventions that reduce impairment, minimize pain and suffering, and prevent death in people with symptomatic health problems

tetanus a sustained muscle contraction that is often caused by a neurotoxin from the bacterium *Clostridium tetani*

thalassemia a genetic disorder characterized by impaired production of hemoglobin, the molecules in red blood cells that carry oxygen

theory of planned behavior the theory that follow-through on implementing plans for a healthier lifestyle is dependent on the individual's perceived self-efficacy and control over the change

theory of reasoned action the theory that follow-through on implementing plans for a healthier lifestyle is dependent on the individual's belief that the outcome of the change will be worth the effort and his or her confidence that others will support the change

thiamine a B vitamin that is necessary for nerve function

thyroid cancer cancer of the thyroid gland in the neck

toxicology the study of the harmful effects that chemicals and other environmental hazards can have on living things

trachoma an infection with the bacterium *Chlamydia trachomatis* that can lead to blindness in people who do not practice good facial hygiene

Trade-Related Aspects of Intellectual Property Rights (TRIPS) an international agreement negotiated through the World Trade Organization that protects patents, copyrights, registered trademarks, and industrial designs across national boundaries

traditional birth attendant (TBA) as a lay midwife who may be able to handle uncomplicated births but does not have the advanced training to safely manage complications

trafficking the crime of arranging for a person to relocate with the intention of forcing that migrant into sex work, debt bondage, slavery, or other types of forced labor

trans fat a liquid oil that has been transformed into a solid fat by using pressure to add hydrogen to it

transgender a person with a gender identity that does not match the sex assigned at birth

transient ischemic attack (TIA) a mini-stroke in which stroke-like symptoms appear temporarily due to ischemia that is not so severe that it causes cell death

transmissibility the ease with which an infectious agent is passed from an infected host to another individual

transtheoretical model the theory that describes individual behavior change as a five-stage process from precontemplation to contemplation, preparation for action, action, and maintenance

traumatic brain injury (TBI) short- or long-term damage arising from a concussion or other form of intracranial injury

trematode a fluke that often has a complex life cycle that involves two different animal hosts

trichomoniasis a sexually transmitted infection caused by *Trichomonas vaginalis*

trichuriasis an intestinal whipworm infestation

trypanosomiasis a tsetse fly-borne infection with *Trypanosoma brucei* parasites that causes often-fatal African sleeping sickness

tuberculosis (TB) an infection caused by the bacterium *Mycobacterium tuberculosis*

type 1 diabetes a form of diabetes in which the body does not produce enough insulin

type 2 diabetes a form of diabetes in which the body develops insulin resistance and stops responding appropriately to insulin even when the hormone is still being produced

typhoid an infection with *Salmonella* Typhi that causes severe diarrhea and a high fever

UNAIDS the Joint United Nations Programme on HIV/AIDS, an entity co-sponsored by ten UN system agencies to advance HIV/AIDS prevention and control

under-5 child a child between birth and the fifth birthday

under-5 mortality rate (U5MR) the number of children who die before their fifth birthdays per 1000 live births

underemployment employment that is involuntarily part-time or does not generate an income that is above the local poverty level

undernutrition malnutrition resulting from deficiencies in the amount of food or types of nutrients eaten or from poor absorption of the nutrients that have been consumed

underweight a condition in which has child has low weight-for-age

UNDP the United Nations Development Programme, which focuses on poverty reduction

unemployment lack of employment for pay despite actively seeking a paid job

UNEP the United Nations Environment Programme, which promotes healthy ecosystems and sustainable use of natural resources

UNFPA the United Nations Population Fund, formerly the UN Fund for Population Activities, which supports reproductive health programs

UNICEF the United Nations Children's Fund, formerly the UN International Children's Emergency Fund, which advocates for children's rights and provides humanitarian assistance for children

unintentional injury an unplanned injury that happens very quickly

unipolar depressive disorder a depressive disorder characterized by depression without cycles of mania

United Nations the world's largest intergovernmental organization

Universal Declaration of Human Rights (UDHR) an international agreement unanimously adopted by the member states of the UN in 1948 that spells out more than two dozen civil, political, economic, social, and cultural human rights

universal health coverage (UHC) a population-level status achieved when everyone has access to high-quality health services and is protected from major health-associated financial shocks

universal precautions the use of barriers like gloves to prevent contact with blood or body fluids

unsaturated fatty acid a fatty acid that contains at least one double bond in the hydrogen chain

urbanicity the degree to which a particular location is urban

urbanization a shift toward more people living in cities and fewer people living in rural areas

USAID the United States Agency for International Development, which is the lead international cooperation agency in the United States

uterine cancer cancer of the endometrium or uterus

vaccination the intentional delivery of a substance into the body in order to stimulate development of immunity against a particular disease

vector control interventions that reduce the size and density of the insect population

vector-borne infection an infection with a human–arthropod–human cycle of infection (or an animal–insect–animal cycle that occasionally affects a human)

vertical program a program that delivers disease-specific clinical services that are not fully integrated into the health system

vertical transmission transmission of a pathogen from an infected pregnant woman to her offspring during pregnancy, delivery, or breastfeeding

VIA visual inspection with acetic acid as a diagnostic test for cervical cancer

violence the use of force or power to threaten or inflict physical, sexual, and psychological harm on another person

virulence the ability of an infectious agent to cause severe disease or death in a host

virus a piece of nucleic acid (DNA or RNA) encased in a shell made of proteins and sometimes also fatty acids

vital statistics population-level metrics about births, deaths, and other life events

vitamin organic compounds that cannot by synthesized by the body

vitamin A a fat-soluble vitamin critical for growth and vision

vitamin A deficiency (VAD) a vitamin deficiency that is a major cause of preventable blindness in children

vitamin C a vitamin essential for collagen formation, iron absorption, immune system function, and cellular health

vitamin D a mineral that is important for bone health because it assists the body with calcium absorption

voluntary counselling and testing (VCT) a process of being tested for HIV or another infection and receiving counseling about risk reduction, treatment referrals, and communication strategies

voluntourism volunteer tourism, travel for the purpose of volunteering

wasting a condition in which a child has low weight-for-height

water, sanitation, and hygiene (WASH) programs that combine improved water and sanitation systems with health education to promote frequent handwashing and consistent use of toilets

water-soluble vitamin a vitamin that is easily dissolved in the body but is not able to be stored in body tissues

wealth the accumulated worth of the household's resources

West Nile virus a mosquito-borne viral infection that can cause neurologic complications

World Bank a multilateral investment bank that makes loans to developing countries

World Health Organization (WHO) a specialized agency of the United Nations that serves as its primary health agency

World Trade Organization (WTO) a United Nations-related organization that negotiates and enforces trade agreements among UN member nations

XDR-TB an extensively drug-resistant tuberculosis strain that does not respond to rifampicin, isoniazid, fluoroquinolones, and at least one second-line injectable TB medication

xerophthalmia a severe dryness of the eye

yaws an endemic treponematosis that causes disfiguring skin lesions

years lived with disability (YLD) a quantitative estimate of the burden to a population from nonfatal health conditions that cause significant impairment and distress

years of life lost (YLL) a quantitative estimate of the burden from premature mortality in a population

yellow fever a vaccine-preventable mosquito-borne viral infection that causes jaundice that turns the skin and eyes of affected people yellow

Zika a mosquito-borne viral infection that is usually asymptomatic but has been linked to an increased risk of microcephaly in babies born to women who contracted the virus during the pregnancy

zinc a mineral that is important for immune function, growth, and child development

zoonosis an infectious disease that usually occurs in animals and only occasionally infects humans

z-score a statistical indicator of how many standard deviations away from the mean an individual's measure is

Index

Page numbers followed by "*f*" indicate figures.